Core
Curriculum
for Oncology
Nursing

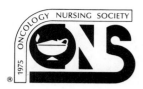

ONCOLOGY NURSING SOCIETY

Core Curriculum for Oncology Nursing

SECOND EDITION

Editors

Jane C. Clark, MN, RN, OCN
Clinical Nurse Specialist, Oncology
Emory University Hospital
Atlanta, Georgia

Rose F. McGee, PhD, RN
American Cancer Society Professor of Oncology Nursing
Nell Hodgson Woodruff School of Nursing
Emory University
Atlanta, Georgia

W.B. SAUNDERS COMPANY
A Division of Harcourt Brace & Company
Philadelphia   London   Toronto   Montreal   Sydney   Tokyo

W.B. SAUNDERS COMPANY
A Division of
Harcourt Brace & Company

The Curtis Center
Independence Square West
Philadelphia, Pennsylvania 19106

Library of Congress Cataloging-in-Publication Data

Core curriculum for oncology nursing / [edited by] Jane C. Clark, Rose
  McGee—2nd ed.
    p. cm.
  ISBN 0-7216-3486-9
  1. Cancer—Nursing. 2. Cancer. I. Clark, Jane C. II. McGee,
  Rose.
  [DNLM: 1. Oncologic Nursing—outlines.   WY 18 C7968]
  RC266.C67 1992   616.99′4′0024613—dc20
  DNLM/DLC   92-11722

Editor: Thomas Eoyang

CORE CURRICULUM FOR ONCOLOGY NURSING   ISBN   0-7216-3486-9

Printed in the United States of America

Last digit is the print number: 9   8   7   6   5   4   3

Contributors

Joyce Alexander, MN, RN, OCN
Clinical Nurse Specialist, Oncology,
Emory University Hospital,
Atlanta, Georgia
Lymphomas

Anne Belcher, PhD, RN
Associate Professor and Professor of Oncology
  Nursing,
University of Maryland School of Nursing,
Baltimore, Maryland
*Factors Affecting Responses to the Risk for or
  Actual Diagnosis of Cancer*

Catherine Bender, MN, RN
Assistant Professor, Graduate Program,
Medical-Surgical Nursing, Oncology,
The University of Pittsburgh;
Liaison to Graduate Nursing Program,
Pittsburgh Cancer Institute,
Pittsburgh, Pennsylvania
Implications of Antineoplastic Therapy for Nursing

Lynne Brophy, BSN, RN, OCN
Staff Nurse, Inpatient Oncology Unit,
Duke University Medical Center,
Durham, North Carolina
*Implications of Biological Response Modifier
  Therapy for Nursing*

Jennifer Dunn Bucholtz, MS, RN
Adjunct Faculty,
Department of Advanced Nursing Science,
University of Delaware,
Newark, Delaware;
Faculty Associate, The Johns Hopkins School of
  Nursing;
Clinical Specialist, Division of Radiation
  Oncology,
The Johns Hopkins Oncology Center,
Baltimore, Maryland
Implications of Radiation Therapy for Nursing

Jane C. Clark, MN, RN, OCN
Clinical Nurse Specialist, Oncology,
Emory University Hospital,
Atlanta, Georgia
*Nursing Management of Responses to the Cancer
  Experience*

Margaret Crowley, BSN, MSEd, RN
Clinical Instructor,
Associate Degree Nursing Program,
School of Allied Health,
Hahnemann University;
Independent Contractor, Wissahickon Hospice;
Staff Nurse, Hematology-Oncology,
University of Pennsylvania Hospital
Philadelphia, Pennsylvania
Primary Prevention in Oncology Nursing Practice

iii

Mary Cunningham, MS, RN

Clinical Instructor,
University of Texas School of Nursing;
Clinical Nurse Specialist—Pain,
Department of Neuro-Oncology,
University of Texas System Cancer Center,
M.D. Anderson Cancer Center,
Houston, Texas
Professional Issues in Cancer Care

Leonita H. Cutright, MSN, RN

Oncology Clinical Specialist,
Memorial Hospital,
Chattanooga, Tennessee
Head and Neck Cancers

Ruth Bope Dangle, MN, RN

Formerly Oncology Clinical Nurse Specialist,
Riverside Methodist Hospitals,
Columbus, Ohio
Cancer Epidemiology

Marilyn Davis, MN, RN, OCN

Instructor, School of Medicine,
University of Colorado Health Sciences Center,
Denver, Colorado
*Secondary Prevention in Oncology Nursing
    Practice*

Katharine Sibley Edmonds, BSN, RN, OCN

Oncology Outpatient Clinic,
St. Vincent's Hospital,
The Joseph and Theresa Bruno Cancer Center,
Birmingham, Alabama
Leukemias

Lynn Erdman, MN, RN, OCN

Director, Cancer Center,
Presbyterian Hospital,
Charlotte, North Carolina
*Nursing Implications of Supportive Therapies in
    Cancer Care*

Nina Entrekin, MN, RN, OCN

Director of Program Development,
American Cancer Society,
Florida Division;
PRN Staff Nurse,
H. Lee Moffitt Cancer Center,
University of South Florida,
Tampa, Florida
Breast Cancer

Joanne Peter Finley, MS, RN

Nurse Educator,
The Johns Hopkins Oncology Center,
Baltimore, Maryland
*Nursing Care of Patients with Metabolic and
    Physiological Oncological Emergencies*

Marie Flannery, MS, RN

Assistant Professor, Clinical Nursing,
University of Rochester School Of Nursing;
Oncology Clinical Nurse Specialist,
University of Rochester Cancer Center,
Rochester, New York
Reproductive Cancers

Mary Magee Gullatte, MN, RN

Clinical Associate Faculty,
Nell Hodgson Woodruff School of Nursing,
Emory University;
Head Nurse, Medical Oncology,
Emory University Hospital,
Atlanta, Georgia
Legal Issues Influencing Cancer Care

Robin Renee Gwin, MN, RN, OCN

Staff Nurse III,
Hematology/Bone Marrow Transplant Unit,
Emory University Hospital,
Atlanta, Georgia
Selected Ethical Issues in Cancer Care

James Halloran, MSN, RN, OCN, ANP

University of Texas School of Public Health,
AIDS Education and Training Center for Texas and
    Oklahoma,
Houston, Texas
HIV-Related Cancers

Jane C. Hunter, MN, RN, OCN
Breast Services Coordinator and Clinical Nurse
   Specialist,
Presbyterian Hospital Cancer Center,
Charlotte, North Carolina
*Nursing Care of Patients with Structural
   Oncological Emergencies*

Judith (Judi) L. Johnson, PhD, RN
Adjuvant Professor,
University of Minnesota;
Nursing Director, Medical-Surgical/Oncology,
North Memorial Medical Center,
Minneapolis, Minnesota
*Dissemination of Information Through Patient and
   Public Education*

Mary Johnson, PhD, RN
Associate Professor, St. Olaf College;
Instructor, Abbott Northwestern Hospital,
Minneapolis, Minnesota
*Dissemination of Information Through Patient and
   Public Education*

Nancy Kane, MS, RN, OCN
Program Director for Oncology Services,
Catholic Medical Center,
Manchester, New Hampshire
Implications of Unproven Methods for Nursing

Susan Leigh, BSN, RN
Cancer Survivorship Consultant,
Tucson, Arizona
Cancer Survivorship Issues

Julena Lind, MN, RN
Interim Chair and Assistant Professor of Nursing,
University of Southern California,
Los Angeles, California
Lung Cancer; Genitourinary Cancers

Alice Longman, EdD, RN, FAAN
Professor, The University of Arizona
College of Nursing,
Tucson, Arizona
Skin Cancer

Maryellen Maguire-Eisen, MSN, RN
Dana Farber Cancer Institute,
Hanover, Massachusetts
Leukemias

Rose F. McGee, PhD, RN
Professor, Nell Hodgson Woodruff School of
   Nursing,
Emory University;
American Cancer Society Professor of Oncology
   Nursing,
Atlanta, Georgia
*Nursing Management of Responses to the Cancer
   Experience*

Deborah Stephens Mills, MN, RN, OCN
Oncology Clinical Nursing Specialist,
Christine LaGuardia Phillips Cancer Center,
Holston Valley Hospital and Medical Center,
Kingsport, Tennessee
Changes in Oncology Health Care Settings

Betty Owens, MS, RN
Neuro-Oncology Nurse Specialist,
Division of Neurosurgery,
University of Colorado
Health Sciences Center,
Denver, Colorado
Neurological Cancers

Ricky Preston, MA, RN
Formerly Director,
Hospice and Home Care,
University of Pensylvania,
Philadelphia, Pennsylvania
*Nursing Management of Responses to the Cancer
   Experience*

Joan Exparza Richters, MN, RN, OCN
Oncology Clinical Nurse Specialist,
Gwinnett Medical Center,
Lawrenceville, Georgia
Selected Ethical Issues in Cancer Care

Paula Trahan Rieger, MS, RN, OCN
Clinical Nurse Specialist,
University of Texas,
M.D. Anderson Cancer Center,
Houston, Texas
*Implications of Biological Response Modifier
Therapy for Nursing*

Marcia Rostad, MS, RN, NS, OCN
Adjunct Faculty, College of Nursing,
University of Arizona;
Pediatric Oncology Clinical Nurse Specialist,
University Medical Center,
Tucson, Arizona
*Nursing Implications of Supportive Procedures in
Cancer Care*

Roberta Anne Strohl, MN, RN
Associate Professor, School of Medicine,
Department of Radiation Oncology,
University of Maryland,
Baltimore, Maryland
*Implications of Diagnosis and Staging on
Treatment Goals and Strategies*
Colorectal Cancers

Thomas J. Szopa, MS, RN, OCN, CETN
Adjunct Assistant Professor of Nursing,
University of New Hampshire,
Durham, New Hampshire;
Clinical Nurse Specialist,
Oncology and Ostomy/Wound Management,
Elliot Hospital,
Manchester, New Hampshire
Implications of Surgical Treatment for Nursing

Linda Tenenbaum, MSN, RN, OCN
Professor, Nursing,
Broward Community College,
Fort Lauderdale, Florida
*Principles of Preparation, Administration, and
Disposal of Antineoplastic Agents*

Deborah L. Volker, MA, RN, OCN
Director of Nursing Staff Development,
The University of Texas,
M.D. Anderson Cancer Center,
Houston, Texas
Standards of Oncology Nursing Practice
*Standards of Oncology Education: Patient, Family,
and Public*
Pathophysiology of Cancer

Jennifer S. Webster, MN, MPH, RN, OCN
Clinical Nurse Specialist,
Bone Marrow Transplant Program,
Emory University Hospital,
Atlanta, Georgia
*Sociodemographic and Attitudinal Changes
Affecting Cancer Care*

Teresa Wikle, BA, BSN, RN, OCN
Bone Marrow Transplant
Nurse Consultant,
Sutter Memorial Hospital,
Sacramento, California
*Implications of Bone Marrow Transplantation for
Nursing*

Preface

Five challenges guided the development of the second edition of the *Core Curriculum for Oncology Nursing:*

- To incorporate the revised core curriculum and revised practice and education standards of oncology nursing
- To explicate the critical nursing roles and responsibilities in the care of people with cancer and their families
- To present new knowledge about the care of people at risk for or with a diagnosis of cancer
- To make a significant contribution to the oncology nursing literature
- To make the process a rewarding experience for the authors, reviewers, and editors

In 1989 the Oncology Nursing Certification Corporation (ONCC) undertook the Role Delineation Study to identify the competencies of the oncology certified nurse. The findings from this study served as the basis for revising the test blueprint for the certification examination in oncology nursing. In addition, the Education Committee of the Oncology Nursing Society (ONS) revised the core curriculum for oncology nursing in 1990.

The second edition of the *Core Curriculum in Oncology Nursing* is divided into sections that are consistent with the major categories of both the test blueprint and the core curriculum. Principal topics within each section were identified as chapters. The ultimate goal was to make the nursing process and the standards of practice and education reality-based through application to each topic. In most cases this approach to presenting nursing knowledge varied with the topic; therefore the format evolved in the course of the development of the book. This evolution often tested the patience and originality of the authors and editors, but the process of deliberation served to enrich both the content and clarity of the text. Background information relevant to each topic is explained under theory; content critical to a thorough, initial evaluation of the patient is presented under assessment; nursing diagnoses commonly associated with each topic are outlined for reference; nursing planning and implementation activities are illustrated based on nursing goals of care; and finally, the outcomes of nursing care for the patient and family are described under evaluation.

The need to update information was a further impetus for a second edition of the *Core Curriculum.* The specifics of each topic have been updated. Some topics have been expanded significantly as is the case with the standards of practice and education, issues in practice and care, pathophysiology of cancer, and biological response modifiers. Furthermore, new topics have been added such as HIV-related malignancies, reproductive cancers, lymphomas, fluid imbalances, antimicrobial therapy, and anaphylaxis. In keeping with the priorities of the ONS, integration of recent knowledge on cancer rehabilitation, resources, and pain management was a goal as well.

The intended use of the book is to provide a reference for oncology nurses at both the generalist and advanced practice levels. Staff nurses on general patient care units, on specialized oncology areas, in the community, and in rehabilitation facilities may use the text as a reference for developing individualized plans of care for people with cancer and their families. Clinical nurse specialists may use the text for developing models for oncology nursing practice and performance review; standards of care; quality assurance programs; or educational programs for staff, clients, families, and the public. Educators may use the text for curriculum development at the generalist and advanced practice levels. Administrators may use the text to justify structure, personnel, and process changes to meet the evolving needs of people at risk for or with a diagnosis of cancer and their families within institutions or the community. The book also is intended to be used as a review for the certification examination in oncology nursing.

If you are new to oncology nursing, we suggest that you begin by reviewing the sections on pathology of cancer, diagnosis and staging of cancer, and treatment of cancer. This review should provide a basis for study of the cancer nursing practice and characteristics of major cancers sections. If you have worked in oncology care, we suggest that you begin by reviewing a section with which you are familiar. This review will give you an idea of the level of content presented and familiarize you with the format of content presentation before proceeding to new content areas. We have attempted to maintain a consistent format throughout the text to provide a template for learning. Topics have been cross-referenced to decrease repetition, and tables have been used to present important material more concisely. At the end of each topic is a bibliography that may be used to augment material presented in the text. All references have been verified by a medical librarian to increase accuracy of the text and to thereby decrease user frustration.

The expertise and commitment of the authors and reviewers who served as contributors to the second edition of the *Core Curriculum* made the work of editing challenging, enlightening, and enjoyable. The outstanding contribution of each individual is to be applauded, and the collective knowledge base of this impressive cadre of oncology nurses served as the quality control in the selection and presentation of content.

We thank the ONS Education Committee and the Board of Directors for the privilege of serving as co-editors for the second edition. The editors of the text have a combined experience in oncology nursing of over 50 years. This longevity in the specialty served to evoke a recurrent question of why their task of editing a core curriculum did not occur in the 1960s versus the 1990s. The knowledge base then was limited to a few oncology nursing texts and no journals. However, the problems associated with editing a seemingly unmanageably large knowledge base is a far better state than the clean slate which existed in the early professional years of the editors. The reader will, however, accept these reflections as a forewarning that not every important reference nor fact could be captured in this edition of the *Core Curriculum*. As you use this book, please accept the challenge to make known to the editors or to the ONS Education Committee suggestions for the next edition. The future of oncology nursing appears to be that of continued phenomenal growth; therefore, feedback is crucial to ensure that subsequent editions exceed the former in promoting "state of the art" quality nursing care on preventive, interventive, and restorative levels.

Jane C. Clark
Rose F. McGee

Contents

Section Three   Pathophysiology of Cancer

Section Four   Cancer Epidemiology

Section Five   Treatment of Cancer

Cancer Nursing Practice

1

Standards of Oncology Nursing Practice

Deborah L. Volker, MA, RN, OCN

I. Definitions.
  A. *Nursing*—the diagnosis and treatment of human responses to actual or potential health problems.
  B. *Standard*—a norm that expresses an agreed-upon level of practice that has been developed to characterize, measure, and provide guidance for achieving excellence.
  C. Components of each standard:
    1. Standard statement.
    2. *Rationale*—explanation of the underlying reason for the standard.
    3. *Structure criteria*—descriptions of the environment and resources needed to achieve desired outcomes.
    4. *Process criteria*—descriptions of the major sequence of events and activities required to obtain desired outcomes.
    5. *Outcome criteria*—descriptions of the end results of nursing actions.

II. Oncology Nursing Society (ONS)/American Nurses' Association (ANA) standards of oncology nursing practice.
  A. Professional practice standards I through VI (Table 1-1).
    1. Professional practice standards relate to:
      a. Theory.
      b. Data collection.
      c. Nursing diagnosis.
      d. Planning.
      e. Intervention.
      f. Evaluation.
    2. The professional practice standards (I through VI) are focused on the 11 high-incidence problem areas common to clients cared for by oncology nurses:
      a. Prevention and early detection.
        (1) Personal risk factors.
        (2) Early detection practices.

Table 1-1
PROFESSIONAL PRACTICE STANDARDS

Standard I: THEORY

The oncology nurse applies theoretical concepts as a basis for decisions in practice.

Standard II: DATA COLLECTION

The oncology nurse systematically and continually collects data about the health status of the client. The data are recorded, accessible, and communicated to appropriate members of the multidisciplinary team.

Standard III: NURSING DIAGNOSES

The oncology nurse analyzes assessment data to formulate nursing diagnoses.

Standard IV: PLANNING

The oncology nurse develops an outcome-oriented care plan that is individualized and holistic. The plan is based on nursing diagnoses and incorporates preventive, therapeutic, rehabilitative, palliative, and comforting nursing actions.

Standard V: INTERVENTION

The oncology nurse implements the nursing care plan to achieve the identified outcomes for the client.

Standard VI: EVALUATION

The oncology nurse regularly and systematically evaluates the client's responses to interventions to determine progress toward achievement of outcomes and to revise the data base, nursing diagnoses, and the plan of care.

From American Nurses' Association & Oncology Nursing Society (1987). *Standards of Oncology Nursing Practice*. Kansas City, Mo: American Nurses' Association.

    b. Information—client's current knowledge about diagnosis, treatment, resources, predictable problems, participation in care (e.g., financial matters, spiritual concerns, hospice).
    c. Coping.
      (1) Past and present coping mechanisms.
      (2) Current ability to mobilize and availability of resources.
      (3) Alternative coping strategies during all phases of care.
    d. Comfort.
      (1) Source and degree of discomfort.
      (2) Method of pain and symptom management.
      (3) Effects of disease and treatment on life-style.
      (4) Outcomes of interventions to alleviate discomfort.
    e. Nutrition.
      (1) Current nutritional status.
      (2) Effects of disease and treatment on nutritional status.
      (3) Past and present nutritional patterns.
    f. Protective mechanisms.
      (1) Immune function.
      (2) Hematopoietic function.
      (3) Integumentary function.
      (4) Sensorimotor function, including level of consciousness and thought processes.

   g. Mobility.
      (1) Level of mobility.
      (2) Potential for sequelae.
   h. Elimination.
      (1) Past and present patterns of elimination.
      (2) Effects of disease and treatment on elimination patterns.
   i. Sexuality.
      (1) Effects of disease and treatment.
      (2) Psychological response to disease and treatment.
      (3) Past and present sexual patterns and functioning.
   j. Ventilation.
      (1) Level of respiratory status.
      (2) Alterations in gas exchange.
      (3) History of exposure to respiratory contaminants.
   k. Circulation.
      (1) Alterations in tissue perfusion.
      (2) Alterations in cardiac output.
3. Purpose of professional standards in oncology nursing:
   a. For the nurse generalist:
      (1) Serves as a guide to provide quality care by:
         (a) Identifying the theoretical basis of practice.
         (b) Applying the nursing process to assure that:
            i. Data collection is systematic, continuous, recorded, and communicated.
            ii. Nursing diagnoses are derived from interpretation of presenting data and are open to revision.
            iii. The plan of care is derived from theoretical principles and stated nursing diagnoses.
            iv. The plan of care reflects priorities and prescribed nursing strategies to achieve health promotion, maintenance, and restoration.
            v. Client/family participation does occur.
            vi. Client/family progress is assessed jointly by the nurse and client/family.
            vii. Client/family evaluation of outcomes directs reassessment and revision of the plan of care.
      (2) Facilitates professional development by:
         (a) Identifying gaps in knowledge base.
         (b) Determining range of practice for which one is prepared.
   b. For oncology nursing practice, promotes development by:
      (1) Providing a basis for the development of performance evaluation instruments.
      (2) Providing a basis for quality assurance.
      (3) Providing the basis and impetus for peer review.
      (4) Generating research questions.
      (5) Stimulating research to validate practice.
      (6) Providing a basis for program evaluation.
      (7) Promoting intradisciplinary and multidisciplinary collaboration.
   c. For client and family, ensures:
      (1) Participation in health restoration, promotion, and maintenance.
      (2) Quality of care consistent with existing standards.

Table 1-2
PROFESSIONAL PERFORMANCE STANDARDS

Standard VII: PROFESSIONAL DEVELOPMENT

The oncology nurse assumes responsibility for professional development and continuing education and contributes to the professional growth of others.

Standard VIII: MULTIDISCIPLINARY COLLABORATION

The oncology nurse collaborates with the multidisciplinary team in assessing, planning, implementing, and evaluating care.

Standard IX: QUALITY ASSURANCE

The oncology nurse participates in peer review and interdisciplinary program evaluation to assure that high-quality nursing care is provided to clients.

Standard X: ETHICS

The oncology nurse uses the Code for Nurses and "A Patient's Bill of Rights" as guides for ethical decision making in practice.

Standard XI: RESEARCH

The oncology nurse contributes to the scientific base of nursing practice and the field of oncology through the review and application of research.

NOTE: A complete statement of the standards may be obtained from Oncology Nursing Society, 501 Holiday Drive, Pittsburgh, PA, 15220 (phone, 412-921-7373).
From American Nurses' Association & Oncology Nursing Society (1987). *Standards of Oncology Nursing Practice*. Kansas City, Mo: American Nurses' Association.

    B. Professional performance standards VII through XI (Table 1-2) relate to:
       1. Professional development.
       2. Multidisciplinary collaboration.
       3. Quality assurance.
       4. Ethics.
       5. Research.

III. Examples of ways oncology nurses apply professional practice and performance standards in clinical settings.
    A. *Example 1*: application of theory (Standard I) to planning care by using Maslow's hierarchy of needs to plan and prioritize interventions for the postlaryngectomy client.
       1. Identify concepts of the Maslow hierarchy of needs theory.
          a. Behavior is directed by a number of basic needs.
          b. Although interrelated, these needs tend to be hierarchical (lower needs must be met before higher needs can be achieved; Figure 1-1).
          c. Needs include:
             (1) Physiological needs.
             (2) Safety and security.
             (3) Love and belonging.
             (4) Esteem and self-esteem.
             (5) Self-actualization.
       2. Use theory to plan and prioritize care measures, beginning with first priority— physiological and safety needs:

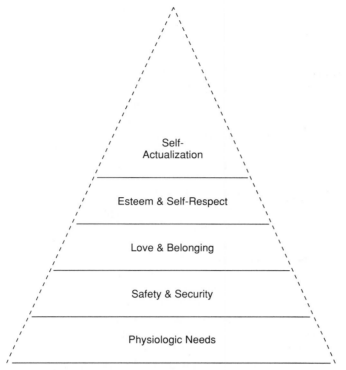

Figure 1-1 Maslow's hierarchy of human needs. *(From Maslow, A.H., 1970. Motivation and personality [2nd ed]. New York: Harper and Row, Inc.)*

   a. Assess:
      (1) Patency of laryngectomy tube.
      (2) Symptoms of respiratory distress.
      (3) Efficacy of respiratory efforts.
      (4) Vital signs and arterial blood gases.
      (5) Secretions.
      (6) Integrity of tissue at operative site.
   b. Assist with coughing and deep breathing.
   c. Suction every 1 to 2 hours and as secretions warrant.
   d. Provide humidification.
   e. Maintain adequate fluid intake.
   f. Maintain nutritional intake (enteral alimentation via nasogastric tube or hyperalimentation).
   g. Keep call light and other communication tools accessible to client.
   h. When appropriate and client is ready to learn, teach:
      (1) Stoma care, suctioning.
      (2) Importance of humidification.
      (3) Alterations in respiratory status that should be reported.
      (4) Measures to prevent aspiration through stoma.
      (5) Significant other how to perform resuscitation through stoma.
      (6) Importance of wearing/carrying identification noting that client breathes through a stoma.
 3. Use theory to order remaining needs; according to Maslow, once the priority needs (physiological and safety) are met, the order of subsequent needs follow the hierarchy; for example:

      a. Impact of the diagnosis and treatment on relationships with family and friends.

      b. Self-esteem.

      c. Sexuality.

      d. Employment.

B. *Example 2*: application of Standard II (Data Collection) and accompanying process criteria to guide new client assessment and requisite documentation of findings.

    1. See Figure 1-2 for example of cancer nursing assessment instrument.

    2. Anticipated outcome: an initial data base is developed, shared with the client as appropriate, recorded, and made readily accessible to the multidisciplinary team.

C. *Example 3*: application of Standard IV (Planning) to guide the development of institution-specific plans of care for the 11 high-incidence problem areas.

    1. See Table 1-3 for example: Impaired Skin Integrity Related to Radiation Therapy.

    2. Relevant outcome criteria. The client:

      a. Lists measures to prevent skin breakdown.

      b. Identifies the signs and symptoms of skin breakdown and infection.

      c. Identifies the appropriate health team member to contact immediately if signs of skin breakdown or infection occur.

      d. Describes measures to manage skin breakdown.

      e. Identifies signs and symptoms to report to health professional.

D. *Example 4*: application of Standard IX (Quality Assurance) as a framework for an institutional quality assurance program.

    1. Use the structure, process, and outcome criteria of each standard as statements of acceptable practice.

    2. Use the 11 high-incidence problems as an outline for identification of indicators (well-defined, measurable dimensions of the quality and appropriateness of an important aspect of the patient's care that can include measurable care processes, clinical events, complications, or outcomes) that require monitoring.

    3. Define indicators.

    4. Determine a threshold (a preestablished aggregate level of performance that should be achieved) for action.

    5. Monitor for occurrences.

    6. Take corrective actions based on findings (Table 1-4 gives an example, using Standard IV, Planning).

E. *Example 5*: application of professional practice and performance standards to education:

    1. Use the standards to form a curricular outline for generalist oncology nursing education, staff development, and continuing education programs.

    2. Use process criteria as learner objectives within an educational program.

    3. Use outcome criteria as patient teaching objectives (Table 1-5).

F. *Example 6*: application of professional practice and performance standards to management:

    1. Both the professional practice and professional performance standards can be used as a framework for development of staff performance evaluation instruments (Table 1-6).

    2. Resource justification. Use structure criteria to:

      a. Address the resources and environment required for the practice of oncology nursing.

Text continued on page 15

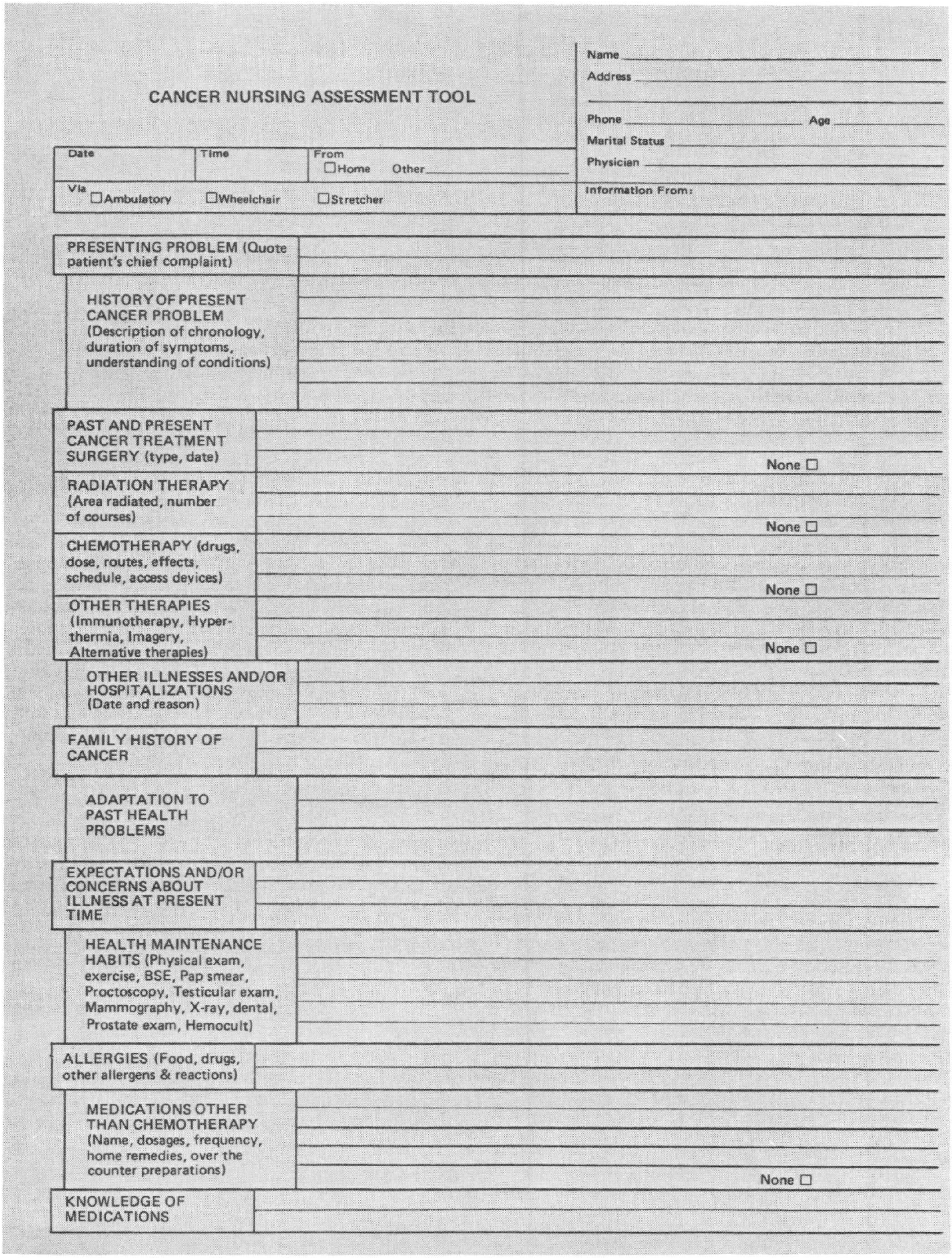

CANCER NURSING ASSESSMENT TOOL

Name _____

Address _____

Phone _____ Age _____

Marital Status _____

Physician _____

Date	Time	From ☐ Home Other _____

Via ☐ Ambulatory   ☐ Wheelchair   ☐ Stretcher

Information From:

PRESENTING PROBLEM (Quote patient's chief complaint)

HISTORY OF PRESENT CANCER PROBLEM (Description of chronology, duration of symptoms, understanding of conditions)

PAST AND PRESENT CANCER TREATMENT SURGERY (type, date)   None ☐

RADIATION THERAPY (Area radiated, number of courses)   None ☐

CHEMOTHERAPY (drugs, dose, routes, effects, schedule, access devices)   None ☐

OTHER THERAPIES (Immunotherapy, Hyperthermia, Imagery, Alternative therapies)   None ☐

OTHER ILLNESSES AND/OR HOSPITALIZATIONS (Date and reason)

FAMILY HISTORY OF CANCER

ADAPTATION TO PAST HEALTH PROBLEMS

EXPECTATIONS AND/OR CONCERNS ABOUT ILLNESS AT PRESENT TIME

HEALTH MAINTENANCE HABITS (Physical exam, exercise, BSE, Pap smear, Proctoscopy, Testicular exam, Mammography, X-ray, dental, Prostate exam, Hemocult)

ALLERGIES (Food, drugs, other allergens & reactions)

MEDICATIONS OTHER THAN CHEMOTHERAPY (Name, dosages, frequency, home remedies, over the counter preparations)   None ☐

KNOWLEDGE OF MEDICATIONS

Figure 1-2 Cancer Nursing Assessment Tool. *(Reprinted from the* Oncology Nursing Forum *with permission from the Oncology Nursing Press. Miaskowski, C.A. & Nielsen, B. [1985]. A cancer nursing assessment tool. Oncol Nurs Forum 12*[6]*, 37-42.)*

NURSING DIAGNOSIS DATA BASE — Complete all blank spaces in the right hand column, then, using the cues in the left hand column, make a statement in each category describing a deviation from normal, if no deviations, check the box stating "Within Normal Limits."

VENTILATORY INTEGRITY shortness of breath, dyspnea on exertion, paroxysmal noctural dyspnea, cyanosis, cough, sputum production, fatigue, tracheostomy, aids to breathing.	Respiratory Rate: Smoking: Breath Sounds: Category WNL ☐
CIRCULATORY INTEGRITY rhythm, pulse deficit, chest pain, palpitations, intermittent elaudication, color of extremities, edema, neck veins, varicosities.	Blood Pressure: Pulse Category WNL ☐
NUTRITION dysphagia, anorexia, stomatitis, nausea, vomiting, weight loss, changes in taste, food preferences, dietary patterns, nutritional supplements, feeding devices, hyperalimentation.	DIET: Food Preparation By: Food Intolerances: Height: Weight: Alcohol Intake: Dentures: Upper ☐ Lower ☐ Both ☐ None ☐ Oral Exam: Category WNL ☐
INTESTINAL INTEGRITY pain, constipation, diarrhea, distention, tarry stools, change in bowel habits, blood per rectum, hemorrhoids, colostomy, ileostomy, appliances, liver breadth, spleenomegaly.	Normal Pattern: Last B.M.: Aids for Bowel Functioning: Hemocult: Bowel Sounds: Category WNL ☐
RENAL - URINARY INTEGRITY frequency, burning, color, hematuria, nocturia, retention, polyuria, incontinence, flank pain, aids to urination, dialysis, appliances, catheter.	 Category WNL ☐
COMFORT Pain Description - location, duration, periodicity, severity, aggravating factors. Relief Measures - medication, biofeedback, meditation, TENS, visual imagery, diversional activity, music therapy	Sleep Pattern: Pain Description: Relief Measures: Category WNL ☐

Figure 1-2 continued

PROTECTIVE MECHANISMS Skin Integrity — change in wart or mole, color, swelling, turgor, abrasions, petechiae, scars, · ulcers, photosensitivity, pruritis, desquammation, temperature, extravasation.	Category WNL ☐
Immune/Hematologic — chills, fever, rigors, petechiae, nosebleeds.	Temperature: Evidence of Bleeding: Evidence of Infection: Blood Values: Hct Hgb Platelets WBC Category WNL ☐
SENSORY - PERCEPTUAL INTEGRITY — orientation, memory loss, personality changes, syncope, vertigo, convulsions, headache, numbness, tingling, alterations in heat and cold sensation.	Level of Consciousness: Pupils: Category WNL ☐
VISION — visual disturbances, diplopia, blurring, tearing.	Eye Glasses? Yes ☐ No ☐ Contact Lenses? Yes ☐ No ☐ Glass Eye? Yes ☐ No ☐ Degree of Visual Acuity: Category WNL ☐
HEARING — tinnitus, vertigo, pain, discharge	Hearing Aid? Yes ☐ No ☐ Degree of Hearing Loss: Category WNL ☐
SPEECH — language barrier, aphasia, dysarthria.	Category WNL ☐
MOBILITY lethargy, gait, muscle weakness, paralysis, deformities, joint swelling, physical tolerance, muscle atrophy, tremors, range of motion, range of ambulation, fractures, set-up at home to assist mobility.	Muscle Strength: RUE LUE RLE LLE Level of Independence: Use of Aids: None☐ Walker ☐ Cane ☐ Wheelchair ☐ Other Category WNL ☐
SEXUAL INTEGRITY menses, contraception, pregnancies, breast changes, gynecomastia, impotency, changes in sexual activity, changes in sexual desire, changes in sexual performance.	LMP: Last Pap Smear: Breast Exam: Testicular Exam: Category WNL☐

Figure 1-2 continued

Figure 1-2 continued on following page

COPING INTEGRITY anxiety, anger, depression, body image changes, affect, self-esteem, stress, role changes, communication patterns, counseling	Spirituality: Ethnic Background: Category WNL □
SOCIAL INTEGRITY	Occupation: Education: Family - Significant Other: With Whom Does Patient Live? Family Support Systems: Impact of Hospitalization on Family: Economic Resources Previous Use of Community Agencies:
ANTICIPATED TEACHING NEEDS (Based on knowledge deficits assessed)	 None □
DISCHARGE PLAN	Anticipated Discharge to: Possible Need for Follow-Up Care (Check all that apply) ACS □ Hospice □ Reach to Recovery □ Ostomy Association □ Laryngectomy Association □ Social Service □ Counseling □ Other: Discharge Plan:

Additional Comments:

Signature_____R.N.

Figure 1-2 continued

Table 1-3

INSTITUTION-SPECIFIC CARE PLAN FOR THE CLIENT WITH AN ALTERATION IN PROTECTIVE
MECHANISMS

STANDARD: Impaired skin integrity related to radiation therapy

Population at Risk:

Patients with cancer treated with external-beam radiation therapy.

Expected Outcomes

1. Patient/caregiver verbalizes rationale for potential or actual impairment of skin integrity.
2. Patient/caregiver identifies/demonstrates measures to control or correct impaired skin integrity.

Nursing Interventions:

1. Assess irradiated skin for color, dryness, moisture, scaling, temperature, tenderness, or itching and note high-risk areas such as skin folds (perineum, axilla), ostomies, tracheostomy. Assess areas of wet desquamation for signs of infection.
2. For areas of dry desquamation, use water-based, soothing, topical ointments (hydrous lanolin, Aquaphor, Aloe Vera) as ordered to control tenderness/dryness of skin. All ointment must be removed from the skin before patient goes to receive radiation therapy. Cornstarch may be used for dry, itchy skin.
3. For areas of wet desquamation, the following measures should be used:
   a. Cleanse area with water or saline solution; pat dry.
   b. Do not use cornstarch.
   c. Keep area moist to promote healing (moisture-permeable dressings, hydrocolloids, hydrogels.)
4. Promote comfort by using:
   a. Bed cradles to keep linen off body.
   b. Convoluted foam mattress or alternating air pressure mattress (bed therapy).
   c. Body positioning and supports; avoid friction when moving patient.
   d. Systemic analgesics as ordered.
5. Implement and teach hygienic measures to prevent contamination and/or infection:
   a. Cleanse area with warm water (no soap).
   b. Protect markings.
   c. Avoid friction when cleaning.
   d. Pat skin dry or blow dry with hair dryer at cool setting.
   e. Expose area to air as much as possible.
6. Provide patient with teaching materials about radiation therapy.
7. Consult with enterostomal therapist about management of ostomies in the radiation field.
8. Teach signs/symptoms of skin changes, indicating those to report to health care team (erythema, scaling, tenderness).
9. Explain rationale and measures to maintain adequate nutritional and fluid status.
10. Discuss rationale and measures to prevent skin irritation/breakdown:
    a. Avoid strenuous activity.
    b. Avoid constricting clothing (belts, garters, restraints, brassieres, ties) over irradiated skin.
    c. Avoid irritating substances (tape, soap, perfume, deodorants, iodine, talcum, rough clothing) on irradiated skin. Shave with electric razor only.
    d. Wear soft, cotton clothing over skin at a radiation port and exit sites.
    e. Avoid hot or cold applications (heating pads, hot water bottles, ice caps) to areas.
    f. Avoid use of oil-based creams, ointments, and lotions that may contain heavy metals.
    g. Avoid sun exposure throughout entire life (wear hats, use sunscreen [SPF (sun protection factor) ≥ 15], or wear protective clothing).
11. Inform patient of signs/symptoms of infection.
12. Document nursing assessment, interventions, and evaluations as appropriate on medical record of patient.

Modified from Standards Development Committee (1991). The University of Texas, M.D. Anderson Cancer Center Division of Nursing, Houston, Texas.

Table 1-4
MONITORING PROJECT: SELF-CARE OF CENTRAL VENOUS ACCESS DEVICES (CVAD)

STANDARD: (statement of acceptable practice).
The patient describes appropriate actions for highly predictable problems and major side effects of the disease or therapy (ANA/ONS, Standard IV, outcome criterion for information).

Indicator

Before discharge with CVAD, 100% of patients (or the designated caregiver) demonstrate ability to manage care of the CVAD independently, including:

a. Performance of heparin flush.
b. Changing heparin cap.
c. Changing dressing.
d. Verbalization of problems that must be reported to the health care team.
e. Verbalization of the phone number to call in the event of a problem.

Threshold for Action

Less than 100%.

Monitoring for Occurrences

For a 1-month period, all patients discharged with a CVAD will be assessed on the above items (a through e) within 24 hours before discharge and reassessed during first return visit to the ambulatory clinic. Results of the assessment will be documented on the CVAD Patient Education Monitoring Tool by the infusion therapy clinical nurse specialist.

Analysis of Findings

Data will be compiled and analyzed by the Information Management Department and submitted to the Oncology Quality Assurance Committee and infusion therapy clinical nurse specialist for review. In the event the threshold for action is reached, a report of the problem analysis, plan for corrective action, and plan for remonitoring will be submitted to the quality assurance department head.

From American Nurses' Association & Oncology Nursing Society (1987). *Standards of Oncology Nursing Practice.* Kansas City, Mo: American Nurses' Association, p. 11.

Table 1-5
APPLICATION OF OUTCOME CRITERIA TO PATIENT EDUCATION

Use of Standards IV and VI outcome criteria for teaching the patient with an alteration in nutritional status related to disease and treatment.

Goal

The patient manages nutrition and hydration in a way that facilitates health and comfort in the presence of disease and treatment (ANA/ONS Standard VI).

Learning Objectives: (ANA/ONS Standard VI)

The patient will:
1. Identify foods that are tolerated and foods that cause discomfort or are distasteful.
2. Describe measures that enhance food intake and retention.
3. List appropriate dietary alternatives to provide sufficient nutrients when foods that were part of the customary diet are no longer tolerated.
4. Describe methods of modifying consistency, flavor, or amounts of nutrients to ensure adequate nutritional intake.
5. Describe dietary modifications compatible with his or her other cultural, social, and ethnic practices.
6. Describe interventions to relieve symptoms (e.g., nausea, vomiting, stomatitis) that interfere with nutritional intake.
7. List foods and fluids that provide optimal comfort during the terminal stage of illness.
8. Identify mechanisms to assess personal nutritional status.

Modified from American Nurses' Association & Oncology Nursing Society (1987). *Standards of Oncology Nursing Practice.* Kansas City, Mo: American Nurses' Association, pp. 11, 12, 15.

Table 1-6
EXCERPTS FROM AN ONCOLOGY STAFF NURSE PERFORMANCE EVALUATION TOOL

STANDARD VII: The oncology nurse assumes responsibility for professional development.

Criteria	Rating* 1	2	3
1. Initiates independent learning activities to increase knowledge of oncology nursing concepts and skills.			
2. Participates in ongoing continuing education activities. Earns _____ continuing education units per year.			
3. Continually updates knowledge of political, cultural, social, and ethical issues related to oncology.			
4. Demonstrates professional responsibility by participation in appropriate professional and community organizations.			
5. Maintains an awareness of personal beliefs and value systems and of effect on client care.			
6. Formally and informally communicates new knowledge with professional colleagues and others.			
7. Adheres to policies and procedures.			
8. Participates in a professional support group as needed.			

Rating scale: 1, performance below standard; 2, performance meets standard; 3, performance exceeds standard.
From American Nurses' Association & Oncology Nursing Society (1987). *Standards of Oncology Nursing Practice*. Kansas City, Mo: American Nurses' Association, pp. 13, 14, 17.

      b. Support the need for time, money, systems, and personnel required for patient care in accordance with the standards (Table 1-7).
  G. *Example 7*: identification of possible research questions.
    1. What are the high-incidence problem areas in oncology nursing practice?
      a. The 11 areas outlined in the standards were identified by oncology nursing experts in 1979.
      b. The 11 areas currently identified have not been tested empirically as reliable measures of the scope of oncology nursing practice.
      c. Each problem area should be tested clinically in a variety of patient populations in a variety of care settings.
    2. Which nursing interventions promote optimal patient outcomes?
      a. Some of the high-incidence areas (e.g., prevention and early detection, comfort, and protective mechanisms) have been targeted by nurse researchers.
      b. Most of the process criteria, however, have not been validated.
    3. Are the highest priority areas for cancer nursing research (listed below) consistent with the standards?
      a. Prevention and early detection (designated as a high-incidence problem area in the standards).
      b. Symptom management (crosscuts a number of the high-incidence problem areas).

Table 1-7
EXAMPLES OF STRUCTURE CRITERIA AND SUGGESTED RESOURCES TO MEET THE CRITERIA

Criteria	Resources
Opportunities are available in the practice setting for professional development (Standard VII).	Continuing education offerings. Relevant professional journals and other current publications. Scheduled time away from work duties to engage in professional development activities.
Oncology nurses are represented on peer review and quality assurance teams that evaluate health care outcomes (Standard IX).	Peer review and quality assurance teams. Oncology nurse representation on peer review and quality assurance teams.
Independent nursing interventions are promoted within the practice setting (Standard V).	Policies, procedures, and standards of care that reflect and support independent nursing interventions. Adequate staffing to allow for implementation of independent nursing interventions. Employee performance standards that support the implementation of independent nursing interventions. Clinical nurse specialist who serves as resource and role model for advanced nursing practice.
Oncology nurses are provided resource material about research in oncology nursing–related interdisciplinary areas (Standard XI).	Professional journals and other relevant publications that feature research-based information. Nursing research committee.

From American Nurses' Association & Oncology Nursing Society (1987). *Standards of Oncology Nursing Practice*. Kansas City, Mo: American Nurses' Association, pp. 13, 17, 19, 20.

    c. Pain control and management (included in the "comfort" high-incidence problem area).
    d. Patient or health education (crosscuts a number of the high-incidence problem areas).
    e. Coping and stress management (coping is designated as a high-incidence problem area).
  4. Do measurement instruments exist for research related to the standards? Although ongoing development is critical, numerous instruments exist that measure a variety of phenomena associated with the high-incidence problems:
    a. Instruments for assessing health and function (e.g., functional status, mental status and level of consciousness, coping, spirituality, sexuality, information-seeking behaviors).
    b. Instruments for assessing clinical problems (e.g., pain, nausea and vomiting, dyspnea, skin integrity, alterations in taste and smell).

BIBLIOGRAPHY

American Hospital Association (1972). *A Patient's Bill of Rights*. Chicago: The Association.
American Nurses' Association (1980). *Nursing: A Social Policy Statement*. Kansas City, Mo: The Association.
American Nurses' Association (1985). *Code for Nurses With Interpretive Statements*. Kansas City, Mo: The Association.
American Nurses' Association & Oncology Nursing Society (1987). *Standards of Oncology Nursing Practice*. Kansas City, Mo: American Nurses' Association.
Dorsett, DS. (1990). Quality of care. In S.L. Groenwald, M.H. Frogge, M. Goodman, and C.H. Yarbro (eds). *Cancer Nursing: Principles and Practice* (2nd ed). Boston: Jones & Bartlett Publishers, pp. 1151-1177.

Frank-Stromborg, M. (1988). *Instruments for Clinical Nursing Research*. Norwalk, Conn: Appleton & Lange.

Funkhouser, S.W. & Grant, M.M. (1989). 1988 ONS survey of research priorities. *Oncol Nurs Forum 16*(3), 413-416.

Maslow, A.H. (1972). *Motivation and Personality* (2nd ed). New York: Harper & Row, Inc.

Miaskowski, C. (1989). Quality assurance issues in oncology nursing. *Cancer 64*(suppl 1), 285-289.

Miaskowski, C.A. & Nielsen, B. (1985). A cancer nursing assessment tool. *Oncol Nurs Forum 12*(6), 37-42.

Miaskowski, C. & Rostad, M. (1990). Implementing the ANA/ONS Standards of Oncology Nursing Practice. *J Nurs Quality Assurance 4*(3), 15-23.

2

Standards of Oncology Education: Patient, Family, and Public

Deborah L. Volker, MA, RN, OCN

I. Definitions.
  A. *Education*—process of inducing measurable changes in knowledge, skills, and attitudes through planned learning activities.
  B. *Standard*—a norm that expresses an agreed-upon level of practice that has been developed to characterize, measure, and provide guidance for achieving excellence.
  C. *Client*—individual, family, group, or community for whom the nurse provides formally specialized services.
  D. *Family*—persons who are related or who represent a significant support group for the client.
  E. *Public*—the people of an organized community.
  F. *Domains of learning*:
      1. *Cognitive*—knowledge and intellectual abilities.
      2. *Psychomotor*—physical skills.
      3. *Affective*—attitudes, values.

II. Purpose and intended outcomes of the standards.
  A. Purposes are to provide comprehensive guidelines for nurses to:
      1. Develop, implement, and evaluate formal and informal patient/family teaching.
      2. Develop, implement, and evaluate formal and informal public education programs.
  B. Intended outcomes are to:
      1. Enhance the quality of patient teaching.
      2. Exemplify the scope of teaching in all phases of cancer care, including prevention, early detection, rehabilitation, and supportive care.
      3. Improve health promotion and care for the public.

III. Format of the standards: descriptive statements, with defining criteria designed to guide the achievement of quality education for the patient/family and public. Each standard includes the following categories:
  A. Nurse.
  B. Resources.

C. Curriculum.
D. Teaching-learning process.
E. Learner.

IV. Statement of standards of oncology education.
  A. Patient/family education (Table 2-1).
  B. Public education (Table 2-2).

V. Examples of application of standards of oncology education to clinical practice.
  A. *Example 1*: use the standards to guide development of standardized patient teaching plans. Table 2-3 presents an example that uses criteria from Standards IV and V.
  B. *Example 2*: use the standards as a framework for quality assurance program to monitor quality of patient/public educational activities.
    1. Monitoring project described in Table 1-4 also illustrates aspects of Standard V of the standards of oncology education—the patient/family apply knowledge, skills, and attitudes to management of actual or potential human responses to the cancer experience.
    2. Relevant criteria for the monitoring project—the patient/family:
      a. Demonstrates psychomotor and coping skills required for self-care (catheter care) (Criterion 4).
      b. Describes signs and symptoms that should be reported to the health care team (Criterion 6).

VI. Examples of application of standards of oncology education to professional education.
  A. *Example 1*: use the standards to form curricular outlines for generalist oncology nursing education, staff development, and continuing education programs. Table

Table 2-1
PATIENT/FAMILY EDUCATION

Standard I: ONCOLOGY NURSE

The oncology nurse at both the generalist and advanced practice levels is responsible for patient/family education related to cancer.

Standard II: RESOURCES

Resources are adequate to achieve the objectives of patient/family education related to cancer care.

Standard III: CURRICULUM

Knowledge, skills, and attitudes related to the management of human responses to cancer are reflected in the educational program for the patient/family facing cancer.

Standard IV: TEACHING-LEARNING PROCESS

Teaching-learning theories are applied to the development, implementation, and evaluation of learning experiences related to cancer care.

Standard V: LEARNERS: THE PATIENT/FAMILY

The patient/family apply knowledge, skills, and attitudes to management of actual or potential human responses to the cancer experience.

NOTE: A complete statement of the education standards (patient/family and public) may be obtained from the Oncology Nursing Society, 501 Holiday Drive, Pittsburgh, PA 15220 (phone, 412-921-7373).
From Oncology Nursing Society (1989). *Standards of Oncology. Education: Patient/Family and Public*. Pittsburgh, Penn: The Society, pp. 1-3.

Table 2-2
PUBLIC EDUCATION

Standard I: ONCOLOGY NURSE

The oncology nurse provides formal and informal cancer-related public education commensurate with personal education and experience.

Standard II: RESOURCES

Resources for public education related to cancer prevention, detection, and control are adequate and appropriate to achieve program objectives.

Standard III: CURRICULUM

Knowledge, skills, and attitudes related to the physical and psychosocial aspects of cancer prevention, early detection, and control are included in public education programs.

Standard IV: TEACHING-LEARNING PROCESS

Teaching-learning theories are applied to the development, implementation, and evaluation of learning experiences related to cancer education for the public.

Standard V: LEARNERS: THE PUBLIC

Personal behaviors and public policy related to cancer prevention, detection, control, rehabilitation, and supportive care are influenced by formal and informal cancer public education.

From Oncology Nursing Society (1987). *Standards of Oncology Education: Patient/Family and Public*. Pittsburgh, Penn: The Society, pp. 1-3.

Table 2-3
TEACHING PLAN FOR THE PATIENT WHO EXPERIENCES THROMBOCYTOPENIA
SECONDARY TO MYELOSUPPRESSIVE CHEMOTHERAPY

RELEVANT STANDARDS: Teaching-learning theories are applied to the development, implementation, and evaluation of learning experiences related to cancer care (Standard IV); the patient/family applies knowledge, skills, and attitudes to management of actual or potential human responses to the cancer experience (Standard V).

Teaching Goal

The patient will demonstrate ability to describe the effect of chemotherapy on platelet production, self-care actions to prevent or diminish bleeding, and signs/symptoms to report to the health care team.

Teaching Plan	Relevant Standard Criteria
1. Assess level of education and ability and readiness of patient to learn.	The nurse collects data systematically from the patient/family and other sources to assess learning needs, readiness to learn, and situational and psychosocial factors influencing learning (Standard IV, Criterion 1).
2. Assess cognitive, affective, and psychomotor learning needs relevant to thrombocytopenia.	Analyzes assessment data to identify cognitive, psychomotor, and affective learning needs (Standard IV, Criterion 2).

3. In collaboration with patient, develop teaching plan based on identified need.
  a. Behavioral objectives.
    (1) Explain the production and function of platelets.
    (2) Describe effect of chemotherapy on platelet production.
	Develops a teaching plan in collaboration with the patient/family that includes: Bases behavioral objectives on identified learning needs.

From Oncology Nursing Society (1987). *Standards of Oncology Education: Patient/Family and Public*. Pittsburgh, Penn: The Society, pp. 7-8.

Table 2-3

Teaching Plan	Relevant Standard Criteria
(3) Explain the relationship between platelet count and risk of bleeding.	
(4) List signs/symptoms of bleeding that should be reported.	
(5) Describe measures to prevent/control bleeding.	
b. Content (select as appropriate):	Content meets identified objectives.
(1) Normal bone marrow function.	
(a) Platelet production.	
(b) Platelet function.	
(2) Impact of chemotherapy.	
(a) Myelosuppression.	
(b) Recovery of cell production.	
(3) Relationship between platelet count and risk of bleeding.	
(4) Signs/symptoms of bleeding:	
Bleeding gums or nose.	
Spontaneous bruising, petechiae.	
Blood in urine or stool.	
Excessive bleeding after venipuncture.	
Hematemesis.	
Hemoptysis.	
Headache, blurred vision.	
Vaginal bleeding.	
Rectal bleeding.	
(5) Measures to prevent bleeding:	
Prolonged pressure at puncture sites.	
No intramuscular injections.	
No medications that contain aspirin.	
Electric razor instead of straight-edged razor.	
No tampons, suppositories, rectal medications or temperatures.	
Extreme caution during manicure or pedicure.	
c. Suggested teaching strategies (select as appropriate):	Teaching strategies and learning experiences promote active participation by the patient/family.
(1) One-to-one discussion.	
(2) Printed booklets.	
(3) Videotapes.	
(4) Chemotherapy class.	
d. Teaching/learning environment: provide environment free of interruption/distraction that promotes patient participation.	Environmental adaptations promote learning.

Table continued on following page

Table 2-3

TEACHING PLAN FOR THE PATIENT WHO EXPERIENCES THROMBOCYTOPENIA
SECONDARY TO MYELOSUPPRESSIVE CHEMOTHERAPY *Continued*

Teaching Plan	Relevant Standard Criteria
e. Evaluation criteria (select as appropriate): evaluation methods include verbalization and demonstration. Upon completion, patient will demonstrate ability to:	Methods and criteria for evaluation (Standard IV, Criterion 3).
(1) Explain normal platelet function.	
(2) Describe the relationship between bone marrow function, platelet count, risk of bleeding.	The patient/family describes behaviors that promote a level of independence appropriate to learning ability (Standard V, Criterion 3) and describes signs and symptoms that should be reported to the health care team (Standard V, Criterion 6).
(3) List signs/symptoms of bleeding to report.	
(4) Demonstrate/describe self-care measures for prevention, detection, and control of bleeding.	
4. Implement teaching plan.	Implements the teaching plan in an environment conducive to learning (Standard IV, Criterion 4).
5. Evaluate ability of patient to meet the selected evaluation criteria via: a. Verbalization. b. Return demonstration.	Collects data from the patient/family and other sources to evaluate achievement of learning objectives, effectiveness and efficiency of instruction, and the need to revise the teaching plan (Standard IV, Criterion 5).
6. Modify plan; reinforce teaching as necessary (e.g., use of written instructions) to reinforce learning, teaching a family member to serve as a resource for the patient.	Modifies teaching-learning process based on evaluation data (Standard IV, Criterion 6).

2-4 provides an example of a lesson plan for teaching the public about prevention and early detection of skin cancers.

    B. *Example 2*: use the standards and criteria as learner objectives for cancer nursing education programs.

VII. Examples of application of standards of oncology education to management.
    A. *Example 1*: the standards and criteria can be incorporated into staff performance evaluation instruments (educator component of the role). See Table 2-5 for an example.
    B. *Example 2*: resource justification. Use standard criteria to:
        1. Address the resources and environment required for patient/family and public education activities.
        2. Support the need for time, money, systems, and personnel required for education in accordance with the standards.

VII. Examples of application of standards of oncology education to research— suggested areas for investigation.

Table 2-4

CONTENT OUTLINE FOR PUBLIC EDUCATION PROGRAM ON PREVENTION AND EARLY
DETECTION OF SKIN CANCERS

RELEVANT STANDARD: Knowledge, skills, and attitudes related to the physical and psychosocial aspects of cancer prevention, early detection, and control are included in public education
programs.

Content Outline	Relevant Criteria
I. Overview of skin cancers: carcinogenesis (how skin cancers arise).	Public education program includes:

II. Risk factors.
  A. Fair, freckled complexion.
  B. Sun exposure.
    1. Recreational.
    2. Occupational.
  C. Chemical exposure.
  D. Radiation exposure.
  E. Scars from previous burns.
	Accurate and current information about principles of carcinogenesis, genetic and environmental risks for cancer (Criterion 1).

III. Signs and symptoms.
  A. Changes in moles; sore that does not heal.
  C. Persistent lump/swelling.
  D. Bleeding from mole, birthmark, freckle.
	Signs and symptoms of common cancers (Criterion 3).

IV. Early detection.
  A. Skin self-examination techniques (National Cancer Institute booklet).
  B. Community agencies for follow-up.
	Community resources for cancer-related information and services (Criterion 6).

V. Prevention.
  A. Minimization of sun exposure.
    1. Avoid sun bathing and use of tanning booths.
    2. Use sunscreens.
    3. Wear protective clothing.
  B. Occupational precautions.
	Methods to modify health behaviors and practices for cancer prevention and health promotion (Criterion 2).

From Oncology Nursing Society (1987). *Standards of Oncology Education: Patient/Family and Public*. Pittsburgh, Penn:
The Society, p. 11.

A. *Example 1*: clinical testing of specific criteria for each standard.
  1. Investigation of various teaching methodologies and the impact on patient learning outcomes (e.g., does the use of interactive videodisk teaching modules improve the ability of the patient to perform self-care activities?).
  2. Investigation of optimal approaches to teaching people with low literacy skills (e.g., what is the effect of using group/classroom learning activities versus one-to-one teaching of self-care activities in the low-literacy population?).
  3. Investigation of the impact of public education programs on the practice of life-style choices that minimize personal risks for cancer (e.g., what is the effect of public education classes on use of sunscreen products?).

Table 2-5

EXCERPT FROM AN ONCOLOGY STAFF NURSE PERFORMANCE EVALUATION TOOL

Standard	Rating* 1	2	3
STANDARD IV: Teaching-learning theories are applied to the development, implementation, and evaluation of learning experiences related to cancer care.			
Criteria—The nurse:			
1. Collects data systematically from the patient/family and other sources to assess learning needs, readiness to learn, and situational and psychosocial factors influencing learning.			
2. Analyzes assessment data to identify cognitive, psychomotor, and affective learning needs.			
3. Develops a teaching plan in collaboration with the patient/family that includes: a. Behavioral objectives based on identified learning needs. b. Content to meet identified objectives. c. Teaching strategies and learning experiences that promote active participation by the patient/family. d. Environmental adaptations to promote learning. e. Methods and criteria for evaluation.			
4. Implements the teaching plan in an environment conducive to learning.			
5. Collects data from the patient/family and other sources to evaluate achievement of learning objectives, effectiveness and efficiency of instruction, and the need to revise the teaching plan.			
6. Modifies teaching-learning process based on evaluation data.			

*Rating scale: 1, performance below standard; 2, performance meets standard; 3, performance exceeds standard.
From Oncology Nursing Society (1987). *Standards of Oncology Education: Patient/Family and Public.* Pittsburgh, Penn: The Society, pp. 7-8.

4. Investigation of the influence of religious, cultural, and ethnic practices on the teaching-learning process (e.g., what cultural characteristics influence the teaching-learning process in the Hispanic population?).

BIBLIOGRAPHY

American Nurses' Association and Oncology Nursing Society (1987). *Standards of Oncology Nursing Practice.* Kansas City, Mo: American Nurses' Association.

Oncology Nursing Society (1989). *Standards of Oncology Education: Patient/Family and Public.* Pittsburgh, Penn: The Society.

3

Factors Affecting Responses to the Risk for or Actual Diagnosis of Cancer

Anne Belcher, PhD, RN

THEORY

I. A variety of factors influence the responses of individuals and their significant others when faced with the risk or actual diagnosis of cancer.
  A. Developmental stage: divided by age groupings that reflect the variety of tasks to be performed as one ages from birth to death.
    1. Early adulthood (18 to 30 years).
      a. Selecting a mate.
      b. Learning to live with a life partner.
      c. Starting a family.
      d. Rearing children.
      e. Managing a home.
      f. Starting a work career.
      g. Finding a social group.
      h. Assuming civic responsibilities.
    2. Middle adulthood (30 to 55 years).
      a. Establishing and maintaining an economic standard of living.
      b. Relating to one's spouse as a person.
      c. Accepting and adjusting to the physiological changes of middle age.
      d. Adjusting to aging parents.
      e. Assisting teenage children to become responsible and happy adults.
      f. Developing adult leisure activities.
    3. Older adulthood (over 55 years).
      a. Adjusting to decreasing physical strength and health.
      b. Adjusting to retirement and reduced income.
      c. Adjusting to the death of a spouse.
      d. Establishing an explicit affiliation with one's age group.
      e. Adapting and adopting flexible social roles.
      f. Maintaining a satisfactory physical living arrangement.

4. The risk or diagnosis of cancer potentially disrupts the achievement of present and future developmental tasks.

B. Socioeconomic level.
   1. Influences not only potential risk factors for disease but also access to preventive health care, treatment, and rehabilitative health care.
   2. Poverty is associated with a constellation of factors that affect the risk for cancer: malnutrition, substandard housing, hopelessness, unemployment, illiteracy, lack of health insurance, and diminished access to health care.

C. Maturational level.
   1. Cancer incidence is bimodal, exhibiting a peak during childhood and exhibiting a sharp rise from childhood to old age.
   2. Physiological changes that occur as a consequence of aging may affect the response of the patient to cancer treatment (see Table 19-3).
   3. Psychosocial changes may also adversely affect the elderly with respect to cancer prevention, early detection, treatment, and rehabilitation motivation and behavior.
      a. The elderly are more likely to assume aches, pains, ill health, and disability are inevitable.
      b. The elderly have fewer relatives and friends to use as lay referral systems to the health care system.
      c. The elderly often have inaccurate or limited access to health information.
      d. The elderly often refrain from working outside the home, limiting the incentives to keep well and the income or insurance coverage required to access the health care system.
      e. The elderly often have negative attitudes about cancer and assume a passive role in decision making about health care decisions.

D. Psychological development.
   1. Evidence exists that supports the value of coping resources such as social support, sense of control, and stress management in adapting to the demands of cancer.
   2. Number, type, and effectiveness of previous coping strategies affect the response to illness demands.
   3. Positive self-concept has a positive effect on adaptation.

E. Education level.
   1. Education affects the ability of the individual to value, access, interpret, and apply information related to the risk or actual diagnosis of cancer.
      a. Lack of education and illiteracy may preclude the individual from awareness of modifications in life-style that may reduce cancer risks or of recommendations for cancer screening.
      b. Lack of education may adversely affect the attitudes the individual has about cancer, treatment, and rehabilitation:
         (1) Stigma of cancer's association with death.
         (2) Fear of contagion.
         (3) Guilt.
         (4) Pain and disfigurement associated with cancer treatment.
         (5) Unpleasant sense of individual vulnerability and mortality.
   2. Education affects the ability of the individual to obtain resources to meet the demands of cancer diagnosis, treatment, and follow-up care.

F. Support systems.
   1. *Family*: a psychosocial group consisting of the client and one or more persons (children and adults) in which a commitment for members to nurture each other exists.

      a. Nuclear.

      b. Extended.

      c. Nontraditional such as single parent or same-sex partners.

  2. *Significant others*: individuals identified by the client with whom a meaningful relationship exists.

      a. Friends.

      b. Lovers.

      c. Distant relatives.

  3. The quality of the relationships shared among family members/significant others affects the responses to the risk or actual diagnosis of cancer.

      a. Interrelationship and interdependence among family members/significant others.

      b. Concern shared about members of the family or significant others.

      c. Degree to which members are helpful and supportive to one another.

      d. Degree to which individual members are allowed and encouraged to act openly and to express their feelings directly.

      e. Degree to which an open expression of anger and aggression is tolerated.

      f. Degree to which individual members are encouraged to be independent, assertive, and self-sufficient.

      g. Developmental status of the individual members and the relationship.

      h. Previous or concurrent stressors and the type and effectiveness of individual and relationship coping strategies.

  4. Roles within supportive relationships.

      a. Roles influence functions, confer power, and govern the relationship.

      b. Changes in role assignment may occur based on the health status of the members and the flexibility of the members to accept or delegate responsibilities.

      c. Role incumbents within the relationship usually do not leave the role; rather they experience increased difficulty in performing role responsibilities.

      d. The permanence of role changes depends on the duration and severity of illness.

  5. Communication styles and patterns.

      a. A composite of the patterns of communications that each member brings to the relationship and of the patterns established within the relationship.

      b. Communication patterns are unique to each relationship and reflect attitudes toward age, gender, role, responsibilities, cultural and ethnic tradition, and conformity to societal norms.

      c. Communication patterns may include body movements such as facial expressions, social distance, body posturing, and eye contact.

      d. Communication patterns may be used to maintain the relationship and to exclude outsiders such as health care providers from the relationship.

  6. Responses of family members/significant others to the diagnosis of cancer.

      a. Psychosocial responses of adults and children: frustration, helplessness, guilt, grief, protectiveness, fear, concealment of emotions, uncertainty, powerlessness, ambivalence, increased need for closeness, and resiliency.

      b. Changes in roles and responsibilities: assumption of nonfamiliar roles or increased responsibilities; shift in levels of dependence/independence; changes in constellation of external reference groups such as church, clubs, social friends, and coworkers; modification of traditions valued in the relationship; and changes in the daily routine.

G. Community resources.

  1. When the demands of illness, treatment, and rehabilitation exceed the resources

of the individual and family/significant others, the community may be able to provide additional materials and services.

   2. Materials and services may include:

      a. Agencies that provide financial counseling.

      b. Financial assistance with needs of daily living such as food, housing, child care, and transportation.

      c. Education and care services sponsored by the National Cancer Institute through the Cancer Information Service (1-800-4-CANCER); American Cancer Society; Corporate Angel Network, Inc., for transportation to a treatment center; Leukemia Society of America; National Hospice Organization; Society for the Right to Die; and the United Cancer Council.

      d. Self-help groups sponsored by the American Cancer Society: CanSurmount, I Can Cope, Reach to Recovery, International Association of Laryngectomies; Make Today Count; Candlelighters; Encore; TOUCH; United Ostomy Association; We Can Do; wellness centers or groups; and the National Coalition for Cancer Survivorship.

II. These factors interact to create individual responses and group responses to the risk of or actual diagnosis of cancer.

DATA COLLECTION

See Table 3-1 on page 29.

ASSOCIATED NURSING DIAGNOSES

   I. Altered role performance.

  II. Ineffective individual coping.

 III. Altered health maintenance.

 IV. Impaired home maintenance management.

  V. Social isolation.

 VI. Altered family process.

VII. Impaired adjustment.

NURSING PLANNING AND IMPLEMENTATION

  I. Developmental tasks.

   A. Assist client and family to identify valued individual and family developmental tasks.

   B. Prioritize developmental tasks with respect to demands imposed by cancer and treatment.

   C. Help client and family identify personal and external resources needed to complete tasks.

   D. Evaluate progress toward task achievement throughout the course of treatment and follow-up care.

 II. Socioeconomic status.

   A. Assist client and family to identify socioeconomic issues complicated by the demands of cancer.

   B. Help to identify personal, family, and community resources available to meet identified socioeconomic needs.

     1. Social Security.

     2. Medicare/Medicaid.

Table 3-1
ASSESSMENT PARAMETERS ON FACTORS AFFECTING RESPONSES TO CANCER

Factor	Assessment Parameters
Developmental stage	Perception of life tasks that have been completed. Perception of immediate life tasks to be accomplished. Perception of how a diagnosis of cancer may affect present and future life goals.
Socioeconomic level	Level of individual and family income and number of persons supported. Insurance benefits (health, disability, and life). Perceived access to health care. Living conditions (type of housing, ownership versus rental, number of occupants, location, and sanitation).
Maturational level	Chronological age. Presence of physiological changes of aging. Motivation to seek cancer-related information. Life-style parameters (living arrangements, stressors, support systems, nutrition, and means of travel).
Psychological development	Previous life stressors. Strategies used to cope with stressors. Perceived effectiveness of previous coping strategies. Individual description of self. Perceived description of self by significant others. Perception of future.
Education level	Level of formal education. Reading level and comprehension. Ability to analyze and synthesize information. Value of education and knowledge about cancer.
Support systems	Identification of significant others within and outside the family. Description of support received and provided. Decision-making process and activities. Perceived demands of cancer and treatment and available supports to meet demands. Knowledge of community resources.

      3. American Cancer Society: Road to Recovery, direct aid for items such as dressings, selected medications, ostomy supplies, and breast prosthesis, depending on division policies.
      4. Vocational rehabilitation.
  C. Evaluate implications of socioeconomic variables on access to care, compliance with treatment plan, ability to assume independence in self-care, and follow-up care.
  D. Refer to appropriate facilities and agencies when planning transitions from one phase of the cancer experience to another.

III. Maturational level.
  A. Assist client and family/significant others to identify maturational strengths available to meet the demands of the cancer experience.
  B. Encourage expression of concerns and issues related to aging and coping with cancer.

C. Reward requests for information and participation in decision making about aspects of care.

IV. Psychological development.
   A. Support client and family/significant others in use of effective coping strategies.
   B. Teach new coping strategies as required by the demands of the illness.
   C. Monitor the changing psychological responses of the client and family/significant others.
   D. Evaluate the psychological development throughout the phases of diagnosis, treatment, rehabilitation, recurrence, survivorship, or death.
   E. Refer to appropriate members of the health team when the complexity or severity of psychological responses interferes with delivery of care, client safety, or rehabilitation or when needs exceed the expertise of the care provider.

V. Educational level.
   A. Provide explanations of procedures, informed consents, treatment, drug information, and follow-up care in language and format appropriate to the educational level of the client and family/significant other.
   B. Present information using a variety of formats: written, pictures, video, computers, or demonstration.
   C. Plan repetition of critical information.
   D. Seek consensual validation that information is heard, interpreted, and applied appropriately.

VI. Support systems.
   A. Provide information about available resources to meet identified needs.
   B. Assist client, family, or significant others to obtain resources as needed.
   C. Evaluate the need for and number, type, and effectiveness of resources used at regular intervals during the cancer experience.

EVALUATION OF CLIENT AND FAMILY OUTCOMES

I. Describe potential effects of cancer, treatment, and rehabilitation on individual developmental tasks, socioeconomic status, psychological development, and relationships with family members and significant others.

II. Discuss individual and relationship strengths and limitations that may affect the response to the cancer experience.

III. Identify potential strengths, needs, and resources within the family and community to meet the demands of the cancer experience.

IV. Access appropriate individual and community resources.

BIBLIOGRAPHY

Dugan, S.O. & Scallion, L.M. (1984). The older adult. In S.N. McIntire & A.L. Cioppa (eds). *Cancer Nursing. A Developmental Approach.* New York: John Wiley & Sons, pp. 225-253.

Edlund, B. & Sneed, N.V. (1989). Emotional responses to the diagnosis of cancer: age-related comparisons. *Oncol Nurs Forum, 16*(5), 691-697.

Frank-Stromborg, M. (1986). The role of the nurse in early detection of cancer: population sixty-six years of age and older. *Oncol Nurs Forum, 13*(3), 66-74.

Frank-Stromborg, M. & Savela, B. (1990). Yellow pages for the cancer nurse. In S.L. Groenwald, M.H. Frogge, M. Goodman, & C.H. Yarbro (eds). *Cancer Nursing: Principles and Practice* (2nd ed). Boston: Jones & Barlett Publishers, pp. 1281-1308.

Frank-Stromborg, M., Wright P.S., Segalla M., & Diekmann, J. (1984). Psychological impact of the "cancer" diagnosis. *Oncol Nurs Forum, 11*(3), 16-22.

Germino, B. (1991). Cancer and the family. In S.B. Baird, R. McCorkle, and M. Grant (eds). *Cancer Nursing: A Comprehensive Textbook.* Philadelphia: W.B. Saunders Co., pp. 38-60.

Gray-Price, H. & Szczesny, S. (1985). Crisis intervention with families of cancer patients: a developmental approach. *Top Clin Nurs* 7(1), 58-70.

Lewis, F.M. (1986). The impact of cancer on the family: a critical analysis of the research literature. *Patient Educ Counseling* 8(3), 269-289.

Lewis, F.M. & Ellison, E.S. (1985). The impact of breast cancer on the family. *Semin Oncol Nurs*, 1(3), 206-213.

McIntire, S.N. (1984). The adult. In S.N. McIntire & A.L. Cioppa (eds). *Cancer Nursing. A Developmental Approach.* New York: John Wiley & Sons, pp. 206-253.

Shields, P. (1984). Communication: A supportive bridge between cancer patient, family, and health care staff. *Nurs Forum* 21(1), 31-36.

Thorne, S. (1985). The family cancer experience. *Cancer Nurs* 8(5), 285-291.

Thorne, S.E. (1988). Helpful and unhelpful communications in cancer care: the patient perspective. *Oncol Nurs Forum* 15(2), 167-172.

Vess, J.D., Moreland, J.R., & Schwebel, A.I. (1985). A follow-up study of role functioning and the psychological environment of families of cancer patients. *J Psychosoc Oncol* 3(2), 1-14.

Welch-McCaffrey, D. (1983). When it comes to cancer, think family. *Nursing* 13(12), 32-35.

4

Primary Prevention in Oncology Nursing Practice

Margaret Crowley, BSN, RN

THEORY

I. Definition of *primary prevention*—risk of cancer is reduced through client behaviors related to:
   A. Eliminating or limiting exposure to causative factors.
   B. Promoting protective factors (including health-promoting activities).

II. Theoretical principles and assumptions.
   A. Recognizing risk factors identifies individuals at higher risk for development of cancer.
   B. Reduction of exposure to carcinogens may reduce cancer development.
      1. Cancer development includes initiating and promoting factors.
      2. Promotion can be reversed.
      3. Avoidance of synergistic effects (alcohol and tobacco, asbestos and tobacco) may decrease incidence.
   C. Changes in life-style may reduce risks of cancer development.
   D. The National Cancer Institute's (NCI) goals for the year 2000 to reduce cancer deaths by 50% include two goals on cancer prevention (Table 4-1), thereby providing the rationale for establishing nursing priorities (e.g., smoking, diet) in cancer prevention.
   E. The public is often skeptical or fatalistic ("everything causes cancer"); therefore nurses should be prepared to discuss both the strengths and weaknesses of existing data sources regarding risks.
      1. Epidemiological studies.
         a. Strengths of epidemiological studies.
            (1) Effects on humans versus animals are shown.
            (2) Types of cancer vary markedly between countries, providing valuable data sources.
            (3) Migrant populations develop the type of cancer characteristic of new locale, providing clues about geographical and social differences.
            (4) Different life-styles such as those of Mormons or nuns in same environment (which controls for environmental variables) result in different cancer incidence.

Table 4-1
NATIONAL CANCER INSTITUTE CANCER CONTROL OBJECTIVES: PREVENTION

Control Factor	Rationale	Year 2000 Objective
Prevention		
Smoking	Causal relationship between smoking and cancer has been scientifically established.	Reduce the percentage of adults who smoke from 34% (in 1983) to 15% or less.
		Reduce the percentage of youths who smoke by age 20 from 36% (in 1983) to 15% or less.
Diet	Research indicates that high-fat and low-fiber consumption may increase the risk for various cancers. In 1983, National Academy of Sciences reviewed research on diet and cancer and recommended a reduction in fat, and more recent studies have led National Cancer Institute to recommend an increase in fiber. Research is underway to verify the causal relationships and to test the impact on cancer incidence.	Reduce average consumption of fat from 40% to 25% or less of total calories.
		Increase average consumption of fiber from 8-12 g to 20-30 g per day.

   b. Weaknesses of epidemiological studies.
      (1) Most studies are correlational; therefore cause cannot be inferred.
      (2) Long lag time between exposure and development of disease (latency) may obscure differences, especially in low-incidence cancers.
      (3) Difficult to incriminate agent when exposure is uniform throughout the population (high-fat diet).
      (4) Difficult to relate occurrence to low exposure (radon).
   2. Whole animal bioassay.
      a. Strengths: can control or measure exposure to specific factors not feasible in humans (dosage, synergistic factors, inhibitors).
      b. Weaknesses:
         (1) Extrapolation of animal studies to humans is limited because of species differences.
         (2) Animal doses often exceed human exposures.
   3. Mutagenesis studies (Ames test).
      a. Strengths:
         (1) All carcinogenic chemicals are mutagenic.
         (2) Mutagenic studies provide faster testing of carcinogens.
      b. Weakness: not all cells transformed in vitro (undergoing mutagenesis) exhibit biological neoplasia (carcinogenesis).

DATA COLLECTION
   I. Identify life-style risk factors:
      A. Tobacco use.
         1. Tobacco is leading carcinogen of recent times.
         2. Strongly linked to lung cancer (risk of cancer is 10 times greater by middle age for smokers versus lifelong non-smokers).

Table 4-2
OCCUPATIONAL CANCER HAZARDS

Agent	Cancer Site or Type	Type of Workers Exposed
Acrylonitrile	Lung, colon	Manufacturers of apparel, carpeting, blankets, draperies, synthetic furs, and wigs
4-Aminobiphenyl	Bladder	Chemical workers
Arsenic and certain arsenic compounds	Lung, skin, scrotum, lymphatic system, hemangiosarcoma of the liver	Workers in the metallurgical industries, sheep-dip workers, pesticide production workers, copper smelter workers, vineyard workers, insecticide makers and sprayers, tanners, miners (gold miners)
Asbestos	Lung, larynx, gastrointestinal (GI) tract, pleural and peritoneal mesothelioma	Asbestos factory workers, textile workers, rubber-tire manufacturing industry workers, miners, insulation workers, shipyard workers
Auramine and the manufacture of auramine	Bladder	Dyestuffs manufacturers, rubber workers, textile dryers, paint manufacturers
Benzene	Leukemia	Rubber-tire manufacturing industry workers, painters, shoe manufacturing workers, rubber cement workers, glue and varnish workers, distillers, shoemakers, plastics workers, chemical workers
Benzidine	Bladder, pancreas	Dyeworkers, chemical workers
Beryllium and certain beryllium compounds	Lung	Beryllium workers, electronics workers, missile parts producers
Bis(chloromethyl)ether (BCME)	Lung	Workers in plants producing anion-exchange resins (chemical workers)
Cadmium and certain cadmium compounds	Lung, prostate	Cadmium production workers, metallurgical workers, electroplating industry workers, chemical workers, jewelry workers, nuclear workers, pigment workers, battery workers
Carbon tetrachloride	Liver	Plastics workers, dry cleaners
Chloromethyl methyl ether (CMME)	Lung	Chemical workers, workers in plants producing ion-exchange resin
Chromium and certain chromium compounds	Lung, nasal sinuses	Chromate-producing industry workers, acetylene and aniline workers, bleachers, glass, pottery, pigment, and linoleum workers
Coal tar pitch volatiles	Lung, scrotum	Steel industry workers, aluminum potroom workers, foundry workers

From U.S. Congress, Office of Technology Assessment, *Assessment of Technologies for Determining Cancer Risks from the Environment,* OTA-H-138 (Springfield, VA: National Technical Information Service, June 1981).

Table 4-2
OCCUPATIONAL CANCER HAZARDS *Continued*

Agent	Cancer Site or Type	Type of Workers Exposed
Coke oven emissions	Lung, kidney, prostate	Steel industry workers, coke plant workers
Dimethyl sulphate	Lung	Chemical workers, drug makers, dyemakers
Epichlorohydrin	Lung, leukemia	Chemical workers
Ethylene oxide	Leukemia, stomach	Hospital workers, research laboratory workers, beekeepers, fumigators
Hematite and underground hematite mining	Lung	Miners
Isopropyl oils and the manufacture of isopropyl oils	Paranasal sinuses	Isopropyl oil workers
Mustard gas	Respiratory tract	Production workers
2-Naphthylamine	Bladder, pancreas	Dye workers, rubber-tire manufacturing industry workers, chemical workers, manufacturers of coal gas, nickel refiners, copper smelters, electrolysis workers
Nickel (certain compounds) and nickel refining	Nasal cavity, lung, larynx	Nickel refiners
Polychlorinated biphenyls (PCBs)	Melanoma	PCBs workers
Radiation, ionizing	Skin, pancreas, brain, stomach, breast, salivary glands, thyroid, GI tract, bronchus, lymphoid tissue, leukemia, multiple myeloma	Uranium miners, radiologists, radiographers, luminous dial painters
Radiation, ultraviolet	Skin	Farmers, sailors, arc welders
Soots, tars, mineral oils	Skin, lung, bladder, GI tract	Construction workers, roofers, chimney sweeps, machinists
Thorium dioxide	Liver, kidney, larynx, leukemia	Chemical workers, steelworkers, ceramic makers, incandescent lamp makers, nuclear reactor workers, gas mantle makers, metal refiners, vacuum tube makers
Vinyl chloride	Liver, brain, lung, hematolymphopoietic system, breast	Plastics factory workers, vinyl chloride polymerization plant workers
Agent(s) not identified	Pancreas	Chemists
	Stomach	Coal miners
	Brain, stomach	Petrochemical industry workers
	Hematolymphopoietic system	Rubber industry workers
	Bladder	Printing pressmen
	Eye, kidney, lung	Chemical workers
	Leukemia, brain	Farmers
	Colon, brain	Pattern and model makers
	Esophagus, stomach, lung	Oil refinery workers

      3. Strongly associated with cancers of mouth, larynx, pharynx, esophagus.
      4. Contributes to development of cancers of bladder, pancreas, kidney, stomach, and liver.
      5. Exposure to environmental tobacco smoke may increase risk of lung cancer.
      6. Smokeless tobacco (chewing tobacco) is associated with cancers of the oral cavity.
   B. Alcohol consumption.
      1. Increases risk of cancer of esophagus, liver, and pharynx.
      2. Has a synergistic effect with tobacco.
   C. Dietary differences.
      1. May increase risk of cancer:
         a. Obesity (breast).
         b. High-fat diet (breast, prostate, colon).
         c. Salt-cured, smoked, and nitrate-cured food (esophagus, stomach).
      2. May decrease risk of cancer:
         a. High-fiber diet (colon).
         b. Diet high in vitamins A and C.
         c. Increased intake of cruciferous vegetables.
   D. Sexual practices associated with a higher cancer incidence include:
         a. Large number of sexual partners.
         b. Early age of sexual activity (uterine, cervix).

II. Identify occupational/physical environmental risks.
   A. Occupational cancer hazards (Table 4-2).
      1. Chemical exposures increase risk of bladder and lung cancer.
      2. Asbestos fibers increase incidence of mesothelioma of lung.
      3. Asbestos fibers and cigarette smoke increase incidence of all types lung cancer (synergistic effects).
      4. Radiation exposure increases incidence of leukemia, breast, and lung cancer.
   B. Carcinogens in the physical environment.
      1. Ultraviolet light (sunlight) exposure increases risk of cancers of skin, including melanoma.
      2. Radiation exposure from naturally occurring radium (radon) decay may increase risk of cancer of lung (data inconclusive).
      3. Secondary exposure (passive smoking) to cigarette smoke may increase risk of cancer of lung.

III. Identify biological risk factors.
   A. Genetic predisposition.
      1. Family history of cancer increases risk (high-risk families).
      2. Daughters of mothers with breast cancer (especially mothers with premenopausal bilateral cancer) have increased risk of breast cancer.
      3. Fair skin (Celtic ancestry) increases risk of skin cancer.
      4. Individuals with familial polyposis or Gardner's syndrome are expected to develop cancer of colon.
      5. Children with retinoblastoma, neuroblastoma, and Wilms' tumor have a genetic predisposition.
   B. Viral exposures.
      1. Chronic hepatitis B infection may lead to liver cancer.
      2. Papilloma virus lesions may progress to squamous cell carcinoma of skin.
      3. Papilloma virus has been associated with cervical cancer.
      4. Epstein-Barr virus is linked to Burkitt's lymphoma and nasopharyngeal cancers.

5. Retrovirus human T-cell lymphotropic virus-1 (HTLV-1) is linked to T-cell leukemia and HTLV-2 to hairy cell leukemia.
6. Human immunodeficiency virus (HIV) is associated with an increased risk of Kaposi's sarcoma, Hodgkin's lymphoma, and B-cell lymphoma.

IV. Identify iatrogenic risks.
   A. Hormonal agents.
      1. Estrogen therapy in menopausal women is associated with endometrial cancer.
      2. Estrogen exposure in the fetus (diethylstilbestrol) is associated with vaginal cancer in adulthood.
      3. Contraceptives may be associated with liver cancer and possibly breast cancer (data are inconclusive).
      4. Anabolic steroids may be associated with liver cancer.
   B. Immunosuppressive agents (organ recipients) increase risk of non-Hodgkin's lymphoma.
   C. Antineoplastic agents (especially alkylating agents, cyclophosphamide, melphalan, and busulfan) increase risk of secondary cancers.

V. Assess combination risk factors to identify subpopulations at greatest risk.
   A. Synergistic effects of carcinogens (alcohol and tobacco).
   B. Hereditary predisposition and life-style choices (pigmented nevi syndrome and sun exposure).

VI. Assess motivation for preventive behavior (health belief model).
   A. Perceived susceptibility—evidence indicates individuals at risk often are unaware of their risks (ask "How likely do you feel you are to develop cancer?").
   B. Perceived severity of respective cancer ("How serious do you think this type of cancer is?").
   C. Perceived benefits of preventive behavior ("Do you think you can decrease your risk by not smoking [or the habit in question]?").
   D. Perceived barriers to preventive action ("What problems do you think you may have in lowering fat content in your diet [or the behavior in question]?").
      1. Deleterious effects of risk behaviors may not be manifest for years (latency); therefore present-versus-future orientation may be a barrier.
      2. Lack of motivation to change life-style may be related to addictive nature of habit in question (smoking, alcohol consumption).
      3. Costs and limited access to care may result in knowledge or resource deficits.

ASSOCIATED NURSING DIAGNOSES
   I. Knowledge deficit related to recognition of risk factors.
   II. Knowledge deficit related to life-style changes to reduce risk of cancer development.

NURSING PLANNING AND IMPLEMENTATION STRATEGIES TO REDUCE CANCER RISK
   I. Personalize risks.
      A. Risk-appraisal questionnaire.
      B. Interviews.
   II. Identify behavioral changes that may reduce cancer risks.
      A. Changing diets.
         1. Avoid overeating, which may contribute to obesity.
         2. Reduce total fat intake from 40% to less than 25% of caloric intake by substituting low-fat for high-fat foods in diet (Table 4-3).

Table 4-3
FOOD GUIDE AT A GLANCE

First Choice	Second Best	Limit
Fats and Oils		Butter, margarine, cooking and salad oils, lard, shortening, mayonnaise, salad dressing
Dairy Foods		
Skim milk: fluid, powdered, and evaporated	Low-fat and part-skim (2%) milk and milk products: yogurt, cottage cheese, frozen yogurt, farmer cheese, ricotta cheese	Whole (homogenized) milk and whole-milk products: yogurt, cottage cheese, ricotta cheese
1% milk	Sherbet	Cream, nondairy creamers
Buttermilk (skim)	Ice milk	Sour cream
Fat-free yogurt		Cream cheese
Cottage cheese (1% fat)		Hard cheeses
Skim farmer cheese		Ice cream
Sapsago cheese		
Parmesan cheese		
Meat and Protein		
Lean veal, fish, poultry (without skin)	Red meat, fat trimmed	Sausage, bacon, luncheon meat, hot dogs, fried meat, fried fish, duck
Legumes (beans, lentils, peas)	Turkey roll	
Egg whites	Lamb	Dry roasted or fried nuts
	Egg yolks	Peanut butter
	Tofu and tempeh	
Bread, Cereals, and Other Starches		
Breads, plain rolls, bagels, cereals, pasta, rice, potatoes	Muffins, tea biscuits, crackers, low-fat cookies	Commercial and "mix" baked goods (doughnuts, croissants, pastries, pies, cakes), fried potatoes, fried rice, potato chips, corn chips, granola
Air-popped corn		
Fruit and Vegetables		
All fresh, frozen, and canned fruit and vegetables without added fat		Coconut
		French fries
		Tempura vegetables
		Avocado
		Olives
Sugar, Alcohol		
Honey, molasses, maple syrup, jams, hard candy	Alcoholic beverages	Chocolate, caramel, toffee, nougat, fudge
Beverages		
Juice (unsweetened)	Drinks containing caffeine (e.g., coffee, tea, hot chocolate, cola)	Drinks made with ice cream or cream
Herbal tea	Sweetened (naturally and artificially) carbonated beverages	
Club soda, seltzer, water		

From Boyar, A.P., Rose, D.P., and Wynder, E.L. (1988). Recommendations for the prevention of chronic disease: the application for breast disease. *Am J Clin Nutr* 48(suppl):896. © American Society for Clinical Nutrition.

Table 4-4

FIBER CONTENT OF COMMONLY USED FOODS

Food	Serving Size	Fiber/Serving (g)	Food	Serving Size	Fiber/Serving (g)
Breads			**Vegetables (cooked)**		
Bran muffins	1 muffin	2.5	Asparagus, cut	½ cup	1.0
Cracked wheat	1 slice	1.0	Beans, string, green	½ cup	1.6
Crisp bread, rye	2 crackers	2.0	Broccoli	½ cup	2.2
Crisp bread, wheat	2 crackers	1.8	Brussel sprouts	½ cup	2.3
French bread	1 slice	0.7	Cabbage, red	½ cup	1.4
Italian bread	1 slice	0.3	Cabbage, white	½ cup	1.4
Mixed grain	1 slice	0.9	Carrots	½ cup	2.3
Pita bread (5 inches)	1 piece	0.4	Cauliflower	½ cup	1.1
Pumpernickel bread	1 slice	1.0	Corn, canned	½ cup	2.9
Raisin bread	1 slice	0.6	Kale, leaves	½ cup	1.4
White bread	1 slice	0.6	Parsnip	½ cup	2.7
Whole wheat bread	1 slice	2.1	Peas	½ cup	3.6
			Potato (without skin)	1 medium	1.4
Pasta and Rice (cooked)			Potato (with skin)	1 medium	2.5
Macaroni	1 cup	1.0	Spinach	½ cup	2.1
Rice, brown	½ cup	1.0	Squash, summer	½ cup	1.4
Rice, polished	½ cup	0.2	Sweet potatoes	½ medium	1.7
Spaghetti (regular)	1 cup	1.1	Turnip	½ cup	1.6
Spaghetti (whole wheat)	1 cup	3.9	Zucchini	½ cup	1.8
Fruits			**Vegetables (raw)**		
Apple (without skin)	1 medium	2.7	Bean sprout, soy	½ cup	1.5
Apple (with skin)	1 medium	3.5	Celery, diced	½ cup	1.1
Apricot (fresh)	3 medium	1.8	Cucumber	½ cup	0.4
Apricot, dried	5 halves	1.4	Lettuce, sliced	1 cup	0.9
Banana	1 medium	2.4	Mushrooms, sliced	½ cup	0.9
Blueberries	½ cup	2.0	Onions, sliced	½ cup	0.8
Cantaloupe	¼ melon	1.0	Pepper, green sliced	½ cup	0.5
Cherries, sweet	10	1.2	Tomato	1 medium	1.5
Dates	3	1.9	Spinach	1 cup	1.2
Grapefruit	½	1.6			
Orange	1	2.6	**Nuts and Snacks**		
Peach (with skin)	1	1.9	Almonds	10 nuts	1.1
Peach (without skin)	1	1.2	Peanuts	10 nuts	1.4
Pear (with skin)	½ large	3.1	Filberts	10 nuts	1.8
Pear (without skin)	½ large	2.5	Popcorn, commercial	1 cup	0.7
Pineapple	½ cup	1.1			
Plums, damson	5	0.9	**Legumes**		
Prunes	3	3.0	Baked beans, tomato sauce	½ cup	8.8
Raisins	¼ cup	3.1			
Raspberries	½ cup	3.1	Chickpeas, cooked	½ cup	3.4
Strawberries	1 cup	3.0	Dried peas, cooked	½ cup	4.7
Watermelon	1 cup	0.4	Kidney beans, cooked	½ cup	7.3
			Lima beans, cooked/canned	½ cup	4.5
Juices					
Apple	½ cup (4 oz)	0.4	Lentils, cooked	½ cup	3.2
Grapefruit	½ cup (4 oz)	0.5	Navy beans, cooked	½ cup	6.0
Grape	½ cup (4 oz)	0.6			
Orange	½ cup (4 oz)	0.5			
Papaya	½ cup (4 oz)	0.8			

From Lanza, E. and Butrum, R. (1986). A critical review of food fiber analysis and data. *J Am Dietetic Assoc 86* (June), 732-740.

3. Increase fiber intake from 8 to 12 g per day to 20 to 30 g per day by eating whole grain cereals, fresh fruits, and vegetables (Table 4-4).
4. Increase intake of foods rich in vitamins A and C.
    a. Foods rich in vitamin A include spinach, carrots, sweet potatoes, peaches, and apricots.
    b. Foods rich in vitamin C include oranges, grapefruit, strawberries, and peppers (red and green).
5. Include cruciferous vegetables in diet: cabbage, broccoli, brussel sprouts, kohlrabi, and cauliflower.
6. Minimize intake of salt-cured, smoked, and nitrite-cured foods (luncheon meat, bacon, hot dogs).

B. Changing life-style.
1. Abstain from tobacco use (Tables 4-5 and 4-6).
2. Eliminate or limit alcohol consumption.
3. Reduce exposure to ultraviolet light in the form of sunlight.
    a. Use sunscreens (SPF 15) when exposed.
    b. Avoid sun during periods of greatest intensity (midday, 11 AM to 1 PM).
    c. Wear protective clothing and hats when working in the sun.

C. Avoiding exposure to HIV virus.
1. Abstinence or a monogamous relationship with a noninfected partner avoids sexual exposure.
2. Limiting the number of sexual partners and choosing partners at low risk for infection reduces chances of exposure.
3. Following safe-sex recommendations limits exposure: avoid exchange of semen, vaginal fluid, or blood between partners (use condom and spermicide for all insertive sexual practices).

Table 4-5
NURSING ACTIVITIES REGARDING SMOKING CESSATION

1. Recognize high-risk individuals:
    a. Adolescent women.
    b. Low socioeconomic groups.
    c. Low education groups.
2. Assess client smoking behaviors:
    a. Number of cigarettes smoked per day.
    b. Length of time as smoker.
    c. Reasons for smoking (habit, addiction, social pressures).
    d. Desire to quit smoking.
    e. Previous attempts to quit.
3. Provide brief, firm advice to:
    a. Identify hazards of tobacco (to self and others).
    b. Counsel on benefits of quitting (immediate and long-term or to unborn child).
    c. Provide relevant reading materials.
4. Identify strategies for quitting (see Table 4-6).
5. Discuss ways to deal with client concerns about smoking cessation: weight gain, cravings, irritability, headache, depression, insomnia.
6. Secure commitment by setting date with client to stop smoking.
7. Monitor client's progress; provide positive reinforcement; avoid blaming for lack of success.
8. Evaluate outcomes frequently: follow up with phone calls, written reminders, or subsequent visits.

Table 4-6

MAJOR BEHAVIOR MODIFICATION STRATEGIES AND SAMPLE ACTIVITIES APPLIED TO SMOKING CESSATION COUNSELING

Strategies	Sample Activities
Adversive techniques	Before quitting, associate smoking with negative consequences (e.g., use rapid smoking without inhaling, snap wrist with rubber band when desire to smoke is felt).
Self-monitoring	Log cigarettes smoked using wrap-sheet around pack, recording time smoked, location and activity while smoking, and importance of cigarette. Identify smoking trigger.
Contingency management/ reinforcement	Plan daily and long-term rewards, often monetary, for taking steps towards quitting.
Stimulus control	Disrupt usual routine. Reduce or eliminate trigger situations (e.g., coffee, alcohol, smoking friends). Spend more time with nonsmoking friends.
Response substitutions	Plan substitutes for smoking in trigger situations (e.g., chew gum, raw vegetables; use deep breathing). Increase positive addictions (e.g., exercise). Discard smoking paraphernalia.
Increase personal commitment to quit	Make a list of quitting benefits. Announce quitting plans to family and friends. Sign a contract with self-specified quit date.
Enlist social support	Quit with a friend. Join a group program. Identify family member as helper.
Anxiety management	Learn meditation or relaxation techniques. Take 5-10 deep breaths when craving smoking. Begin regular exercise program.
Coping response training/ cognitive rehearsal	Think positively. Practice ways of turning down offered cigarettes. Have plans for common trigger situations. Rehearse nonsmoking coping response for anticipated barriers. Use mental imagery, picturing self as nonsmoker.

From Risser, N.L. (1987). Prevention of lung cancer: stopping smoking. *Semin Oncol Nurs 3,* 231.

    4. Avoiding intravenous (IV) drug use eliminates exposure from needle/syringe contamination; using sterile needles/syringes reduces risk.
    5. Preventing pregnancy in infected women avoids exposure to fetus.
    6. Avoiding anal-receptive intercourse and multiple sexual partners among male homosexuals reduces risk.
  D. Modifying workplace behavior.
    1. Recognize carcinogens in the workplace.
    2. Minimize exposure through use of proper safety equipment and procedures.
  E. Adopting health promotion behaviors.
    1. Exercise (minimum of 20 minutes twice a week).
    2. Balanced diet.
    3. Stress management.

III. Mutually develop plan to minimize risk.

IV. Obtain commitment (date to begin, follow-up, reminder system).

 V. Revise plan based on feedback.

EVALUATION OF CLIENT OUTCOMES

I. Identify risk factors related to life-style, occupation, genetics, and the environment.

II. List ways to limit risk factors.

III. Discuss health-promoting and risk-reduction practices.

IV. Identify resources and programs for cancer prevention: *Tobacco Free Young America*, *Taking Control, Nutrition, Common Sense and Cancer* (American Cancer Society), *Quit, for Good* (National Institutes of Health).

BIBLIOGRAPHY

American Cancer Society (1990). *Cancer Facts and Figures—1990*. Atlanta: The Society.

Baird, S.B. (ed) (1991). *A Cancer Source Book for Nurses* (6th ed). Atlanta: American Cancer Society.

Beck, S., Breckenridge, S., Potterf, S., Wallace, S., Ware, J., Asay, E., & Giles, R.T. (1988). The family high-risk program: targeted cancer prevention. *Oncol Nurs Forum, 15*(3), 301-306.

Committee on Diet, Nutrition and Cancer of National Academy of Sciences (1985). Executive Summary. In P. Greenwald, A.G. Ershow, & W.D. Novelli (eds). *Cancer, Diet and Nutrition: A Comprehensive Sourcebook*. Chicago: Marqis Who's Who, pp. 34-44.

Doll, R. & Peto, R. (1985). The causes of cancer and quantitative estimates of avoidable risks of cancer in the United States today. In P. Greenwald, A.G. Ershow, & W.D. Novelli (eds). *Cancer, Diet and Nutrition: A Comprehensive Sourcebook*. Chicago: Marqis Who's Who, pp. 3-24.

Donehower, M.G. (1987). Malignant complications of AIDS. *Oncol Nurs Forum 14*(1), 57-64.

Gianella, A. (1985). Teaching cancer prevention and detection. *Cancer Nurs 8*(suppl 1), 9-16.

Glasel, M. (1985). Cancer prevention: the role of the nurse in primary and secondary cancer prevention. *Cancer Nurs 8*(suppl 1), 5-8.

Groopman, J. & Browder, S. (1989). Cancer in AIDS and other immunodeficiency states. In V.T. DeVita, Jr., S. Hellman, & S.A. Rosenberg (eds). *Cancer Principles & Practice of Oncology*, vol 2. Philadelphia: J.B. Lippincott, pp. 1953-1959.

Harley, N.H. & Harley, J.H. (1990). Potential lung cancer risk from indoor radon exposure, *CA 40*(5), 265-275.

Heusinkveld K.B.(1991). Preventive oncology. In S.B. Baird, R. McCorkle, & M. Grant (eds). *Cancer Nursing: A Comprehensive Textbook*. Philadelphia: W.B. Saunders Co., pp. 143-154.

Howley, P. (1989). Principles of carcinogenesis: viral. In V.T. DeVita, Jr, S. Hellman, & S.A. Rosenberg (eds). *Cancer Principles & Practice of Oncology*, vol 1 (3rd ed). Philadelphia: J.B. Lippincott.

Love, R.R. & Olsen, S.J. (1985). An agenda for cancer prevention in nursing practice. *Cancer Nurs 8*(6), 329-338.

McNally, J.C., Stair, J.C., & Somerville, E.T. (eds). (1985). *Guidelines for Cancer Nursing Practice*. Orlando, Fla: Grune & Stratton.

Office of Technology Assessment (1982). *Cancer Risk: Assessing and Reducing the Dangers in our Society*. Boulder, Colo: Westview Press.

Oncology Nursing Society (1989). *Standards of Oncology Education*. Pittsburgh: The Society.

Pitot, H.C. (1989). Principles of carcinogenesis: chemical. In V.T. DeVita, Jr., S. Hellman, & S.A. Rosenberg (eds). *Cancer Principles & Practice of Oncology,* vol 1 (3rd ed). Philadelphia: J.B. Lippincott, pp. 116-135.

White, L.N. (1986). Cancer prevention and detection; from twenty to sixty-five years of age. *Oncol Nurs Forum 13*(2), 59-64.

Secondary Prevention in Oncology Nursing Practice

Marilyn Davis, MS, RN

Individual Cancer Risk Appraisal

THEORY

I. Definitions.
   A. *Secondary prevention*—defining and identifying high-risk groups and groups with precursor stages of cancer.
   B. *Risk*—the likelihood that exposure to a certain factor will influence the chance of developing a particular cancer based on the national average.
   C. *Absolute risk*—a measure of occurrence of cancer as gauged by incidence (new cases) or mortality (deaths) attributable to that cancer.
   D. *Relative risk*—an estimation of increase in probability of development of a certain cancer based on amount of exposure to the associated risk factor(s). The higher the relative risk factor, the greater is the risk of development of a specific cancer.
   E. *Attributable risk*—the amount of preventable disease, allowing for a calculation of incidence of the disease likely to occur in the absence of all identified risk factors (suggests areas for development of education programs designed to prevent or minimize exposure to risk factors).

II. Rationale.
   A. Local and/or systemic treatment modalities have not demonstrated the capability to cure most cancers; therefore prevention and early detection strategies have gained increasing importance.
   B. To achieve the National Cancer Institute's (NCI) goal of a 50% reduction in cancer mortality by the year 2000 (Table 5-1), early detection efforts must be intensified.
   C. Dramatic increases in survival are achieved when cancer is detected early and appropriate therapy is instituted effectively.
   D. Present efforts are focused on education of both populations at risk for development of specific cancers and health care professionals.
   E. Quantification of risk profiles improves efficiency and decreases costs of screening.

Table 5-1

NATIONAL CANCER INSTITUTE CANCER CONTROL OBJECTIVES: SCREENING

Control Factor	Rationale	Year 2000 Objective
Screening		
Breast	Effectiveness of breast screening in reducing mortality has been scientifically established	Increase the percentage of women ages 50-70 who have annual physical breast examination and mammography from 45% for physical examination alone and 15% for mammography to 80% for each
Cervical	Effectiveness of cervical screening in reducing mortality has been scientifically established	Increase the percentage of women who have a Pap smear every 3 yr to 90% from 79% (ages 20-39) and to 80% from 57% (ages 40-70 yr)

From National Cancer Institute 1988. *Cancer* 62, 1852.

DATA COLLECTION

  I. Individual risk appraisal—early-detection physical examination guidelines are built on the epidemiological data base that suggests general, cancer site–specific, and individual variables (instruments and computer programs to quantify risks have been developed and are cited in the literature):

    A. Age—incidence increases with age; majority of malignant diseases occur in the over-65 age group.

    B. Sex—more common in males than females.

    C. Race—in the United States highest male incidence in blacks, then in whites, then Hawaiians; female Hawaiians exhibit the highest incidence, followed by whites, then blacks.

    D. Geography—major differences in incidence and mortality exist in different parts of the world; migratory data demonstrate adoption of the cancer pattern of the area to which migration occurs, suggesting environmental and life-style variables.

    E. Socioeconomic environment variables.

      1. Urbanization and pollution are associated with increased incidences of cancer.

      2. Tobacco use is higher among socioeconomically disadvantaged.

      3. More advanced disease presentations are seen in rural communities and lower socioeconomic groups.

  II. Physical examination—early detection of cancer in the asymptomatic or symptomatic individual is facilitated through the mechanism of a cancer-related checkup; American Cancer Society guidelines suggest:

    A. Cancer checkup every 3 years for asymptomatic individuals under 40 years of age.

    B. Annual checkups for those over 40 years of age.

    C. Symptomatic individuals should seek medical evaluation; "Cancer's Seven Warning Signals (CAUTION)," as published by the American Cancer Society, are:

      1. *C*hange in bowel or bladder habits.

      2. *A* sore that will not heal.

      3. *U*nusual bleeding or discharge.

      4. *T*hickening or lump in breast or elsewhere.

      5. *I*ndigestion or difficulty swallowing.

6. *O*bvious change in wart or mole.
7. *N*agging cough or hoarseness.

III. For both the asymptomatic and symptomatic individuals, a comprehensive data base is developed:
   A. History.
      1. Age, sex, race, date and place of birth, occupation, next of kin, insurance coverage.
      2. Reason for seeking examination; if symptomatic, use STOP framework:

a. *S*ymptom	Location and severity.
b. *T*ime	When does the symptom occur, and how long does it last?
c. *O*ther	What aggravates symptom? What relieves symptom?
d. *P*reconceptions	What does the individual think is happening?

      3. Previous state of health.
      4. Previous cancer.
      5. Allergies.
      6. Present state of health.
         a. Daily medications.
         b. Diet.
         c. Elimination.
         d. Habits—smoking, exercise, alcohol, sexual.
      7. Family medical history.
      8. Family cancer history.
   B. Review of systems—general.
      1. Weight—present, usual, recent gain/loss.
      2. Performance status—present and previous level of activity; note any weakness, fatigue, malaise.
      3. Neurological—headache; seizures; vertigo; visual disturbances; sensory, motor, or cognitive deficits.
      4. Endocrine—sweating, tachycardia, palpitations, flushing.
      5. Hematologic—bruising, petechiae, purpura, prolonged bleeding.
      6. Lymphatic—lymphadenopathy.
      7. Musculoskeletal—pain, stiffness, limitation of movement.
      8. Respiratory—cough, pain, dyspnea, hemoptysis, shortness of breath.
      9. Cardiac—hypertension, dyspnea, orthopnea, chest pain.
      10. Head and neck—pain, tenderness, dysphagia, difficulty chewing, hoarseness, discharge.
      11. Gastrointestinal—appetite, pain, nausea, vomiting, change in bowel pattern.
      12. Gynecological—discharge, abnormal bleeding, pain, enlargement of abdominal girth, bloating.
      13. Urinary tract and bladder—hematuria, change in urinary pattern.
      14. Integumentary—changes in warts or moles, new lesions.
   C. Site-specific examination.
      1. Skin

a. Inspection	Sun-exposed areas, including face, chest, back, arms, legs, followed by scalp, mucous membranes, interdigital webs, axillae, and soles of the feet. Note mole distribution and description; irregularity and asymmetry; patient report of any sensation, change in color, size, or bleeding.

b. Cancer detection tests	Biopsy and histology of suspicious lesions (small lesions are excised; large lesions require punch or incisional biopsy for tissue diagnosis).

2. Breast
   a. Clinical breast examination — Inspection and palpation of breasts, supraclavicular and infraclavicular nodes, and axillae. Note tenderness, masses, dimpling, cutaneous nodules, asymmetry
   b. Cancer detection tests — Mammograms, sonograms, needle or excision biopsy.
3. Female genitalia
   a. Inspection — Note masses, asymmetry, lesions.
   b. External palpation — Note masses, tenderness, shape and consistency of ovaries, uterus, lower abdominal region.
   c. Pelvic and rectal examination — Note mucosal integrity and color, lesions, bleeding, discharge, constriction, nodules, masses.
   d. Cancer detection tests — Needle, excisional, or conization biopsy of abnormal areas; endometrial washings or biopsy if warranted; cervical and vaginal Papanicolaou (Pap) smears; colposcopy.
4. Male genitalia
   a. Inspection — Note masses, asymmetry, lesions, cutaneous nodules.
   b. External palpation — Note tenderness, masses, consistency, contour, shape of scrotum, scrotal contents (testes, epididymis), inguinal lymph nodes.
   c. Digital rectal examination
      (1) Prostate gland — Palpate for masses, tenderness, nodules, size, texture, and firmness.
      (2) Rectum — Note masses, constriction, tenderness.
   d. Cancer detection tests — Needle biopsy of suspicious prostatic tissue with or without ultrasound guidance; needle aspiration or biopsy of other suspicious lesions or nodules except testis (if indicated, an inguinal orchiectomy is performed).
5. Oral cavity
   a. Inspection — Color and integrity of mucous membranes, tongue.
   b. Oral examination — Note color, lesions, masses, tenderness.
   c. Cancer detection tests — Histological confirmation by biopsy of suspicious lesion.

   D. Biological markers and laboratory tests (Table 5-2).

ASSOCIATED NURSING DIAGNOSES

I. Knowledge deficit regarding individual risk assessment.

II. Anxiety related to conceptions or misconceptions regarding risk factor detection and early detection.

III. Fear related to cancer and/or treatment.

NURSING PLANNING AND IMPLEMENTATION

I. Apply known risk data to identify subpopulations at risk.

II. Conduct individual risk appraisals and provide immediate feedback to the individual.

III. Schedule risk appraisal monitoring and reminder system; secure commitment from the individual.

IV. Report risk factors identified in individual risk appraisal to appropriate referral service.

V. Teach self-examination (breast, testicular, skin, oral, neck).

VI. Initiate public education on early detection in workplace and schools.

VII. Coordinate community resources to foster public values regarding health maintenance and early detection.

EVALUATION OF CLIENT OUTCOMES

I. Identify risk factors and plan for follow-up.

II. List seven warning signals of cancer.

III. List procedure and symptoms to report in self-care examinations (breast, testicular, vulvar, skin, neck, nodes).

IV. Identify resources for cancer education and information (American Cancer Society [ACS] and NCI cancer answer lines).

V. Describe components of ACS Cancer-Related Checkup that will be requested in future health care follow-up. *Text continued on page 54*

Table 5-2
SELECTED LABORATORY TESTS IN THE DIAGNOSIS, MANAGEMENT, AND FOLLOW-UP OF CANCER

In general, an isolated normal, elevated, or decreased laboratory value is not an absolute in the diagnosis and management of a specific malignancy. Rather, laboratory values add to the clinical diagnostic, management, and evaluative process. Institutional reference ranges may vary significantly with different methods and standardization modes.

Name	Specimen and Reference Range	Clinical Information*	Comments
Tumor Markers			
Acid phosphatase	Serum total Males: 2.5-11.7 U/L Females: 0.3-9.2 U/L	↑ in prostatic cancer (↑ in 5% with tumor confined to prostate gland, 20% with regional extension of tumor and 80% with bone metastases)	In males, 50% of acid phosphatase is prostatic. Remainder is from liver, disintegrating platelets, and erythrocytes. Transient rise possible after transurethral resection of prostate or biopsy. Generally not influenced by digital prostate examination. Usually falls within several weeks of institution of successful hormonal manipulation in advanced prostate cancer
	Tartrate: inhibited fraction Males: 0.2-3.5 U/L Females: 0-0.8 U/L	↑ some primary bone malignancies, multiple myeloma	
Alkaline phosphatase	Serum adult: 4-13 U/dl (King-Armstrong) 1.5-4.5 U/dl (Bodansky) 0.8-2.3 U/dl (Bessey-Lowry)	↑ in metastatic cancer to bone and liver, osteogenic sarcoma, myeloma, and Hodgkin's lymphoma with bone involvement	May also be elevated in conditions of increased bone metabolism such as healing fractures, renal disease, and liver disease

* ↑, Elevated; ↓, decreased.   *Table continued on following page*

Table 5-2
SELECTED LABORATORY TESTS IN THE DIAGNOSIS, MANAGEMENT, AND FOLLOW-UP
OF CANCER *Continued*

Name	Specimen and Reference Range	Clinical Information*	Comments
Tumor Markers *Continued*			
Alpha fetoprotein (AFP)	Serum <30 ng/ml	↑ in 70% of hepatocellular cancers, in choriocarcinoma, teratoma, embryonal cell tumors of testis and ovary, some pancreatic, stomach, colon, and lung tumors. Not in pure seminomas without teratomatous component	Oncofetal protein synthesized in the liver. Useful in monitoring tumor response to treatment
Carcinoembryonic antigen (CEA)	Plasma Nonsmokers: 0-5 ng/ml Smokers: 0-10 ng/ml	↑ in 70% of colon cancers. Also seen in lung, pancreas, stomach, breast, head and neck, and prostate malignancies. ↑ in 20% of heavy smokers	Helpful in monitoring response to therapy or indicating disease recurrence
Chorionic gonadotropin (beta subunit) (β-hCG)	Serum or plasma Males and nonpregnant females: <5.0 IU/L	↑ in a hydatidiform mole, choriocarcinoma, testicular teratoma, ectopic hCG production by some cancers of the pituitary gland, stomach, pancreas, lung, colon, and liver	Serial determinations helpful in monitoring response to treatment or early detection of recurrence
Pancreatic oncofetal antigen (POA)	Serum	Positive in large percentage of pancreas tumors.	
Placental alkaline phosphatase (PAP)	Serum (Regan isoenzyme)	↑ in a variety of tumors, only half of which demonstrate ↑ serum alkaline phosphatase. ↑ in 40% of seminomas	Ectopic synthesis may be of value in monitoring tumor response to treatment
Hormones			
Adrenocorticotropic hormone (ACTH)	Plasma Highest in morning; lowest at bedtime.	↑ in ectopic ACTH-producing tumors (lung, particularly small cell), adrenal carcinoma, adenoma	Paraneoplastic syndrome usually accompanied by hypokalemia, hyperglycemia, lethargy, confusion, nausea and vomiting with absence of classic Cushing's syndrome manifestations
Androstendione	Serum Male: 107 ± 25 ng/dl Female: 151 ± 38 ng/dl	↑ in ectopic ACTH-producing tumors, ovarian tumors	Produced in adrenals and gonads. Precursor in biosynthesis of androgens and estrogens

Table 5-2
SELECTED LABORATORY TESTS IN THE DIAGNOSIS, MANAGEMENT, AND FOLLOW-UP
OF CANCER *Continued*

Name	Specimen and Reference Range	Clinical Information*	Comments
Hormones *(continued)*			
Antidiuretic hormone (ADH)	Plasma	↑ in brain tumors (primary or secondary). ↑ in systemic malignancies with ectopic ADH production	Inappropriate secretion of ADH is paraneoplastic syndrome, occurring most frequently in small cell carcinoma of lung. Hyponatremia in the presence of excessive urinary sodium is generally found
Calcitonin	Fasting serum or plasma Male: <100 pg/ml Female: <25 pg/ml	↑ in medullary carcinoma of the thyroid, some lung and breast tumors, carcinoids, colon cancer and GI malignancies	To confirm diagnosis of medullary carcinoma, calcium or pentagastric stimulation test performed
Estrogens, total	Serum Adult Male: 40-115 ng/L Adult Female: 61-350 ng/L	↑ in estrogen-producing ovarian tumors, some testicular tumors, and adrenal cortical tumors	
Estrogen (estradiol) receptor assay	0.5-1.0 g of tissue Negative: <3.0 fmol/mg protein Borderline: 3-10 fmol/ mg protein Positive: >10 frmol/mg protein	60% of breast cancers are characterized by estrogen receptors	Useful for identifying breast tumors most likely to respond to endocrine manipulation
Glucagon	Plasma	↓ in some pancreatic neoplasms	
Growth hormone (hGH)	Serum or plasma Male: <2 ng/ml Female: <10 ng/ml	↑ in ectopic secretion by some stomach and lung tumors	
Parathyroid hormone (hPTH)	Fasting serum	↑ squamous cell or epidermoid lung cancers and renal cell producing a ectopic hyperparathyroidism	Ectopic tumor produces PTH. May be associated with hypercalcemia
Progesterone	Serum Male: 0.12-0.3 ng/ml Nonpregnant female: 0-30 ng/ml	↑ in some ovarian tumors, molar pregnancy	
Progesterone receptor assay	1 gr of tissue Normal: ≤5 fmol/mg protein Positive: >10 fmol/mg protein		May be useful in predicting tumors likely to respond to endocrine manipulation

Table continued on following page

Table 5-2
SELECTED LABORATORY TESTS IN THE DIAGNOSIS, MANAGEMENT, AND FOLLOW-UP
OF CANCER *Continued*

Name	Specimen and Reference Range	Clinical Information*	Comments
Hormones *(continued)*			
17-Ketogenic steroids	24-hour acidified urine Male: 5-23 mg/d Female: 3-15 mg/d	↑ in adrenal adenoma and carcinoma, ectopic adrenocorticotropic hormone (ACTH) syndrome	
17-Ketosteroids	24-hour urine Male: 8-22 Female: 6-15	↑ in adrenal tumors, testicular tumors, interstitial cell tumors, androgenic ovarian tumors	
Testosterone	Serum Adult male: 572 ± 135 ng/dl Nonpregnant females: 37 ± 10 ng/dl	↑ some adrenocortical tumors, gonadotropin-producing extragonadal tumors	Fall to castration level following adequate hormonal manipulation in advanced prostatic cancer
Blood Chemistries			
Calcium	Fasting serum Adult: 8.4-10.2 mg/dl	↑ in 9% of malignancies with bone involvement (mainly breast, lung, and kidney). Also in multiple myeloma, lymphomas, leukemias, squamous cell carcinoma of the lung, cancer of the kidney, esophagus, pancreas, liver, and bladder	Hypercalcemia occurs in about 10% of patients with cancer, some of whom will have no bony involvement
Cholesterol	Serum, plasma Fasting ≥12 hr Adults: 140-210 mg/dl	↓ in 16% of malignancies with bone involvement. ↑ in some prostatic, liver, and pancreatic malignancies	
Ferritin	Serum Male: 15-200 mg/dl Female: 12-150 mg/dl	↑ in acute myeloblastic and lymphoblastic leukemias, some Hodgkin's lymphomas, and breast cancers	Main iron storage protein in body
Glucose	Serum Adult: 70-105 mg/dl	↑ in pheochromocytoma, glucagonoma; pancreatic malignancies. May be ↑ in presence of islet cell tumor, carcinoma of the adrenal gland, and stomach, and fibrosarcoma	

Table 5-2
SELECTED LABORATORY TESTS IN THE DIAGNOSIS, MANAGEMENT, AND FOLLOW-UP
OF CANCER *Continued*

Name	Specimen and Reference Range	Clinical Information*	Comments
Blood Chemistries (*continued*)			
Uric acid	Serum Male: 4.2-8 mg/dl Female: 3.2-7.3 mg/dl	↑ in some disseminated malignancies. ↓ in some neoplasms, including Hodgkin's lymphoma, multiple myeloma, and bronchogenic carcinoma	Monitor while on cytotoxic therapy
Enzymes			
Amylase	Serum Adult: 56-190 IU/L	↑ in some lung and ovarian tumors	
Amylase isoenzymes	Serum	↑ in some bronchogenic or serous ovarian tumors	
Lactic dehydrogenase (LDH) and LDH isoenzymes	Serum Ranges are highly method-dependent, i.e.: 1. Pyruvate to lactate (210-420) 2. Lactate to pyruvate (45-90)	↑ in extensive carcinomatosis and malignant processes (about 50% of cancer patients have alterations in LDH patterns) ↑ in 90% of patients with acute leukemia	LDH helpful when elevated in nonseminomatous germ cell tumors of the testis. ↑ With massive platelet destruction and in lymphomas and lymphocytic leukemias. LDH may be ↑ in carcinoma of the prostate
Leucine aminopeptidase (LAP)	Serum 14-4 U/L	↑ in 60% of patients with pancreatic carcinoma with liver metastases	
Lysozyme	Serum 4.0-13.0 mg/L	↑ in acute monocytic or myelomonocytic leukemia and chronic myeloid leukemia	
Serum gamma glutamyl transpeptidase (SGGT)	Serum Males: 6-37 mU/ml Females: 4-24 mU/ml	↑ in some cases of renal cell carcinoma and liver metastases	Elevation may precede findings on liver scan
Serum glutamic oxaloacetic transaminase (SGOT)	Serum Adult: 5-40 U/ml	↑ in about 50% of patients with liver metastases or infiltration	
Serum glutamic pyruvic transaminase (SGPT)	Serum Adult: 5-35 U/ml	↑ in some liver carcinomas	

Table continued on following page

Table 5-2
SELECTED LABORATORY TESTS IN THE DIAGNOSIS, MANAGEMENT, AND FOLLOW-UP
OF CANCER *Continued*

Name	Specimen and Reference Range	Clinical Information*	Comments
Proteins (immunoglobulins are produced by lymphocytes and plasma cells. They are fractionated into major components by electrophoresis.)			
Immunoglobulin A (IgA)	Serum Adult: 60-330 mg/dl	Slight polyclonal ↑ in some malignancies of breast, and monoclonal ↑ in IgA myeloma	Approximately 15% of total immunoglobulins. Protects mucosal surfaces as first line of defense against microorganisms
Immunoglobulin D (IgD)	Serum Adult: 0-15 mg/dl	Slight monoclonal ↑ in IgD myeloma	About 1% of immunoglobulins. Physiological function unknown. May receive or differentiate on lymphocytic surfaces. 90% of multiple myelomas are of IgD type, and almost all patients will have Bence Jones urinary proteins
Immunoglobulin E (IgE)	Serum Adult: 0.01-0.04 mg/dl	Slight monoclonal ↑ in IgE myeloma. Slight ↑ in certain advanced stage neoplasms	About 1% of immunoglobulins. Functions in severe allergic reactions
Immunoglobulin G (IgG)	Serum Adult: 550-1900 mg/dl	Slight monoclonal ↑ in IgG myeloma	Accounts for 75% of total immunoglobulins. Produces antibodies to bacteria, fungi, viruses, and toxins. Occurs as second line immune response after IgM. Involved in passive immunization of the newborn
Immunoglobulin M (IgM)	Serum Adults: 45-145 mg/dl		Approximately 10% of immunoglobulins. First antibody to respond to bacteria and bacteria toxins
Haptoglobin (Hp)	Serum Adult: 30-160/dl	May be ↑ in cancer, particularly with metastases, and in lymphomas	Produced by liver. Single result of limited value. Serial determinations suggested

Table 5-2
SELECTED LABORATORY TESTS IN THE DIAGNOSIS, MANAGEMENT, AND FOLLOW-UP
OF CANCER *Continued*

Name	Specimen and Reference Range	Clinical Information*	Comments
Hematology			
Leukocyte count (white blood cell count, WBC)	Whole blood Adult male: 3,900-10,600/mm³ Adult female: 3,500-11,000/mm³	↑ in hematological malignancies, and myeloproliferative disorders	Some expressions of leukemia show normal or ↓ WBC. Life span of leukocytes in peripheral circulation is 6-8 hr

Differential count
  Neutrophils
    Segmented
    Bands
	
	56%
	3%
		↑ in a wide range of myeloproliferative disorders. May be ↑ in widespread malignancies. ↓ in aplastic anemia, marrow replacement of tumor	% of total WBC. Neutrophils active in phagocytosis

Lymphocytes	34%	↑ in lymphocytic leukemias. May be ↑ in Hodgkin's disease and malignancies	Antibody production
Monocytes	4%	↑ in monocytic leukemia	Stimulate plasmacytes to produce immunoglobulins
Eosinophils	2.5%	May be ↑ in chronic myelogenous leukemia, Hodgkin's disease, metastatic malignancies	Release granules of serotonin, histamine, and heparin. Allergic responses
Basophils	0.5%	May be ↑ in chronic myelogenous leukemia, Hodgkin's disease	Control blood viscosity. Granules contain heparin
Platelet count	Whole blood Adults: 150,000-400,000/mm³	↑ myeloproliferative disorders. May be ↑ in advanced malignancies. May be ↓ in leukemias, tumors metastatic to bone marrow	Life span 6-10 days in peripheral circulation
Hematocrit	Whole blood Adult males: 42%-52% Adult females: 37%-47%	↑ in anemia associated with many malignant processes, leukemias	Erythrocyte life span approximately 120 days. Result may be falsely low if drawn in recumbent patient
Hemoglobin	Whole blood Adult males: 13.5-17.5 g/dl Adult females: 12.0-16.0 g/dl	↑ in anemia associated with many malignant processes, leukemias	Results may be falsely high in dehydration

Cancer Screening

THEORY

I. Definitions.

A. *Screening*—an organized service using a specialized test and/or standardized physical examination procedure designed to identify unrecognized disease among asymptomatic and/or high-risk populations.

B. *Screening test*—examination with demonstrated effectiveness in identifying a condition requiring further evaluation or intervention earlier than would be done without screening.

C. *Sensitivity* of a screening test—ability to identify presence (positivity) of the target condition; high sensitivity diminishes the incidence of false-positive results:

$$\frac{\text{Number positive when disease is present}}{\text{Number positive + Number negative when disease is present}}$$

D. *Specificity* of a screening test—ability to confirm absence (negativity) of the target condition; high specificity results in fewer false-negative results:

$$\frac{\text{Number negative when disease is absent}}{\text{Number positive + Number negative when disease is absent}}$$

E. *Positive predictive value* of a screening test—calculation that reflects efficiency in producing true or correct positive results:

$$\frac{\text{Number positive when disease is present}}{\text{Number positive when disease is absent + Number positive when disease is present}}$$

F. *Reliability*—a measure of the capacity of a test to produce the same result upon retest.

II. Rationale.

A. The application of screening is most efficiently instituted when:

1. The disease is prevalent.
2. The disease is of serious consequences and is considered serious by screenees.
3. The screening test has demonstrated effectiveness in detecting a specific cancer earlier than without screening.
4. The screening test has few false-positive results, minimizing the economic and psychological cost of further testing when disease is absent.
5. A treatment is available that, if initiated early or in the asymptomatic stage, is more effective than treatment initiated after symptoms occur.
6. The screening test is acceptable to the screenee (minimal cost, discomfort, inconvenience, or risk).

B. Maximal potential for secondary prevention is to quantify risks (health history, risk profiles) and selectively screen groups at highest risk, thereby improving efficiency and decreasing costs.

C. For some cancers, entire populations are at risk (women over 30 for breast cancer, over-50 population for colon cancer) and should be screened.

D. Nurses constitute the largest body of health care professionals and are practicing in all types of health care settings; therefore nurses have the potential to minimize cancer morbidity and mortality by facilitating early detection of cancer among individuals and groups.

E. NCI goals for the year 2000, with respect to screening, establish breast and cervical screening as priorities in reducing cancer mortality and morbidity (Table 5-1).

DATA COLLECTION*

I. Breast.
  A. Screening tests.
    1. Clinical examination.
      a. Sensitivity estimates range from 45% to 87%.
      b. Specificity uncertain.
    2. Mammography.
      a. Sensitivity ranges from 71% to 75%.
      b. Specificity reported between 94% to 99%.
    3. Breast self-examination (Figure 5-1).
      a. Sensitivity reported as low (26% to 34%).
      b. Training may improve results.
      c. Specificity uncertain.
  B. Recommendations.
    1. Clinical examination.
      a. Every 3 years from ages 20 to 40.
      b. Annually after age 40.
    2. Mammography.
      a. Baseline between ages 35 to 39.
      b. Every 1 to 2 years between ages 40 to 49.
      c. Yearly after the age of 50.
      d. May conclude at age 75 if no pathology ever demonstrated.
      e. Family history of breast cancer suggests need for earlier age baseline and compliance with interval testing.
    3. Breast self-examination: monthly, beginning at age 20.

II. Prostate.
  A. Screening tests.
    1. Digital rectal examination.
      a. Sensitivity and specificity not established.
      b. Accessibility of gland to palpation limited.
      c. Cost effective procedure.
    2. Transrectal ultrasound.
      a. Sensitivity and specificity not established.
      b. High incidence of false-positive results.
      c. Role in screening remains investigational.
    3. Serum tumor markers (see Table 5-2).
      a. Prostatic acid phosphatase sensitivities reported from 20% to 45%.
      b. Prostatic-specific antigen highly sensitive, but limited specificity, ranging from 38% to 56%.
      c. Not recommended for routine screening.
  B. Recommendation: annual digital rectal examination beginning at age 40.

III. Colon/rectum.
  A. Screening tests.
    1. Digital rectal examination.
      a. Sensitivity and specificity low.
      b. Limited access.

---

*The ACS and the Clinical Preventive Services (CPS) recommendations were used to compile the review of the effectiveness of screening tests for specific sites and recommendations for screening.

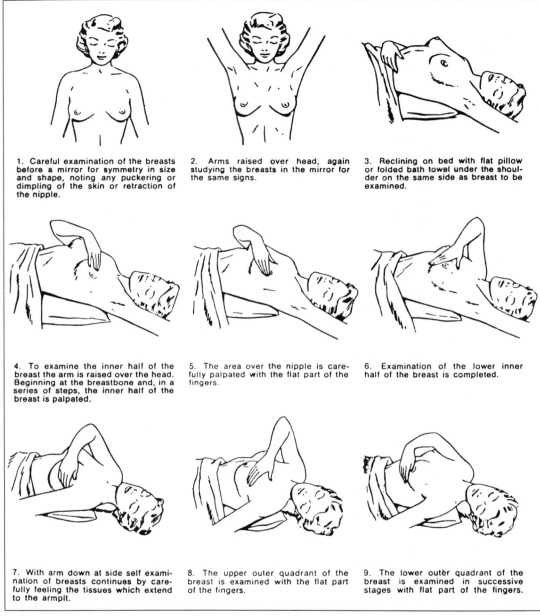

1. Careful examination of the breasts before a mirror for symmetry in size and shape, noting any puckering or dimpling of the skin or retraction of the nipple.

2. Arms raised over head, again studying the breasts in the mirror for the same signs.

3. Reclining on bed with flat pillow or folded bath towel under the shoulder on the same side as breast to be examined.

4. To examine the inner half of the breast the arm is raised over the head. Beginning at the breastbone and, in a series of steps, the inner half of the breast is palpated.

5. The area over the nipple is carefully palpated with the flat part of the fingers.

6. Examination of the lower inner half of the breast is completed.

7. With arm down at side self examination of breasts continues by carefully feeling the tissues which extend to the armpit.

8. The upper outer quadrant of the breast is examined with the flat part of the fingers.

9. The lower outer quadrant of the breast is examined in successive stages with flat part of the fingers.

Figure 5-1 Technique of breast self-examination. *(From American Cancer Society.)*

    2. Fecal occult blood testing (Table 5-3).
        a. Sensitivity not established; many false positive results (see Table 5-3 for dietary and medication instructions).
        b. Sensitivity and specificity may be higher with costly quantitative hemoglobin/stool measurements.
    3. Sigmoidoscopy—longer and more flexible instruments improve sensitivity but increase costs.

Table 5-3
OCCULT BLOOD TESTING FOR GASTROINTESTINAL DISEASE: CLIENT INSTRUCTIONS

Guaiac Slide Tests (hemoccult, coloscreen)

Procedure: Client smears feces on slides and returns to laboratory or physician's office.
Preparation: For 48 hours before first stool specimen collection:
1. Avoid the following foods—red meat, turnips, horseradish, melons.
2. Avoid the following drugs and vitamins—vitamin C (>250 mg/day), aspirin, anti-inflammatory drugs, iron supplements.
3. Include the following foods—well-cooked poultry and fish, bran, peanuts, popcorn, cooked fruits and vegetables.
Precautions: Do not collect specimen while menstruating or bleeding from hemorrhoids; protect slide from heat or light.

Colocare Test

Procedure: Client places a test pad in the toilet and records color changes that indicate results.
Preparation: 1. No dietary, fruit, or vegetable restrictions are required.
2. Follow red meat and vitamin C restrictions as above.

  B. Recommendations.
1. Annual digital rectal examination beginning at age 40 years.
2. Annual fecal occult blood testing beginning at age 50.
3. Sigmoidoscopy every 3 to 5 years beginning at age 50.
4. Known risk factors suggest need for periodic screening.

IV. Cervix.
  A. Screening tests.
1. Pap smear.
a. Sensitivity not determined.
b. Specificity may be greater than 90%.
2. Cervicography.
  B. Recommendations.
1. Annual Pap smears for all women who are or have been sexually active or who are age 18 or older.
2. Pap smears may be performed less frequently at the discretion of the clinician after three or more consecutively normal annual smears.

V. Lung.
  A. Screening tests.
1. Chest x-ray examination—low yield in asymptomatic population.
2. Sputum cytology—lower yield than chest x-ray examination.
  B. Recommendations.
1. Screening by routine chest radiography or sputum cytology not recommended.
2. Smoking cessation efforts promoted instead.

VI. Skin.
  A. Screening tests.
1. Physical examination of the skin—no convincing sensitivity and specificity estimates.

2. Skin self-examination (Figure 5-2).
  B. Recommendations.
    1. Complete skin examination incorporated into periodic physical examination.
    2. Monthly self-examination of skin.

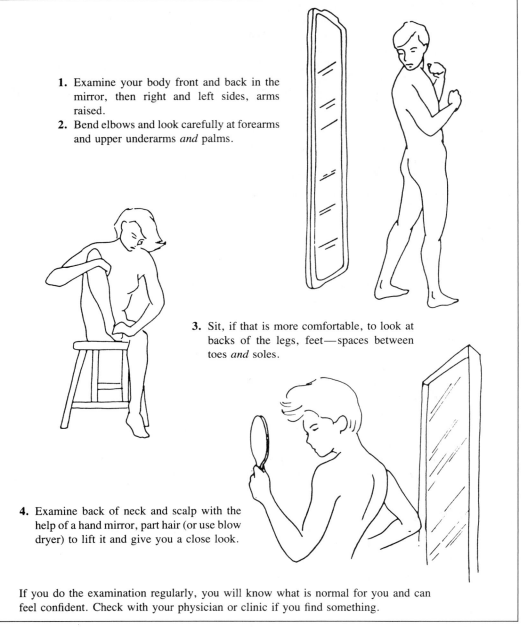

1. Examine your body front and back in the mirror, then right and left sides, arms raised.
2. Bend elbows and look carefully at forearms and upper underarms *and* palms.

3. Sit, if that is more comfortable, to look at backs of the legs, feet—spaces between toes *and* soles.

4. Examine back of neck and scalp with the help of a hand mirror, part hair (or use blow dryer) to lift it and give you a close look.

If you do the examination regularly, you will know what is normal for you and can feel confident. Check with your physician or clinic if you find something.

Figure 5-2 Your skin self-examination. *(From American Cancer Society.)*
The best time to do this simple monthly examination is after a bath or shower. Use a full-length and a hand mirror so that you can check any moles, blemishes, or birthmarks from the top of your head to your toes, noting anything new—a change in size, shape, or color or a sore that does not heal.

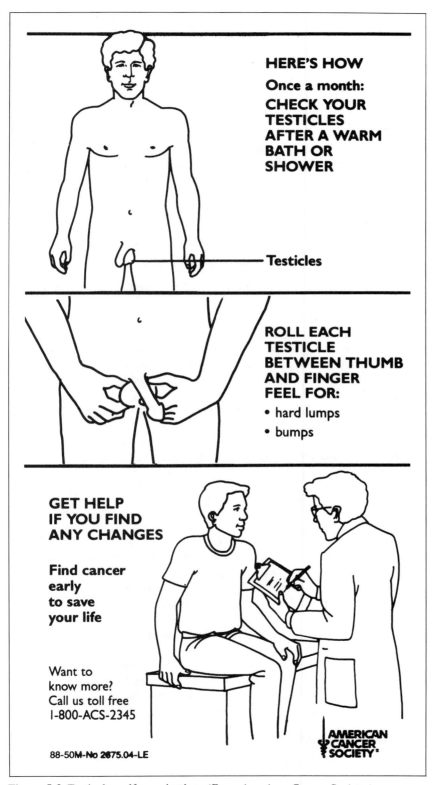

Figure 5-3 Testicular self-examination. *(From American Cancer Society.)*

      3. Complete skin examination on routine basis for individuals with personal or family history of skin cancer, precursor lesions, or increased sun exposure.

      4. Measures to minimize needless sun exposure encouraged.

VII. Testicle.
  A. Screening test.
    1. Clinical palpation of testes.
    2. Testicular self-examination (Figure 5-3).
  B. Recommendations.
    1. Annual clinical testicular examination.
    2. Monthly testicular self-examination beginning with onset of puberty.
    3. Periodic screening for men with history of cryptorchidism, orchiopexy, or testicular atrophy.

ASSOCIATED NURSING DIAGNOSES

I. Knowledge deficit regarding recommended screening procedures.

II. Anxiety related to possible findings of screening tests.

III. Health seeking behavior deficit related to perceived barriers.

NURSING PLANNING AND IMPLEMENTATION

I. Lessen perceived and actual barriers.
  A. Target high-risk groups (elderly, socioeconomically disadvantaged) within respective community (nursing homes, urban areas) to ensure access.
  B. Recruit community representatives to act as liaisons to facilitate participation and follow-up.
  C. Facilitate resource allocation to provide low cost and/or reimbursement for screening tests.
  D. Provide education to clarify misconceptions about perceived risk (e.g., low radiation risks with improved mammography techniques).

II. Facilitate perceived and actual benefits of screening.
  A. Provide teaching to minimize false-positive results for stool occult blood tests (dietary, medications); see Table 5-3.
  B. Teach and monitor self-examination procedures.
  C. Personalize risk by using health history and risk profiles.
  D. Maximize quality control of screening tests (low false-negative results and low false-positive results).
  E. Use media resources to publicize benefits of early detection.
  F. Collect data to evaluate quality control of screening:
    a. Number screened.
    b. Proportion of population screened once, twice, or more.
    c. Detected prevalence of preclinical disease.
    d. Cost per case.
    e. Proportion of positive findings brought to diagnosis and treatment.
    f. Predictive value of positive tests (proportion positive found to have cancer).
    g. Costs of follow-up of false-positive findings.

EVALUATION OF CLIENT OUTCOMES

I. Discuss recommendations for screening and early detection.

II. Describe self-examination procedures and recommendations.

III. Identify personal high-risk factors.

BIBLIOGRAPHY

Baird, S.B., McCorkle, R. & Grant, M. (1991). *Cancer Nursing: A Comprehensive Textbook.* Philadelphia: W.B. Saunders Co.

Bates, B. & Hockelman, R.A. (1983). *A Guide to Physical Examination* (3rd ed). Philadelphia: J.B. Lippincott.

Casciato, D.A. & Lowitz, B.B. (1983). *Manual of Bedside Oncology.* Boston: Little, Brown, & Co.

Cohen, R.F., & Frank-Stromberg, M. (1990). Cancer risk and assessment. In S.L. Groenwald, M.H. Frogge, M. Goodman & C.H. Yarbo (eds). *Cancer Nursing: Principles and Practices* (2nd ed). Boston: Jones & Bartlett Publishers, pp. 103-118.

Frank-Stromborg, M. (1991). Evaluating cancer risks. In S.B. Baird, R. McCorkle & M. Grant (eds). *Cancer Nursing: A Comprehensive Textbook.* Philadelphia: W.B. Saunders Co., pp. 155-189.

Jaffe, M.S. & Skidmore, L.C. (1984). *Diagnostic and Laboratory Cards for Clinical Use.* Bowie, Md: Robert J. Brady.

Olsen, J.J. & Frank-Stromberg, M. (1991). Cancer screening and early detection. In S.B. Baird, R. McCorkle & M. Grant (eds). *Cancer Nursing: A Comprehensive Textbook.* Philadelphia: W.B. Saunders Co., pp. 190-218.

Otto, S.E. (ed). (1991). *Oncology Nursing.* St Louis: Mosby-Year Book.

Tietz, N.W. (1983). *Clinical Guide to Laboratory Tests.* Philadelphia: W.B. Saunders Co.

U.S. Preventive Services Task Force (1989). *Guide to Clinical Preventive Services: An Assessment of the Effectiveness of 169 Interventions.* Baltimore: Williams & Wilkins.

Wallach, J.B. (1978). *Interpretation of Diagnostic Tests: A Handbook Synopsis of Laboratory Medicine* (3rd ed). Boston: Little, Brown & Co.

6

Dissemination of Information Through Patient and Public Education

Judith (Judi) L. Johnson, PhD, RN
Mary Johnson, PhD, RN

THEORY

I. Education of the public and client/significant other facing cancer involves two types of education—health education and patient education.
   A. *Health education*—the process of assisting individuals, acting separately and collectively, to make informed decisions on matters affecting individual, family, and community health.
   B. *Patient education*—a series of structured or nonstructured experiences designed to help patients and significant others voluntarily:
      1. Cope with the crisis responses to the diagnosis of cancer.
      2. Cope with long-term adjustments to disease and treatment.
      3. Cope with symptoms.
      4. Gain information about sources of prevention, diagnosis, and care.
      5. Develop needed self-care skills.
      6. Develop attitudes to maintain or regain health.

II. Rationale for education of persons at-risk for or living with a diagnosis of cancer.
   A. Teaching is an integral part of adaptation and is a part of total health care.
   B. Planned education experiences ensure that important health-related information is available and presented in a consistent manner.
   C. Education prepares the public and client/significant others with knowledge and skills for participation in decision making and self-care.
   D. Educational experiences give the public and clients/significant others the opportunity to exchange ideas, discuss problems, and develop solutions with each other and health care providers.
   E. Educational experiences strengthen the concept of partnership among the public, clients, significant others, and health care providers.

III. Theoretical principles of teaching and learning.
   A. Human factors.
      1. Learning occurs when people perceive a need to learn something.

     a. Needs identified by health care providers may not be consistent with needs identified by the public or client/significant other.

     b. Learner-identified needs should receive priority.

     c. Motivation for learning comes when a gap exists between what people know and what they want to know.

     d. Learning should be problem centered rather than subject centered.

  2. Learning is influenced by accumulated life experiences.

  3. Learning is influenced by trust, mutual respect, acceptance of differences, and freedom of expression.

  4. Learning does not always occur because teaching has been done; therefore learning must be reinforced.

B. Organizational factors.

  1. Public and client/significant other teaching is a component of the job description of registered nurses in cancer care.

  2. Public and client/significant other education programs are supported and recognized by medical and administrative personnel.

C. Physical factors

  1. The learning environment focuses the attention of the public or client/significant other on learning: privacy, adequate space, comfortable seating, adequate lighting, and minimal distractions.

  2. Time is required for learning to take place.

D. Educational materials and methods factor.

  1. Materials selected for use are sensitive to developmental, educational, and socioeconomic status and to cultural and spiritual attitudes and beliefs of the public target group or client/significant other.

  2. Methods used in education engage the public and client/significant other in the learning process.

     a. Teaching-learning requires human interaction.

     b. People learn better when more than one of their senses are stimulated.

  3. Materials and methods are selected based on the objectives of the learning experience and the learning styles of the public or client/significant other.

DATA COLLECTION

I. Pertinent personal history.

A. Developmental level: age, sensory and mental changes associated with aging, self-esteem, ego strength, and past life experiences.

B. Sociocultural background: values, customs, beliefs, communication patterns, and roles.

C. Socioeconomic status.

D. Intellectual status: vocabulary and language skills, extent of formal education, concrete and abstract thinking skills, and problem-solving skills.

E. Spiritual orientation: beliefs in higher being and roles of higher being in the lives of individuals.

F. Social support systems: types, patterns of use, adequacy, and value to individual.

II. Responses to disease and treatment.

A. Physical responses: presence of physical responses that alter comfort levels can result in a decrease in both motivation and receptiveness to learning.

  1. Presence of fever, lack of sleep, weakness, fatigue, nausea, vomiting, and pain.

  2. Changes in physical or mental parameters related to medications to control physical responses.

    B. Emotional responses: intense positive and negative responses can result in a decrease in receptiveness to learning.
      1. Presence of anxiety, depression, anger, fear, and distrust.
      2. Changes in emotional parameters related to medications to control disease and physical responses to disease and treatment.
    C. Stage of adaptation: responses such as disbelief, developing awareness, reorganization, resolution, and identity changes influence the content and timing of and the methods used for education.

ASSOCIATED NURSING DIAGNOSES

  I. Knowledge deficit.

 II. Self-care deficit.

III. Role disturbance.

IV. Impaired individual coping.

 V. Impaired family coping.

NURSING PLANNING AND IMPLEMENTATION

  I. Develop outcome goals for the educational experience.
    A. Include the learners in goal development.
    B. Identify goals that are congruent with the interdisciplinary treatment plan.
    C. State goals in realistic and measurable terms.
    D. Prioritize goals in collaboration with the learners and health care providers.
    E. Assign a time frame for achievement of goals.

 II. Determine content and experiences that contribute to goal achievement.
    A. Review current literature related to the knowledge, skills, or attitudes that are a part of the established goals.
    B. Review literature related to the experiences that are most effective in assisting the learner to achieve established goals.

III. Select materials and methods to guide the learner to goal achievement.
    A. Obtain and review educational materials specific to the established goals.
      1. Resources for existing public and client/significant other cancer education are available from the:
        a. American Cancer Society.
        b. National Cancer Institute.
        c. Leukemia Society of America.
        d. American Lung Association.
        e. Pharmaceutical companies.
        f. Hospital equipment companies.
        g. Cancer Information System (1-800-4-CANCER).
      2. User-developed materials may be developed using the following guidelines:
        a. Direct content to one person.
        b. Use short words, sentences, and paragraphs.
        c. Select descriptive nouns and active verbs for headings.
        d. Choose a large uppercase, and lowercase typeface.
        e. Use illustrations to complement copy.
        f. Write a caption for each illustration.
        g. Use black type on a white background.
    B. Select materials appropriate to the intellectual status, reading level, and cultural and socioeconomic backgrounds of the learner.

C. Select methods determined the most effective in teaching specific content, skills, or attitudes within the specific phase of the cancer experience.

IV. Develop a plan for evaluating the effectiveness of the teaching and learning.
  A. Determine the level of measurement to evaluate achievement of the goal such as accuracy, increasing approximations to the behavior, number of behaviors, persistence, or originality.
  B. Define the method(s) to use to evaluate achievement: direct observation of behavior, oral questioning, written tests, and self-reports.
  C. Determine the methods for evaluating the efficacy of teaching style and methods, and the appropriateness of content.
  D. Establish the time frames for evaluation.
  E. Define a process for documentation of achievement of outcomes, provision of feedback to learners, and revision of the teaching-learning plans based on evaluation data.

EVALUATION OF PUBLIC, PATIENT, AND FAMILY OUTCOMES

I. Oncology Nursing Society Standards of Oncology Education: the public:
  A. Demonstrates positive attitudes about cancer and individuals experiencing cancer.
  B. Describes life-style choices that minimize personal risks for cancer and promote health.
  C. Participates in cancer screening activities.
  D. Identifies a course of action for early detection when signs and symptoms of cancer are discovered.
  E. Identifies sources of cancer information, care, rehabilitation, and support care in the community.
  F. Describes the political process for accomplishing social changes to minimize environmental and life-style risks for cancer and to benefit individuals experiencing cancer.

II. Oncology Nursing Society Standards of Oncology Education: the patient and significant other:
  A. Describe the illness, goals, and plan of therapy, potential risks and benefits, and available alternative therapies.
  B. Assume an active role in decision making and identification of needs with respect to the development, implementation, and evaluation of the plan of care.
  C. Describe behaviors that promote a level of independence appropriate to age, developmental stage, learning ability, resources, personal preference, prognosis, and physical ability.
  D. Demonstrate psychomotor and coping skills required for self-care.
  E. Describe signs and symptoms that should be reported to the health care team.
  F. Discuss affective and interpersonal responses to cancer treatment and care.
  G. Identify community resources available for health promotion and cancer care.

BIBLIOGRAPHY

American Nurses' Association/Oncology Nursing Society (1987). *Standards of Oncology Nursing Practice.* Kansas City, Kan: American Nurses' Association.

Bille, D.A. (ed) (1981). *Practical Approaches to Patient Teaching.* Boston: Little Brown & Co.

Blumberg, B.D. & Johnson, J. (1990). Teaching strategies: the patient. In S.L. Groenwald, M.H. Frogge, M. Goodman, & C.H. Yarbro (eds). *Cancer Nursing: Principles and Practice.* Boston: Jones & Bartlett Publishers, pp. 1246-1255.

Fernsler, J.I. (1991). Developing strategies for public education in cancer. In S.B. Baird, R. McCorkle, & M. Grant (eds). *Cancer Nursing: A Comprehensive Textbook.* Philadelphia: W.B. Saunders Co. pp. 932-943.

Gordon, M. (1987). *Nursing Diagnosis: Process and Application* (2nd ed). New York: McGraw-Hill.

Johnson, J. & Blumberg, B.D. (1984). A commentary on cancer patient education. *Health Educ Q 10* (special suppl), 7-18.

Johnson, J. & Flaherty, M. (1980). The nurse and cancer patient education. *Semin Oncol 7*,63-70.

Morra, M.E. (1991). Developing strategies for patient education in cancer. In S.B. Baird, R. McCorkle, & M. Grant (eds). *Cancer Nursing: A Comprehensive Textbook*. Philadelphia: W.B. Saunders Co., pp. 944-956.

Oncology Nursing Society (1989). *Standards of Oncology Education: Patient/Family and Public*. Pittsburgh: Author.

Rankin, S.H. & Stalling, K.D. (1990). *Patient Education: Issues, Principles, and Practices* (2nd ed). Philadelphia: J.B. Lippincott.

Redman, B.K. (1984). *The Process of Patient Education*. St. Louis: C.V. Mosby.

Redman, B.K. (1987). Teaching the patient and family or significant other. In C. Ziegfeld (ed) *Core Curriculum for Oncology Nurses*. Philadelphia: W.B. Saunders Co., pp. 353-359

Rorden, J. (1987). *Nurses as Health Teachers: A Practical Guide*. Philadelphia: W.B. Saunders Co.

Nursing Management of Responses to the Cancer Experience

Jane C. Clark, MN, RN, OCN
Rose F. McGee, PhD, RN
Ricky Preston, MA, RN

COPING

Grief

THEORY

I. Definition: changes in thinking, feelings, and behaviors that occur as a direct consequence of an actual or perceived loss of a loved person, valued object, status, or identity.

II. Risk factors.
   A. Disease and treatment related:
      1. Diagnosis with a poor prognosis, uncertain outcome, or likelihood of recurrence.
      2. Perceived or actual changes in body structure and/or function such as cachexia, amputation, alopecia, or cognitive dysfunction.
   B. Situational:
      1. Loss of persons through divorce, death, or separation.
      2. Loss of external objects such as pets, home, or possessions.
   C. Life-style:
      1. Status losses such as failure, demotion, firing, retirement, or bankruptcy.
      2. Perceived or actual loss of social support.
   D. Developmental—aging.

III. Standard medical therapy.
   A. Pharmacological management with sedatives, antidepressants, and mood elevators.
   B. Individual or family psychotherapy.
   C. Behavioral interventions such as self-help groups or relaxation.
   D. Occupational or recreational therapy.
   E. Spiritual counseling.

IV. Potential sequelae of prolonged grief.
   A. Dysfunctional grief responses:
      1. Failure to complete the normal grief response within a year or a time span proportional to the meaning of the loss.
      2. Anticipatory grief responses that result in resolution before the actual loss.
   B. Behavioral disorders such as manic-depressive states, hysteria, obsessive-compulsive behavior, and suicidal ideation or attempts.
   C. Abnormal social behavior such as drug or alcohol addiction, juvenile delinquency, or excessive generosity.
   D. Somatic illness such as gastrointestinal ulcers or colitis.

DATA COLLECTION

I. History.
   A. Presence of risk factors.
   B. Presence of defining physical and psychosocial characteristics of grief:
      1. Shock and disbelief—emotional and physical immobility and denial of loss.
      2. Developing awareness—crying, angry outbursts, shortness of breath, choked feelings, sighing, flashes of anguish, retelling the story, painful dejection, changes in eating and sleeping patterns, or decrease in libido.
      3. Bargaining and restitution—idealizing the loss and contracting for reprieval or deliverance.
      4. Accepting the loss—reliving past experiences, preoccupation with the lost object, crying, somatic symptoms, fight or flight responses, dreams, or nightmares.
      5. Resolving the loss—establishing new relationships, planning for the future, recalling rich memories or past experiences, affirming oneself, and resuming previous roles.

II. Pattern of grief response.
   A. Duration.
   B. Previous losses and patterns of resolution.
   C. Sociocultural factors that influence the grief response.
   D. Potential strengths and weaknesses that may facilitate or impede the grief process such as personality traits, coping patterns, spiritual beliefs, patterns of family interactions, and availability of resources.
   E. Presence or potential for cumulative losses.

III. Perceived meaning of the loss(es) sustained to the client and family.

IV. Perceived impact of grief response on mood, relationships, and activities of daily living, work, or school.

ASSOCIATED NURSING DIAGNOSES

I. Dysfunctional grieving.

II. Anticipatory grieving.

III. Altered role performance.

IV. Altered family processes.

V. Sleep pattern disturbances.

VI. Self-esteem disturbance.

NURSING PLANNING AND IMPLEMENTATION

I. Interventions to minimize risk of occurrence and severity of dysfunctional grief.
   A. Use interpersonal relationship skills appropriate to the stage of the grief process:
      1. Encourage talking about perceived or actual loss(es).
      2. Actively listen to subjective responses to loss(es).
      3. Provide nonjudgmental atmosphere to facilitate expression of negative emotions and minimize feelings of guilt.
      4. Validate perceptions of responses.
      5. Facilitate establishment of personal goals.
      6. Give permission to grieve and to resolve the loss.
   B. Institute measures to facilitate coping:
      1. Teach relaxation techniques.
      2. Encourage participation in support groups.
      3. Refer for counseling as indicated.
      4. Give permission to resume past roles and establish new relationships.
   C. Identify means to channel energy constructively.

II. Interventions to maximize client safety and comfort.
   A. Advocate avoidance of conditions that block resolution of grief process: oversedation, closed communications, and social isolation.
   B. Implement suicidal prevention precautions if overt or covert evidence of suicidal ideations are manifest.
   C. Report critical changes to physician:
      1. Oversedation.
      2. Withdrawal or social isolation.
      3. Extreme emotional reactions—anger, guilt, depression, or hostility.
      4. Developmental regression.
      5. Overt or covert evidence of suicidal ideations.

III. Interventions to monitor for complications related to the grief process.
   A. Weight changes—gain or loss.
   B. Changes in sleep, rest, or eating patterns.
   C. Decline in physical and psychosocial functioning.

IV. Interventions to enhance adaptation/rehabilitation.
   A. Encourage expression of anticipatory grief.
   B. Provide bereavement care to assist to resolve secondary losses, attend to unfinished business, and incorporate loss into life.
   C. Allow client and family to experience the discomforts of the loss within a supportive environment.
   D. Provide anticipatory socialization by teaching about loss and role playing.
   E. Encourage referral for psychotherapy as indicated.

V. Interventions to incorporate client and family in care.
   A. Use teaching aids on grief and loss.
   B. Complete family assessments.
   C. Provide family counseling and bereavement care.

EVALUATION OF CLIENT AND FAMILY OUTCOMES

I. Identify perceived losses, significance of losses, and adaptive coping strategies.

II. Discuss stages of the normal grief response.

III. Identify institutional and community resources to deal with losses.

IV. Describe personal strengths and resources for dealing with losses.

Anxiety

THEORY

I. Definition: state of feeling apprehensive in response to a nonspecific or unidentifiable threat.

II. Risk factors.
   A. Disease related:
      1. Uncertainty of prognosis and/or social stigma of diagnosis.
      2. Inadequate symptom control—pain or insomnia.
      3. Associated complications—sepsis or hypoglycemia.
      4. Progression—paraneoplastic syndrome and cachexia.
   B. Treatment related:
      1. Prolonged regimen and/or hospitalization.
      2. Intensive therapy—combination therapy, bone marrow transplantation, and mutilative surgery.
      3. Untoward or side effects—alopecia or immunosuppression.
      4. Termination of therapy.
   C. Life-style and/or situational:
      1. Disease-related losses—health, status, finances, and social interaction.
      2. Withdrawal from narcotics, alcohol, or barbiturates.
      3. Exposure to new situations.
      4. Excessive intake of caffeine and/or nicotine.
   D. Developmental:
      1. Low self-esteem or intense fears in childhood.
      2. Blocked expectations, needs, or goals.

III. Principles of medical management.
   A. Psychotherapy—individual and/or family.
   B. Behavioral interventions—self-help groups and relaxation exercises.
   C. Medications—antianxiety drugs such as benzodiazepines or antidepressants.
   D. Diversional therapy—occupational and/or recreational.

IV. Potential sequelae of anxiety.
   A. Psychosomatic illnesses—gastric ulcers, colitis, or obesity.
   B. Behavioral changes—acting out or eating disturbances.
   C. Physical symptoms—nausea, vomiting, and headaches.
   D. Mental disturbances—panic or paranoia.
   E. Cognitive dysfunction—loss of memory, disorientation, or problems with concentration and decision making.
   F. Transmission of anxiety to others.

DATA COLLECTION

I. History.
   A. Presence of risk factors.
   B. History of defining characteristics of anxiety:
      1. Physical—flushing, sweating, tenseness, tremors, pacing and overactivity or immobility, changes in weight (gain or loss), changes in sleep patterns (insomnia, hypersomnia, early morning awakening), shortness of breath, vom-

iting, diarrhea, fatigue, muscle aches, feelings of heaviness, headaches, dry mouth, palpitations, decreased hearing and/or visual acuity.
2. Psychosocial—irritability, feeling "keyed up" or irritable, changes in perceptual field (hypervigilant or narrowly focused), tendency to cry easily, self-doubt and blaming, problems with problem solving and decision making, regressive or assaultive behavior, compulsiveness.
C. Patterns of anxiety—onset; frequency; severity; associated symptoms; precipitating, aggravating, and alleviating factors.
D. Perceived effectiveness of previous responses to anxiety (some anxiety responses are constructive or motivational, whereas others are destructive)—patterns of responses may include overactivity, inactivity, abusive behavior, or somatization.
E. Perceived impact of anxiety on client/family—physical, economic, life-style, interpersonal, work, or school.

II. Physical findings.
A. Flushing, sweating, and dilated pupils.
B. Hyperactivity such as tenseness, tremors, jerky movements, pacing, or hypoactivity.
C. Sighing respirations and/or shortness of breath.
D. Disheveled dress and inappropriate affect.
E. Pressured speech, blocking, overtalking, focusing on one recurring thought, and blaming self and/or others.

III. Laboratory findings.
A. Increased blood sugar level.
B. Increased epinephrine level.

ASSOCIATED NURSING DIAGNOSES

I. Fatigue.

II. Ineffective individual coping.

III. Altered nutrition.

IV. Sleep pattern disturbance.

V. Anticipatory grief.

NURSING PLANNING AND IMPLEMENTATION

I. Interventions to minimize risk and severity of anxiety.
A. Discuss unmet needs that may contribute to anxiety.
B. Explore similarities between present situation and successfully resolved problems of the past.
C. Provide information about the anticipated course of the disease and treatment to limit threat of the unknown.
D. Use diversion or relaxation techniques as appropriate.

II. Interventions to maximize client safety during anxiety.
A. Provide safe, supportive, and predictable environment.
B. Walk with client if pacing.
C. Assist with self-care as needed.
D. Accept symptoms, and listen attentively.
E. Allow to ventilate thoughts and feelings.
F. Refrain from making demands or forced decision making during high-anxiety states.

G. Speak slowly, calmly, and directly to client.
H. Set limits to minimize risks to client.
I. Provide positive feedback if alternative coping lessens anxiety.
J. Be attentive to requests but avoid fostering dependency.

III. Interventions to monitor for complications related to anxiety and/or treatment.
   A. Observe for indications of panic attacks—decreased level of orientation, hallucinations, hypotension, pallor, or rage.
   B. Observe for untoward effects of antianxiety drugs—dry mouth, drowsiness, or depression.
   C. Observe for seizures or other symptoms of withdrawal or abrupt discontinuance of antianxiety or antidepressive drugs.

IV. Interventions to involve client and family in exploring maladaptive coping mechanisms.
   A. Discuss possible secondary gains of anxious behavior.
   B. Teach strategies such as diversion techniques to minimize focusing on somatic or emotional responses to anxiety.
   C. Discuss interference with daily functioning attributed to maladaptive responses such as overeating or overactivity.
   D. Report critical changes in client assessment parameters to the physician:
      1. Panic attacks.
      2. Avoidance behaviors such as denial, projection, and rationalization.
      3. Suicidal attempts or verbalization of suicidal ideations.
      4. Untoward effects of antianxiety drug therapy.
      5. Abrupt discontinuance of antianxiety drugs.

V. Interventions to enhance adaptation/rehabilitation.
   A. Promote sleep with comfort measures or medications as ordered by physician.
   B. Limit or discontinue alcohol, caffeine, and nicotine intake.
   C. Implement strategies to manage side effects of antianxiety and/or antidepressant therapy:
      1. Dry mouth—increase fluid intake, chew sugarless gum, and provide frequent mouth care.
      2. Constipation—high-fiber diet (see "Constipation").
      3. Blurred vision—generally passes; advise not to change glasses.
      4. Drowsiness—generally passes; caution about operating mechanical equipment or driving.
      5. Dizziness—avoid rapid movements of head and change positions slowly.

VI. Interventions to incorporate client and family in care.
   A. Assist to identify feelings of anxiety, to ventilate feelings, and to seek support.
   B. Instruct client and family in recreational/diversional/creative outlets for emotional energy.
   C. Provide information on community resources such as crisis intervention hotlines, I Can Cope, or CanSurmount.
   D. Provide opportunity to explore cultural/religious aspects of responses to illness, loss, or death.

EVALUATION OF CLIENT AND FAMILY OUTCOMES
I. Identify anxiety-provoking situations and associated responses.
   A. Identify sources of anxiety.
   B. Initiate interactions with others to ventilate feelings of anxiety.

C. Identify functional and dysfunctional responses.

D. Discuss disease and prognosis accurately and comfortably.

II. Participate in anxiety-reducing techniques.

A. Plan to omit or limit alcohol, caffeine, and nicotine intake.

B. Describe methods to decrease feelings of anxiety.

C. Perform positive feedback strategies for functional coping.

D. Identify support systems within the family and community.

E. Describe means to channel energy constructively.

Depression

THEORY

I. Definition: a state of being sad, discouraged, gloomy, or in low spirits, which may vary from a transient mood alteration to a psychiatric illness with suicidal ideation.

II. Risk factors.

A. Disease related and/or treatment related, especially during critical points such as:

1. Diagnosis.
2. Prolonged or difficult treatment.
3. Recurrence or progression.
4. Termination of treatment.
5. Terminal stage of the disease process.

B. Situational and/or developmental:

1. Perceived or actual loss of personal control.
2. Lack of perceived or actual social support.
3. Cumulative crises in family or related to the illness.
4. Financial burden of disease, treatment, or lost wages.
5. Changes in social roles and relationships.
6. Biological vulnerability, especially family history of manic depression.
7. Psychological makeup, especially low self-esteem or pessimism.

III. Standard medical therapy.

A. Treatment of underlying condition.

B. Individual or group psychotherapy.

C. Mood altering drugs—sedatives, tranquilizers, or antidepressants.

D. Stress reduction techniques—hypnosis, biofeedback, or relaxation exercises.

E. Electroshock therapy.

F. Occupational or recreational therapy.

IV. Potential sequelae of depression.

A. Somatic changes related to changes in appetite or sleep patterns.

B. Interference with role functioning at home, school, or work.

C. Suicidal ideation and/or attempts.

D. Psychotic behaviors—delusions, hallucinations, paranoia, manic attacks, phobias, depersonalization, or obsessive-compulsiveness.

E. Transmission of depression to significant others.

DATA COLLECTION

I. History.

A. Presence of risk factors.

B. Presence of defining characteristics of depression—fatigue, muscle aches, feelings of heaviness, loss of interest in work, school, sex, or social activities, frequent somatic complaints or hypochondriasis with symptoms worse in the morning, feelings of being tense or "jerky," or preoccupation with trivia or feelings of depression.

  C. Patterns of symptoms of depression—onset, frequency, severity, associated symptoms, and precipitating, aggravating, and alleviating factors.

  D. Perceived meaning of symptoms to client and family.

  E. Perceived impact of depression on client and family and perceived effectiveness of strategies to relieve symptoms.

II. Physical findings.
  A. Flat affect, lack of spontaneity, minimal eye contact, and slumped posture.
  B. Slow speech or minimal verbalizations.
  C. Inactivity or agitated behavior.
  D. Agitation (rare, but may herald suicidal attempts, especially after being withdrawn and passive).

III. Psychosocial findings.
  A. Crying, labile emotions, or verbalization of hopelessness.
  B. Self-reproach, pessimism, or guilt.
  C. Refusal of treatment or to follow health recommendations.
  D. Problems with word finding or decision making.

IV. Laboratory and diagnostic findings.
  A. Changes in cortisol levels.
  B. Cognitive changes revealed on psychometric testing.

ASSOCIATED NURSING DIAGNOSES

  I. Self-esteem disturbances.

 II. Hopelessness.

III. Anger.

IV. Powerlessness.

 V. Sleep pattern disturbances.

VI. Altered role performance.

NURSING PLANNING AND IMPLEMENTATION

  I. Interventions to minimize risk of symptom occurrence and/or severity of depression.
  A. Give client and family control by informing of diagnosis, treatment, or changes and by offering choices in treatment and self-care when possible.
  B. Spend quality time with client—listen and accept feelings nonjudgmentally.
  C. Foster communications between client, family, and health team by formulating a list of concerns, arranging care conferences, or other strategies.
  D. Give permission to express feelings and to ask for help.
  E. Validate feelings, goals, and self-perceptions as appropriate.
  F. Assist client and family to redefine goals, values, and view of self in terms of the reality of the disease, treatment, and resources.
  G. Assist to focus on the present and short-term, attainable goals.
  H. Initiate spiritual, occupational, or psychological referrals as indicated.

 II. Interventions to maximize client safety and comfort.
  A. Attend to dietary and mobility needs if extremely withdrawn or apathetic.

B. Consider all discussions of suicide as serious and report to necessary personnel to assure client safety.

C. Monitor and report reactions to antidepressants, sedatives, or other drugs that may enhance depression.

D. Caution client against:
  1. Abrupt discontinuance of antidepressants, for they should be tapered.
  2. Use of alcohol while taking mood-altering drugs.

E. Report critical changes in client assessment parameters to physician:
  1. Marked changes in mood or interactions, either withdrawal or agitation.
  2. Untoward responses to medications.
  3. Weight changes—loss or gain of 10% or more of weight.
  4. Cognitive and/or physiological changes related to insomnia that impede functioning or progress.

III. Interventions to monitor responses to depression and treatment.
  A. Monitor physiological changes that may explain somatic complaints.
  B. Monitor for side effects or adverse reactions to antidepressants.
  C. Observe for symptoms of withdrawal of antidepressants.

IV. Interventions to enhance adaptation/rehabilitation.
  A. Teach client/family energy conservation strategies.
  B. Provide positive reinforcement for behaviors that approximate goal achievement.
  C. Assist with problem solving and information gathering.
  D. Accept verbalized anger or negative feelings; do not personalize.
  E. Assist client to manage side effects of antidepressants:
    1. Dry mouth—increase fluid intake, chew sugarless gum, and perform frequent mouth care.
    2. Constipation—initiate bowel program.
    3. Blurred vision—generally resolves; advise not to change glasses.
    4. Dizziness—avoid changing positions rapidly.
    5. Drowsiness—generally resolves; caution against use of mechanical devices and driving.

V. Interventions to incorporate client and family in care.
  A. Initiate referral to self-help or support groups as indicated.
  B. Inform of telephone hotlines for crisis intervention.
  C. Teach alternate coping strategies such as muscular relaxation or use of music or recreational therapy.
  D. Assist to channel energy constructively by participating in health care, verbalizing negative feelings, and instituting health promotion activities.

EVALUATION OF CLIENT AND FAMILY OUTCOMES

I. Describe personal risk factors for depression.

II. List strategies to decrease risks or complications of depression.

III. Identify personal, family, community, and professional resources to meet crises of cancer experience or depressed state.

IV. Discuss situations that require professional intervention.
  A. Acute changes in ability to control physical and/or psychological responses.
  B. Rapid deterioration in physical status.
  C. Overt or covert indications of suicidal ideation or attempts.

Fear

THEORY

I. Definition: state of feelings of uneasiness related to an identifiable threat or danger; such a state may be adaptive or maladaptive.

II. Risk factors.
  A. Physical changes associated with the illness or treatment—loss of body part or alopecia.
  B. Situational changes—hospitalization or institutionalization.
  C. Developmental changes:
    1. Age-related fears:
      a. Birth to 2 years—loud noises and falling.
      b. Ages 2 to 6 years—dark and being lost.
      c. Ages 7 to 8 years—failure and being disliked.
      d. Ages 9 to 10 years—death, failing grades, animals, and heights.
      e. Ages 11 to 12 years—being alone, rejection, and loss of parents.
      f. Young adult—disfigurement and disapproval by peers.
      g. Middle-age adult—loss of status or persons.
      h. Older adult—institutionalization, desertion, and death.
    2. Threat to self-esteem—abandonment and rejection.
  D. Life-style changes:
    1. Immigration, divorce, or poverty.
    2. Interference with basic human needs or safety.
    3. Blocked goals or expectations.
  E. Universal fears—death or perception of cancer as uniformly fatal or uncontrollable.

III. Standard medical therapy.
  A. Behavioral interventions—desensitization, biofeedback, relaxation, hypnosis, and guided imagery.
  B. Psychotherapy.
  C. Self-help or support group participation.

IV. Potential sequelae of fear.
  A. Neurotic anxiety—anxiety out of proportion to stimulus.
  B. Panic—pallor, cognitive dysfunction, or disorientation.
  C. Chronic illness—asthma, gastrointestinal ulcers, or sexual dysfunction.
  D. Psychological or social dysfunction such as acting out or anger.

DATA COLLECTION

I. History.
  A. Verbalized fears.
  B. Past fears and responses.
  C. Appropriateness of fear to stimulus and to developmental level.
  D. Changes in gastrointestinal or genitourinary functioning—vomiting, diarrhea, or urinary frequency.
  E. Insomnia and/or nightmares.

II. Physical findings.
  A. Facial flushing or pallor.
  B. Tremor.
  C. High-pitched and/or trembling voice.

    D. Tense body posturing.

    E. Increased blood pressure, pulse, and/or respiration.

    F. Diaphoresis.

    G. Syncope.

    H. Somatic changes—parasthesias, palpitations, or tingling.

  III. Psychosocial findings.

    A. Verbalization of fears—real fear may differ from identified threat.

    B. Preoccupation with fears, although stressor is removed.

    C. Expressed feelings of loss of control.

    D. Repeated questioning about diagnosis, treatment, and/or prognosis.

  IV. Laboratory findings—nonspecific.

ASSOCIATED NURSING DIAGNOSES

  I. Powerlessness.

 II. Anger.

III. Hostility.

NURSING PLANNING AND IMPLEMENTATION

  I. Interventions to minimize risk of occurrence or severity of fear.

    A. Remove stimulus or remove client from stimulus situation.

    B. Provide quiet, supportive environment.

    C. Provide physical support with touch as tolerated.

    D. Avoid invasion of personal space.

    E. Give permission to express fears, feelings.

    F. Accept fears as real.

    G. Use simple, direct statements and soothing tones to allay feelings of uneasiness.

    H. Provide thorough orientation to environment and to changes.

    I. Keep client and family informed of illness, treatment, and prognosis.

 II. Interventions to maximize client safety and comfort.

    A. Provide consistency in personnel, plan of care, and approach.

    B. Promote emotionally nonthreatening environment.

    C. Report critical changes in client assessment parameters to physician:

      1. Distorted fears.

      2. Panic attacks.

      3. Physiological changes.

III. Interventions to enhance adaptation/rehabilitation.

    A. Encourage expression of feelings.

    B. Assist to clarify distortions and misperceptions.

    C. Focus on capabilities and effective coping rather than perceived ineffectiveness.

    D. Teach use of activities such as exercise, reading, and music to rechannel energy and diffuse fear.

    E. Identify community resources to deal with disabling or persistent fears.

IV. Interventions to incorporate client and family in care.

    A. Assist to discuss fears and to identify confrontational strategies.

    B. Teach alternative coping strategies such as relaxation or thought stopping.

    C. Provide client education about age-related fears.

    D. Provide client education about irrational fears of cancer and/or death.

EVALUATION OF CLIENT AND FAMILY OUTCOMES

I. Discuss fears.

II. Identify factors that intensify and alleviate fears.

III. Differentiate real from imagined fears.

IV. Identify alternative coping strategies.

V. List personal and professional resources to confront fears.

Powerlessness

THEORY

I. Definition: perception that one's own action will not significantly affect an outcome; a perceived lack of control over a current situation or immediate happening.

II. Risk factors.
   A. Disease related:
      1. Physiological loss of control as a result of carcinogenesis.
      2. Physiological demands of illness.
      3. Perceived loss of part of self.
      4. Lack of knowledge about disease process or health status.
      5. Chronic nature of cancer.
   B. Treatment related:
      1. Physical side effects of treatment modalities of cancer.
      2. Psychosocial side effects of disease and treatment for cancer.
      3. Lack of knowledge about the course, demands of, and prognosis related to treatment.
   C. Situational:
      1. Controls imposed by the health care environment.
      2. Life-style of helplessness.
      3. Ineffective interpersonal interactions.
      4. Loss of ability to manage own health care that necessitates hospitalization.
      5. Loss of control in decision-making matters.
      6. Relinquishing of prior roles to others.

III. Standard medical therapy.
   A. Incorporation of client/family into decision making about care.
   B. Professional counseling.

IV. Potential sequelae of prolonged powerlessness.
   A. Despair.
   B. Helplessness.
   C. Hopelessness.

DATA COLLECTION

I. History.
   A. Presence of risk factors for powerlessness.
   B. Presence of subjective defining characteristics of powerlessness:
      1. Verbal expressions of having no control over a situation or outcome.
      2. Verbal expressions of dissatisfaction or frustration with progress.
   C. Presence of objective defining characteristics of powerlessness:
      1. Nonparticipation in care or decision making when opportunities are provided.
      2. Reluctance to express feelings.

3. Apathy.
4. Dependence on others for care.
    D. Perceived impact of powerlessness on activities on daily living, life-style, relationships, work or school, role responsibilities, and mood.
II. Psychosocial examination.
    A. Presence of psychological responses to powerlessness—irritability, resentment, anger, and guilt.
    B. Perceived or actual changes in valued role performance.

ASSOCIATED NURSING DIAGNOSES

I. Hopelessness.

II. Knowledge deficit.

III. Ineffective individual coping.

IV. Altered role performance.

NURSING PLANNING AND IMPLEMENTATION

I. Interventions to minimize the risk of occurrence, severity, or complications of powerlessness.
    A. Provide client and family with adequate information to participate in decision making about care.
    B. Encourage client and family to ask questions about care, treatment plans, and prognosis.
    C. Identify factors that contribute to powerlessness for individual client and family.
    D. Provide consistent communications about changes in health status and self-care demands.
    E. Encourage client and family to express feelings related to living with cancer.
    F. Maintain personal articles, call light, and telephone within reach of client unless contraindicated by safety needs.

II. Interventions to monitor for complications related to powerlessness.
    A. Elicit subjective responses of client and family about satisfaction with amount of information received, quality of interpersonal communications, and opportunities for participating in decision making.
    B. Assess level of participation in decision-making and information-seeking activities.

III. Interventions to incorporate client and family in care.
    A. Seek opinions and suggestions about care from the client and family members.
    B. Reinforce participative behaviors in decision making by the client and family members.
    C. Make client and family responsible for portions of care as appropriate for condition.

IV. Report critical changes in client assessment parameters to physician.
    A. Powerlessness that compromises the ability of the client and family to participate in decision making and self-care.
    B. Verbal expressions of despair or intention of self-harm.

EVALUATION OF CLIENT AND FAMILY OUTCOMES

I. Describe personal risk factors for powerlessness.

II. Participate in measures to minimize the risk of occurrence, severity, and complications of powerlessness.

III. Report signs, symptoms, and complications of powerlessness to a member of the health care team.

IV. List changes in the condition of the client that require professional assistance in management.
   A. Lack of motivation to participate in self-care activities.
   B. Verbal expressions of intention to harm self.

COMFORT

Pain

THEORY

I. Definition: an unpleasant sensory and emotional experience associated with actual or potential tissue damage or described in terms of such damage.
   A. Acute pain:
      1. Pain of short duration, usually considered less than 6 months.
      2. Cause of pain usually is known.
      3. Intensity of pain ranges from mild to severe.
   B. Chronic pain:
      1. Pain of prolonged duration, usually greater than 6 months.
      2. Cause of pain may or may not be known.
      3. Pain has not responded to treatment or has not subsided after healing.
      4. Intensity of pain ranges from mild to severe.

II. Risk factors.
   A. Disease related:
      1. Infiltration of nerves, bone, soft tissues, or retroperitoneum by tumor.
      2. Compression of tissues and nerves by tumor growth.
      3. Localized tissue necrosis resulting from tumor invasion.
      4. Stimulation of pain receptors resulting from distention of normal tissues as in effusions or edema.
      5. Concurrent conditions such as arthritis, dysmenorrhea, or musculoskeletal disease.
   B. Treatment related:
      1. Invasive diagnostic and treatment procedures.
      2. Acute complications of cancer therapies such as stomatitis, localized infection, inflammation of tissues within radiation treatment fields, or opportunistic infections.
      3. Long-term complications of cancer therapies such as adhesions and phantom-limb pain after surgery or fibrosis and compression of nerves after radiation therapy.
   C. Life-style related:
      1. Overactivity.
      2. Immobility.
      3. Improper body alignment.
      4. Anxiety or stress precipitated by the impact of cancer on activities of daily living, role performance, relationships, communications patterns, and economic factors.

III. Standard medical therapy.
   A. Treatment of underlying cause.
   B. Treatment of pain (Figure 7-1).

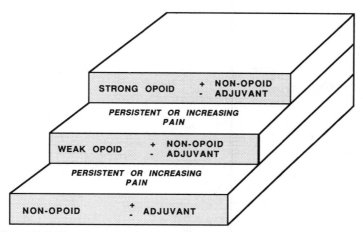

Figure 7-1 Treatment of pain: World Health Organization analgesic ladder.

1. Analgesics (Table 7-1).
   a. Nonnarcotics.
   b. Narcotics.
2. Adjuvant pharmacological therapy.
   a. Antidepressants.
   b. Anticonvulsants.
   c. Psychostimulants.
   d. Tranquilizers.
3. Behavioral interventions—physical or occupational therapy, biofeedback, hypnosis, guided imagery, relaxation techniques, and music, play, or art therapy.
4. Radiation therapy.
5. Surgical interruption of pain pathways (Table 7-2).

IV. Potential sequelae of prolonged pain.
   A. Depression, anger, social withdrawal.
   B. Failure to participate in activities of daily living, treatment plan, sexual activity,

---

Table 7-1

MAIN GROUPS OF ANALGESICS

---

1. Nonnarcotics or nonsteroidal antiinflammatory drugs (NSAIDs)—work primarily at the peripheral nervous system level:
   a. Over the counter (OTC)—mainly aspirin (ASA), acetaminophen (Tylenol), and ibuprofen (Advil, Nuprin, 200 mg tablets).
   b. Prescription, e.g., ibuprofen (Motrin), naproxen (Naprosyn), and indomethacin (Indocin).
2. Narcotics or opioids—work primarily at the central nervous system level:
   a. Narcotic agonists, e.g., morphine, meperidine (Demerol), hydromorphone (Dilaudid), levorphanol (Levo-Dromoran), oxymorphone (Numorphan), and codeine.
   b. Narcotic agonist-antagonists, e.g., pentazocine (Talwin), nalbuphine (Nubain), butorphanol (Stadol), and buprenorphine (Buprenex).

Modified from McCaffery, M. and Beebe, A. (1989). *Pain: Clinical Manual for Nursing Practice.* St. Louis: C.V. Mosby Co., p. 54.

Table 7-2
SURGICAL INTERVENTIONS FOR PAIN

Type	Procedure	Examples of Application
Neurotomy	Destruction of peripheral nerve.	Chest wall pain.
Rhizotomy	Sectioning of preganglionic sensory nerve root fibers.	Pain associated with lung, head, and neck. Visceral pain.
Cordotomy	Interruption of ascending pain and temperature fibers in the anterolateral spinal cord.	Visceral or somatic pain. Unilateral pain.
Myelotomy	Interruption of pain and temperature fibers.	Intractable pain. Bilateral pain. Pain in perineum, pelvis, lower extremities, and abdomen.
Sympathectomy	Interruption or removal of a portion of the sympathetic nervous system.	Visceral pain.

Modified from Carson, B.S. (1987). Neurologic and neurosurgical approaches to cancer pain. In D.B. McGuire & C.H. Yarbro (eds). *Cancer Pain Management*. Orlando: Grune & Stratton, Inc., pp. 223-243.

roles, problem solving, decision making, and home, work, or school responsibilities.
   C. Substance abuse—alcohol, tobacco, or drugs.
   D. Distrust of health care professionals.
   E. Use of pain for secondary gains.
   F. Fatigue.

DATA COLLECTION
   I. History.
      A. Presence of risk factors for pain.
      B. Presence of defining characteristics of pain.
      C. Patterns of pain—onset, location, duration, quality, frequency, severity, associated symptoms, and precipitating, aggravating, and alleviating factors.
      D. Types and effectiveness of self-care measures in relieving pain.
      E. Perceived meaning of pain to client and family.
      F. Impact of pain on activities of daily living, life-style, comfort, relationships, work, school, and role responsibilities, and mood.
      G. Pain tolerance—level of pain client is willing to endure.
   II. Physical examination.
      A. Guarding behavior.
      B. Facial mask of pain.
      C. Changes in muscle tone.
      D. Increased blood pressure, pulse rate, or respiratory rate.
      E. Pupillary dilation.
   III. Psychosocial examination.
      A. Behavioral expressions of pain—crying, pacing, rocking, social withdrawal, or restlessness.

B. Narrowed focus.

C. Distortion of time.

D. Presence of associated psychosocial responses—depression, anxiety, or fear.

ASSOCIATED NURSING DIAGNOSES

I. Pain.

II. Sleep pattern disturbance.

III. Impaired physical mobility.

IV. Alteration in elimination: constipation.

V. Self-care deficit.

VI. Alteration in nutrition.

VII. Social isolation.

NURSING PLANNING AND IMPLEMENTATION

I. Interventions to minimize the risk of occurrence, severity, and complications of pain.
   A. Measures to promote physical comfort:
      1. Maintain proper body alignment.
      2. Use special equipment—beds, assistive devices, or mattress protectors.
      3. Apply heat or cold.
      4. Minimize noxious environmental stimuli—heat, light, noise, or touch.
   B. Measures to promote relaxation:
      1. Massage—superficial, pressure, or vibration.
      2. Deep breathing exercises.
      3. Guided imagery of pleasant or soothing experiences.
      4. Hypnosis.
   C. Measures to provide distraction:
      1. Cutaneous stimulation.
      2. Humor.
      3. Reading or watching television or videotapes.
      4. Occupational therapy.
      5. Music therapy.
   D. Measures to promote psychological comfort:
      1. Communicate belief in pain experience.
      2. Demonstrate respect for client and family responses to the pain experience.
      3. Encourage client and family participation in decisions related to pain management.
      4. Confront maladaptive efforts of client to manage or cope with pain.
      5. Discuss concerns and advocate use of adjuvant pharmacological therapies as ordered by physician.
      6. Commit to remain with client if pain unrelieved and to continue to try to control pain.
   E. Measures to decrease exacerbation of pain response:
      1. Administer analgesics early in the pain experience to avoid severe pain.
      2. Administer pain medications on a regular schedule determined by the peak action and duration of medications, needs of client, and orders of the physician.
      3. Schedule pain-inducing activities or procedures to occur during peak analgesic effect.
   F. Measures to decrease complications of pain management regimens:
      1. Initiate bowel regimen upon initiation of narcotic therapy.

Date _____

Patient's Name _____ Age _____ Room _____

Diagnosis _____ Physician _____

Nurse _____

I. Location: (Patient or nurse mark drawing.)

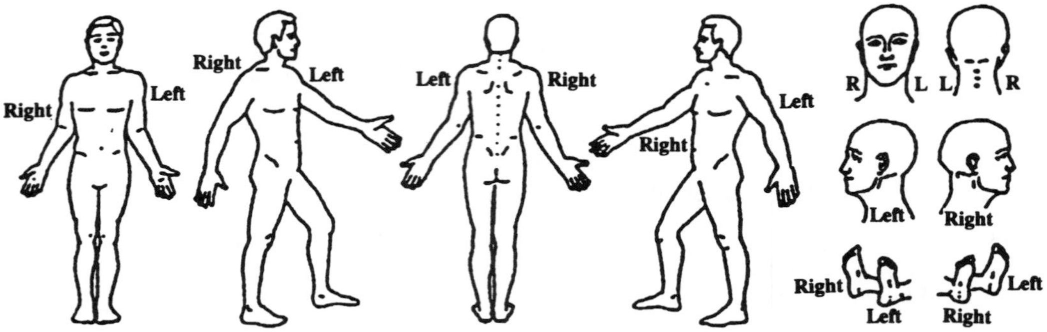

II. Intensity: (Patient rates the pain.) Scale used _____
Present _____
Worst pain gets _____
Best pain gets _____
Acceptable level of pain _____

III. Quality: (Use patient's own words, e.g., prick, ache, burn, throb, pull, sharp.) _____

IV. Onset, duration, variations, rhythms: _____

V. Manner of expressing pain: _____
_____
_____

VI. What relieves the pain? _____
_____
_____

VII. What causes or increases the pain? _____

VIII. Effects of pain: (Note decreased function, decreased quality of life.)
Accompanying symptoms (e.g., nausea) _____
Sleep _____
Appetite _____
Physical activity _____
Relationship with others (e.g., irritability) _____
Emotions (e.g., anger, suicidal, crying) _____
Concentration _____
Other _____
IX. Other comments: _____
X. Plan: _____

Figure 7-2 Initial Pain Assessment Tool and Flow Sheet. *(From McCaffery, M., & Beebe, A. [1989]. Pain: Clinical Manual for Nursing Practice. St. Louis: C.V. Mosby Co., pp. 21, 27.)*

Patient _____ Date _____
Pain rating scale used* _____
Purpose: To evaluate the safety and effectiveness of the analgesic(s).
Analgesic(s) prescribed _____

Time	Pain Rating	Analgesic	R	P	BP	Level of Arousal	Other†	Plan & Comments

*Pain rating: a number of different scales may be used. Indicate which scale is used and use the same one each time. For example, 0–10 (0 = no pain, 10 = worst pain).

†Possibilities for other columns: bowel function, activities, nausea and vomiting, other pain relief measures. Identify the side effects of greatest concern to patient, family, physician, nurses.

Figure 7-2 continued

    2. Implement preventive measures to prevent or minimize side effects of narcotic therapy—antiemetics, antacids, and environmental safety precautions.

  II. Measures to promote a team approach to pain management.
    A. Include client and family in planning pain management strategies.
    B. Serve as a client advocate in encouraging behaviors that convey the client experience to the health care team.
    C. Suggest administration of combinations of narcotic and nonnarcotic medications as indicated.
    D. Suggest changes in dosage or frequency, not both, when adjustments to the pain regimen to meet client needs are warranted.
    E. Assess components of the pain experience and adequacy of relief measures systematically (Figure 7-2).
    F. Consult with professional who practices nonpharmacological methods of pain control.

 III. Implement strategies to monitor for complications related to pain management regimen.
    A. Respiratory status—decrease in respiratory rate greater than eight breaths per minute; increase in partial pressure of carbon dioxide (PCO_2) level, and decrease in ventilatory volume.
    B. Central nervous system—changes in levels of sedation, euphoria, coordination during activity, and mood.
    C. Cardiovascular—hypotension.
    D. Gastrointestinal status—decreased motility and strength of contractions.
    E. Genitourinary status—increased tone and amplitude of contractions.
    F. Dermatological status—vasodilation of cutaneous vessels; increased temperature of skin; flushing of face, neck, and thorax; sweating; and pruritus.

 IV. Report critical changes in client assessment parameters to physician.
    A. Marked subjective changes in characteristics of the pain experience.
    B. Occurrence of significant side effects of pain management regimen:
      1. Marked decrease in level of consciousness.
      2. Respiratory depression less than eight breaths per minute.
      3. Constipation, urinary retention, or vomiting uncontrolled by recommended measures.

EVALUATION OF CLIENT AND FAMILY OUTCOMES

  I. Describe personal risk factors for pain associated with cancer or treatment.

 II. Identify physiological, psychosocial, and cultural factors that influence the perception of pain and acceptance of treatment.

 III. Describe the impact of pain on activities of daily living, role performance, work or home responsibilities, self-concept, and comfort.

 IV. Define the goals of pain management as determined jointly by the client and care team.

  V. Participate in strategies to minimize the potential complications of pain management techniques.

 VI. List situations that require professional assistance with pain management:
    A. Pain unrelieved with usual pain management regimen.
    B. Acute changes in the character of pain.
    C. Unrelieved complications of pain management regimen.

Insomnia

THEORY

I. Definition: inability to go to sleep, stay asleep, or sleep long enough, uninterrupted, to feel rested and relaxed on awakening.

II. Risk factors.
   A. Disease related:
      1. Presence of symptoms related to tumor invasion such as obstruction, pain, fever, shortness of breath, pruritus, and fatigue.
      2. Presence of paraneoplastic syndromes with increased corticosteroid production.
   B. Treatment related:
      1. Presence of symptoms related to surgery such as pain.
      2. Sleep-cycle disruption related to frequent monitoring activities by health care team.
      3. Administration of medications that alter sleep cycle such as narcotics, caffeine, sedatives, and steroids.
      4. Presence of symptoms related to chemotherapy and/or supportive therapy administration such as frequency of voiding with hydration before chemotherapy or increased fluid intake with antibiotic or nutritional support therapy; frequency of vomiting; and/or depression.
      5. Changes in sleep environment or routines with hospitalization.
   C. Life-style related:
      1. Increased physical and/or psychological stress.
      2. Decreased physical activity.

III. Standard medical therapy.
   A. Sedatives or hypnotics to induce and maintain sleep.
   B. Drugs or treatments to control physical or psychological symptoms of disease or treatment.

IV. Potential sequelae of prolonged insomnia.
   A. Changes in mental status and cognitive ability.
   B. Fatigue.

DATA COLLECTION

I. History.
   A. Usual patterns of sleep:
      1. Usual time to retire.
      2. Routines before retiring such as bathing, eating, warm milk, and relaxation.
      3. Usual length of time needed to go to sleep.
      4. Awakening episodes during the night and early morning.
         a. Perceived causes such as noises, nightmares, need to void, presence of symptoms.
         b. Perceived difficulty in returning to sleep.
      5. Usual time to awaken.
      6. Subjective responses to sleep periods.
      7. Quantity and quality of rest/sleep periods during daytime.
   B. Changes in sleep-rest patterns since diagnosis of or treatment for cancer.
   C. Perceptions of significant others about the quantity and quality of sleep by client.
   D. Review of prescription and nonprescription medication use.

    E. Impact of insomnia on activities of daily living, mood, relationships with others, cognitive function, ability to perform self-care, and interest in life.

    F. Presence of restlessness, irritability, lethargy, fatigue, apathy, decreased concentration, attention span, and problem-solving ability.

II. Physical examination.

    A. Mild, fleeting nystagmus, ptosis of eyelids, and dark circles under eyes.

    B. Expressionless face.

    C. Frequent yawning and changes in position.

    D. Thickness of speech, mispronunciation, or incorrect word usage.

III. Psychosocial examination.

    A. Presence of depression.

    B. Presence of anxiety.

    C. Presence of situational stressors significant for client.

ASSOCIATED NURSING DIAGNOSES

I. Sleep pattern disturbance.

II. Activity intolerance.

III. Fatigue.

IV. Altered role performance.

V. Altered thought process.

NURSING PLANNING AND IMPLEMENTATION

I. Institute measures to promote a restful sleep environment.

    A. Straighten or provide clean bed linens.

    B. Encourage use of usual clothing worn at bedtime such as gowns, pajamas, underwear, or no clothing.

    C. Decrease or increase environmental stimuli such as lighting, music, and presence of significant other per client preference.

    D. Establish preferred room temperature.

II. Institute measures to increase relaxation before bedtime.

    A. Encourage bathing, snack and/or warm milk, back rub, positioning, reading or watching television, progressive muscle relaxation, or imagery.

    B. Avoid intake of stimulants such as caffeine or alcohol before bedtime.

III. Institute nursing measures to control or minimize occurrence and severity of physical symptoms (see section on specific symptom).

IV. Plan nursing care requirements to decrease interruptions during sleep periods.

V. Institute interventions to monitor for complications related to insomnia.

    A. Assess perceived quantity and quality of sleep each day.

    B. Assess perceptions of client about relationships with significant others, ability to perform roles, and mood states.

    C. Assess perceptions of significant others about relationship with client, performance of roles by client, and mood state.

VI. Interventions to incorporate client and family in care.

    A. Teach stress management techniques.

    B. Teach effective bedtime routine.

    C. Teach signs and symptoms related to complications of insomnia to report to a member of health care team.

EVALUATION OF CLIENT AND FAMILY OUTCOMES

I. Describe personal risk factors for insomnia.

II. Report signs, symptoms, and complications of insomnia to a member of the health care team.

III. Participate in measures to minimize the risk of occurrence, severity, and complications of insomnia.

IV. List changes that require professional assistance in management—insomnia that interferes with the ability of the client to function at desired level.

Pruritus

THEORY

I. Definition: itching.

II. Risk factors.
   A. Disease related:
      1. Hematological malignancies such as lymphoma, leukemia, myeloma, and Hodgkin's disease.
      2. Solid tumors such as melanoma, inflammatory breast cancer, and lung cancer.
      3. Liver and kidney disease.
      4. Fluid and electrolyte imbalances such as dehydration and hypercalcemia.
      5. Infection such as candidiasis.
      6. Allergic reaction to foods, clothing, and medications.
   B. Treatment related:
      1. Wound healing after surgery.
      2. Local skin reactions within radiation therapy fields.
      3. Allergic reactions to antineoplastic medications, immunotherapy, or other substances.
      4. Local tissue response at immunotherapy injection sites.
   C. Life-style related:
      1. Dry atmospheric conditions.
      2. Anxiety.

III. Standard medical therapy.
   A. Treatment of underlying condition.
   B. Antihistamines.
   C. Tranquilizers.
   D. Steroids.
   E. Antiprostaglandins.
   F. Sequistra agents.

IV. Potential sequelae of prolonged itching.
   A. Impaired skin integrity.
   B. Infection.
   C. Bleeding.
   D. Sleep disturbances.

DATA COLLECTION

I. History.
   A. Review of previous therapy for cancer.
   B. Review of prescription and nonprescription medications.
   C. Presence of underlying systemic disease (renal failure, biliary disease, diabetes.)

    D. Pattern of pruritus—incidence, frequency, severity, alleviating factors, and aggravating factors.

    E. Impact of pruritus on life-style, comfort, and activities of daily living.

II. Physical examination.

    A. Scratch marks on skin.

    B. Erythema of the skin.

    C. Excoriation of the skin.

    D. Thickening of the skin.

    E. Dryness of the skin.

    F. Vaginal discharge.

    G. Deposits of urea or bilirubin on skin surface.

III. Potential laboratory findings.

    A. Elevated white blood count.

    B. Elevated uric acid levels.

    C. Elevated blood urea nitrogen (BUN) and/or creatinine levels.

    D. Abnormal liver function studies.

    E. Elevated glucose levels.

IV. Psychosocial examination.

    A. Presence of anxiety.

    B. Changes in self-concept.

ASSOCIATED NURSING DIAGNOSES

  I. Alteration in comfort.

 II. Impaired skin integrity.

III. Sleep pattern disturbance.

IV. Body image disturbance.

NURSING PLANNING AND IMPLEMENTATION

  I. Interventions to minimize the risk of occurrence and severity of pruritus.

    A. Measures to maintain skin hydration:

      1. Encourage fluid intake of more than 3000 ml per day.

      2. Use water-soluble skin emollients on damp skin.

      3. Provide a humidified environment.

    B. Measures to prevent vasodilation:

      1. Maintain a cool environment.

      2. Encourage use of cool baths or showers.

      3. Encourage avoidance of beverages containing alcohol and caffeine.

      4. Use distraction and relaxation techniques to reduce anxiety.

 II. Measures to decrease risk of complications of pruritus.

    A. Cut fingernails short and smooth.

    B. Encourage frequent and thorough handwashing.

    C. Use alternative methods of skin stimulation:

      1. Pressure.

      2. Massage.

      3. Vibration.

      4. Cool temperature.

    D. Avoid tight clothing.

E. Avoid irritating fabrics (corduroy or wool) or substances (detergents or harsh soaps).

III. Interventions to monitor for complications related to pruritus.
   A. Conduct skin assessment each week or with a change in symptomatology.
   B. Assess for signs and symptoms of infection (fever, purulent drainage, painful, and reddened sites).

IV. Interventions to monitor client response to symptom management.
   A. Monitor subjective reports of the client of changes in the pattern of pruritus.
   B. Monitor changes in level of comfort and sleep pattern.
   C. Monitor changes in condition of skin.
   D. Monitor compliance with measures to decrease severity of itching and to reduce incidence of complications.

V. Interventions to incorporate client and family in care.
   A. Teach handwashing techniques.
   B. Teach measures to decrease risk of occurrence or severity of pruritus.
   C. Teach signs and symptoms related to complications of pruritus to report to health care team.

VI. Report critical changes in client assessment parameters to the physician.
   A. Presence of signs and symptoms of infection.
   B. Presence of signs and symptoms of impaired skin integrity.

EVALUATION OF CLIENT AND FAMILY OUTCOMES

I. Describe personal risk factors for pruritus.

II. Report signs, symptoms, and complications of pruritus to a member of the health care team.

III. Participate in measures to minimize the risk of occurrence, severity, and complications of pruritus.

IV. List changes that require professional assistance in management—infection or impaired skin integrity.

Hiccups

THEORY

I. Definition: abrupt, intermittent, repeated, and involuntary spasms of the diaphragm causing a sound ("hic") that results from the vibration of closed vocal cords as air rushes suddenly into the lungs.

II. Risk factors resulting in the irritation of the phrenic nerve between the spinal cord and the terminal ramifications on the undersurface of the diaphragm.
   A. Disease related:
      1. Primary or metastatic tumors compressing the phrenic nerve.
      2. Central nervous system tumors.
      3. Infection of the peritoneum.
      4. Uremia.
      5. Hiatal hernia.
      6. Alcoholism.
      7. Intestinal obstruction.

    B. Treatment related:
      1. Surgery involving the diaphragm.
      2. Radiation therapy to a field containing the phrenic nerve.
      3. Intraperitoneal chemotherapy.
    C. Situational:
      1. Exposure to cold.
      2. Ingestion of liquids of extreme temperatures.
      3. Anxiety.

III. Standard medical therapy.
    A. Medications—calcium channel blockers, amitriptyline, metoclopramide, chlorpromazine, and barbituates.
    B. Abdominal decompression.
    C. Nasal or oral irritation.
    D. Phrenic nerve crush.
    E. Phrenic nerve block.

IV. Potential sequelae of prolonged hiccups.
    A. Fatigue.
    B. Sleep pattern disturbances.
    C. Inability to eat.
    D. Aspiration.
    E. Increased intracranial pressures.
    F. Wound dehiscence.
    G. Vomiting.

DATA COLLECTION

I. History.
    A. Presence of personal risk factors for hiccups.
    B. Pattern of hiccups—onset; frequency; duration; and predisposing, aggravating, and alleviating factors.
    C. Perceived meaning of hiccups to client and family.
    D. Impact of hiccups on activities of daily living, life-style, comfort, relationships, work, school, or role responsibilities, and mood.

II. Physical examination—rate and force of hiccups.

III. Psychosocial examination—anxiety.

ASSOCIATED NURSING DIAGNOSES

I. Ineffective breathing pattern.

II. Social isolation.

III. Fatigue.

IV. Sleep pattern disturbance.

V. Fear.

NURSING PLANNING AND IMPLEMENTATION

I. Interventions to decrease the risk of occurrence, severity, and complications of hiccups.
    A. Modify dietary intake to:
      1. Avoid foods that produce flatus.
      2. Avoid foods served at extreme temperatures.

    B. Instruct client in stress reduction techniques.

    C. Encourage client to sit in an upright position for 30 to 60 minutes after meals.

    D. Instruct client in nonpharmacological measures to manage hiccups:

        1. Rebreathing own air from a paper bag.

        2. Holding breath while taking a large swallow of water.

        3. Swallowing a spoonful of granulated sugar unless contraindicated by condition.

        4. Applying finger pressure to the eyes through closed lids for several minutes.

II. Interventions to maximize client safety.

    A. Teach client and family positioning to use during severe hiccups to decrease the risk for aspiration should vomiting occur.

    B. Encourage to avoid eating during periods of severe hiccups.

III. Report critical changes in client assessment parameters to physician.

    A. Prolonged, intractable hiccups lasting longer than 48 hours or occurring more than 12 times per minute.

    B. Signs and symptoms of wound dehiscence.

    C. Signs and symptoms of aspiration.

EVALUATION OF CLIENT AND FAMILY OUTCOMES

  I. Describe personal risk factors for hiccups.

  II. Report signs and symptoms of persistent hiccups to a member of the health care team.

III. Participate in strategies to minimize the risk of occurrence, severity, and complications of hiccups.

IV. List changes in the condition of the client that require professional assistance in management.

    A. Adverse changes in the character or pattern of hiccups.

    B. Weight loss greater than 10% of body weight.

    C. Presence of signs and symptoms of complications of hiccups.

NUTRITION

Dysphagia

THEORY

  I. Definition: difficulty in swallowing, usually accompanied by a sensation of material lodging in the esophagus.

  II. Risk factors.

    A. Disease related:

        1. Infiltration or impingement of the esophagus by tumor.

        2. Impingement of the esophagus by fluid accumulation.

        3. Loss of vocal cord sphincter control.

        4. Loss of innervation to the esophagus.

    B. Treatment related:

        1. Surgical procedures that impair ability to hold food in mouth, lateralize, masticate, form a bolus, move bolus through the oropharynx, or move bolus through the esophagus.

        2. Increased cellular destruction of normal cells of oral cavity and esophagus from effects of chemotherapy such as 5-fluorouracil (5-FU).

3. Increased cellular destruction of normal cells of oral cavity and esophagus from immediate effects of radiation therapy to field that includes the oral cavity and esophagus.
4. Fibrosis and stenosis associated with the long-term effects of radiation therapy to field that includes the oral cavity and esophagus.
5. Changes in character of oral secretions related to chemotherapy or radiation therapy before bone marrow transplant.

C. Life-style related—emotional responses to disease and/or treatment.
D. Iatrogenic related:
1. Psychotropic medications may impair gag reflex and thus affect swallowing.
2. Anticholinergic agents.

III. Standard medical therapy.
A. Treatment for underlying disease such as nodal radiation therapy, antifungal and antibacterial medications, and laser therapy.
B. Endoscopic dilation.
C. Steroids.
D. Alternative pathway for nutrition such as feeding tube or gastrostomy tube.
E. Medications to decrease pain and anxiety related to swallowing.

IV. Potential sequelae of prolonged dysphagia.
A. Decreased nutritional intake.
B. Weight loss.
C. Fluid and electrolyte imbalances.
D. Inability to control secretions.
E. Avoidance of attempts to swallow.

DATA COLLECTION

I. History.
A. Review of previous therapy for cancer.
B. Presence of underlying systemic disease such as infection, tumor infiltration, or stroke.
C. Patterns of dysphagia—incidence, frequency, alleviating factors, aggravating factors.
D. Perceived significance of dysphagia to client/significant other.
E. Impact of dysphagia on life-style, comfort, and activities of daily living.

II. Physical examination.
A. Ability of client to swallow food or liquids of various consistencies.
B. Ability to hold food in mouth and lateralize food for chewing.
C. Ability to masticate.
D. Ability to propel food to oropharynx with tongue.
E. Objective responses to attempts to swallow—drooling, gagging, coughing, pain, aspiration, or regurgitation.
F. Weight.

ASSOCIATED NURSING DIAGNOSES

I. Alteration in nutrition: less than body requirements.

II. Fear.

III. Impaired skin integrity.

IV. Impaired swallowing.

NURSING PLANNING AND IMPLEMENTATION

I. Interventions to minimize the risk of occurrence, severity, or complications of dysphagia.
   A. Measures to increase ease and effectiveness of swallowing:
      1. Position client in upright position.
      2. Tilt head forward, chin pointing to chest.
      3. Stimulate steps in swallowing that client is unable to initiate independently:
         a. Open mouth—apply light pressure on chin; stroke digastric muscle beneath the chin; touch lips with a spoon.
         b. Bring lips together—stroke lips with spoon or finger; apply manual pressure to close the upper and lower lips.
         c. Stimulate salivary secretion—allow client to see food or fluids; serve foods and liquids at extreme temperatures to stimulate sensation; stimulate salivary glands with application of ice.
         d. Swallowing—provide an environment free of distractions; ice sternal notch and rub the back of the neck; encourage multiple swallows with each attempt.
   B. Provide appropriate assistive devices such as straws, plunger spoon to place food in pharynx, asepto syringe, or pastry tube.
   C. Institute measures to decrease pain with swallowing such as using soft or pureed foods, cutting foods in small pieces, and administering local anesthetics to oral cavity and esophagus.
   D. Consult with speech therapist for additional techniques for individual client situation.

II. Interventions to maximize safety.
   A. Be physically present when client is attempting to swallow.
   B. Explain measures to manage difficulties in swallowing before occurrence.
   C. Implement strategies to decrease fear and anxiety associated with attempts to swallow such as relaxation techniques.

III. Interventions to monitor for complications related to dysphagia.
   A. Maintain daily dietary intake record.
   B. Weigh daily.
   C. Assess for signs and symptoms of dehydration—decreased skin turgor, dryness in mouth, increased temperature.

IV. Interventions to monitor client response to symptom management.
   A. Monitor subjective reports of the client/significant other of changes in the pattern of dysphagia.
   B. Monitor compliance with measures to decrease severity of dysphagia.
   C. Monitor subjective reports of client/significant other of psychological responses to attempts to swallow.

V. Interventions to incorporate client and family in care.
   A. Teach techniques to increase ease of swallowing.
   B. Teach emergency techniques should aspiration or regurgitation occur with attempts to swallow.
   C. Teach signs and symptoms related to complications of dysphagia to report to a member of the health care team.

VI. Report critical changes in client assessment parameters to physician.
   A. Presence of weight loss greater than 10% of body weight.
   B. Presence of signs and symptoms of infection.
   C. Presence of signs and symptoms of an obstructed airway.

EVALUATION OF CLIENT AND FAMILY OUTCOMES

I. Describe personal risk factors for dysphagia.

II. Report signs, symptoms, and complications of dysphagia to a member of the health care team.

III. Participate in measures to minimize the risk of occurrence, severity, and complications of dysphagia.

IV. Demonstrate competence in emergency techniques for aspiration, regurgitation, and airway obstruction associated with dysphagia.

V. Identify resources in the community to assist with rehabilitation.

VI. List changes in the condition of the client that require professional assistance in management.
   A. Aspiration.
   B. Airway obstruction.
   C. Weight loss greater than 10% of body weight.
   D. Dehydration.

Nausea and Vomiting

THEORY

I. Definition.
   A. *Nausea*—an unpleasant sensation associated with an inclination to vomit.
   B. *Vomiting*—a forceful explusion of gastric contents through the mouth.

II. Risk factors.
   A. Disease related:
      1. Primary or metastatic tumor of the central nervous system that includes the vomiting center.
      2. Obstruction of a portion of the gastrointestinal tract by primary or metastatic tumor.
      3. Increased intracranial pressure from a tumor or intracranial bleeding.
      4. Food toxins, infection, or motion sickness.
      5. Metabolic abnormalities such as hyperglycemia, hyponatremia, or hypercalcemia.
      6. Renal or hepatic dysfunction.
   B. Treatment related:
      1. Stimulation of the true vomiting center through the cellular by-products of increased cellular destruction associated with cancer therapies.
      2. Stimulation of the chemoreceptor trigger zone and the true vomiting center by antineoplastic agents such as cisplatin, nitrogen mustard, doxorubicin, and dacarbazine.
      3. Stimulation of the true vomiting center through afferent pathways by radiation therapy to fields that include the gastrointestinal tract and result in inflammation, edema, and irritation.
      4. Side effects of medications such as digitalis, morphine, antibiotics, vitamins, or iron.
      5. Side effects of concentrated nutritional supplements.
   C. Situational.
      1. Increased levels of tension, stress, or anxiety without adequate coping strategies.

    2. Noxious visual or olfactory stimuli.

    3. Conditioned response to cancer care facilities, treatments, or personnel.

III. Standard medical therapy.
    A. Treatment of underlying disease.
    B. Antiemetics such as prochlorperazine (Compazine) or metoclopramide (Reglan).
    C. Behavioral interventions such as progressive muscle relaxation, imagery, distraction, and self-hypnosis.
    D. Fluid and electrolyte replacement.

IV. Potential sequelae of prolonged nausea and vomiting.
    A. Fluid and electrolyte imbalances such as dehydration and hypokalemia.
    B. Esophageal tears.
    C. Weight loss related to nutritional deficiencies.
    D. Aspiration.
    E. Noncompliance with treatment plan.

DATA COLLECTION

I. History.
    A. Presence of risk factors for nausea and vomiting.
    B. Presence of defining characteristics of nausea and vomiting—unpleasant sensation in back of throat, esophagus, or stomach and expulsion of gastric contents.
    C. Patterns of nausea and vomiting—onset, frequency, severity, associated symptoms, precipitating factors, aggravating factors, and alleviating factors.
    D. Effectiveness of previous self-care strategies in relieving nausea and vomiting.
    E. Characteristics of emesis.
    F. Perceived meaning of nausea and vomiting to client and family.
    G. Impact of nausea and vomiting on activities of daily living, life-style, comfort, relationships, work, school, role responsibilities, and mood.

II. Physical examination.
    A. Sweating, salivation, and circumoral pallor.
    B. Coolness of skin.
    C. Decreased pulse, increased depth of respirations, and increased blood pressure.
    D. Decreased muscle strength.

III. Psychosocial examination.
    A. Anxiety.
    B. Fear.

ASSOCIATED NURSING DIAGNOSES

I. Alteration in nutrition: less than body requirements.

II. Fear.

III. Fluid volume deficit.

IV. Altered role performance.

NURSING PLANNING AND IMPLEMENTATION

I. Interventions to minimize the risk of occurrence, severity, or complications of nausea and vomiting.
    A. Modify environment to decrease stimuli by lowering lighting, limiting noise, and avoiding exposure to noxious sights and smells.
    B. Maintain a cool, well-ventilated environment.

    C. Modify diet to include bland foods served at room or chilled temperature.

    D. Provide client relief from food preparation responsibilities.

    E. Decrease activity level and suddenness of movement during periods of increased nausea and vomiting.

    F. Replace fluids lost with high-caloric, electrolyte-rich, cool liquids such as Gatorade, Popsicles, and soft drinks.

    G. Provide comfort measures during nauseous periods or after vomiting subsides such as a cool cloth to the forehead or back of the neck, change of clothing or bedding as needed, relaxation exercises, soothing music, and rest.

    H. Administer antiemetics around the clock per physician's order during periods of increased risk for nausea or vomiting.

II. Interventions to maximize safety.

    A. Position client during vomiting episode to decrease risks of aspiration.

    B. Have emesis basin within reach.

    C. Provide assistance with ambulation as needed for clients who are weak or experiencing sedative effects from antiemetics.

    D. Keep side rails up for clients experiencing sedative effects from antiemetics.

III. Interventions to monitor for complications related to nausea and vomiting.

    A. Assess for signs and symptoms of dehydration each day—decreased skin turgor, dryness in mouth, and increased temperature.

    B. Monitor intake, urinary output, including volume and color, and intake/output ratio each day.

    C. Monitor level of pain associated with vomiting or intake of fluid and food.

    D. Assess character of emesis for critical changes in force of expulsion, frequency, volume, color, or consistency.

    E. Assess vital signs and level of consciousness after each episode of vomiting.

IV. Interventions to monitor client response to symptom management.

    A. Monitor subjective reports of the client and family of changes in the pattern of nausea, vomiting, or character of emesis.

    B. Monitor compliance with measures to decrease incidence and severity of nausea and vomiting.

V. Interventions to incorporate client and family in care.

    A. Teach positioning techniques to decrease risk of aspiration.

    B. Teach administration of antiemetics around the clock during periods of increased risk of nausea and vomiting.

    C. Teach side effects of antiemetics.

    D. Teach comfort and relaxation strategies.

VI. Report critical changes in client assessment parameters to physician.

    A. Presence of adverse changes in pattern of nausea or vomiting.

    B. Presence of signs and symptoms of aspiration, dehydration, or associated pathology.

EVALUATION OF CLIENT AND FAMILY OUTCOMES

I. Describe personal risk factors for nausea and vomiting.

II. Report signs, symptoms, and complications of nausea and vomiting to a member of the health care team.

III. Participate in measures to minimize the risk of occurrence, severity, and complications of nausea and vomiting.

IV. Demonstrate competence in self-care techniques for management of nausea and vomiting.

V. List changes in the condition of the client that require professional assistance in management.
   A. Presence of adverse changes in pattern of nausea and vomiting.
   B. Weight loss greater than 10% of body weight.
   C. Presence of signs and symptoms of dehydration.
   D. Presence of signs and symptoms of bleeding.

Taste Alterations

THEORY
   I. Definition: an actual or perceived change in taste sensations.
   A. *Hypogeusesthesia*—a decrease in taste sensations.
   B. *Dysgeusia*—a distorted sensation of taste.

  II. Risk factors.
   A. Disease related:
      1. Invasion of oral cavity, nasal passages, or tongue by tumor.
      2. Excretion of noxious substances by the tumor that modifies taste sensations.
      3. Oral infections—candidiasis.
   B. Treatment related:
      1. Surgical removal of the tongue, interruption of the olfactory nerve, and variation of the normal airway (tracheostomy).
      2. Radiation induced:
         a. Destruction of the taste buds at doses greater than 1000 rads.
         b. Dryness of mouth.
         c. Loss of taste for foods.
      3. Chemotherapy-induced changes in taste:
         a. Lowered threshold for bitter tastes.
         b. Increased threshold for sweet tastes.
         c. Metallic or medicine taste.
   C. Life-style related:
      1. Poor oral hygiene.
      2. Nutritional deficiencies—decreased levels of zinc, nickel, copper, niacin, and vitamin A.
   D. Developmental—age-induced degeneration of the taste buds.

 III. Standard medical therapy—nutritional supplement replacements.

  IV. Potential sequelae of prolonged taste alterations.
   A. Anorexia.
   B. Decreased dietary intake.
   C. Weight loss.

DATA COLLECTION
   I. History.
   A. History of risk factors.
   B. Subjective description of changes in tastes.
   C. Impact of taste changes on desire for food.
   D. Impact of taste changes on dietary intake.

II. Physical findings.
   A. Oral assessment:
      1. Erythema or desquamation of mucous membranes of oral cavity.
      2. Interruption in integrity of mucous membranes or structures of oral cavity.
      3. Presence of signs and symptoms of infection.
   B. Weight loss.

III. Laboratory findings.
   A. Decreased levels of albumin.
   B. Decreased levels of zinc, copper, and nickel.
   C. Decreased levels of niacin.
   D. Decreased levels of vitamin A.

ASSOCIATED NURSING DIAGNOSES

I. Alteration in nutrition: less than body requirements.

II. Altered oral mucous membranes.

NURSING PLANNING AND IMPLEMENTATION

I. Interventions to minimize risk of occurrence and severity of taste alterations.
   A. Institute measures to increase sensitivity of taste buds:
      1. Increase use of flavorings and spices in foods.
      2. Serve foods warm to increase aroma.
      3. Increase fluid intake with meals.
      4. Encourage oral hygiene before and after meals.
   B. Institute measures to decrease aversiveness of selected foods or food groups:
      1. Add increased sweeteners to foods.
      2. Marinate red meats in sweet juices.
      3. Offer meat-protein substitutes such as peanut butter, eggs, or cheese.
   C. Institute measures to increase salivation:
      1. Serve liquids with meals.
      2. Use artificial saliva.

II. Interventions to monitor for complications related to taste alterations.
   A. Weigh client at regular intervals.
   B. Maintain a dietary intake record each day.

III. Interventions to incorporate client and family in care.
   A. Instruct client and family in dietary modifications to enhance or modify the taste of foods.
   B. Consult with dietician for dietary instruction.

EVALUATION OF CLIENT AND FAMILY OUTCOMES

I. Describe the personal risk factors for changes in taste sensations.

II. Report signs and symptoms of taste sensations to health care team.

III. Participate in measures to minimize the effects of taste changes on joy of eating and dietary intake.

IV. Report significant weight loss (of more than 10% of total body weight) to health care team.

Xerostomia

THEORY

I. Definition: dryness of the mouth.

II. Risk factors.
   - A. Disease related:
     1. Primary tumor involvement of salivary gland.
     2. Metastatic tumor involvement of salivary gland.
     3. Obsessive-compulsive or anxiety state.
     4. Other diseases such as diabetes, infection, or candidiasis.
   - B. Treatment related:
     1. Surgical removal of the salivary gland.
     2. Radiation therapy with salivary gland in field.
     3. Pharmacological therapy for symptom management: antihistamines, atropine, diuretics, analgesics, and antiemetics.
   - C. Life-style related:
     1. Alcohol ingestion.
     2. Nicotine ingestion.

III. Standard medical therapy.
   - A. Artificial saliva.
   - B. Dental prophylaxis: periodic cleaning and fluoride treatment.
   - C. Prophylactic oral antimicrobial therapy.

IV. Potential sequelae of prolonged xerostomia.
   - A. Impaired oral mucous membrane integrity.
   - B. Difficulty chewing, swallowing, and speaking.
   - C. Dental caries.
   - D. Inadequate digestion of starches.

DATA COLLECTION

I. History.
   - A. Review of previous therapy for cancer.
   - B. Review of prescription and nonprescription medications.
   - C. Pattern of xerostomia—incidence, frequency, alleviating factors, and aggravating factors.
   - D. Impact of xerostomia on food taste, intake, digestion, and communication.

II. Physical examination.
   - A. Dry, shiny mucous membranes of oral cavity.
   - B. Thick, scanty saliva.
   - C. Difficulty in chewing and swallowing.
   - D. Difficulty in speaking.

III. Laboratory findings—decreased pH of oral secretions.

IV. Psychosocial examination.
   - A. Presence of fear.
   - B. Presence of anxiety.

ASSOCIATED NURSING DIAGNOSES

I. Alteration in comfort.

II. Altered oral mucous membrane.

III. Altered nutrition: less than body requirements.

NURSING PLANNING AND IMPLEMENTATION

I. Interventions to minimize the risk of occurrence and severity of xerostomia.
   A. Measures to increase salivary flow:
      1. Offer tart, warm foods and liquids such as hot tea with lemon or sugarfree lemon candy.
      2. Suggest chewing sugarfree Gatorgum.
      3. Apply moderate pressure to sternal notch.
      4. Massage the back of the neck.
   B. Measures to provide moisture to oral mucosa:
      1. Moisten foods with liquids and sauces such as gravy, cream, or soups.
      2. Sip liquids with meals.
      3. Keep container with preferred fluids near client.
      4. Rinse oral cavity with water every 2 hours while awake.
      5. Use artificial saliva.
      6. Use room humidifier if not contraindicated by other conditions.
   C. Measures to decrease risk of complications of xerostomia:
      1. Encourage strict oral hygiene protocol before and after meals.
         a. Remove debris with soft-bristled toothbrush and nonirritating dentifrice.
         b. Rinse oral cavity with water.
      2. Avoid physical, chemical, and thermal irritants such as poorly fitting dental prosthetics; alcohol and tobacco; hot liquids; and hot, spicy, or course foods.

II. Interventions to monitor for complications related to xerostomia.
   A. Examine oral cavity (Figure 7-3) each week or as symptomatology changes.
   B. Encourage periodic dental examinations.

III. Interventions to incorporate client and family in care.
   A. Teach oral hygiene protocol and oral assessment guidelines.
   B. Teach measures to decrease risk of occurrence or severity of xerostomia.
   C. Teach signs and symptoms related to complications of xerostomia to report to member of health care team.

IV. Report critical changes in client assessment parameters to physician.
   A. Presence of signs and symptoms of infection.
   B. Presence of signs and symptoms of altered oral mucous membrane integrity.
   C. Weight loss of more than 10 pounds.

EVALUATION OF CLIENT AND FAMILY OUTCOMES

I. Describe personal risk factors for xerostomia.

II. Report signs, symptoms, and complications of xerostomia to a member of the health care team.

III. Participate in measures to minimize the risk of occurrence, severity, and complications of xerostomia.

IV. List changes that require professional assistance in management—infection or lesions of the oral cavity, weight loss greater than 10 pounds, or dental caries.

Category	Voice	Swallow	Lips	Tongue	Saliva	Mucous membranes	Gingiva	Teeth, Dentures, or denture bearing area
Tools for Assessment	Auditory assessment	Observation	Visual/palpatory	Visual/palpatory	Tongue blade	Visual assessment	Tongue blade and visual assessment	Visual assessment
Methods of Measurement	Converse with patient	Ask patient to swallow. To test gag reflex, gently place blade on back of tongue and depress	Observe and feel tissue	Feel and observe appearance of tissue	Insert blade into mouth, touching the center of the tongue and the floor of the mouth	Observe appearance of tissue	Gently press tissue with tip of blade	Observe appearance of teeth or denture bearing area
1 (Numerical and descriptive rating) 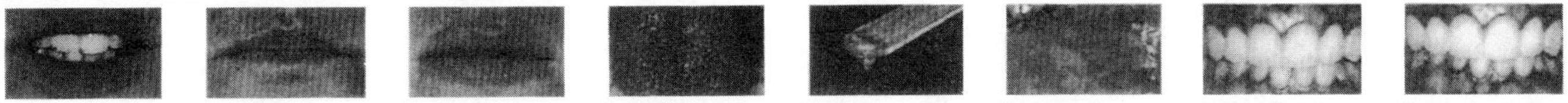	Normal	Normal swallow	Smooth and pink and moist	Pink and moist and papillae present	Watery	Pink and moist	Pink and stippled and firm	Clean and no debris
2 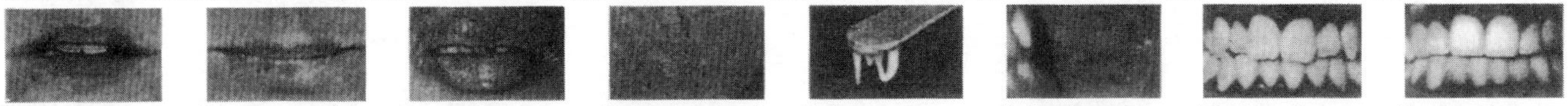	Deeper or raspy	Some pain on swallow	Dry or cracked	Coated or loss of papillae with shiny appearance with or without redness	Thick or ropy	Reddened or coated (increased whiteness) without ulcerations	Edematous with or without redness	Plaque or debris in localized areas (between teeth if present)
3 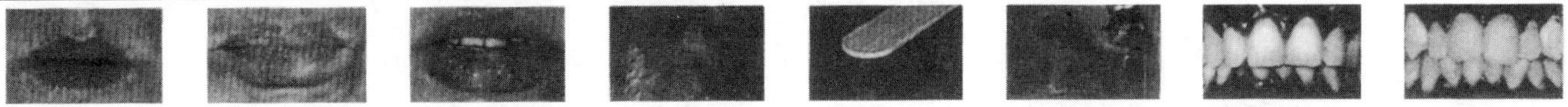	Difficulty talking or painful	Unable to swallow	Ulcerated or bleeding	Blistered or cracked	Absent	Ulcerations with or without bleeding	Spontaneous bleeding or bleeding with pressure	Plaque or debris generalized along gum line or denture bearing area

Figure 7-3 Conducting an oral examination. (*Courtesy June Eilers, RN, MSN, University of Nebraska Medical Center, Omaha, Nebraska and Halbrand, Inc., Willoughby, Ohio.*)

Anorexia

THEORY

I. Definition: loss of appetite.

II. Risk factors.
   A. Disease related:
      1. False sense of satiety created by metastatic process.
      2. Tumor by-products from tumor lysis.
      3. Dysphagia.
      4. Metastatic obstruction by tumor.
      5. Concurrent renal or hepatic disease.
      6. Concurrent physical responses to the disease—pain, fatigue.
   B. Treatment related:
      1. Side effects of radiation, chemotherapy, or biotherapy—dry mouth, nausea and vomiting, mucositis, changes in taste.
      2. Changes in structure related to oral surgery and/or prophylactic dental procedures.
      3. Side effects of medications—narcotics, antibiotics, iron.
      4. Changes in daily meal patterns and food offerings.
   C. Situational:
      1. Psychogenic reactions to the cancer experience—anxiety, fear, depression.
      2. Noxious visual, auditory, or olfactory stimuli.
      3. Changes in activity level.

III. Standard medical therapy.
   A. Treatment of underlying cause.
   B. Appetite stimulants.
   C. Vitamins.
   D. Nutritional supplementation.

IV. Potential sequelae of prolonged anorexia.
   A. Fluid and electrolyte imbalances.
   B. Weight loss.
   C. Weakness, lethargy.
   D. Alteration in tissue repair and wound healing.
   E. Decreased activity level.

DATA COLLECTION

I. History.
   A. Review of previous self-care strategies to relieve anorexia.
   B. Previous dietary patterns and history of anorexia.
   C. Recent treatment and anticipated side effects.
   D. Perceived significance of anorexia to client/significant other.
   E. Impact of anorexia on fluid and electrolyte status.
   F. Pattern of anorexia—onset; frequency; severity; associated symptoms; precipitating, aggravating, and alleviating factors.
   G. Associated socioemotional factors influencing appetite.

II. Physical examination.
   A. Weight loss.
   B. Poor skin turgor, dry mouth, decreased urinary output, and other indications of dehydration or electrolyte imbalance.

III. Psychosocial examination.
1. Psychological responses—fear, anger, anxiety, depression.
2. Noxious stimuli in the environment.
3. Influence of ethnicity or social patterns on intake changes.

ASSOCIATED NURSING DIAGNOSES

I. Alteration in nutritional intake: less than body requirements.

II. Fluid volume deficit.

III. Impaired skin integrity.

NURSING PLANNING AND IMPLEMENTATION

I. Interventions to minimize the risk of occurrence, severity, or complications of anorexia.
   A. Measures to increase caloric and nutritional value of oral intake:
      1. Offer frequent, nutritionally dense meals in small servings throughout the day.
      2. Maximize food intake during periods of greatest appetite, usually breakfast.
      3. Advise to minimize fluid intake before and with meals.
      4. Maximize client choices and access to favorite foods within dietary restrictions.
   B. Measures to promote comfort and ease while eating:
      1. Administer pain medications, if needed, 30 to 60 minutes before meals.
      2. Assist with oral care, as needed, before and after meals.
      3. Plan activities to allow for adequate rest before meal time.
      4. Position client in comfortable position with ready access to food.
      5. Minimize noxious stimuli in the environment—sounds, sights, odors.

II. Interventions to monitor for complications related to anorexia.
   A. Maintain daily dietary intake record.
   B. Weigh daily.
   C. Assess for signs and symptoms of dehydration—decreased skin turgor, dryness in mouth, increased temperature.
   D. Monitor for signs and symptoms of electrolyte imbalance.
   E. Note indications of skin breakdown, dehiscence, or delayed wound healing.

III. Interventions to monitor client response to symptom management.
   A. Monitor subjective reports of the client/significant other of changes in patterns of eating.
   B. Monitor compliance with measures to facilitate high-caloric, high-protein nutritional intake.
   C. Monitor subjective reports of client/significant other of psychological responses to interventions to facilitate dietary intake.

IV. Interventions to incorporate client and family in care.
   A. Encourage significant others to provide favorite foods, within dietary restrictions.
   B. Teach significant others methods to enhance caloric and protein content of diet.
   C. Teach signs and symptoms of dehydration, delayed wound healing, and malnutrition.
   D. Assist client and family not to become so fixated on dietary intake that efforts are counterproductive in terms of facilitating nutrition.

V. Report critical changes in client assessment parameters to physician.
   A. Presence of weight loss greater than 10% of body weight.
   B. Presence of signs and symptoms of dehydration and/or malnutrition.

VI. Interventions to enhance adaptation and rehabilitation.
   A. Provide written and/or audiovisual materials on nutrition.
   B. Initiate referral to dietitian for nutritional assessment and intervention as indicated.

EVALUATION OF CLIENT AND FAMILY OUTCOMES

I. Describe personal risk for complications related to loss of appetite.

II. Report signs, symptoms, and complications of anorexia to a member of the health care team.

III. Participate in measures to minimize the risk of occurrence, severity, and complications of anorexia.

IV. Identify resources in the community to assist with nutrition.

V. List changes in the condition of the client that require professional assistance in management.
   A. Weight loss greater than 10% of ideal body weight.
   B. Dehydration.
   C. Changes in skin integrity or wound healing.

PROTECTIVE MECHANISMS

Leukopenia

THEORY

I. Definition: a quantitative decrease in the total number of white blood cells (neutrophils, monocytes, lymphocytes, eosinophils, and basophils) to less than 3000 cells/mm^3.

II. Risk factors.
   A. Disease related:
      1. Decreased production of white blood cells (WBCs) related to primary malignant disease of the marrow, tumor invasion of marrow, genetically transmitted deficiencies, and age.
      2. Increased consumption of WBCs related to infection without adequate marrow replacement.
      3. Increased destruction of WBCs associated with autoimmune diseases, hypersplenism, viral and bacterial infections, and antigen-antibody reactions.
   B. Treatment related:
      1. Chemotherapy—destruction of rapidly dividing normal hematopoietic cells and malignant cells results in a decrease in the production of WBC precursors and ultimately mature WBCs.
      2. Radiation therapy—destruction of rapidly dividing normal hematological cells within the radiation treatment fields that include areas of increased hematopoietic activity (pelvis, sternum, and proximal ends of the long bones) results in a decrease in the production of WBC precursors and ultimately mature WBCs.

3. Other pharmacological agents such as phenothiazines, alcohol, selected antibiotics, diazepam, indomethacin, and antithyroid drugs may inhibit WBC production.

III. Standard medical therapy.
   A. Prophylactic and empirical antimicrobial and antifungal therapy.
   B. Granulocyte transfusions.
   C. Avoidance of pharmacological agents that inhibit WBC production or function.
   D. Colony-stimulating factor therapy (see Chapter 23).

IV. Potential sequelae of prolonged leukopenia.
   A. Increased risk of infection.
   B. Changes in activities of daily living such as work, leisure, and self-care practices.
   C. Septic shock.
   D. Organ system damage.
   E. Death.

DATA COLLECTION

I. History.
   A. Review of previous type of and length of time since cancer treatment.
   B. Review of prescription and nonprescription medications.
   C. Impact of leukopenia on life-style and self-care.

II. Physical examination.
   A. Localized symptoms of infection such as redness, swelling, pain, and pus; classic symptoms may not be present with severe leukopenia.
   B. Fever or hypothermia.
   C. Generalized symptoms of infection such as fatigue or malaise, increased pulse and respirations, and decreased blood pressure.
   D. Site-specific symptomatology of infection such as cough, abnormal breath sounds, oral pain, back pain, burning, urgency, and frequency of urination, or rectal discomfort with bowel elimination.

III. Psychosocial examination.
   A. Perceptions of meaning of leukopenia for client and family.
   B. Effects of leukopenia on life-style and activities of daily living.

IV. Laboratory findings.
   A. WBC less than 3000 cells/mm³.
   B. Absolute granulocyte count (AGC) less than 500 cells/mm³
      (AGC = Total WBC × [% segs + % bands]).

ASSOCIATED NURSING DIAGNOSES

I. Potential for infection.

II. Knowledge deficit related to self-care.

III. Altered role performance.

NURSING PLANNING AND IMPLEMENTATION

I. Notify physician of WBC less than 500 cells/mm³.

II. Institute measures to decrease risk of exposure to endogenous organisms in clients with leukopenia.
   A. Handwashing before and after meals and after urination or bowel movement.

B. Consistent personal hygiene measures:
   1. Bathing with an antimicrobial soap with attention to areas of skin folds.
   2. Oral care to remove debris, moisten oral cavity, and decrease trauma to mucosal surfaces.
   3. Perineal care after urination and bowel movements.

III. Institute measures to decrease risk of exposure to exogenous organisms.
   A. Instruct all persons having direct contact with client in handwashing techniques with an antimicrobial soap.
   B. Limited exposure to sources of large numbers of microbes such as pets, raw, unpeeled fruits and vegetables, fresh-cut flowers in standing water, humidifiers, and immunizations.
   C. Avoid large crowds of people within enclosed environments and persons at risk for or with communicable and/or infectious diseases.
   D. Plan nursing care assignments to decrease risks of cross-contamination (private rooms or protective isolation).
   E. Maintain aseptic techniques when performing invasive procedures.

IV. Institute interventions to monitor for complications.
   A. Assess all sites of invasive procedures for evidence of infection.
   B. Assess skin and mucosal surfaces for breaks in natural barriers to micro-organisms.
   C. Monitor for signs and symptoms of septic shock (see Chapter 9).

V. Initiate interventions to incorporate client and family in care.
   A. Teach measures to decrease risk of complications of leukopenia.
   B. Teach signs and symptoms related to complications of leukopenia to report to a member of the health care team.

VI. Report critical changes in client assessment parameters to physician.
   A. Presence of marked decrease or increase in temperature, blood pressure, respirations, or pulse.
   B. Presence of breaks in the natural barriers to microorganisms.

EVALUATION OF CLIENT AND FAMILY OUTCOMES

I. Describe personal risk factors for leukopenia.

II. Participate in measures to minimize the risk of infection from endogenous and exogenous sources.

III. Report significant changes in condition to health care team.
   A. Temperature greater than 101° F.
   B. Localized or site-specific symptoms of infection without fever.
   C. Exposure to communicable disease such as chickenpox or measles.
   D. Significant loss of integrity of skin and mucous membranes.

IV. Identify community resources available for management of emergency situations.

Thrombocytopenia

THEORY

I. Definition: a quantitative decrease in the number of circulating platelets.

II. Risk factors.
   A. Disease related:

1. Decreased production of platelets related to primary malignant disease of marrow, tumor invasion of marrow, or genetically transmitted platelet deficiencies.
2. Increased consumption of platelets related to disseminated intravascular coagulation associated with malignancy.
3. Increased destruction of platelets related to bacterial or viral infection or autoimmune responses.

B. Treatment related:
1. Chemotherapy—destruction of rapidly dividing normal hematopoietic cells and malignant cells results in a decrease in the production of platelet precursors and ultimately mature platelets.
2. Radiation therapy—destruction of rapidly dividing normal hematopoietic cells within radiation treatment fields that include areas of increased hematopoietic activity (pelvis, sternum, and proximal ends of long bones) results in a decrease in the production of platelet precursors and ultimately mature platelets.
3. Supportive therapy—dilutional decrease in the number of circulating platelets may occur with massive blood transfusions, extracorporeal circulation, exchange transfusions, and fluid therapy.
4. Other pharmacological agents such as thiazides, alcohol, and estrogens may inhibit platelet production.

III. Standard medical therapy.
   A. Platelet transfusions.
   B. Avoidance of pharmacological agents that inhibit platelet production and/or function.

IV. Potential sequelae of prolonged thrombocytopenia.
   A. Increased risk of bleeding.
   B. Anemia.
   C. Changes in activities of daily living such as work, leisure, and self-care practices.

DATA COLLECTION

I. History.
   A. Review of previous therapy for cancer.
   B. Review of prescription and nonprescription medications.
   C. Impact of thrombocytopenia on life-style and self-concept.

II. Physical examination.
   A. Petechiae, bruising, and ecchymoses.
   B. Active bleeding from the gums, nose, bladder, bowel, or vagina.
   C. Active bleeding from sites of invasive procedures:
      1. Surgical procedures.
      2. Venous and arterial access.
      3. Diagnostic tests such as bone marrow and liver biopsies and lymphangiograms.
      4. Enemas, rectal temperatures, urethral catheterization, and oral suctioning.

III. Laboratory findings.
   A. Platelet count less than $150,000/mm^3$.
   B. Prolonged bleeding times (prothrombin time [PT] and partial thromboplastin time [PTT]).

IV. Psychosocial examination.
   A. Perceptions of meaning of thrombocytopenia for client and family.
   B. Effects of thrombocytopenia on life-style, activities of daily living, and self-concept.

ASSOCIATED NURSING DIAGNOSES

I. Potential for injury.

II. Knowledge deficit related to self-care with thrombocytopenia.

III. Disturbance in self-concept related to petechiae, bruising, and ecchymoses of thrombocytopenia.

IV. Altered oral mucous membrane.

NURSING PLANNING AND IMPLEMENTATION

I. Notify physician of platelet count less than 50,000/mm^3 or presence of active bleeding.

II. Institute measures to decrease risk of complications of thrombocytopenia.
   A. Institute bleeding precautions:
      1. Avoid use of sharp objects such as razors or knives.
      2. Avoid invasive procedures such as enemas, catheterizations, intramuscular injections, and rectal temperatures.
      3. Apply direct pressure for 5 minutes to all needle puncture sites.
      4. Institute bowel program to decrease risk of constipation.
      5. Avoid Valsalva maneuver and straining with bowel movements or blowing nose.
      6. Use soft toothbrush and gentle friction for mouth care; avoid use of fine dental floss.
   B. Institute safety measures:
      1. Assist with self-care, activities of daily living, and ambulation as needed.
      2. Place bed in low position and side rails up at all times.

III. Institute interventions to monitor for complications related to thrombocytopenia.
   A. Assess skin for evidence of increased petechiae, bruising, or ecchymoses, especially on the extremities.
   B. Assess all sites of invasive procedures for evidence of bleeding.
   C. Assess client for evidence of bleeding from internal sources:
      1. Blood in stool.
      2. Hematuria.
      3. Intracranial hemorrhage:
         a. Changes in level of consciousness.
         b. Restlessness.
         c. Headache.
         d. Changes in pupillary response.
         e. Seizures.
         f. Widening of pulse pressure.
         g. Focal changes such as visual disturbances, ataxia, and affective changes.

IV. Initiate interventions to incorporate client and family in care.
   A. Teach measures to decrease risk of complications of thrombocytopenia.
   B. Teach signs and symptoms related to complications of thrombocytopenia to report to a member of the health care team.
   C. Report critical changes in client assessment parameters to physician:
      1. Presence of bruising or bleeding from any site.
      2. Presence of signs and symptoms of internal bleeding.

EVALUATION OF CLIENT AND FAMILY OUTCOMES

I. Describe personal risk factors for thrombocytopenia.

II. Report signs, symptoms, and complications of thrombocytopenia to a member of the health care team.

III. Participate in measures to minimize the risk of complications of thrombocytopenia.

IV. List changes that require professional assistance in management—active bleeding from any site.

V. Identify community resources available for management of emergency situations.

Stomatitis, Esophagitis, or Mucositis

THEORY

I. Definition.
   A. *Mucositis*—generalized inflammation of mucous membranes.
   B. *Esophagitis*—inflammation of mucous membranes of the esophagus.
   C. *Stomatitis*—inflammation of the mucous membranes of the oral cavity.

II. Risk factors.
   A. Disease related—infiltration of mucous membranes of the gastrointestinal tract by primary or metastatic tumor.
   B. Treatment related:
      1. Local reactions of mucous membranes to surgical manipulation.
      2. Administration of cancer chemotherapeutic agents that destroy the normal rapidly dividing cells of the mucous membranes—antimetabolites, antibiotics, steroids.
      3. Radiation therapy that includes the head and neck, chest, or abdomen in treatment fields.
      4. Graft-versus-host disease.
      5. Immunosuppression.
   C. Life-style related:
      1. Inadequate oral hygiene practices.
      2. Dehydration.
      3. Exposure to chemical irritants—mouthwashes, tobacco, alcohol.
      4. Exposure to physical irritants—extreme temperatures of foods, high fiber foods, poor-fitting dentures.

III. Standard medical therapy.
   A. Prophylactic antibacterial, antifungal, and antiviral agents.
   B. Systemic and/or topical analgesics—viscous lidocaine (Xylocaine), diphenhydramine (Benadryl).
   C. Tucks compresses, sitz baths.
   D. Topical protective agents.
   E. Dietary and vitamin supplements.
   F. Systemic and/or local antiinflammatory agents—oral steroids or steroid enemas.
   G. Antidiarrheal medications.

IV. Potential sequelae of prolonged stomatitis, esophagitis, or mucositis.
   A. Impaired integrity of the mucous membranes.
   B. Infection.
   C. Difficulty swallowing.

    D. Difficulty speaking.

    E. Inadequate nutritional intake or absorption.

    F. Diarrhea.

    G. Pain.

    H. Bleeding.

DATA COLLECTION

  I. History.

    A. Review of previous therapy for cancer.

    B. Review of medications.

    C. Review of exposure to chemical or physical irritants.

    D. Review of oral hygiene practices.

    E. Pattern of mucositis—incidence; frquency; precipitating, alleviating, and aggravating factors.

    F. Impact of stomatitis, esophagitis, or mucositis on life-style, comfort, nutrition, and activities of daily living.

  II. Physical examination (see Figure 7-3).

    A. Redness, swelling, tenderness of mucous membranes.

    B. Diminished taste sensations.

    C. Burning sensation.

    D. Pain.

    E. Changes in the character of the stool.

    F. Changes in the character of saliva.

    G. Presence of white patches on mucous membranes.

ASSOCIATED NURSING DIAGNOSES

  I. Alteration in comfort: pain.

  II. Alteration in nutrition: less than body requirements.

  III. Impaired communication.

  IV. Impaired skin integrity.

  V. Body image disturbance.

NURSING PLANNING AND IMPLEMENTATION

  I. Interventions to minimize the risk of occurrence and severity of mucositis.

    A. Measures to decrease inflammation of mucous membranes:

      1. Encourage oral and perineal hygiene measures.

      2. Encourage fluid intake of greater than 3000 ml/day.

      3. Avoid exposure to chemical and/or physical irritants.

    B. Measures to increase comfort:

      1. Topical protective agents—antacids, kaolin-containing substances, oral paste (Orabase).

      2. Sitz baths.

      3. Increased frequency of oral hygiene, using soft toothbrush or sponge swab.

      4. Systemic or topical analgesics.

    C. Measures to decrease risk of complications of mucositis:

      1. Modify dietary intake to bland, soft, liquid, high-caloric, high-protein foods.

      2. Encourage oral and perineal hygiene measures.

      3. Provide privacy for perineal hygiene measures.

    4. Develop alternate means of communicating—magic slate, cards, using direct and short answers.

II. Interventions to monitor for complications related to mucositis.
    A. Conduct oral and perineal assessment daily or with change in symptomatology.
    B. Assess for signs and symptoms of infection.
    C. Monitor intake and output.

III. Interventions to monitor client response to symptom management.
    A. Monitor subjective reports of the client of changes in the pattern of mucositis.
    B. Monitor changes in level of comfort.
    C. Monitor changes in integrity of the mucous membranes.
    D. Monitor compliance with measures to decrease severity of mucositis and to reduce the incidence of complications.

IV. Interventions to incorporate client and family in care.
    A. Teach oral and perineal hygiene measures.
    B. Teach measures to decrease risk of occurrence or severity of mucositis.
    C. Teach signs and symptoms of complications of mucositis to report to health care team.

V. Report critical changes in client assessment parameters to physician.
    A. Presence of signs and symptoms of infection.
    B. Presence of signs and symptoms of impaired skin integrity.

EVALUATION OF CLIENT AND FAMILY OUTCOMES

I. Describe personal risk factors for mucositis.

II. List signs, symptoms, and complications of mucositis to report to the health care team.

III. Discuss measures to minimize the risk of occurrence, severity, and complications of mucositis.

IV. List situations that require professional assistance in management.
    A. Temperature elevations greater than 101° F.
    B. Significant changes in nutritional intake.
    C. Poorly controlled symptom management—diarrhea, discomfort.

Delirium

THEORY

I. Definition: a tempory state of impaired mental functioning.

II. Risk factors—most clients with cancer have multiple interacting causes for delirium.
    A. Disease related:
        1. Primary or metastatic tumors to the central nervous system.
        2. Fluid and electrolyte disturbances such as hypercalcemia and hypoglycemia.
        3. Infection.
        4. Failure of organs such as the liver or kidneys.
        5. Cerebral hypoxia from respiratory compromise.
    B. Treatment related:
        1. Medications such as narcotics, steroids, anticholinergics, and chemotherapeutic agents that cross the blood-brain barrier.
        2. Intrathecal medications.
        3. Cranial irradiation.

    C. Life-style related:
       1. Anxiety.
       2. Fear.
       3. Environmental changes.

III. Standard medical therapy.
    A. Treatment of underlying condition.
    B. Early psychiatric consultation.
    C. Neuroepileptics.

IV. Potential sequelae of prolonged delirium.
    A. Physical or mental harm to clients, family, or staff.
    B. Sleep disturbances.
    C. Social isolation.

DATA COLLECTION

I. History.
    A. Review of risk factors.
    B. Pattern of changes in mood, behaviors, and sleep patterns.
    C. Impact of delirium on activities of daily living, interactions with family and significant others, life-style, and family, work, or community responsibilities.

II. Physical examination.
    A. Disheveled appearance.
    B. Tachycardia.
    C. Tachypnea.
    D. Asterixis.
    E. Moist, cold skin.

III. Psychosocial examination.
    A. Altered level of consciousness.
    B. Labile emotional state.
    C. Inappropriate behavioral responses.
    D. Hallucinations.
    E. Disorientation to person, time or place.

IV. Laboratory findings—consistent with underlying condition.

ASSOCIATED NURSING DIAGNOSES

I. Potential for injury.

II. Alteration in thought process.

III. Sleep pattern disturbance.

NURSING PLANNING AND IMPLEMENTATION

I. Interventions to maximize safety for the client, family, and staff.
    A. Maintain bed in lowest position with side rails up.
    B. Keep environment quiet and well lit.
    C. Encourage short, frequent contacts with familiar, nonthreatening persons.
    D. Avoid confrontation behaviors with combative client.
    E. Talk to client in calm, reassuring manner.
    F. Call for assistance in management.

II. Interventions to decrease risks of complications of delirium.
    A. Reorient client to person, place, and time as needed.

    B. Avoid sensory overload.
    C. Provide clock, calendar, and familiar objects.
III. Interventions to monitor for complications related to delirium.
    A. Evaluate sleep patterns of client.
    B. Monitor number and length of personal contacts with client.
    C. Conduct mental status assessment daily of changes in symptoms.
    D. Assess for signs and symptoms of progressive delirium—agitation, delusions,
        and hallucinations.
IV. Interventions to incorporate client and family in care.
    A. Teach family measures to decrease incidence of delirium and risks of compli-
        cations.
    B. Assist family to alter environment to promote safety.
    C. Encourage client to participate in self-care activities as condition permits.

EVALUATION OF CLIENT AND FAMILY OUTCOMES

  I. Describe personal risk factors for delirium.

 II. Report signs and symptoms of delirium to a member of the health care team.

III. Participate in measures to minimize the severity and complications of delirium for
      the client and family.

IV. List changes in the condition of the client that require professional assistance in
      management.
    A. Deteriorating mental status.
    B. Inability to provide care or safety for client within present setting.

 V. Identify community resources for support and services for client and family.

MOBILITY

Fatigue

THEORY

  I. Definition: a feeling of weariness, tiredness, or temporary loss of physical or emo-
      tional energy to respond to sensory or motor stimuli.

 II. Risk factors.
    A. Disease related:
        1. Anemia.
        2. Fever.
        3. Tumor necrosis.
        4. Metastasis.
        5. Hypokalemia.
    B. Treatment related:
        1. Anemia-related fatigue associated with cancer therapy—surgery, radiation
            therapy, chemotherapy, and biotherapy.
        2. Intake of antihypertensives, narcotics, sedatives, and hypnotics.
    C. Life-style related:
        1. Sleep disturbances.
        2. Stress.
        3. Inadequate nutritional intake for metabolic needs.

   4. Intake of alcohol, caffeine, and nicotine.
   5. Inadequate exercise.
III. Standard medical therapy.
   A. Treatment of underlying condition.
   B. Sedatives.
   C. Antidepressants.
   D. Professional counseling.
IV. Potential sequelae of prolonged fatigue.
   A. Social isolation.
   B. Immobility.
   C. Inability to engage in self-care activities independently.
   D. Depression.

DATA COLLECTION

   I. History.
   A. Presence of risk factors.
   B. Subjective complaints of fatigue or desire for rest and sleep.
   C. Review of prescription and nonprescription medications.
   D. Pattern of fatigue—incidence, severity, aggravating and alleviating factors, and course.
   E. Impact of fatigue on activities of daily living.
   F. Perceptions of the relationship of fatigue to the cancer experience.

   II. Physical findings.
   A. Rounded shoulders.
   B. Tired facial features.
   C. Yawning.

III. Psychosocial examination.
   A. Depression.
   B. Impaired concentration and problem-solving ability.
   C. Emotionally labile or irritable.
   D. Disinterest in surroundings.

IV. Laboratory data.
   A. Decreased hematocrit or hemoglobin levels.
   B. Abnormal blood glucose level.
   C. Abnormal electrolyte values or hormone levels.

ASSOCIATED NURSING DIAGNOSES

   I. Impaired physical mobility.

   II. Sleep pattern disturbance.

III. Alteration in nutrition: less than body requirements.

NURSING PLANNING AND IMPLEMENTATION

   I. Interventions to minimize energy expenditure.
   A. Prioritize activities of daily living to allow for independence in client-valued activities, pacing of activities, and rest periods.
      1. Encourage client to rest when fatigued.
      2. Pace activities in relationship to energy levels.

3. Assist client in delegating nonessential activities to others.
4. Reduce environmental stimuli.
B. Provide assistance with activities of daily living as needed—bathing, grooming, toileting, feeding, and mobility.

II. Interventions to minimize effects of associated conditions—anemia, depression, and insomnia.

III. Interventions to monitor for complications related to fatigue.
A. Evaluate mental status of client on a regular schedule.
B. Assess changes in sleep patterns.
C. Monitor physical and mental abilities to meet demands of living.

IV. Strategies to incorporate client and family in care.
A. Prepare client and family for potential fatigue expected as an effect of cancer or treatment.
B. Teach energy conservation measures.
C. Teach client and family how to use assistive devices.
D. Encourage client to document patterns of fatigue over time.
E. Teach client and family stress reduction strategies.
F. Describe signs and symptoms related to complications of fatigue to report to health care team.

V. Report critical changes in client assessment parameters to physician—unexplained or sudden increase in fatigue.

EVALUATION OF CLIENT AND FAMILY OUTCOMES

I. Describe personal risk factors for fatigue.

II. Describe expected duration of fatigue.

III. Report signs and symptoms of fatigue to health care team.

IV. Participate in measures to conserve energy, participate in valued activities, and achieve adequate rest.

V. Identify resources within the health care system and community to assist with activities of daily living.

Activity Intolerance

THEORY

I. Definition: inability, physiologically or psychologically, to endure or tolerate an increase in activity.

II. Risk factors.
A. Disease related:
1. Compromise of the cardiovascular or respiratory systems as a result of primary or metastatic cancer.
2. Concurrent cardiovascular, respiratory, musculoskeletal, neurological, hepatic, or renal disease.
B. Treatment related:
1. Surgical treatment resulting in short-term or long-term cardiovascular or respiratory compromise.
2. Acute and long-term consequences of radiation therapy—anemia, fatigue, or pulmonary fibrosis.

3. Acute and long-term consequences of chemotherapy—anemia, fatigue, cardiotoxicity, pulmonary fibrosis, or neurological toxicities.
4. Acute consequences of biotherapy—fatigue, malaise, and fever.

C. Situational:
1. Depression.
2. Lack of motivation.
3. Sedentary life-style.
4. Hospitalization.
5. Multiple stressors.

D. Medications—narcotics and sedatives.

III. Standard medical therapy.
A. Treatment of underlying cause and contributing factors.
B. Physical therapy for increased strength and endurance exercises.

IV. Potential sequelae of prolonged activity intolerance.
A. Inability to perform activities of daily living.
B. Changes in role responsibilities.
C. Tachycardia.
D. Dyspnea.

DATA COLLECTION

I. History.
A. Patterns of activity.
B. Changes in ability to perform activities over time.
C. Resources used in past to accommodate decrease in activity tolerance and perceived effectiveness.

II. Physical examination after activity.
A. Changes in strength and rate of pulse that fails to return to pre-activity parameters 3 minutes after resting.
B. Failure to increase or actual decrease in blood pressure with activity.
C. Excessive increase or decrease in respiratory rate with activity.
D. Pallor or cyanosis.
E. Dizziness.
F. Changes in mental status—confusion.

III. Psychosocial examination.
A. Depression.
B. Fear.
C. Social isolation.
D. Lack of motivation.

IV. Laboratory data.
A. Decreased hemoglobin or hematocrit levels.
B. Decreased pulmonary function study results.
C. Electrolyte abnormalities.
D. Abnormalities in cardiac function.
E. Increased BUN or creatinine levels.

ASSOCIATED NURSING DIAGNOSES

I. Activity intolerance.

II. Diversional activity deficit.

III. Impaired home maintenance management.

IV. Self-care deficit.

V. Self-esteem disturbance.

NURSING PLANNING AND IMPLEMENTATION

I. Interventions to maximize safety for client.
  A. Place needed materials within reach of client.
  B. Encourage use of assistive devices for ambulation or activities of daily living.

II. Interventions to minimize risks, severity, or consequences of activity intolerance.
  A. Assess factors that contribute to activity intolerance.
  B. Institute measures to modify factors that contribute to activity intolerance:
    1. Provide adequate rest periods during day and uninterrupted rest at night.
    2. Implement strategies to control associated symptoms—pain, nausea, vomiting, diarrhea, or depression.
    3. Instruct client in isometric exercises.
  C. Use personal incentives to encourage activity:
    1. Discuss potential incentives with client and family.
    2. Elicit participation from client in negotiating realistic activity goals over time.
    3. Plan a purpose for each activity goal.
    4. Provide positive feedback for accomplishment of goals.

III. Interventions to monitor client response to increased activity.
  A. Physiological parameters (Table 7-3).
  B. Subjective responses to activity.

Table 7-3
PHYSIOLOGICAL RESPONSES TO ACTIVITY: EXPECTED AND ABNORMAL

	Pulse	Blood Pressure	Respirations
Resting			
Normal	60-90	<140/90	<20
Abnormal	>100	>140/90	>20
Immediately after Activity			
Normal	↑ Rate ↑ Strength	↑ Systolic	↑ Rate ↑ Depth
Abnormal	↓ Rate ↓ Strength Irregular rhythm	Decrease or no change in systolic	Excessive ↑ ↓ Rate
3 Min after			
Normal	Within six beats of resting pulse		
Abnormal	More than seven beats of resting pulse or complaints of confusion, incoordination, dyspnea, pallor		

From Carpenito, L.J. (1983). *Nursing Diagnosis: Application to Clinical Practice*. Philadelphia: J.B. Lippincott Co.

IV. Report critical changes in client assessment parameters to physician.
   A. Persistent tachycardia after significant rest period.
   B. Persistent dyspnea unresolved with rest.
   C. Chest pain with activity.
   D. Syncopal episodes with activity.

EVALUATION OF CLIENT AND FAMILY OUTCOMES

   I. Describe personal risk factors for activity intolerance.

   II. Participate in measures to achieve a balance between energy expenditure and restoration.

   III. List signs and symptoms of activity intolerance that require professional assistance for management—marked decrease in ability to tolerate activity.

   IV. Identify community resources available to assist with activities of daily living and home maintenance.

ELIMINATION

Constipation

THEORY

   I. Definition: the infrequent passage of hard stool, often associated with abdominal and rectal pain.

   II. Risk factors.
   A. Disease related:
      1. Obstruction of bowel by tumor.
      2. Fluid and electrolyte imbalances—dehydration, hypercalcemia, and hypokalemia.
      3. Immobility.
   B. Treatment related:
      1. Manipulation of intestines during surgery.
      2. Surgical trauma to neurogenic pathways to intestines and/or rectum.
      3. Neurotoxic effects of cancer chemotherapeutic agents such as vincristine and vinblastine (Velban).
      4. Nutritional deficiencies such as decreased fiber, roughage, and fluid intake.
      5. Side effects of pharmacological agents such as narcotics, analgesics, anticholinergics, and antacids.
   C. Situational:
      1. Lack of privacy.
      2. Interference with usual bowel program.
      3. Failure to respond to defecation reflex because of pain, fatigue, or social activities.
   D. Developmental—aging.

   III. Standard medical therapy.
   A. Surgical correction of obstructive disease.
   B. Correction of fluid and electrolyte imbalances.
   C. Enemas or irrigations.
   D. Medications such as laxatives, stool softeners, and suppositories.
   E. Increased fiber in diet.

IV. Potential sequelae of constipation.
  A. Fecal impaction.
  B. Paralytic ileus.
  C. Intestinal obstruction.
  D. Laxative dependence.

DATA COLLECTION

  I. History.
  A. Presence of risk factors.
  B. History of defining characteristics of constipation:
    1. Change in usual patterns of bowel elimination such as decreased frequency, hard stool, abdominal cramping, and increased use of laxatives.
    2. Change in factors contributing to bowel elimination such as activity level, fluid intake, and intake of dietary roughage and fiber.
    3. History of constipation and/or laxative use.
    4. Anxiety regarding bowel patterns.
  C. Gastrointestinal symptoms—nausea, vomiting, and anorexia.
  D. Pattern of occurrence of constipation—onset, frequency, severity, associated symptoms, precipitating, aggravating, and alleviating factors.
  E. Perceived effectiveness of self-care measures to relieve constipation.
  F. Perceived impact of constipation on comfort, activities of daily living, and mood.

 II. Physical findings.
  A. Decreased or absent bowel sounds.
  B. Flatulence.
  C. Abdominal distention.
  D. Fecal impaction.

ASSOCIATED NURSING DIAGNOSES

  I. Alteration in comfort.

 II. Anxiety.

III. Ineffective individual coping.

NURSING PLANNING AND IMPLEMENTATION

  I. Interventions to minimize risk and severity of constipation.
  A. Institute measures to maintain bowel elimination patterns:
    1. Encourage at least 3000 ml of fluid intake each day.
    2. Modify diet as tolerated to include high fiber and roughage, with fresh fruits, vegetables, whole grains, and dried beans.
    3. Maintain or increase physical activity level.
    4. Establish a daily bowel program.
  B. Implement effective interventions usually used by client to alleviate constipation and not contraindicated by health status.
  C. Initiate prophylactic bowel regimen with narcotic therapy.

 II. Interventions to maximize client safety.
  A. Check for impaction if symptoms warrant.
  B. Avoid digital rectal examinations if client is neutropenic and/or thrombocytopenic.

III. Interventions to monitor for complications related to constipation.
  A. Assess for interference with deep breathing related to abdominal distention.

    B. Monitor indicators of social withdrawal related to flatulence.

    C. Monitor untoward responses to symptom management:
       1. Abdominal cramping or diarrhea with laxatives.
       2. Rectal emptying and aggravation of constipation with enemas.
       3. Inadequate fluid intake for effectiveness of stool softeners.

    D. Report critical changes to physician:
       1. Abdominal distention.
       2. Fecal impaction.
       3. Bleeding.
       4. Absence of bowel sounds.

IV. Implement strategies to enhance adaptation and rehabilitation.

    A. Encourage avoidance of laxative abuse with combination of laxatives and stool softeners.

    B. Emphasize dietary control of constipation with foods high in fiber such as celery, bran, and whole wheat breads.

    C. Advise adoption of a daily fluid intake of 3000 ml.

    D. Advise adoption of a daily bowel program:
       1. Daily schedule for evacuation such as after meals when gastrocolic reflexes are active.
       2. Privacy.
       3. Medications such as stool softeners or expanders; avoidance of laxatives if possible.
       4. Enemas or irrigation procedures if necessary.

V. Interventions to incorporate client and family in care.

    A. Teach to control constipation through fluid intake, dietary control, and activity level.

    B. Inform of hazards of laxative dependence.

    C. Instruct to limit use of gas-producing foods such as cabbage, beans, green peppers, and onions in meal planning.

EVALUATION OF CLIENT AND FAMILY OUTCOMES

I. Identify personal risk factors for constipation.

II. Identify usual bowel pattern and practices.

III. Participate in strategies to decrease risk of constipation.

IV. Discuss signs and symptoms of constipation to report to health care team.

V. List situations related to constipation that require professional intervention.

    A. Constipation unrelieved by usual methods.

    B. Severe pain or bleeding with bowel movement.

    C. Adverse reactions to medications or measures used to treat constipation.

Diarrhea

THEORY

I. Definition: an increase in the quantity, frequency, or fluid content of stool that is different from the usual pattern of bowel elimination.

II. Risk factors.

    A. Disease related:
       1. Obstruction of bowel from intrinsic or extrinsic tumor.

   2. Intestinal bacteria or viruses.
   3. Graft-versus-host disease in which immunocompetent cells of the allogeneic donor marrow recognize normal gastrointestinal cells as "foreign" and initiate an immune reaction that leads to cell destruction of target tissues in gut.
   4. Food intolerance.
  B. Treatment related:
   1. Fluid malabsorption syndrome associated with resection of significant portions of bowel.
   2. Increased cellular destruction in bowel lumen from effects of radiation therapy on normal cells in treatment fields that include the gastrointestinal tract.
   3. Increased cellular destruction in bowel lumen from effects of chemotherapy such as 5-FU on normal cells.
   4. Medications such as antibiotics, antacids, or laxatives.
   5. Nutritional therapies such as tube feedings and dietary supplements.
   6. Fecal impaction.
  C. Life-style related:
   1. Increased stress and anxiety in presence of inadequate coping strategies.
   2. Changes in usual dietary habits such as increases in dietary fiber.

III. Standard medical therapy.
  A. Antidiarrheal or antispasmodic medications such as bismuth subsalicylate (Pepto-Bismol), loperamide (Immodium), or activated attapulgite (Kaopectate).
  B. Modification of associated therapy such as radiation, chemotherapy, nutritional supplements, or antibiotics.
  C. Treatment of associated conditions such as *Clostridium difficile* or graft-versus-host disease.
  D. Decompression or surgery for bowel obstruction.
  E. Manual disimpaction if WBC and platelet count permit.

IV. Potential sequelae of prolonged diarrhea.
  A. Dehydration.
  B. Electrolyte imbalances such as hypokalemia or hyponatremia.
  C. Weakness and fatigue.
  D. Impaired skin integrity of perineal area.
  E. Decreased social interaction.

DATA COLLECTION

 I. History.
  A. Review of previous therapy for cancer.
  B. Review of prescription and nonprescription medications.
  C. Usual bowel pattern—frequency, color, amount, odor, and consistency of stool.
  D. Recent changes in factors contributing to usual bowel elimination patterns:
   1. Increased levels of stress.
   2. Dietary changes that increase bowel motility such as fiber and roughage, fruit juices, coffee, alcohol, fried foods, or fatty foods.
  E. Known food or medication intolerance.
  F. Presence of flatus, cramping, abdominal pain, urgency to defecate, recent weight loss, decreased urinary output of 500 ml less than intake.

 II. Physical examination.
  A. Hyperactive bowel sounds.
  B. Hard stool in rectum.
  C. Perineal irritation.

III. Psychosocial examination.
   A. Presence of fear.
   B. Presence of anxiety.
   C. Complaints of isolation.

ASSOCIATED NURSING DIAGNOSES

I. Alteration in fluid and electrolyte balance.

II. Impaired skin integrity.

III. Alteration in nutrition: less than body requirements.

NURSING PLANNING AND IMPLEMENTATION

I. Interventions to minimize the risk of occurrence and severity of diarrhea.
   A. Modify dietary intake to avoid foods client can not tolerate.
   B. Decrease fiber and roughage.
   C. Encourage smaller meals eaten more frequently.

II. Implement strategies to decrease bowel motility.
   A. Serve foods and liquids at room temperature.
   B. Avoid coffee and alcohol.
   C. Avoid spicy, fried, or fatty foods and food additives.
   D. Teach strategies to modify stress response such as relaxation, distraction, or imagery.

III. Interventions to maximize client safety.
   A. Monitor level of weakness and fatigue.
   B. Provide assistance with ambulation and activities of daily living as indicated.

IV. Interventions to monitor for complications related to diarrhea.
   A. Assess the character of bowel movement each day or with a change in symptoms.
   B. Assess perineal area each day or with a change in symptoms.
   C. Monitor intake and output ratio.
   D. Monitor for subtle changes in client affect, neuromuscular responses, activity level, and cognitive status as cues for potential electrolyte imbalances.
   E. Monitor for changes in skin turgor.
   F. Report significant changes in condition or symptomatology to physician.

V. Interventions to incorporate client and family in care.
   A. Teach perineal hygiene program, including cleansing perineal area with mild soap, rinsing thoroughly, patting area dry, and applying a skin barrier after each bowel movement.
   B. Teach dietary modifications to minimize diarrhea.
   C. Teach signs and symptoms related to complications of diarrhea to report to a member of the health care team.

EVALUATION OF CLIENT AND FAMILY OUTCOMES

I. Describe personal risk factors for diarrhea.

II. Participate in measures to decrease the risk or occurrence, severity, and complications of diarrhea.

III. List situations that require professional assistance in management:
   A. Changes in usual bowel pattern that persist for more than 72 hours and are unrelieved with usual interventions.
   B. Presence of signs and symptoms of complications of diarrhea.

Incontinence

THEORY

I. Definition: involuntary escape of urine from the lower urinary tract or stool from the lower gastrointestinal tract to a degree that is socially or hygienically unacceptable to the client.

II. Risk factors.
   A. Disease related:
      1. Lack of a conscious sensation to evacuate the bladder or bowel such as in clients with congenital abnormalities or spinal cord severance at the level of bladder or bowel control.
      2. Loss of sensation of bladder or bowel distention such as in clients with diabetic neuropathy.
      3. Loss of the ability to inhibit bladder or bowel evacuation such as in clients with primary or metastatic tumors in the cerebral cortex, stroke, or Parkinson's disease.
      4. Loss of reflex contractions of the bladder or bowel such as in clients with paraplegia.
      5. Obstruction of the bladder or bowel by an intrinsic or extrinsic tumor, enlarged prostate, or fecal impaction.
      6. Metabolic abnormalities such as hyperglycemia, hypokalemia, or hypercalcemia.
      7. Infection of bladder or bowel.
      8. Dementia.
   B. Treatment related:
      1. Surgical interruption of neural pathways that control bladder and bowel function such as in an anterior-posterior resection or prostatectomy.
      2. Immediate (inflammation) and long-term (fibrosis) effects of radiation therapy to fields that include the bladder and bowel.
      3. Fistula formation as a complication of surgery or radiation therapy.
      4. Antineoplastic agents with known neurological complications such as vincristine and vinblastine.
      5. Improper placement of urinary catheter.
      6. Side effect of medications such as tranquilizers, sedatives, diuretics, or laxatives.
   C. Life-style related—denial of urge or delay in evacuation of bladder or bowel.

III. Standard medical therapy.
   A. Treatment of underlying disease.
   B. Surgical correction such as urethral suspension or lengthening, or implantable incontinence devices.
   C. Medications such as propantheline bromide (Pro-Banthine), oxybutynin (Ditropan), and bethanechol (Urecholine).
   D. Bladder and/or bowel training program.

IV. Potential sequelae of prolonged incontinence.
   A. Perineal irritation or excoriation.
   B. Embarrassment.
   C. Changes in role responsibilities and life-style.

DATA COLLECTION

I. History.
   A. Presence of risk factors for incontinence.

    B. Presence of defining characteristics of incontinence—complaint of hygienically or socially unacceptable loss of urine or stool.

    C. Type of incontinence—bladder or bowel.

    D. Patterns of incontinence—onset, frequency, severity, associated symptoms, precipitating factors, aggravating factors, and alleviating factors.

    E. Effectiveness of previous self-care strategies in relieving incontinence.

    F. Perceived meaning of incontinence to client and family.

    G. Impact of incontinence on activities of daily living, life-style, comfort, relationships, work, school, and role responsibilities, and mood.

II. Physical examination.

    A. Involuntary escape of urine or stool.

    B. Protrusion of bladder or bowel into vagina (females).

    C. Presence of impaction.

    D. Presence of enlarged prostate (males).

    E. Presence of irritation or excoriation of perineal area.

    F. Presence of foul odor.

III. Diagnostic tests.

    A. Urinalysis, culture and sensitivity to rule out infection.

    B. Stool culture and sensitivity to rule out infection.

    C. Urometrics to evaluate neuromuscular factors.

    D. Cystoscopy or colonoscopy.

ASSOCIATED NURSING DIAGNOSES

I. Impaired skin integrity.

II. Alteration in self-concept.

III. Sleep pattern disturbance.

IV. Altered role performance.

V. Social isolation.

NURSING PLANNING AND IMPLEMENTATION

I. Interventions to minimize the risk of occurrence, severity, or complications of incontinence.

    A. Rearrange environment to limit barriers to toilet, such as reduce distance with use of bedside commode or clear a pathway to toilet.

    B. Have client wear clothing that may be removed quickly.

    C. Clean perineum after each voiding or bowel movement with a mild soap, rinse thoroughly, and pat dry.

    D. Use a skin barrier or protectant as needed.

    E. Encourage open discussion of the impact of incontinence on client and family.

       1. Bladder incontinence:

          a. Establish schedule for voiding such as every 2 hours.

          b. Assume normal position for voiding if possible, such as sitting for females and standing for males.

          c. Use techniques to stimulate voiding as needed such as icing and brushing the perineal area and groin or using running water.

          d. Void as soon as urge is felt.

          e. As stream of urine starts, shut off stream by contracting perineal muscles for 5 seconds, then relax muscles, and continue voiding.

          f. Limit fluid intake after 6:00 PM.

  2. Bowel incontinence:
   a. Establish schedule for bowel evacuation such as each morning after break-fast.
   b. Use techniques to stimulate bowel evacuation such as digital stimulation, glycerin suppository, or drinking coffee.
   c. Evacuate bowel as soon as urge is felt.
 F. Use internal or external incontinence devices such as catheters as a last resort to manage incontinence.

II. Interventions to maximize safety.
 A. Encourage use of assistive devices as needed to maintain normal position when voiding.
 B. Rearrange environment to decrease barriers to toilet facilities.
 C. Clean accidental loss of urine and stool from environment immediately.

III. Interventions to monitor for complications related to incontinence.
 A. Assess perineal skin integrity each day.
 B. Monitor intake, urinary output (including volume and color), and intake/output ratio each day.
 C. Assess psychological responses of client and family to incontinence.

IV. Interventions to monitor response of client to symptom management.
 A. Monitor subjective reports of the client and family of changes in the pattern of incontinence.
 B. Monitor compliance with measures to decrease incidence and severity of incontinence.

V. Interventions to incorporate client and family in care.
 A. Teach pelvic muscle strengthening exercises.
 B. Teach proper use of materials and devices to control incontinence.
 C. Teach signs and symptoms related to complications of incontinence to report to member of the health care team.

VI. Report critical changes in client assessment parameters to physician.
 A. Presence of adverse changes in pattern of incontinence.
 B. Presence of signs and symptoms of infection or impaction.

EVALUATION OF CLIENT AND FAMILY OUTCOMES

 I. Describe personal risk factors for incontinence.

 II. Report signs, symptoms, and complications of incontinence to a member of the health care team.

 III. Participate in measures to minimize the risk of occurrence, severity, and complications of incontinence.

 IV. Demonstrate competence in self-care techniques for management of incontinence.

 V. List changes in the condition of the client that require professional assistance in management.
 A. Presence of adverse changes in pattern of incontinence.
 B. Presence of signs and symptoms of infection or impaction.

SEXUALITY

Self-Esteem Disturbances

THEORY

I. Definition: a subjective assessment of low personal worth or ability to accomplish goals.

II. Risk factors.
   A. Treatment related:
      1. Diagnosis with a poor prognosis, uncertain outcome, or likelihood of recurrence.
      2. Perceived or actual changes in body structure and/or function such as cachexia, amputation, alopecia, or cognitive dysfunction.
   B. Disease related:
      1. Psychiatric disorders.
      2. Ineffective individual coping.
   C. Developmental:
      1. Deprivation related to achievement of developmental tasks.
      2. Blocking of developmental task achievement.
   D. Situational:
      1. Status losses such as job, economic, or role changes.
      2. Perceived or actual loss of social support.
      3. Inability to set or achieve goals.

III. Standard medical therapy.
   A. Preventive and reconstructive procedures to minimize disease and treatment effects.
   B. Prosthetic devices.
   C. Antianxiety and antidepressant medications.
   D. Behavioral interventions such as self-help groups or relaxation techniques.
   E. Individual or group psychotherapy.

IV. Potential sequelae of self-esteem disturbances.
   A. Depression.
   B. Suicide.
   C. Role abandonment or ineffectiveness.
   D. Social isolation or withdrawal.

DATA COLLECTION

I. History
   A. Presence of risk factors.
   B. Presence of defining characteristics of low self-esteem.
   C. Pattern of self-esteem disturbances—onset, frequency, severity, associated symptoms, and precipitating, aggravating, and alleviating factors.
   D. Significance of changes in self-esteem to client and significant others.
   E. Effectiveness of self-care strategies to adapt to or modify changes in self-esteem.
   F. Impact of changes in self-esteem on mood, relationships, activities of daily living, and roles and responsibilities within the family, community, work, or school.

II. Physical findings.
   A. Neglect of self-care, grooming.
   B. Weight gain or loss.

    C. Cognitive dysfunction such as decreased attention span and difficulty with problem solving, concentration, and/or decision making.

    D. Minimal eye contact.

III. Psychosocial findings.

    A. Evaluates self as unable to deal with events.

    B. Expressions of self-doubt, self-negation, or fears of rejection.

    C. Hesitancy or discomfort in social interactions or new situations.

    D. Rejection of positive feedback and exaggeration of negative feedback about self.

    E. Rationalization of personal failures.

    F. Hypersensitivity to criticism.

ASSOCIATED NURSING DIAGNOSES

  I. Ineffective individual coping.

 II. Ineffective family coping.

III. Family: potential for growth.

IV. Role performance disturbance.

NURSING PLANNING AND IMPLEMENTATION

   I. Interventions to maximize client safety.

    A. Report covert evidence of suicidal intentions to physician.

    B. Teach family members critical signs and symptoms to report to physician.

  II. Interventions to minimize risk of occurrence and severity of disturbances in self-esteem.

    A. Provide opportunity for client to discuss perceived threats to self-esteem.

    B. Allow client to describe changes in behavior and perceptions as a result of cancer and treatment.

    C. Give permission to grieve and to resolve perceived losses.

    D. Assist client to establish realistic goals for self-care, return to roles and responsibilities, expected course of disease, and treatment plan.

    E. Provide positive reinforcement for participation in self-care, decision making, and progress toward goal achievement.

III. Interventions to enhance adaptation and rehabilitation.

    A. Provide literature and resource referrals to community services such as I Can Cope, Reach to Recovery, National Cancer Institute Information Service, and American Cancer Society Resource, Information, and Guidance Program.

    B. Initiate discharge planning that facilitates reintegration into home, community, work, and/or school settings.

IV. Interventions to incorporate client and family in care.

    A. Teach use of restorative devices and rehabilitative services.

    B. Seek client and family input about home care referrals as needed for continued follow-up and care.

    C. Teach client and family strategies to detect and manage self-destructive behaviors.

  V. Report critical changes in client self-esteem or sequelae to physician.

    A. Covert or overt evidence of suicidal ideations.

    B. Self-destructive behaviors.

    C. Self-neglect that hinders adaptation or rehabilitation.

EVALUATION OF CLIENT AND FAMILY OUTCOMES

I. Describe personal risk factors for disturbances in self-esteem.

II. Participate in strategies to minimize the risk of disturbances in self-esteem.

III. Identify community resources to address threats to self-esteem.

IV. List community emergency resources for critical changes in perceived self-esteem.

Body Image

THEORY

I. Definition: self-perception of one's body structure and function as dynamic and different from all others (one component of self-concept).

II. Risk factors.
   A. Actual or perceived changes in body structure or function related to:
      1. Disease such as cachexia or cognitive dysfunction.
      2. Treatment such as alopecia or amputation.
      3. Development or maturation such as dependency or aging.
   B. Perceived rejection or negative responses to one's body or functioning by significant others and/or professionals.

III. Standard medical therapy.
   A. Preventive and reconstructive procedures to minimize disease or treatment effects.
   B. Prosthetic devices.
   C. Medications such as antianxiety drugs or antidepressants.
   D. Behavioral interventions such as self-help groups or relaxation therapy.
   E. Psychotherapy either as an individual or as part of a group.

IV. Potential sequelae of disturbed body image.
   A. Depression.
   B. Suicide.
   C. Role abandonment or ineffectiveness.
   D. Social isolation or withdrawal.

DATA COLLECTION

I. Presence of risk factors.

II. Physical, cognitive, and psychosocial assessment of defining characteristics of body-image changes.
   A. Physical changes:
      1. Neglect or compulsive attention to self-care or grooming.
      2. Weight gain or loss.
      3. Insomnia or hypersomnia.
   B. Cognitive changes:
      1. Decreased attention span.
      2. Problems with concentration.
      3. Difficulty with problem solving and decision making.
   C. Psychosocial changes:
      1. Anorexia or increased appetite.
      2. Dysfunctional grieving (see "Grief").
      3. Expressions of self-doubt, self-negation, or fear of rejection.
      4. Hesitancy or discomfort in social interactions—avoidance of intimacy or social contact.

5. Self-destructive behaviors such as self-neglect or alcoholism.
6. Sexual dysfunction such as impotence or frigidity.
7. Refusal to look at or to assume responsibility for changed body part or function (to view mastectomy incision, care for stoma, or wear prosthesis).

ASSOCIATED NURSING DIAGNOSES

I. Ineffective family or individual coping.

II. Potential for injury.

III. Sleep pattern disturbances.

IV. Family coping: potential for growth.

NURSING PLANNING AND IMPLEMENTATION

I. Interventions to minimize risk of occurrence or severity of body-image disturbance.
   A. Provide opportunity to discuss perceived losses and meaning to self and significant others.
   B. Give permission to grieve and to resolve losses.
   C. Allow to ventilate negative emotions such as anger and guilt.
   D. Monitor professional/significant other responses that imply rejection of the client or negative reactions to body changes.

II. Interventions to maximize client safety.
   A. Monitor and report reactions to drug therapy, such as with a central nervous system depressant that may enhance suicidal potential.
   B. Monitor covert evidence of suicidal intentions such as preoccupation with will or funeral arrangements or sequestration of drugs.
   C. Discuss adverse effects of self-destructive behaviors with client and/or health care team.
   D. Report critical changes to physician:
      1. Overt or covert evidence of suicidal ideations.
      2. Self-destructive behaviors.
      3. Self-neglect that hinders adaptation or rehabilitation.

III. Interventions to enhance adaptation/rehabilitation—prepare client and family for changes in structure or function.
   A. Assure participation in informed consent procedures.
   B. Initiate referral to client services such as United Ostomy Association, Reach to Recovery, or International Association of Laryngectomees.
   C. Assess readiness to view changes and/or to assume responsibility for self-care.
   D. Adapt teaching to client readiness.
   E. Support client and family during initial viewing of changes:
      1. Provide literature and resource referrals such as I Can Cope, Reach to Recovery, National Cancer Institute Information Line, or American Cancer Society Information Services.
      2. Initiate discharge planning that facilitates reintegration into work or school system.

IV. Interventions to incorporate client and family in care.
   A. Teach use of restorative devices and rehabilitative procedures.
   B. Observe client and family return demonstrations of self-care.
   C. Initiate home care referrals as needed for follow-up and rehabilitative care.
   D. Teach client and family strategies to detect and manage self-destructive behaviors.
   E. Use active listening and nonjudgmental acceptance to facilitate discussion of

concerns such as intimacy, resumption of sexual activity, and explanations to significant others.

EVALUATION OF CLIENT AND FAMILY OUTCOMES

  I. Identify perceived losses, significance, and adaptive coping strategies.

  II. Discuss plans for social reintegration and role performance.

  III. Identify community resources to deal with changes, institute restorative measures, and achieve maximal functioning.

  IV. List emergency resources to deal with self-destructive behaviors.

  V. Identify opportunities for personal growth such as volunteering to participate in self-help or support groups or patient-to-patient visitation programs.

Alopecia

THEORY

  I. Definition: the loss of hair (scalp, facial, axillary, pubic, and body).

  II. Risk factors.
    A. Treatment that has an affinity for rapidly dividing cells will damage hair follicles, causing temporary or permanent hair loss.
    B. Radiation therapy greater than 4500 rads may cause permanent hair loss in the area being treated.
    C. Hair loss associated with chemotherapy generally is temporary.
    D. Chemotherapeutic agents vary in the potential to cause alopecia; doxorubicin (Adriamycin), methotrexate, and cyclophosphamide (Cytoxan) have high potential.
    E. The severity of hair loss increases with high doses of chemotherapeutic agents and increased doses of radiation therapy over a decreased number of treatments.
    F. Chemotherapy and radiation therapy given simultaneously have an additive effect.

  III. Standard medical therapy.
    A. Scalp hypothermia.
    B. Scalp tourniquets.

  IV. Potential sequelae of alopecia.
    A. Increased heat loss through scalp.
    B. Impaired self-concept.
    C. Decreased sexual and social interaction.

DATA COLLECTION

  I. Pertinent personal history.
    A. Patterns of hair growth.
    B. Usual hair care practices that may damage hair and facilitate loss—frequent shampooing, use of permanents, color, rinses, blow dryers, heated rollers, and curling irons.
    C. Perceptions of client before and after hair loss about self-concept, body image, perceived sexuality, and responses of significant others, social, and work acquaintances to hair loss.

II. Physical examination.
   A. Decreased thickness of hair.
   B. Changes in texture of hair.
   C. Complete hair loss.

III. Psychosocial examination.
   A. Anger.
   B. Anxiety.
   C. Decreased social interaction.

ASSOCIATED NURSING DIAGNOSES

I. Altered sexuality patterns.

II. Impaired social interactions.

III. Social isolation.

IV. Ineffective individual coping.

V. Body image disturbance.

VI. Situational low self-esteem.

NURSING PLANNING AND IMPLEMENTATION

I. Interventions to minimize the risk of symptom occurrence and severity of alopecia.
   A. Provide anticipatory guidance related to hair loss:
      1. Provide information related to hair loss and regrowth:
         a. Loss occurs over a period of days to weeks.
         b. Regrowth usually occurs 6 to 8 weeks after completion of therapy.
         c. Color and texture of regrown hair may be different from hair growth before loss.
      2. Encourage client to obtain scarves, turbans, caps, and/or wigs before hair loss.
   B. Initiate measures to decrease hair loss:
      1. Wash hair less frequently with a mild or dry shampoo.
      2. Avoid the use of permanents, hair coloring, excessive use of blow dryers, curling irons, heated rollers, and brushes.

II. Implement strategies to enhance adaptation and rehabilitation.
   A. Identify community and personal resources such as insurance companies and the American Cancer Society for financial assistance with head coverings.
   B. Refer to Look Good, Feel Better program of the American Cancer Society.
   C. Encourage discussion of responses to alopecia among client, significant others, and members of the health care team.

EVALUATION OF CLIENT AND FAMILY OUTCOMES

I. Identify personal risk factors for alopecia.

II. Describe patterns of hair loss and potential for hair regrowth.

III. Discuss potential effects of alopecia on self-concept, body image, sexuality, and social interaction.

IV. Discuss measures to prevent, minimize, and/or adapt to alopecia.

V. Identify community resources and insurance benefits available.

Sexual Dysfunction

THEORY

 I. Definition: the state in which an individual experiences a change in sexual function that is viewed as unsatisfying, unrewarding, or inadequate.

 II. Risk factors.
    A. Disease related:
       1. Primary or metastatic tumor of the genitourinary system—cancers of the endometrium, cervix, vagina, vulva, testicle, or penis.
       2. Concurrent disease—venereal disease, chronic renal failure, diabetes mellitus, hyperthyroidism, arthritis, and peripheral vascular disease.
       3. Hormone deficiencies.
       4. Inadequate control of associated symptoms of disease and treatment—pain, nausea, vomiting, anxiety, depression, fear, fatigue, or numbness.

Table 7-4
FEMALE SEXUAL PROBLEMS CAUSED BY CANCER TREATMENT

Treatment	Low Sexual Desire	Less Vaginal Moisture	Reduced Vaginal Size	Painful Intercourse	Trouble Reaching Orgasm	Infertility
Chemotherapy	Sometimes	Often	Sometimes	Often	Rarely	Often
Pelvic radiation therapy	Rarely	Often	Often	Often	Rarely	Often
Radical hysterectomy	Rarely	Often*	Often	Rarely	Rarely	Always
Radical cystectomy	Rarely	Often*	Always	Sometimes	Rarely	Always
Abdominoperineal (A-P) resection	Rarely	Often*	Sometimes	Sometimes	Rarely	Sometimes
Total pelvic exenteration with vaginal reconstruction	Sometimes	Always	Sometimes	Sometimes	Sometimes	Always
Radical vulvectomy	Rarely	Never	Sometimes	Often	Sometimes	Never
Conization of the cervix	Never	Never	Never	Rarely	Never	Rarely
Oophorectomy (removal of one tube and ovary)	Rarely	Never*	Never*	Rarely	Never	Rarely
Oophorectomy (removal of both tubes and ovaries)	Rarely	Often*	Sometimes*	Sometimes*	Rarely	Always
Mastectomy or radiation to the breast	Rarely	Never	Never	Never	Rarely	Never
Anti-estrogen therapy for breast or uterine cancer	Sometimes	Often	Sometimes	Sometimes	Rarely	Always
Androgen therapy	Never	Never	Never	Never	Never	Uncertain

From *Sexuality and Cancer: For the Woman Who Has Cancer and Her Partner* (1988). Atlanta: American Cancer Society.
*Vaginal dryness and size changes should not occur if one ovary is left in or if hormone replacement therapy is given.

Table 7-5
MALE SEXUAL PROBLEMS CAUSED BY CANCER TREATMENT

Treatment	Low Sexual Desire	Erection Problems	Lack of Orgasm	Dry Orgasm	Weaker Orgasm	Infertility
Chemotherapy	Sometimes	Rarely	Rarely	Rarely	Rarely	Often
Pelvic radiation therapy	Rarely	Sometimes	Rarely	Rarely	Sometimes	Often
Retroperitoneal lymph node dissection	Rarely	Rarely	Rarely	Often	Sometimes	Often
Abdominoperineal (A-P) resection	Rarely	Often	Rarely	Often	Sometimes	Sometimes*
Radial prostatectomy	Rarely	Often	Rarely	Always	Sometimes	Always
Radical cystectomy	Rarely	Often	Rarely	Always	Sometimes	Always
Total pelvic exenteration	Rarely	Often	Rarely	Always	Sometimes	Always
Partial penectomy	Rarely	Rarely	Rarely	Never	Rarely	Never
Total penectomy	Rarely	Always	Sometimes	Never	Sometimes	Usually*
Orchiectomy (removal of one testicle)	Rarely	Rarely	Never	Never	Never	Rarely†
Orchiectomy (removal of both testicles)	Often	Often	Sometimes	Sometimes	Sometimes	Always
Hormone therapy for prostate cancer	Often	Often	Sometimes	Sometimes	Sometimes	Always

From *Sexuality and Cancer: For the Man Who Has Cancer and His Partner* (1988). Atlanta: American Cancer Society.
*Artificial insemination of a spouse with the man's own semen may be possible.
†Infertile only if remaining testicle is not normal.

    B. Treatment related:
        1. Effects of cancer treatment (Tables 7-4 and 7-5).
        2. Medications (Table 7-6).
    C. Situational:
        1. Absence of sexual partner.
        2. History of physical or psychosocial abuse.
        3. Lack of privacy—hospitalization.
        4. Financial, work, school, religious, or family stressors.
        5. Alcohol ingestion.
    D. Developmental:
        1. Ineffective or absent role models.
        2. Aging (Table 7-7).
        3. Lack of knowledge.

III. Standard medical therapy.
    A. Hormonal therapy:
        1. Estrogen replacement for vaginal lubrication and maintenance of elasticity.
        2. Testosterone replacement for enhancement of libido.
    B. Surgical reconstruction of organs associated with sexual response.
    C. Prosthetic devices for cosmetic reconstruction—penile prosthesis, testicular prostheses, and breast implants.

Table 7-6
DRUGS THAT ALTER SEXUAL BEHAVIOR

Drug	Probable Effects
Antihypertensives	Produce vasodilation and decreased cardiac output; depress central nervous system
Guanethidine (Esimil)	Cause impotence in men and decreased vaginal lubrication in women
Reserpine (Serpasil)	
Mecamylamine (Inversine)	
Trimethaphan (Arfonad)	
Spironolactone (Aldactone)	
Methyldopa (Aldomet)	
Phenoxybenzamine (Dibenzyline)	
Clonidine (Catapres)	
Propranolol (Inderal)	
Pargyline (Eutonyl)	
Antidepressants	Peripheral blockage of nervous innervation of sex glands
Imipramine (Tofranil)	May have positive effect since they decrease depression
Desipramine (Norpramin, Pertofrane)	
Amitryptyline (Elavil)	
Nortriptyline (Aventyl)	
Protriptyline (Vivactil)	
Phenelzine sulfate (Nardil)	
Tranylcypromine sulfate (Parnate)	
Antihistamines	Block parasympathetic nervous innervation of sex glands
Diphenhydramine (Benadryl)	
Promethazine (Phenergan)	
Chlorpheniramine (Chlor-Trimeton)	
Antispasmodics/Anticholinergics	Inhibit parasympathetic innervation of sex glands
Methantheline (Banthine)	
Glycopyrrolate (Robinul)	
Hexocyclium (Tral)	
Poldine (Nacton)	
Diphenoxylate hydrochloride with atropine (Lomotil)	
Sedatives and Tranquilizers	Block autonomic innervation of sex glands
Chlorpromazine (Thorazine)	May have positive effect because they produce tranquilization and relaxation
Prochlorperazine (Compazine)	May have negative effect influencing libido
Thioridazine (Mellaril)	
Mesoridazine (Serentil)	
Chlordiazepoxide (Librium)	

Table 7-6
DRUGS THAT ALTER SEXUAL BEHAVIOR *Continued*

Drug	Probable Effects
Diazepam (Valium)	
Phenoxybenzamine (Dibenzyline)	
Chlorprothixene (Taractan)	
Haloperidol (Haldol)	
Oral Contraceptives	Remove fear of pregnancy
Alcohol	In small amounts, may increase libido
	In large amounts, impairs neural reflexes involved in erection and ejaculation
	Chronic use may cause impotence
Narcotics	Central sedation causes impotence in chronic users
Cancer Chemotherapy Agents	Possible temporary sterility or neurotoxicity in males, causing impotence
Estrogen	Suppresses sexual function in males
Diuretics Ethacrynic acid (Edecrin)	Chronic use may cause impotence
Furosemide (Lasix)	

From Carpenito, L.J. (1983). *Nursing Diagnosis: Application to Clinical Practice.* Philadelphia: J.B. Lippincott Co.

Table 7-7
DEVELOPMENTAL STAGES AND SEXUAL TASKS

Stage	Sexual Task
Infancy	Gender identity
Childhood	Pleasure-pain associated with organs and eliminative functions; masturbation takes place with resulting shame or acceptance; secondary sex characteristics become evident
Adolescence	Mastery over impulse control; acceptance of conflict between moral proscriptions and sexual urges; handling new physiological functions (menses for girls and ejaculation for boys)
Young adulthood	Sexual adequacy and performance plus fertility concerns and questions related to parenting
Middle adulthood	For the female, menopause and resulting vasomotor changes, atrophy of breasts, reduction of clitoral size, and loss of vaginal lubrication; for the male, delay on attaining an erection, a reduced compulsion to ejaculate, episodic impotence, possible prostatitis.
Old age	Reduced vitality, fear of incompetence or injury (coital coronary); fear of being viewed as "dirty old person"; unavailability of a partner (widowhood); limited physical capacity and reduced options.

Modified from Johnson, B.L., and Gross, J. (eds). *Handbook of Oncology Nursing.* © 1992. Boston: Jones and Bartlett Publishers.

    D. Salvage procedures before treatment—sperm banking or protection of ovaries by suturing outside radiation treatment field.

    E. Counseling.

    F. Control of associated symptoms of disease and treatment.

IV. Potential sequelae of prolonged sexual dysfunction.

    A. Depression

    B. Anxiety.

    C. Loss of intimacy.

    D. Decreased self-esteem.

DATA COLLECTION

I. History.

    A. Presence of risk factors for sexual dysfunction.

    B. Presence of defining characteristics of sexual dysfunction:

        1. Verbalization of problem.

        2. Alterations in achieving perceived sex role.

        3. Actual or perceived limitation imposed by disease and/or treatment.

        4. Inability to achieve sexual satisfaction.

        5. Alteration in relationship with partner.

        6. Changes in desire for sexual expression.

    C. Previous sexual patterns and preferences:

        1. Preferred sexual roles and relationships.

        2. Perceptions of self as a sexual being.

        3. Perceived perceptions of others related to self as a sexual being.

        4. Preferred sexual behaviors:

            a. Types.

            b. Frequency.

            c. Satisfaction.

    D. Reproductive history:

        1. Age at onset of sexual activity.

        2. Menstrual history (females).

        3. Number, sex, and age of children.

        4. Previous difficulty with reproduction—amenorrhea, anovulation, decreased viability of sperm, or impotence.

        5. Previous complications of pregnancy—spontaneous abortion, premature delivery, eclampsia, or fetal abnormalities.

        6. Types and length of contraceptive use.

II. Physical findings.

    A. Presence of reproductive structures and organs.

    B. Presence of signs and symptoms that affect sexual health.

III. Psychosocial findings.

    A. Perceptions of self as a male or female.

    B. Relationships with others of the same and opposite sex.

    C. Characteristics of previous relationships.

    D. Presence of psychological responses that affect sexual health.

IV. Laboratory and diagnostic data.

    A. Decreased hormone levels.

    B. Ultrasound.

    C. Abdominal x-ray examinations.

ASSOCIATED NURSING DIAGNOSES

I. Altered role performance.

II. Activity intolerance.

III. Anticipatory grieving.

IV. Self-esteem disturbance.

NURSING PLANNING AND IMPLEMENTATION

I. Interventions to minimize risk of occurrence, severity, or complications of sexual dysfunction.
  A. Give permission for client and partner to express sexual concerns:
    1. Elicit sexual concerns of both the client and partner if available.
    2. Listen nonjudgmentally to expressed concerns.
    3. Encourage continued communication among client, partner, and health care team about sexual concerns or problems throughout diagnosis, treatment, rehabilitation, and survivorship or death.
  B. Provide information related to potential effects of disease and treatment on sexual health (see Tables 7-4 and 7-5).
  C. Make specific suggestions about strategies to adapt to changes in sexuality imposed by disease and/or treatment:
    1. Decreased libido:
      a. Encourage discussion of feelings with partner.
      b. Identify settings, people, and activities that increase sexual desire such as being at home with partner during evening hours, watching a romantic movie, looking at erotic pictures, fantasizing about a sexual adventure, or keeping a sexual interest diary.
      c. Communicate above information to partner.
      d. Discuss use of hormone supplements as ordered by physician.
    2. Vaginal dryness:
      a. Encourage systemic or local hormone replacement therapy unless contraindicated by diagnosis.
      b. Discuss type and length of foreplay activity.
      c. Identify foreplay activities that are effective in increasing arousal.
      d. Communicate preferences to partner.
      e. Use water-based, colorless, nonperfumed lubricant at the entrance of the vagina and on the glans of the penis as needed.
    3. Decreased vaginal length and caliber:
      a. Use vaginal dilator to maintain or increase length and caliber of vagina:
        (1) Select time of day when client and her partner, if desired, will have 15 minutes of uninterrupted time.
        (2) Lubricate dilator with a water-based gel.
        (3) Lying down, gently insert the dilator into the full length of the vagina.
        (4) When the dilator is placed comfortably in the vagina, leave inserted for 10 minutes.
        (5) Remove and wash the dilator with soap and water.
      b. Encourage communication of desires and feelings to partner.
      c. Discuss surgical options for vaginal modification or reconstruction.
    4. Erection problems:
      a. Discuss potential effects of disease and treatment on erectile function with health care team and partner.
      b. Seek treatment for psychological symptoms that may affect erectile function—anxiety or depression.

  c. Suggest diagnostic evaluation of erectile and ejaculatory capability:
   (1) If patient is able to achieve an erection:
    (a) Increase the length of time of foreplay.
    (b) Discuss options to increase arousal and excitement.
   (2) If patient is unable to achieve an erection:
    (a) Discuss options of penile prothesis (Table 7-8).
    (b) Counsel client and partner about alternative methods of giving and receiving sexual pleasure.
5. Painful intercourse:
 a. Plan sexual activity during time when pain is least severe.
 b. Modify positions during intercourse to decrease pressure on painful area and provide increased flexibility of movement and control to client.
 c. Identify relaxing activities before intercourse.
 d. Suggest increasing length of foreplay to achieve adequate arousal.
 e. Focus on feelings that are pleasurable.
6. Difficulty reaching orgasm:
 a. Discuss potential effects of disease or treatment on ability to achieve orgasm with health care team and partner.
 b. Experiment with strategies to increase excitement:
  (1) Positioning.
  (2) Hand-held vibrators.
  (3) Increased length of foreplay.
  (4) Start-stop technique to build sexual excitement.
  (5) Achievement of as firm an erection as possible before orgasm (males).
 c. Communicate strategies that increase excitement to partner.

Table 7-8
A COMPARISON OF INFLATABLE AND SEMIRIGID PENILE PROSTHESES

Factor	Type of Prosthesis	
	Semirigid	**Inflatable**
Ease of concealment	May need special briefs; noticeable in locker room or at public urinal	No problem, although self-contained version may not lie down completely
Size of erection	Some loss of length and thickness	Normal thickness, some loss of length (self-contained version cannot add thickness)
Function during sexual intercourse	80%-90% of patients satisfied	80%-90% of patients satisfied
Infection during healing	Occurs in 1%-2% of patients	Occurs in 1%-2% of patients
Prosthesis erodes through spongy tissue inside penis	In less than 5% of patients	No problems
Prolonged pain after healing	Rare	Rare
Need to repair prosthesis	Rare	5%-15% reoperation rates
Usual hospital stay*	2-4 days	2-5 days
Total costs*	$6,000-$10,000	$10,000-$12,000

*Based on the authors' experiences in 1987 with surgery performed with patient under a general anesthetic.
From *Sexuality and Cancer: For the Man Who Has Cancer and His Partner* (1988). Atlanta: American Cancer Society.

7. Infertility:
    a. Discuss desires for children with client and partner.
    b. Discuss options of sperm banking and ovarian salvage procedures before definitive therapy.
    c. Provide specific information about adoption options and procedures with client and partner.
  D. Refer client and partner to appropriate care provider for intensive therapy in situations in which sexual concerns or problems existed before the diagnosis of cancer or are long standing or in which treatment exceeds the expertise or available time of the primary care providers.

II. Interventions to monitor for complications related to sexual dysfunction.
  A. Assess sexual health parameters before, during, and after treatment at regular intervals:
    1. Perceptions of self as a sexual being.
    2. Perceptions of others as related to self as sexual being.
    3. Behavioral expressions of and satisfaction with sexuality.
  B. Monitor client for adverse psychological responses to disease or treatment that may affect sexual health.
  C. Monitor for uncontrolled symptoms associated with disease, treatment, or complications.

III. Interventions to incorporate client and partner in care.
  A. Include partner in assessment of the quality of individual sexual health and the sexual relationship, discussions of potential effects of disease and treatment, and strategies to minimize potential effects.
  B. Encourage continued open communications between the client and partner as changes occur in sexual health.

EVALUATION OF CLIENT AND FAMILY OUTCOMES

I. Describe personal risk factors for sexual dysfunction.

II. Discuss perceived changes in sexual attitudes, behaviors, and function with partner and health care team.

III. Participate in measures to minimize the risk of occurrence, severity, and complications of sexual dysfunction.

IV. Participate in measures to maintain a positive self-concept, body image, and sense of control.

V. Demonstrate competence in new self-care techniques for management of sexual dysfunction.

VI. Describe alternate methods of sexual expression and intimacy.

VII. List changes in sexual function that require professional assistance in management.

VENTILATION

Dyspnea

THEORY

I. Definition: a subjective sensation of difficulty in breathing and the reaction to the sensation.

II. Risk factors.
   A. Disease related:
      1. Conditions that increase metabolic demands such as fever, anemia, or infection.
      2. Cerebral metastasis that affects respiratory center.
      3. Metastatic effusions in the pleural space, cardiac space, or abdominal cavity that compromise lung expansion, gas exchange, or blood flow to the lungs.
      4. Coexisting cardiac or pulmonary disease that compromises lung expansion, gas exchange, or blood flow to the lungs.
      5. Tumors that impinge on the respiratory tree and decrease the flow of air to the lungs.
   B. Treatment related:
      1. Surgical procedures associated with general anesthesia.
      2. Incisional pain that may compromise lung expansion.
      3. Immediate (pneumonitis) and long-term (fibrosis) effects of radiation therapy to fields including the lungs.
      4. Antineoplastic agents with known pulmonary or cardiac toxicities such as bleomycin, doxorubicin (Adriamycin), and cyclophosphamide (Cytoxan).
      5. Anaphylactic reactions to antineoplastic agents and biological response modifiers.
   C. Life-style related:
      1. Emotional responses such as fear or anxiety to disease and/or treatment.
      2. Tobacco abuse.
      3. Exposure to pulmonary toxic substances in the work place such as asbestos, coal dust, and benzene.
   D. Iatrogenic related:
      1. Pneumothorax secondary to placement of central catheters, fine needle aspirations, cardiocentesis, or thoracentesis.
      2. Anaphylactic reaction to medications.

III. Standard medical therapy.
   A. Treatment of underlying disease with radiation therapy, antifungal and antibacterial medications, and chemotherapy.
   B. Pharmacological agents to increase air flow to lungs such as bronchodilators, theophylline, or aminophylline.
   C. Pharmacological agents to decrease local inflammation and swelling such as steroids.
   D. Pharmacological agents to decrease pain and anxiety.
   E. Exercises to increase respiratory muscle strength and endurance.

IV. Potential sequelae of prolonged dyspnea.
   A. Hypoxia.
   B. Anxiety.
   C. Fear.
   D. Panic.

DATA COLLECTION

I. History.
   A. Presence of risk factors.
   B. Presence of defining characteristics of dyspnea—subjective complaints of client related to difficult, labored, or uncomfortable breathing and anxiety, fear, or panic.
   C. Patterns of dyspnea—onset, frequency, severity, associated symptoms, precipitating factors, aggravating factors, and alleviating factors.
   D. Effectivensss of previous self-care strategies in relieving dyspnea.
   E. Impact of dyspnea on activities of daily living, life-style, comfort, relationships, work, school, and role responsibilities, and mood.

II. Physical examination.
   A. Respiratory rate, depth, and effort.
   B. Use of accessory muscles with breathing.
   C. Nasal flaring.
   D. Cyanosis.
   E. Clubbing of digits.

III. Diagnostic tests.
   A. Since symptom is a subjective response, abnormal laboratory findings may or may not be present.
   B. Abnormal arterial blood gas levels.

ASSOCIATED NURSING DIAGNOSES

I. Impaired gas exchange.

II. Ineffective breathing pattern.

III. Activity intolerance.

IV. Sleep pattern disturbance.

V. Altered oral mucous membranes.

NURSING PLANNING AND IMPLEMENTATION

I. Interventions to minimize the risk of occurrence, severity, or complications of dyspnea.
   A. Measures to increase ease and effectiveness of breathing:
      1. Position client in upright position.
      2. Lean client forward with arms resting on table or knees.
      3. Have client roll shoulders forward.
      4. Encourage client to take slow, deep breaths.
      5. Inhale through nose and exhale through pursed lips.
      6. Exhale two times as long as inhale.
      7. Use diaphragm when breathing.
   B. Elevate head of bed 45 degrees at all times.
   C. Provide diversional activities.
   D. Plan activities throughout the day to limit energy expenditure.
   E. Implement strategies to decrease fear and anxiety associated with dyspnea such as relaxation techniques.

II. Interventions to maximize safety.
   A. Encourage use of assistive devices as needed for ambulation and activities of daily living.

    B. Rearrange environment to decrease energy expenditure:
1. Place items within reach.
2. Slide rather than lift items.
3. Sit rather than stand to do activities.
4. Use handles instead of lifting when carrying items.

    C. Keep side rails up on bed at all times.

III. Interventions to monitor for complications related to dyspnea.
    A. Assess level of consciousness and mental status each day.
    B. Monitor intake, urinary output, including volume and color, and intake/output ratio each day.
    C. Assess heart rate and rhythm, presence of chest heaviness or discomfort, and perfusion in extremities.

IV. Interventions to monitor client response to symptom management.
    A. Monitor subjective reports of the client and family of changes in the pattern of dyspnea.
    B. Monitor compliance with measures to decrease incidence and severity of dyspnea.
    C. Monitor subjective reports of client and family of psychological responses to dyspnea.

V. Interventions to incorporate client and family in care.
    A. Teach positioning techniques.
    B. Teach emergency care techniques and resources available in community for emergency care.
    C. Teach signs and symptoms related to complications of dyspnea to report to a member of the health care team.

VI. Report critical changes in client assessment parameters to physician.
    A. Presence of significant changes in client perception of dyspnea.
    B. Presence of signs and symptoms of decreased oxygen to major organ systems such as chest pain, decrease in level of consciousness, or decrease in urinary output.

EVALUATION OF CLIENT AND FAMILY OUTCOMES

I. Describe personal risk factors for dyspnea.

II. Report signs, symptoms, and complications of dyspnea to a member of the health care team.

III. Participate in measures to minimize the risk of occurrence, severity, and complications of dyspnea.

IV. Demonstrate competence in emergency techniques to treat severe dyspnea and/or panic.

V. List changes in the condition of the client that require professional assistance in management.
    A. Marked change in subjective severity of dyspnea as perceived by the client.
    B. Presence of new symptoms that could alter the treatment plan such as a productive cough or pain.

Airway Obstruction

THEORY

I. Definition: state in which an individual is unable to move air through the respiratory tract because of occlusion.

II. Risk factors.
   A. Disease related:
      1. Obstruction of airway by primary or metastatic tumor.
      2. Swelling of laryngeal tissues related to anaphylaxis.
      3. Tracheobronchial infection.
      4. Fracture of trachea or larynx.
      5. Subcutaneous emphysema of the neck or upper chest.
   B. Treatment related:
      1. Surgical manipulation of tissues surrounding the tracheobronchial tree.
      2. Radiation-induced inflammation from therapy to the head, neck, or chest.
   C. Situational:
      1. Lodging of food in tracheobronchial tree.
      2. Collapse of tracheobronchial tree from trauma.

III. Standard medical therapy.
   A. Back blows, manual thrusts, and finger sweeps.
   B. Suctioning.
   C. Tracheostomy.
   D. Pharyngeal or endotracheal airway.
   E. Laser therapy.

IV. Potential sequelae of prolonged airway obstruction.
   A. Anoxia.
   B. Organ damage.
   C. Death.

DATA COLLECTION

I. History.
   A. Presence of risk factors for airway obstruction.
   B. Presence of defining characteristics of airway obstruction—progressive shortness of breath and effective or ineffective cough, with or without sputum.

II. Physical examination.
   A. Abnormal breath sounds (rales or rhonchi).
   B. Changes in rate (tachypnea) or depth of respirations.
   C. Pallor to deep cyanosis.
   D. Inability to speak.
   E. Severe dyspnea.
   F. Use of sternocleidomastoid and trapezius muscles to breathe.

III. Psychosocial examination—cognitive or perceptual impairment.

IV. Laboratory data—abnormal blood gas values.

ASSOCIATED NURSING DIAGNOSES

I. Ineffective airway clearance.

II. Impaired gas exchange.

III. Anxiety.

IV. Fear.

NURSING PLANNING AND IMPLEMENTATION

I. Interventions to minimize the risk of occurrence, severity, or complications of airway obstruction.
  A. Teach clients turning, coughing, and deep breathing before surgical procedures.
  B. Evaluate respiratory status and effort of clients at risk for airway obstruction at frequent and scheduled intervals.
  C. Institute strategies to manage tracheobronchial secretions effectively.
  D. Encourage sitting position for eating and adequate chewing of food before swallowing.

II. Interventions to monitor for complications related to airway obstruction.
  A. Assess urinary output.
  B. Assess neurological status at scheduled intervals—orientation, response to commands, information and thought processing, and intactness of cranial nerves.
  C. Assess cardiovascular status—rate, rhythm, and presence of chest pain.

III. Interventions to incorporate client and family in care—teach family members emergency procedures for airway obstruction.

IV. Report critical changes in client assessment parameters to physician—progressive objective or subjective respiratory distress.

EVALUATION OF CLIENT AND FAMILY OUTCOMES

I. Describe personal risk factors for airway obstruction.

II. Participate in measures to minimize the risk of occurrence, severity, and complications of airway obstruction.

III. Report signs of airway obstruction immediately to a member of the health care team.

IV. Demonstrate competence in emergency management of airway obstruction.

V. Identify community resources for managing airway obstruction emergencies.

CIRCULATION

Anemia

THEORY

I. Definition: a quantitative or qualitative deficiency in the number of circulating red blood cells needed to meet the oxygenation needs of normal tissues.

II. Risk factors.
  A. Disease related:
    1. Decreased production of red blood cells related to primary malignant disease of the marrow, tumor invasion of marrow, or genetically transmitted red cell deficiencies.
    2. Decreased production of red blood cells related to nutritional deficiencies such as decreased intake, absorption, or utilization of iron, vitamin K, folic acid, or vitamin B_{12}.
    3. Decreased production of red blood cells related to acute or chronic renal disease and associated decrease in the production and release of erythropoietin.

4. Increased destruction or sequestration of red blood cells related to autoimmune disorders associated with malignancy.

B. Treatment related:
1. Radiation therapy—destruction of rapidly dividing normal hematopoietic cells within radiation treatment fields that include areas of increased hematopoietic activity results in a decrease in the production of red blood cell precursors and ultimately mature red blood cells.
2. Chemotherapy—destruction of rapidly dividing normal hematopoietic cells and malignant cells results in a decrease in the production of red cell precursors and ultimately mature red blood cells.
3. Supportive therapy—dilutional decrease in the number of circulating red blood cells may occur with fluid therapy.
4. Other pharmacological agents such as benzene or selected antibiotics may result in a decrease in the production of red blood cells.

III. Standard medical therapy.
A. Red blood cell transfusions (see Chapter 26).
1. Whole blood for volume replacement.
2. Packed red blood cells for quantitative red cell replacement.
B. Nutritional supplements such as vitamins, iron, and folic acid.
C. Avoidance of pharmacological agents that inhibit red cell production and/or maturation.

IV. Potential sequelae of prolonged anemia.
A. Decreased oxygenation of peripheral tissues.
B. Increased risk for injury.
C. Changes in activities of daily living such as work, leisure, and self-care activities.

DATA COLLECTION

I. History.
A. Review of previous therapy for cancer.
B. Review of prescription and nonprescription medications.
C. History of headache, vertigo, tinnitus, palpitations, hypersensitivity to cold, dyspnea on exertion, and insomnia.
D. History of acute or chronic blood loss by stool, urine, emesis, menses, nasopharynx, or site of invasive procedures.
E. Impact of anemia on life-style.

II. Physical examination.
A. Pallor of skin, nail beds, conjunctivae, and circumoral tissues.
B. Active bleeding from the gums, nose, bladder, bowel, and vagina or site of invasive procedures.
C. Increase in pulse, respirations, and pulse pressure and/or a decrease in blood pressure.

III. Psychosocial examination.
A. Perceptions of meaning of anemia for client and family.
B. Effects of anemia on life-style, activities of daily living, and self-concept.

IV. Laboratory data.
A. Decreased hemoglobin and hematocrit levels.
B. Decreased red blood cell indices.
C. Decreased reticulocyte count.
D. Decreased iron, total iron-binding capacity (TIBC), vitamins B_{12} and K, and/or folic acid levels.

ASSOCIATED NURSING DIAGNOSES

I. Potential for injury.

II. Knowledge deficit related to self-care.

III. Disturbance in self-concept.

NURSING PLANNING AND IMPLEMENTATION

I. Notify physician of marked decrease in hemoglobin or hematocrit levels or marked changes in symptomatology associated with anemia.

II. Institute measures to decrease risk of complications of anemia.
   A. Institute safety precautions:
      1. Avoid sudden level changes in position such as from lying to sitting or sitting to standing.
      2. Assist with ambulation and self-care activities as needed.
      3. Place bed in low position and side rails up at all times.
      4. Avoid hazardous activities such as driving if syncopal episodes are present.
   B. Provide a nutritionally balanced diet and/or supplements.

III. Institute interventions to monitor for complications related to anemia.
   A. Assess skin for evidence of inadequate oxygenation such as pallor, decreased capillary refill, or prolonged redness.
   B. Assess blood pressure in lying, sitting, and standing positions.
   C. Assess client for evidence of side effects of therapy for anemia:
      1. Fluid volume excess from red cell transfusions.
      2. Constipation related to iron supplements.

IV. Initiate interventions to incorporate client and family in care.
   A. Teach measures to decrease risk of complications of anemia.
   B. Teach signs and symptoms related to complications of anemia or treatment to report to a member of the health care team.

V. Report critical changes in client assessment parameters to physician.
   A. Changes in the number or frequency of syncopal episodes.
   B. Presence of signs and symptoms of bleeding.
   C. Marked subjective changes in client discomfort from anemia.

EVALUATION OF CLIENT AND FAMILY OUTCOMES

I. Describe personal risk factors for anemia.

II. Report signs, symptoms, and complications of anemia or treatment for anemia to a member of the health care team.

III. Participate in measures to minimize the risk of complications of anemia.

IV. List changes that require professional assistance in management—active bleeding from any site and acute changes in severity of symptoms of anemia.

V. Identify community resources available for management of emergency situations.

Fluid Imbalance: Edema

THEORY

I. Definition: an excessive accumulation of fluid within interstitial spaces.

II. Risk factors.
   A. Disease related:

  1. Concurrent cardiac, renal, or liver disease.
  2. Tumor infiltration of vascular or lymph channels.
  3. Allergic response.
 B. Treatment related:
  1. Surgical disruption of vascular or lymphatic channels.
  2. Radiation therapy:
   a. Inflammation of tissues within the treatment field.
   b. Fibrosis of lymphatic channels within the treatment field.
  3. Medications such as estrogen.
 C. Life-style related:
  1. Increased dietary sodium.
  2. Inadequate dietary protein.
 D. Iatrogenic related:
  1. Plasma expanders.
  2. Intravenous fluid therapy.
  3. Blood component therapy.

III. Standard medical therapy.
 A. Treatment of underlying disease.
 B. Diuretics.
 C. Albumin replacement.
 D. Electrolyte replacement.
 E. Medications such as diuretics or tranquilizers.
 F. Mechanical pumps.
 G. Consults with occupational and physical therapy.

IV. Potential sequelae of prolonged edema.
 A. Increased risk of infection.
 B. Impaired skin integrity.
 C. Impaired circulation.
 D. Electrolyte imbalances.
 E. Impaired physical mobility.
 F. Increased risk of injury related to sensory changes.
 G. Changes in self-concept, body image, and self-esteem.

DATA COLLECTION

 I. History.
 A. Presence of risk factors for edema.
 B. Patterns of edema—onset, frequency, location, severity, precipitating, aggra-vating and alleviating factors, and associated factors.
 C. Impact of edema on activities of daily living, life-style, comfort, relationships, roles and responsibilities within the family, community, work, or school, and mood.
 D. Perceived significance of edema in relation to disease and treatment.

 II. Physical findings.
 A. Local changes:
  1. Swelling—circumference of involved extremity is 4 cm greater than unin-volved extremity at a specific body landmark.
  2. Warmth and/or coolness of skin over edematous area.
  3. Sensory changes—numbness, tingling, or pain.
 B. Motor changes:
  1. Limited range of motion.
  2. Pain on movement.

   C. Circulatory changes:
     1. Diminished peripheral pulses in involved extremity.
     2. Discoloration of effected extremity.
     3. Nail blanching.
III. Psychosocial findings.
   A. Anxiety.
   B. Perceived changes in body image.
   C. Fear.
   D. Changes in mobility, independence in activities of daily living, and social interactions.
IV. Laboratory data.
   A. Abnormal serum electrolyte values.
   B. Increased BUN and serum creatinine levels.
   C. Decreased serum protein and albumin values.

ASSOCIATED NURSING DIAGNOSES
I. Impaired skin integrity.
II. Impaired physical mobility.
III. Activity intolerance.
IV. Self-care deficit.
V. Alteration in comfort.
VI. Sleep pattern disturbance.

NURSING PLANNING AND IMPLEMENTATION
I. Interventions to maximize client safety.
   A. Wear loose protective clothing on extremity such as gloves, long-sleeved shirt, or slacks.
   B. Avoid irritants to edematous skin areas.
   C. Avoid restrictive jewelry on involved extremity.
   D. Test temperatures of bath water and cooking utensils with uninvolved extremity before contact with involved extremity.
II. Institute measures to minimize the risk of occurrence and severity of edema.
   A. Avoid invasive or constrictive procedures such as venipunctures or blood pressure measurements in involved extremity.
   B. Elevate edematous extremities above the apex of the heart while at rest.
   C. Limit fluid intake as ordered by physician.
   D. Institute progressive exercises of involved extremity.
   E. Develop a skin care protocol for edematous areas.
   F. Assist with activities of daily living as needed.
III. Implement interventions to monitor for complications related to edema.
   A. Weigh client daily.
   B. Evaluate the intactness, color, and temperature of skin over edematous area.
   C. Assess the presence and quality of peripheral pulses over edematous areas.
   D. Assess temperature, pulse rate, respiratory rate, and blood pressure.
   E. Evaluate level of mobility and range of motion at regular intervals.
   F. Report adverse changes in electrolyte levels as ordered by physician.
   G. Monitor client perceptions of impact of edema on self-concept, body image, and sexuality.

IV. Report critical changes in client assessment parameters to physician.
   A. Presence of signs and symptoms of infection.
   B. Acute changes in the intactness, color, or temperature of skin over edematous areas.
   C. Diminished or absence of peripheral pulses in edematous extremity.

V. Implement strategies to incorporate client and family in care.
   A. Teach appropriate use of compression equipment.
   B. Teach self-care measures to protect edematous areas.

EVALUATION OF CLIENT AND FAMILY OUTCOMES

I. Identify personal risk factors for development of edema.

II. Participate in measure to decrease the risk for and complications of edema.

III. Report signs and symptoms of edema and sequelae to health care team.

IV. List institutional and community resources available to assist with management of edema.

Fluid Imbalance: Effusion

THEORY

I. Definition: excessive accumulation of fluid within a body space. Primary sites for effusions include:
   A. Pleural space.
   B. Pericardial space.
   C. Peritoneal cavity.

II. Risk factors.
   A. Disease related:
      1. Pleural effusion—cancer of the lung or breast or metastatic disease to the pleural space from other site-specific cancers.
      2. Pericardial effusion:
         a. Cancer of lung, colon, or breast, sarcoma, lymphoma, or leukemia.
         b. Tuberculosis, rheumatic fever, myxedema, or trauma.
      3. Peritoneal effusion—cancer of the ovary, endometrium, breast, colon, pancreas, or stomach.
      4. Coexisting pulmonary, cardiac, or liver disease.
   B. Treatment related:
      1. Previous radiation therapy to chest, thorax, or abdomen.
      2. Surgical modification of venous or lymphatic channels.

III. Standard medical therapy (Table 7-9).

IV. Potential sequelae of progressive effusions.
   A. Pleural effusion—dyspnea.
   B. Pericardial effusion—cardiac tamponade (see Chapter 8).
   C. Peritoneal effusion—discomfort, early satiety, decreased bladder capacity, bowel obstruction, electrolyte imbalance, infection, and impaired skin integrity.

DATA COLLECTION

I. History.
   A. Presence of risk factors.
   B. Perceived meaning of effusion symptoms to client and family.
   C. Effectiveness of self-care strategies in relieving symptoms of effusions.

Table 7-9
STANDARD MEDICAL THERAPY FOR EFFUSIONS

Pleural Effusion	Pericardial Effusion	Peritoneal Effusion
←	Treatment of Underlying Disease	→
Thoracentesis	Pericardiocentesis	Paracentesis
Insertion of chest tubes	Pericardiectomy	Diuretics
Instillation of sclerosing agents such as:	Pericardial window	Peritoneovenous shunt
Nitrogen mustard	Instillation of sclerosing agents such as:	Instillation of intraperitoneal chemotherapy such as:
Bleomycin	Nitrogen mustard	5-FU
Thiotepa	Cisplatin	Bleomycin
5-FU	Tetracycline	Thiotepa
Radioactive colloidal materials	Bleomycin	Nitrogen mustard
Pleurectomy	Thiotepa	Instillation of radioactive or colloid materials intraperitoneally
Pleuroperitoneal shunting	External radiation therapy	

Table 7-10
FINDINGS ASSOCIATED WITH EFFUSIONS

Pleural Effusion	Pericardial Effusion	Peritoneal Effusion
Physical		
Dyspnea	Dyspnea	Abdominal distention
Cough	Cough	Presence of fluid wave
Chest pain	Chest pain	Bulging flanks
Fever	Muffled heart sounds	Weight gain
Dullness to chest percussion	Weak or absent apical pulse	Dyspnea
Absent breath sounds	Hiccups	Orthopnea
	Narrowing pulse pressure	Tachypnea
	Peripheral edema	Edema of lower extremities
Psychosocial		
Anxiety	Anxiety	Anxiety
Restlessness	Agitation	Restlessness
Laboratory/Diagnostic		
Positive cytology	Echocardiogram	Positive cytology
Chest x-ray examination	Chest x-ray examination	Abdominal x-ray examination
	Electrocardiogram	CT scan
	Computed tomographic (CT) scan	
	Positive cytology	

Table 7-11

NURSING PLANNING AND INTERVENTIONS FOR CLIENTS WITH EFFUSIONS

Categories of Interventions	Pleural Effusion	Pericardial Effusion	Peritoneal Effusion
Interventions to maximize safety for the client	Encourage use of assistive devices and personnel for ambulation. Teach client and family safety measures associated with oxygen therapy—no smoking or flames.	Encourage energy conservation strategies. Teach client and family safety measures associated with oxygen therapy—no smoking or flames.	Implement skin care protocol for edematous areas. Encourage use of assistive devices or personnel for ambulation. Avoid skin contact with temperature extremes such as hot water bags.
Interventions to minimize risk of occurrence, severity, of complications of effusions	Elevate head of bed 45 degrees. Encourage use of energy conservation techniques. Teach relaxation techniques. Provide distraction. Suggest wearing loose clothing. Maintain cool environmental temperature.	Elevate head of bed 45 degrees. Encourage use of energy conservation techniques. Teach relaxation techniques. Suggest wearing loose clothing. Maintain cool environmental temperature. Assist with activities of daily living as needed.	Modify diet to decrease sodium intake and increase protein intake. Encourage maintenance of high Fowler's position. Avoid restrictive clothing. Assist client with activities of daily living.
Interventions to monitor for complications related to effusions or treatment	Monitor respiratory rate, depth, and effort. Assess lung fields for adventitious breath sounds. Evaluate skin color of extremities. Monitor transcutaneous oxygen levels. Assess changes in characteristics of pain.	Monitor for peripheral edema. Monitor for distended neck veins. Assess heart rate, rhythm, and regularity. Evaluate skin color of extremities. Assess mental status. Assess changes in characteristics of pain.	Measure abdominal girth and circumference of extremities daily. Weigh client daily. Assess subjective changes in fullness, bloating, and abdominal pressure. Monitor electrolyte values as ordered by physician. Assess temperature at regular intervals. Evaluate daily nutritional intake.
Interventions to incorporate client and family in care	Teach strategies to modify symptoms of pleural effusions. Instruct about situations that require immediate professional assistance for management.	Solicit client directives about activities in which assistance is needed. Teach signs and symptoms to report to care provider.	Teach to select foods low in salt and high in protein. Solicit client directives about activities in which assistance is needed.
Critical changes in client parameters to report to physician	Report acute adverse changes in respiratory rate, depth, or adventitious lung sounds. Report acute adverse changes in mental status. Report adverse changes in arterial blood gas values as ordered by physician.	Report acute respiratory distress. Report fever. Report acute changes in characteristics of pain.	Report acute respiratory distress. Report fever. Report acute changes in characteristics of pain.

D. Impact of effusion symptoms on activities of daily living, life-style, comfort, relationships, work, school, and role responsibilities, and mood.

II. Physical findings (Table 7-10).

III. Psychosocial findings (Table 7-10).

IV. Laboratory and diagnostic data (Table 7-10).

ASSOCIATED NURSING DIAGNOSES

I. Impaired physical mobility.

II. Sleep pattern disturbance.

III. Decreased cardiac output.

IV. Impaired breathing pattern.

V. Self-care deficit.

NURSING PLANNING AND IMPLEMENTATION (Table 7-11).

EVALUATION OF PATIENT AND FAMILY OUTCOMES

I. Describe personal risk factors for specific effusions.

II. Report signs and symptoms of effusions to a member of the health care team.

III. Participate in strategies to decrease the severity of symptoms of specific effusions.

IV. List changes in the condition of the client that require professional assistance in management.

BIBLIOGRAPHY

Barale, K. (1991). Nutritional support. In S.B. Baird, M.G. Donehower, V. Stalsbroten, & T.B. Ades (eds). *A Cancer Source Book for Nurses*. (6th ed). Atlanta: The American Cancer Society.

Benner, P. (1991). Stress and coping with cancer. In S.B. Baird, R. McCorkle, & M. Grant (eds). *Cancer Nursing: A Comprehensive Textbook*. Philadelphia: W.B. Saunders Co., pp. 717-741.

Burns, N. & Holmes, B.C. (1991). Alterations in body image. In S.B. Baird, R. McCorkle, & M. Grant (eds). *Cancer Nursing: A Comprehensive Textbook*. Philadelphia: W.B. Saunders Co., pp. 821-830.

Carnevali, D.L. & Reiner, A.C. (1990). *The Cancer Experience: Nursing Diagnosis and Management*. Philadelphia: J.B. Lippincott Co.

Carpenito, L.J. (1983). *Nursing Diagnosis: Application to Clinical Practice*. Philadelphia: J.B. Lippincott Co.

Chamorro, T. (1991). Cancer and sexuality. In S.B. Baird, M.G. Donehower, V. Stalsbroten, & T.B. Ades (eds). *A Cancer Source Book for Nurses*. (6th ed). Atlanta: The American Cancer Society, pp. 141-149.

Clark, J.C. (1990). Psychosocial dimensions: The patient. In S.L. Groenwald, M.H. Frogge, M. Goodman, & C.H. Yarbro (eds). *Cancer Nursing: Principles and Practice* (2nd ed). Boston: Jones & Bartlett Publishers, pp. 346-364.

Cooper, C.L. (ed) (1984). *Psychosocial stress and cancer*. New York: John Wiley & Sons.

Coyle, N. & Foley, K.M. (1991). Alterations in comfort: pain. In S.B. Baird, R. McCorkle, & M. Grant (eds). *Cancer Nursing: A Comprehensive Textbook*. Philadelphia: W.B. Saunders Co., pp. 782-805.

Donehower, M.G. (1991). Symptom management. In S.B. Baird, M.G. Donehower, V. Stalsbroten, & T.B. Ades (eds). *A Cancer Source Book for Nurses*. (6th ed). Atlanta: The American Cancer Society, pp. 100-110.

Donoghue, M., Nunnally, C., & Yasko, J.M. (1982). *Nutritional Aspects of Cancer Care*. Reston, Va: Reston Publishing Co.

Dudas, S. (1990). Altered body image and sexuality. In S.L. Groenwald, M.H. Frogge, M. Goodman, & C.H. Yarbro (eds). *Cancer Nursing: Principles and Practice* (2nd ed). Boston: Jones & Bartlett Publishers, pp. 581-593.

Fanslow, J. (1991). Pain management. In S.B. Baird, M.G. Donehower, V. Stalsbroten, & T.B. Ades (eds). *A Cancer Source Book for Nurses*. (6th ed). Atlanta: The American Cancer Society, pp. 111-120.

Ferszt, G. & Barg, F.K. (1991). Psychosocial support. In S.B. Baird, M.G. Donehower, V. Stalsbroten, & T.B. Ades (eds). *A Cancer Source Book for Nurses*. (6th ed). Atlanta: The American Cancer Society, pp. 150-158.

Gobel, B.H. (1990). Bleeding. In S.L. Groenwald, M.H. Frogge, M. Goodman, & C.H. Yarbro (eds). *Cancer Nursing : Principles and Practice* (2nd ed). Boston: Jones & Bartlett Publishers, pp. 467-484.

Griffiths, M.J., Murray, K.H., & Russo, P.C. (1984). *Oncology Nursing: Pathophysiology, Assessment, and Intervention*. New York: Macmillan Publishing Co.

Holland, J.C. & Massie, M.J. (1988). Psychiatric management of anxiety in patients with cancer. Chicago: Upjohn Co.

Hughes, J. (1986). Denial in cancer patients. B.A. Stroll (ed). *Coping With Cancer Stress*. Boston: Martinus Nijhoff Publishers, pp. 63-70.

Hughes, J. (1986). Depression in cancer patients. In B.A. Stroll (ed). *Coping With Cancer Stress*. Boston: Martinus Nijhoff Publishers, pp. 53-62.

Jacobs, M.M. & Geels, W. (eds). (1985). *Signs and Symptoms in Nursing: Interpretation and Management*. Philadelphia: J.B. Lippincott Co.

Jalowiec, A. & Dudas, S. (1991). Alterations in patient coping. In S.B. Baird, R. McCorkle, & M. Grant (eds). *Cancer Nursing: A Comprehensive Textbook*. Philadelphia: W.B. Saunders Co., pp. 806-820.

Johnson, B.L. & Gross, J. (eds). (1985). *Handbook of Oncology Nursing*. New York: John Wiley & Sons.

Kaye, P. (1989). *Notes on Symptom Control in Hospice and Palliative Care*. Essex, Conn: Hospice Education Institute, pp. 139-146.

Klemm, P.R. & Hubbard, S.M. (1990). Infection. In S.L. Groenwald, M.H. Frogge, M. Goodman, & C.H. Yarbro (eds). *Cancer Nursing: Principles and Practice* (2nd ed). Boston: Jones & Bartlett Publishers, pp. 442-466.

Krebs, L.U. (1990). Sexual and reproductive dysfunction. In S.L. Groenwald, M.H. Frogge, M. Goodman, & C.H. Yarbro (eds). *Cancer Nursing: Principles and Practice* (2nd ed). Boston: Jones & Bartlett Publishers, pp. 563-580.

Lamb, M.A. (1991). Alterations in sexuality and sexual functioning. In S.B. Baird, R. McCorkle, & M. Grant (eds). *Cancer Nursing: A Comprehensive Textbook*. Philadelphia: W.B. Saunders Co., pp. 821-830.

Lang-Kummer, J.M. (1990). Hypercalcemia. In S.L. Groenwald, M.H. Frogge, M. Goodman, & C.H. Yarbro (eds). *Cancer Nursing: Principles and Practice* (2nd ed). Boston: Jones & Bartlett Publishers, pp. 520-534.

Lydon, J., Purl, S., & Goodman, M. (1990). Integumentary and mucous membrane alterations. In S.L. Groenwald, M.H. Frogge, M. Goodman, & C.H. Yarbro (eds). *Cancer Nursing: Principles and Practice* (2nd ed). Boston: Jones & Bartlett Publishers, pp. 594-643.

McCaffery, M. & Beebe, A. (1989). *Pain: Clinical Manual for Nursing Practice*. St. Louis: C.V. Mosby Co.

McGee, R.F. (1990). Overview of psychosocial dimensions. In S.L. Groenwald, M.H. Frogge, M. Goodman, & C.H. Yarbro (eds). *Cancer Nursing: Principles and Practice* (2nd ed). Boston: Jones & Bartlett Publishers, pp. 341-345.

McGuire, D.B. & Sheidler, V.R. (1990). Pain. In S.L. Groenwald, M.H. Frogge, M. Goodman, & C.H. Yarbro (eds). *Cancer Nursing: Principles and Practice* (2nd ed). Boston: Jones & Bartlett Publishers, pp. 385-441.

McGuire, D.B. & Yarbro, C.H. (eds). (1987). *Cancer Pain Management*. Orlando, Fla: Grune & Stratton.

McNally, J.C., Somerville, E.T., Miaskowski, C., & Rostad, M. (eds). (1991). *Guidelines for Oncology Nursing Practice* (2nd ed). Philadelphia: W.B. Saunders Co.

Moore, L.M. & Ruccione, K. (1990). Late effects of cancer treatment. In S.L. Groenwald, M.H. Frogge, M. Goodman, & C.H. Yarbro (eds). *Cancer Nursing: Principles and Practice* (2nd ed). Boston: Jones & Bartlett Publishers, pp. 669-688.

Nail, L.M. (1990). Fatigue. In S.L. Groenwald, M.H. Frogge, M. Goodman, & C.H. Yarbro (eds). *Cancer Nursing: Principles and Practice* (2nd ed). Boston: Jones & Bartlett Publishers.

National Institute of Mental Health (undated). *Depression: what you need to know*. Rockville, Md: U.S. Department of Health and Human Services.

North American Nursing Diagnosis Association (1989). *Taxonomy 1 With Official Diagnosis Categories*. St. Louis: NANDA.

Piper, B.F. (1991). Alterations in energy: the sensation of fatigue. In S.B. Baird, R. McCorkle, & M. Grant (eds). *Cancer Nursing: A Comprehensive Textbook*. Philadelphia: W.B. Saunders Co., pp. 894-908.

Snyder, M. (1985). *Independent Nursing Interventions*. New York: John Wiley & Sons.

Szeluga, D.J., Groenwald, S.L., & Sullivan, D.K. (1990). Nutritional disturbances. In S.L. Groenwald, M.H. Frogge, M. Goodman, & C.H. Yarbro (eds). *Cancer Nursing: Principles and Practice* (2nd ed). Boston: Jones & Barlett Publishers, pp. 495-519

Varricchio, C.G., Miller, N., & Pazdur, M. (1990). Edema and effusions. In S.L. Groenwald, M.H. Frogge, M. Goodman, & C.H. Yarbro (eds). *Cancer Nursing: Principles and Practice* (2nd ed). Boston: Jones & Bartlett Publishers, pp. 546-562.

Zerwekh, J. (1991). Supportive care for the dying patient. In S.B. Baird, R. McCorkle, & M. Grant (eds). *Cancer Nursing: A Comprehensive Textbook*. Philadelphia. W.B. Saunders Co., pp. 875-884.

8

Nursing Care of Patients with Structural Oncological Emergencies

Jane C. Hunter, MN, RN, OCN

Increased Intracranial Pressure

THEORY

I. Pathophysiology.
- A. The intracranial cavity is a nonexpandable chamber that contains:
  1. Brain tissue.
  2. Vascular tissue.
  3. Cerebrospinal fluid.
- B. An increase in intracranial pressure can result when the volume of any of the three components increases.
- C. Primary or metastatic tumors within the intracranial cavity can result in increased intracranial pressure by:
  1. Displacement of brain tissue.
  2. Edema of brain tissue.
  3. Obstruction of cerebrospinal fluid flow.
  4. Increased vascularity associated with tumor growth.

II. Principles of medical management.
- A. Diagnostic tests:
  1. Computerized tomography (CT) scan.
  2. Magnetic resonance imaging (MRI).
  3. Cerebral angiography—determines if impression from CT scan or MRI is a vascular abnormality or tumor.
  4. Myelography—determines if drop metastases are present.
  5. CT-guided needle biopsy—obtains a tissue diagnosis without open craniotomy.
- B. Nonpharmacological interventions:
  1. Surgery:
     - a. Complete resection of primary tumor or single brain metastasis.
     - b. Tumor bulk reduction with decompression:
       - (1) Provides symptomatic relief.

      (2) Is contraindicated with multiple, small intracranial tumors.

      (3) Is treatment of choice for tumors causing spinal cord compression.

    c. Shunt placement—provides an alternate pathway for cerebrospinal fluid.

  2. Radiation therapy:

    a. Primary treatment or palliative treatment for metastatic disease, depending on radiosensitivity of tumor.

    b. Adjuvant treatment with either surgery or chemotherapy.

    c. Investigational therapy:

      (1) Stereotactic radiosurgery with gamma knife to treat small, focal tumors.

      (2) Adjuvant treatment with hypothermia.

C. Pharmacological interventions:

  1. Chemotherapy for primary or metastatic tumor.

    a. Most antineoplastic agents do not cross blood-brain barrier; nitrosoureas and procarbazine are exceptions.

    b. Regional drug delivery such as intra-arterial, intrathecal, or intratumor drug administration circumvents blood-brain barrier.

  2. Corticosteroids.

    a. Used to decrease inflammation.

    b. Begins before therapy and may be tapered.

    c. May require maintenance doses for residual tumor or dependence from long-term use.

  3. Osmotherapy.

    a. Used to decrease the amount of fluid in the brain tissue.

    b. Mannitol may be used.

  4. Fluid restriction.

  5. Anticonvulsants—used prophylactically to prevent seizures.

DATA COLLECTION

I. Identification of clients at risk.

  A. Clients with cancers of the lung, breast, testicles, thyroid, stomach, or kidney or melanoma.

  B. Clients with primary tumors of brain or spinal cord.

  C. Clients with a diagnosis of leukemia or neuroblastoma.

II. Physical examination—signs and symptoms depend on volume and location of abnormality.

  A. Early signs and symptoms:

    1. Headaches:

      a. Early morning headache may be bilateral and located in occipital or frontal areas.

      b. Headache may be initiated or aggravated by Valsalva maneuver, coughing, or bending.

    2. Gastrointestinal—loss of appetite, nausea, and occasional vomiting.

    3. Neurological—blurred vision and decreased visual fields resulting from papilledema.

  B. Late signs and symptoms:

    1. Cardiovascular—bradycardia and widening pulse pressure.

    2. Respiratory—slow, shallow respirations; tachypnea; and Cheyne-Stokes respirations.

    3. Neurological—decreased ability to concentrate; decreased level of consciousness; personality changes; hemiplegia; hemiparesis; seizures; and pupillary changes.

ASSOCIATED NURSING DIAGNOSES

I. Alteration in tissue perfusion: cerebral.

II. Alteration in sensory perception.

III. Alteration in thought processes.

IV. Ineffective breathing pattern.

V. Impaired verbal communication.

VI. Impaired physical mobility.

NURSING PLANNING AND IMPLEMENTATION

I. Interventions to maximize safety for the client.
  A. Maintain bed rest with increasing intracranial pressure and progressive symptoms.
  B. Keep bed in lowest position and side rails elevated.
  C. Develop a daily schedule of activities with appropriate rest periods.
  D. Use assistive devices as needed.

II. Interventions to decrease severity of symptoms associated with increased intracranial pressure.
  A. Instruct client to avoid Valsalva maneuver:
    1. Administer stool softeners as ordered by physician to prevent constipation.
    2. Administer antiemetics as ordered by physician to prevent vomiting.
    3. Implement measures to control discomfort from headaches (see Chapter 7).
    4. Instruct client to be passive during turning and repositioning.
  B. Implement measures to decrease stress:
    1. Maintain a calm environment.
    2. Minimize external stimulation—light, noise, touch, and temperature extremes.
    3. Encourage calmness during interactions between client and others.
    4. Teach stress reduction strategies to client and family.
  C. Monitor activities and positioning to minimize increased intracranial pressure:
    1. Elevate head of bed 30 degrees to promote venous drainage.
    2. Avoid isometric muscle contractions.
    3. Avoid positions that rotate the head or extend or flex the neck.
    4. Avoid lying in prone position or activities that exert pressure on the abdomen.

III. Interventions to monitor for sequelae of increased intracranial pressure.
  A. Monitor blood pressure for widening pulse pressure; pulse for decrease in rate; and respirations for changes in rate, pattern, or effort.
  B. Assess for changes in levels of consciousness with each client contact.
  C. Monitor for sensory or motor changes—changes in visual acuity, pupil reactions, verbal expression, decrease in muscle strength, coordination, and movement.
  D. Assess for presence of associated symptoms such as nausea, vomiting, and headache.

IV. Interventions to enhance adaptation and rehabilitation.
  A. Assist client and family to set realistic goals to maintain optimal activity and self-care levels within limitations imposed by disease.
  B. Assist client and family to assess physical environment in acute care setting and home and make appropriate changes to promote safety:
    1. Encourage having major living area on ground level in home.
    2. Remove scatter rugs from floors.
    3. Encourage use of rubber-soled, tie-on shoes and assistive devices as needed.

4. Orient client to time and place as needed.
C. Refer to appropriate supportive services:
1. Physical therapy for activity program and use of assistive devices.
2. Social services for support, financial evaluation, and community services.

EVALUATION OF CLIENT AND FAMILY OUTCOMES

I. Identify signs and symptoms of increased intracranial pressure to report to health care team.

II. Participate in strategies to maximize safety for the client within the acute care setting and at home.

III. Participate in decision making regarding treatment and subsequent care needs.

IV. Describe community resources available for rehabilitation or support.

Spinal Cord Compression

THEORY

I. Pathophysiology.
   A. Spinal cord is a cylindrical body of nervous tissue that occupies the upper two thirds of the vertebral canal.
   B. Spinal cord has motor, sensory, and autonomic functions.
   C. Compression of the spinal cord may occur as a result of tumor invasion of the vertebrae and subsequent collapse on the spinal cord; tumor invasion of the spinal canal and resulting increased pressure; or primary tumors of the spinal cord.
   D. Compression of the spinal cord can result in minor changes in motor, sensory, and autonomic function to complete paralysis (see Chapter 36).

II. Principles of medical management.
   A. Diagnostic tests:
      1. Spinal x-ray examinations—show bone abnormalities or soft-tissue masses but do not indicate epidural metastases.
      2. Bone scan—identifies metastases to vertebral bodies.
      3. Myelogram—used as standard test for diagnosis and location of epidural cord compression.
      4. CT scan and MRI.
   B. Nonpharmacological interventions:
      1. Radiation therapy:
         a. Used as most common treatment for epidural metastases and cord compression.
         b. Used alone when no evidence of spinal instability and tumor is known to be radiosensitive.
         c. Given over several weeks to a total dose of 3000 to 4000 rads.
      2. Surgery:
         a. Used if tumor is not responsive to radiation therapy.
         b. Used if recurrent tumor is in an area previously treated with radiation therapy.
         c. Used to decompress area by laminectomy or resection of a vertebral body.
      3. Surgery followed by radiation therapy.
   C. Pharmacological interventions:
      1. Steroids:
         a. Reduce spinal cord edema and pain.
         b. May have oncolytic effect on certain tumors.

2. Antineoplastic agents:
   a. Used as an adjuvant treatment to radiation and/or surgery for tumors responsive to antineoplastics such as lymphomas, germ cell tumors, and neuroblastoma.
   b. Used if recurrence of tumor occurs at a site of previous surgery or radiation therapy.
   c. Used as treatment of choice in children and infants since radiation therapy can inhibit growth.
3. Analgesics—more than 95% of patients with spinal cord compression have pain (see Chapter 7).

DATA COLLECTION

I. Identification of clients at risk.
   A. Cancers that have a natural history for metastasizing to the bone—breast, lung, prostate, kidney, and myeloma.
   B. Cancers that metastasize to the spinal cord—lymphoma, seminoma, and neuroblastoma.
   C. Primary cancers of the spinal cord—ependymoma, astrocytoma, and glioma.

II. Pertinent history.
   A. Type of primary tumor.
   B. Time since onset of symptoms, and level and degree of compression.

III. Physical examination—presenting signs and symptoms vary with the location and severity of the compression.
   A. Early signs and symptoms:
      1. Neck or back pain.
      2. Motor weakness or dysfunction.
      3. Loss of sensation for light touch, pain, or temperature.
      4. Sexual impotence.
   B. Late signs and symptoms:
      1. Loss of sensation for deep pressure and position.
      2. Incontinence or retention of urine or stool.
      3. Paralysis.
      4. Muscle atrophy.

ASSOCIATED NURSING DIAGNOSES

I. Alteration in comfort: pain.

II. Impaired physical mobility.

III. Alteration in sensory perception.

IV. Alteration in bowel and bladder elimination.

V. Sexual dysfunction.

VI. Potential impaired skin integrity.

NURSING PLANNING AND IMPLEMENTATION

I. Interventions to maximize safety for the client.
   A. Mobilize client according to findings of stable or unstable spine (Table 8-1).
   B. Instruct client and family to assess pressure and temperature of objects coming in contact with areas of compromised feeling or sensation of the client.

Table 8-1
MOBILITY INTERVENTIONS

Unstable Spine	Stable Spine
Place sandbags on either side of the head to limit movement.	Initiate range-of-motion exercises after physical therapy evaluation and with a physician order.
Use cervical collar to support cervical spine.	Instruct client/family in isometric exercises.
Support head and neck during all movement.	Provide personal assistance with ambulation.
Use no pillows.	Instruct client/family in use of assistive devices with ambulation.
Maintain alignment when turning or positioning.	Maintain proper alignment while in bed, turning, or positioning.
Use a log roll, pull sheet, or transfer board when turning or positioning.	
Place client on special bed as indicated: Stryker frame or circoelectric bed.	

II. Interventions to decrease the severity of symptoms associated with spinal cord compression.
    A. Assist client to positions of comfort with maintenance of proper body alignment.
    B. Institute nonpharmacological methods of pain control (see Chapter 7).
    C. Institute a bowel and bladder program (Table 8-2).

III. Interventions to monitor for sequlae of spinal cord compression or treatment.
    A. Monitor for progression of motor or sensory deficits every 8 hours (Table 8-3):
        1. Decrease in muscle strength.
        2. Decrease in coordination.
        3. Decrease in perception of temperature, touch, and position.
    B. Monitor bowel and bladder elimination patterns and effectiveness:
        1. Record intake and output every 8 hours.
        2. Palpate for bladder distention if interval between voiding increases.
        3. Record frequency and characteristics of stool with each bowel movement.
        4. Conduct gentle digital rectal examination to check for impaction if no bowel movement within 3 days.
    C. Assess changes in location, character, and associated aggravating and alleviating factors of pain.

IV. Interventions to enhance adaptation and rehabilitation.
    A. Inform client and family of changes in the condition of the client.
    B. Initiate a consult with physical and occupational therapy as soon as spine has been stabilized.
    C. Assist client to maintain a safe level of independence within the limitations imposed by the cord compression.
    D. Encourage client and family to express concerns about the effect of residual limitations on activities of daily living and life-style.

EVALUATION OF CLIENT AND FAMILY OUTCOMES

    I. Lists signs and symptoms that should be reported to the health care team—changes in bowel or bladder patterns, characteristics of pain, sensory and motor function, skin integrity, or sexual function.

    II. Describes strategies to minimize sequelae of spinal cord compression and treatment.

Table 8-2
ELEMENTS OF A BOWEL AND BLADDER PROGRAM

Bowel Program	**Bladder Program**
Provide high-fiber diet: 15–30 g of fiber/day.	Include foods in diet to maintain urinary pH of less than 7.
Offer oral intake of 3000 ml fluid/day.	
Use bedside commode or toilet for all bowel movements.	Avoid foods that produce alkaline urine such as citrus fruits.
Schedule bowel movement at same time each day.	Schedule times for voiding—every 2-3 hr.
Offer a hot drink 30 min before scheduled bowel movement.	Palpate bladder after voiding to evaluate retention.
Use stool softeners such as mineral oil or dioctyl sodium sulfosuccinate (DSS).	Monitor fluid intake.
	Decrease fluid intake after 7:00 PM.
Monitor for signs and symptoms of fecal impaction.	Monitor for signs and symptoms of urinary tract infection.
If laxatives are needed:	*If catheterization is needed:*
Use stimulant to defecation such as a glycerin suppository.	Teach client/family intermittent self-catheterization.
Use chemical stimulant such as bisacodyl (Dulcolax), castor oil, senna concentrate (Senokot), or cascara.	

Table 8-3
ASSESSMENT OF MOTOR AND SENSORY FUNCTIONS

Function	**Assessment Techniques**
Muscle strength	Upper extremities: ask client to grip your finger as firmly as possible. Lower extremities: ask client to resist plantar flexion of his/her feet.
Coordination of hands and feet	Ask client to touch each finger to his/her thumb in rapid sequence. Ask client to turn hand over and back as quickly as possible. Ask client to tap your hand as quickly as possible with the ball of each foot.
Sensory perception	Touch client along length of extremities and trunk with the blunt and sharp end of a safety pin and ask client to identify as either "sharp" or "dull." Ask client to report the sensation of touch when touched with a wisp of cotton. Move one of the client's fingers and ask if the finger is being moved up or down. Touch skin of client with test tube of hot water and then cold water; ask the client to describe the temperature.

III. Participates in rehabilitation program designed to assist client and family to adapt to residual limitations associated with spinal cord compression.

IV. Identifies community resources available for assistance and support.

Superior Vena Cava Syndrome

THEORY

I. Pathophysiology.
   A. The superior vena cava (SVC) is a thin-walled major vessel that carries venous drainage from the head, neck, upper extremities, and the upper thorax to the heart.
   B. The SVC is located in the mediastinum and is surrounded by the rigid structures of the sternum, trachea, and vertebrae and the aorta, right bronchus, lymph nodes, and pulmonary artery.
   C. The SVC is a low-pressure vessel that is easily compressed; compression can occur from direct tumor invasion, enlarged lymph nodes, or a thrombus within the vessel.
   D. When obstruction of the SVC occurs, venous return to the heart from the head, neck, thorax, and upper extremities is impaired:
      1. Venous pressure increases.
      2. Cardiac output decreases.

II. Principles of medical management.
   A. Goals of treatment include treatment of the underlying cause and of presenting symptoms.
   B. Treatment and prognosis are determined by the histological diagnosis of the primary tumor.
   C. Diagnostic tests:
      1. Chest x-ray examination—positive findings associated with superior vena cava syndrome (SVCS) include mass, pleural effusion, and mediastinal widening.
      2. CT scan.
      3. Additional tests to determine the histological diagnosis of the primary condition—bronchoscopy, bone marrow biopsy, mediastinoscopy, thoracentesis, sputum specimen, and needle biopsy of palpable lymph nodes.
   D. Nonpharmacological interventions:
      1. Radiation therapy—the primary treatment for SVCS if client has non-small cell cancer of the lung or a histological diagnosis cannot be made.
      2. Removal of central venous catheter in catheter-induced SVCS if the thrombus cannot be lysed with urokinase or streptokinase.
   E. Pharmacological interventions:
      1. Antineoplastic therapy alone in clients who have had previous mediastinal radiation therapy.
      2. Antineoplastic therapy in conjunction with radiation therapy.
      3. Steroids.
      4. Diuretics.
      5. Thrombolytic therapy.

DATA COLLECTION

I. Identification of clients at risk.
   A. Presence of lymphoma involving the mediastinum, germ cell tumors, cancers of the lung and breast, and Kaposi's sarcoma.

B. Presence of central venous catheters and pacemakers.

C. Previous radiation therapy to the mediastinum.

D. Associated conditions such as histoplasmosis, benign tumors, and aortic aneurysm.

II. Physical examination.

A. Early signs and symptoms of SVCS:
1. Facial swelling upon arising in the morning.
2. Redness and edema in conjunctivae and around the eyes.
3. Swelling of the neck and arms.
4. Neck and thoracic vein distention.
5. Dyspnea.
6. Nonproductive cough.
7. Hoarseness.
8. Cyanosis.
9. Stridor.

B. Late signs and symptoms of SVCS:
1. Headache.
2. Irritability.
3. Visual disturbances.
4. Dizziness.
5. Changes in mental status.

III. Evaluation of laboratory data—assess available laboratory data against previous and normal values for arterial blood gases, electrolytes, kidney function, CBC, and coagulation studies.

ASSOCIATED NURSING DIAGNOSES

I. Ineffective airway clearance.

II. Decreased cardiac output.

III. Alteration in tissue perfusion.

IV. Anxiety.

NURSING PLANNING AND IMPLEMENTATION

I. Interventions to maximize safety for the client.

A. Provide for environmental safety—bed in low position, side rails up, and call light and personal items within reach.

B. Avoid venipunctures, intravenous fluid administration, or measurement of blood pressure in the upper extremities.

C. Take blood pressure in lower extremities.

D. Assist client with ambulation as needed.

E. Remove rings and restrictive clothing.

II. Interventions to decrease severity of symptoms associated with SVCS.

A. Elevate head of bed to decrease dyspnea.

B. Instruct client to avoid Valsalva maneuver or other activities that cause straining.

C. Apply pressure to sites of invasive procedures in the upper body.

D. Space care activities to decrease energy expenditure.

E. Maintain lower extremities in a dependent position.

F. Explain care procedures in clear, simple terms to decrease anxiety.

G. Reassure client that close monitoring will occur.

H. Encourage client to ask questions about care measures and/or changes in condition.

III. Interventions to monitor for sequelae of SVCS or treatment.
   A. Assess for progressive respiratory distress:
      1. Increased respiratory rate with stridor.
      2. Increased anxiety.
      3. Presence of adventitious breath sounds.
      4. Increased subjective complaints of difficulty breathing.
   B. Monitor for signs of progressive edema:
      1. Increased swelling in face, arms, or neck.
      2. Increased venous distention of neck or thorax.
   C. Monitor for changes in tissue perfusion:
      1. Decreased or absent peripheral pulses.
      2. Decrease in blood pressure—systolic pressure less than 90 mm Hg.
      3. Pale or cyanotic skin of the face, extremities, or nail beds.
   D. Assess for changes in neurological/mental status:
      1. Decrease in orientation to person, place, and time.
      2. Increased confusion.
      3. Presence of lethargy.
      4. Increased dizziness or blurred vision.
      5. Increase in severity of headaches.
   E. Monitor for signs and symptoms of anticoagulant therapy—petechiae, ecchymoses, bleeding of gums, nose, urinary tract, or gastrointestinal system.
   F. Monitor for signs and symptoms of steroid therapy—weakness of involuntary muscles, mood swings, steroid-induced glycosuria, dyspepsia, or insomnia.

IV. Interventions to enhance adaptation and rehabilitation from SVCS.
   A. Reassure client that changes in physical appearance will subside as SVCS resolves.
   B. Assist client to plan activities that include continued treatment of disease and management of possible side effects of treatment.
   C. Explain changes in status to client and family after each assessment.

EVALUATION OF CLIENT AND FAMILY OUTCOMES

   I. Identify critical signs and symptoms to report to the health care team.

   II. Describe plans for continued follow-up care.

   III. Participate in decision making about care, discharge planning, and life activities.

   IV. Identify community resources and services for assistance and support.

Cardiac Tamponade

THEORY

   I. Pathophysiology.
      A. The pericardium is a two-layered sac surrounding the heart.
         1. The space between the two layers is the pericardial cavity.
         2. The cavity normally is filled with 50 ml of fluid.
      B. An increase in the intrapericardiac pressure may occur due to:
         1. Fluid accumulation in the pericardial sac.
         2. Direct or metastatic tumor invasion to the pericardial sac.
         3. Fibrosis of the pericardial sac related to radiation therapy.
      C. As intrapericardiac pressure increases:
         1. Left ventricular filling decreases.
         2. The ability of the heart to pump decreases.

3. Cardiac output decreases.
4. Impaired systemic perfusion occurs.

II. Principles of medical management.
   A. Diagnostic tests:
      1. Chest x-ray examination—enlarged pericardial silhouette.
      2. CT scan—pleural effusion, masses, or pericardial thickening.
      3. Echocardiography (ECHO)—most precise diagnostic test; two echoes are seen with tamponade.
      4. Electrocardiography (ECG)—tachycardia, premature contractions, and electrical alternans.
      5. Pericardiocentesis and cytology of fluid:
         a. Bloody fluid associated with positive cytology.
         b. Cytology has a significant false-negative rate.
   B. Nonpharmacological interventions:
      1. Pericardiocentesis—temporary removal of excess pericardial fluid.
      2. Pericardial window—surgical opening of the pericardium to allow fluid drainage.
      3. Total pericardectomy—removal of the pericardial sac for clients with constrictive or chronic pericarditis.
      4. Radiation therapy—radiation to radiosensitive tumors of the pericardium; contraindicated in radiation pericarditis.
   C. Pharmacological interventions:
      1. Pericardial sclerosis—instillation through a pericardial catheter of chemicals (tetracycline, thiotepa, nitrogen mustard, 5-fluorouracil [5-FU], causing inflammation and subsequent fibrosis.
      2. Systemic antineoplastic therapy—treatment of primary tumor may be associated with a pericardiocentesis.
      3. Corticosteroids—temporary reduction of inflammation of constrictive pericarditis.

DATA COLLECTION

I. Identification of clients at risk.
   A. Clients with cancers of the lung, breast, and gastrointestinal tract, leukemia, Hodgkin's or nonHodgkin's lymphoma, sarcoma, or melanoma.
   B. Clients who have received more than 4000 rads of radiation to a field in which the heart is included.

II. Physical examination.
   A. Early signs and symptoms:
      1. Retrosternal chest pain relieved by leaning forward and intensified when lying supine.
      2. Dyspnea.
      3. Cough.
      4. Muffled heart sounds.
      5. Weak or absent apical pulse.
      6. Anxiety and agitation.
      7. Hiccups.
   B. Late signs and symptoms:
      1. Tachycardia.
      2. Tachypnea.
      3. Decreased systolic pressure and rising diastolic pressure (narrowing pulse pressure).

4. Pulsus paradox greater than 10 mm Hg.
5. Increased central venous pressure (CVP).
6. Altered levels of consciousness.
7. Oliguria.
8. Peripheral edema.

III. Evaluation of laboratory data—review laboratory data and compare to previous values and normal parameters.
   A. Arterial blood gas (ABG) values.
   B. Electrolyte values.

ASSOCIATED NURSING DIAGNOSES

 I. Decreased cardiac output.

 II. Ineffective breathing pattern.

III. Alteration in tissue perfusion.

IV. Alteration in comfort: pain.

 V. Anxiety.

NURSING PLANNING AND IMPLEMENTATION

 I. Interventions to maximize safety for the client.
   A. Assist client with activities of daily living and ambulation as needed.
   B. Keep bed in low position and with side rails up.

 II. Interventions to decrease severity of symptoms associated with cardiac tamponade.
   A. Elevate head of bed to position of comfort to minimize shortness of breath.
   B. Monitor response to oxygen therapy as ordered by physician.
   C. Institute nonpharmacological measures to relieve pain (see Chapter 7).
   D. Plan care activities to minimize energy expenditure and allow for rest periods.
   E. Explain procedures to client and family to decrease anxiety.

III. Interventions to monitor for sequelae of cardiac tamponade.
   A. Monitor blood pressure, pulse, respirations for narrowing pulse pressure, paradoxical pulse, arrhythmias, and respiratory distress.
   B. Maintain an accurate intake and output record.
   C. Assess level of consciousness for changes in behavior, orientation, and awareness.
   D. Monitor subjective complaints of the client about pain and shortness of breath.
   E. Assess character and amount of drainage from pericardial catheter, if present.
   F. Assess catheter site for signs and symptoms of infection.
   G. Evaluate extremities for peripheral edema.

IV. Interventions to enhance adaptation and rehabilitation.
   A. Encourage client and family to communicate concerns about condition and treatment to a member of the health care team.
   B. Include client and family in planning and implementation of care if health status permits and participation is not stressful to client and family.

EVALUATION OF CLIENT AND FAMILY OUTCOMES

 I. Identify signs and symptoms to be reported to the health care team.

 II. Describe the effects of cardiac tamponade or treatment on activities of daily living and life-style.

III. Discuss need and plans for continued follow-up.

IV. Identify community resources available for assistance and support.

V. List strategies to minimize effects of treatment on health status and life-style.

BIBLIOGRAPHY

Bell, D.R., Woods, R.L., & Levi, J.A. (1986). Superior vena caval obstruction: a 10-year experience. *Med J Aust 145*(11-12), 566-568.

Buzaid, A.C., Garewal, H.S., & Greenberg, B.R. (1989). Managing malignant pericardial effusion. *West J Med 150*(2), 174-179.

Carpenito, L.J. (1989). *Nursing Diagnosis: Application to Clinical Practice* (3rd ed). Philadelphia: J.B. Lippincott Co.

Chernecky, C.C. & Ramsey, P.W. (1984). *Critical Nursing Care of the Client With Cancer*. Norwalk, Conn: Appleton-Century-Crofts, pp. 81-94.

Delaney, T.F. & Oldfield, E.H. (1989). Spinal cord compression. In V.T. DeVita, Jr., S. Hellman, S.A. Rosenberg (eds). *Cancer: Principles & Practice of Oncology* (3rd ed), Philadelphia: J.B. Lippincott Co., pp. 1978-1985.

Dietz, K.A. & Flaherty, A.M. (1990). Oncologic emergencies. In S.L. Groenwald, M.H. Frogge, M. Goodman, & C.H. Yarbro (eds). *Cancer Nursing Principles and Practice* (2nd ed). Boston: Jones & Bartlett, pp. 644-668.

Donoghue, M. (1983). Spinal cord compression. In J.M. Yasko (ed). *Guidelines for Cancer Care: Symptom Management*, Reston, Va: Reston Publishing Co. pp. 353-357.

Gilkey S. & Reyes, C.V. (1985). Cardiac tamponade in lung cancer. *J Surg Oncol 28*(4), 301-303.

Gribbin, M.E. (1990). Could you detect these oncological crises? *RN 53*(6), 36-42.

Hiller, G. (1987). Cardiac tamponade in the oncology patient. *Focus Crit Care 14*(4), 19-23.

Kalia, S. & Tintinalli, J.E. (1984). Emergency evaluation of the cancer patient. *Ann Emerg Med 13*(9), 723-730.

Levin, V.A., Sheline, G.E., & Gutin, P.H. (1989). Neoplasms of the central nervous system. In V.T. DeVita, Jr., S. Helman, & S.A. Rosenberg (eds). *Cancer: Principles & Practice of Oncology* (3rd ed), Philadelphia: J.B. Lippincott Co., pp. 1557-1611.

Longmore, W. (1986). Cardiopulmonary emergencies in cancer. *Top Emerg Med 8*(2), 25-43.

Miaskowski, C. (1991). Oncologic emergencies. In S.B. Baird, R. McCorkle & M. Grant (eds). *Cancer Nursing: A Comprehensive Textbook*. Philadelphia: W.B. Saunders Co., pp. 885-893.

Nieto, A.F. & Doty, D.B. (1986). Superior vena cava obstruction: clinical syndrome, etiology, and treatment. *Curr Probl Cancer 10*(9), 441-484.

Pass, H.I. (1989). Treatment of malignant pleural and pericardial effusions. In V.T. DeVita, Jr., S. Hellman, S.A. Rosenberg (eds). *Cancer Principles & Practice of Oncology,* (3rd ed). Philadelphia: J.B. Lippincott Co., pp. 2317-2327.

Schenk, E. (1985). The patient with neurologic problems: increased intracranial pressure. In B.C. Long & W.J. Phipps (eds). *Essentials of Medical-Surgical Nursing: A Nursing Process Approach*. St. Louis: C.V. Mosby Co. pp. 371-376.

Sculier, J.P. & Feld, R. (1985). Superior vena cava obstruction syndrome: Recommendations for management. *Cancer Treat Rev 12*(3), 209-218.

Walsh-Essig, E., Farley, H.F., & Wyper, M.A. (1985). The patient with cardiovascular problems. In B.C. Long & W.S. Phipps (eds). *Essentials of Medical-Surgical Nursing: a Nursing Process Approach*. St. Louis: C.V. Mosby Co. pp. 679-686.

Yahalom, J. (1989). Superior vena cava syndrome. In V.T. DeVita, Jr., S. Hellman, & S.A. Rosenberg (eds). *Cancer: Principles & Practice of Oncology* (3rd ed). Philadelphia: J.B. Lippincott Co., pp. 1971-1977.

9

Nursing Care of Patients with Metabolic and Physiological Oncological Emergencies

Joanne Peter Finley, MS, RN

Disseminated Intravascular Coagulation

THEORY

I. Hemostasis is maintained through a balanced system of thrombosis and fibrinolysis (Figure 9-1).
   A. The process of thrombosis is initiated through disruption of the endothelial membrane and/or tissue injury.
      1. Disruption of the endothelial membrane activates a cascade of clotting factors in the intrinsic pathway, resulting in coagulation.
      2. Tissue injury causes the release of tissue thromboplastin into the circulation and the activation of the extrinsic pathway, resulting in coagulation.
      3. Reactions that occur in the intrinsic and extrinsic pathways of coagulation are combined in a final common pathway.
   B. Fibrinolysis, the process by which the reactions that result in clotting are inhibited and developed clots are destroyed, is initiated by the formation of the fibrin clot.
      1. Plasmin is an enzyme that digests the components of the clot.
      2. The products of this reaction, fibrin-split products (FSPs) or fibrin-degradation products (FDPs), are released into the circulation and function as anticoagulants.
      3. FDPs are gradually cleared from the circulation in the reticuloendothelial system (RES).

II. Pathophysiology
   A. Definition of disseminated intravascular coagulation (DIC): the inappropriate, accelerated, and systematic activation of the coagulation cascade, resulting in simultaneous hemorrhage and thrombosis.
   B. In the presence of an underlying condition such as infection, malignancy, or trauma, the intrinsic and/or extrinsic pathway of the clotting cascade is triggered,

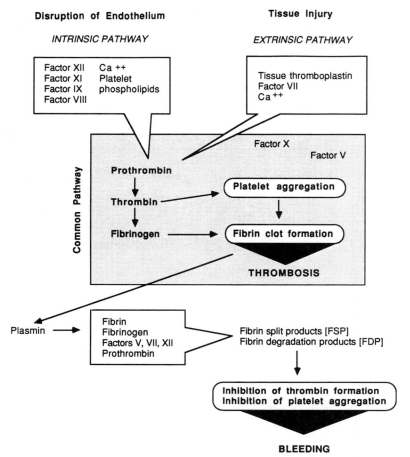

Figure 9-1 Physiology of thrombosis and fibrinolysis.

thrombosis is accelerated, and fibrin clots are formed and deposited in the microcirculation.

C. The consumption of coagulation factors is greater than the ability of the body for replacement; therefore coagulation is inhibited.

D. In addition, fibrinolysis is initiated; FDPs are not removed effectively from the circulation, and an accumulation of anticoagulant substances occurs.

III. Principles of medical management.

A. Diagnostic tests (Table 9-1).

B. Medical management of DIC is targeted to treatment of the underlying, predisposing condition(s); replacement of coagulation factors and platelets; and inhibition of the coagulation process:

1. Treatment of the underlying, predisposing condition such as chemotherapy for malignancy or antibiotics for infection.

2. Replacement of coagulation factors and platelets.

a. Blood component therapy for abnormal hematological parameters or active bleeding (see Chapter 26):

(1) Cryoprecipitate provides fibrinogen and factor VIII.

(2) Platelets.

(3) Fresh frozen plasma provides plasma, fibrinogen, and other clotting

Table 9-1
LABORATORY RESULTS WITH DISSEMINATED INTRAVASCULAR COAGULATION

Laboratory Test	Findings
Prothrombin time (PT)	Increased
Partial thromboplastin time	Increased
Thrombin time	Increased
Fibrinogen	Decreased
Platelet count	Decreased
Fibrin-split products	Increased
Hematocrit/hemoglobin	Decreased

factors; use of fresh frozen plasma may aggravate DIC since clotting factors are present.
   (4) Red blood cells.
   b. Plasmapheresis to replace coagulation factors.
   3. Inhibition of the coagulation or fibrinolytic process.
      a. Plasmapheresis removes triggers of coagulation.
      b. Acetylsalicylic acid (ASA) prevents clotting.
      c. Heparin interferes with thrombin production:
         (1) Use is considered controversial except in acute progranulocytic leukemia (APL).
         (2) Goal is to maintain partial thromboplastin time (PTT) at 1½ to 2 times normal levels.
         (3) Primary side effect is bleeding.
      d. ε-Aminocaproic acid (EACA) inhibits fibrinolysis:
         (1) Usually given with heparin.
         (2) Primary side effect is clotting.
      e. Antithrombin III inhibits procoagulants and fibrinolytic process.

DATA COLLECTION
   I. Identification of clients at risk.
      A. History of cancer—prostate, breast, colon, or leukemia.
      B. History of cancer treatment—surgery, radiation, and chemotherapy.
      C. Trauma, burns, or shock.
      D. Infection and sepsis.
      E. Pregnancy and obstetrical complications.
      F. Presence of liver disease.
      G. Recent blood transfusion or hemolytic transfusion reaction.

   II. Physical examination.
      A. Skin—petechiae, ecchymosis, purpura, acral cyanosis (gray coloration of feet, palms, cheeks, and ears), pallor, and bleeding from sites of invasive procedures.
      B. Gastrointestinal—abdominal distention, decreased bowel sounds, and positive guaiac stool test.
      C. Genitourinary—hematuria and decreased urinary output.
      D. Respiratory—dyspnea, hemoptysis, and tachypnea.

E. Neurological—restlessness, confusion, and lethargy.
F. Musculoskeletal—joint pain, stiffness, and positive Homans' sign.
G. Cardiovascular—tachycardia and diminished peripheral pulses

III. Evaluation of laboratory data (see Table 9-1).

ASSOCIATED NURSING DIAGNOSES
I. Altered tissue perfusion.

II. Impaired skin integrity.

III. Potential for injury.

IV. Alteration in comfort.

NURSING PLANNING AND IMPLEMENTATION
I. Interventions to maximize safety for the client.
   A. Place bed in low position and side rails up.
   B. Clear pathways in room and hallways.
   C. Provide assistance as needed for activities of daily living.

II. Interventions to decrease severity of symptoms associated with DIC.
   A. Apply direct pressure to sites of active bleeding.
   B. Elevate sites of active bleeding if possible.
   C. Apply pressure dressings or sandbags to sites of active bleeding.

III. Interventions to monitor for sequelae of DIC and treatment.
   A. Monitor for signs and symptoms of progressive DIC:
      1. Tachycardia, hypotension, and cool, clammy, cyanotic skin.
      2. Anuria.
      3. Decreased mental status to coma.
      4. Changes in location, severity, or responses to pain.
      5. Changes in the depth, rate, or difficulty of respirations.
   B. Monitor for signs and symptoms of fluid overload.

IV. Interventions to monitor response of client to medical management.
   A. Monitor sites and amount of bleeding:
      1. Weigh dressings.
      2. Count peripads.
      3. Measure bloody drainage.
      4. Hematest urine, stool, and emesis.
   B. Monitor changes in laboratory values and report significant changes to physician.
   C. Assess tissue perfusion parameters—color, temperature, peripheral pulses.
   D. Monitor psychosocial responses of client and family to critical illness.

V. Interventions to enhance adaptation and rehabilitation.
   A. Provide information about planned therapy and response to treatment at regular intervals.
   B. Listen to concerns and fears of client and family.

VI. Interventions to incorporate client and family in care.
   A. Instruct client and family about critical signs and symptoms to report to health care team—new sites of bleeding, changes in color of stool or urine, subjective changes in respiratory effort and effectiveness, and changes in mental status.
   B. Instruct client and family to save all urine, stool, and emesis.
   C. Instruct client and family in measures to prevent bleeding.

EVALUATION OF CLIENT AND FAMILY OUTCOMES

I. Identify personal risk factors for development of DIC.

II. List critical signs and symptoms of DIC that should be reported immediately to the health care team.

III. Describe self-care measures to maximize personal safety.

Septic Shock

THEORY

I. Pathophysiology.
   A. Septicemia is a systemic response to pathogenic microorganisms and associated endotoxins in the blood.
   B. Septic shock is manifested by hemodynamic instability and alterations in cellular metabolism caused by septicemia (Figure 9-2).

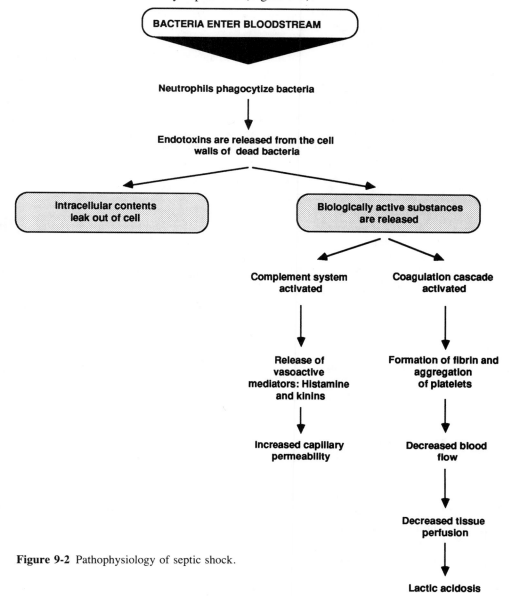

Figure 9-2 Pathophysiology of septic shock.

C. Gram-negative bacteria (*Escherchia coli, Klebsiella pneumoniae,* and *Pseudomonas aeruginosa*) are the most common cause of sepsis.
D. Other organisms include fungi (*Candida* and *Aspergillus*), gram-positive bacteria, anaerobes, viruses, and protozoa.
E. Most infections arise from endogenous flora of the client.
F. Untreated bacteremia in neutropenia clients is fatal; septic shock is associated with a 50% to 70% mortality rate.
G. Mortality is associated with causative organism, site of infection, and the level and duration of neutropenia.

II. Principles of medical management.
   A. Diagnostic tests:
      1. Blood culture—aerobic and anaerobic.
      2. Chest x-ray examination.
      3. Cultures of urine, throat, stool, sputum, and central venous catheters.
      4. Complete blood count.
      5. Prothrombin time (PT)/PTT.
      6. Arterial blood gas values.
   B. Nonpharmacological interventions:
      1. Fluid resuscitation—crystalloids (normal saline solution or lactated Ringer's solution) and colloids (albumin).
      2. Blood component therapy:
         a. Red blood cells.
         b. Granulocyte transfusions may be used if fever persists after broad-spectrum antibiotic and antifungal therapy when prolonged neutropenia is expected.
         c. Therapeutic benefit of granulocyte transfusions is controversial.
      3. Oxygen therapy progressing to ventilatory support as needed.
      4. Central catheter or implantable port removal.
   C. Pharmacological interventions:
      1. Empiric antibiotics for first fever spike in neutropenia clients.
      2. If fever persists after 3- to 5-day course of antibiotics, antifungal therapy (amphotericin) may be initiated; rigors are major side effect.
      3. Steroids.
      4. Naloxone-opiate antagonist—inhibits β-endorphins and transiently increases blood pressure.
      5. Dopamine—vasopressor that increases cardiac contractility, peripheral vascular resistance, and renal blood flow.

DATA COLLECTION
I. Identification of clients at risk.
   A. Neutropenia less than 1000 cells/mm^3.
   B. Age greater than 65 years.
   C. Prosthetic devices such as multilumen catheters, feeding tubes, and tracheostomy tubes.
   D. Malnutrition.
   E. Loss of skin or mucosal integrity.

II. Pertinent history.
   A. Recent chemotherapy, radiation therapy, or steroid therapy.
   B. Diagnosis of cancer such as leukemia, lymphoma, and multiple myeloma.
   C. Chronic disease such as diabetes mellitus and hepatic or renal disease.
   D. Splenectomy.
   E. Recent hospitalization.

III. Physical examination.
   A. Early signs and symptoms:
      1. Typical signs and symptoms of infection may be absent.
      2. Earliest signs—anxiety, restlessness, confusion, and decreased level of consciousness.
      3. Tachypnea, rales, rhonchi, and wheezes.
      4. Tachycardia and widening pulse pressure.
      5. Warm, flushed skin.
      6. Chills and fever.
      7. Anorexia.
   B. Late signs and symptoms:
      1. Disorientation and lethargy.
      2. Dyspnea, cyanosis, and increased pulmonary congestion.
      3. Tachycardia, thready pulse, and narrowing pulse pressure.
      4. Cool, clammy skin.
      5. Decreased or absent urinary output.

IV. Evaluation of laboratory data.
   A. Positive blood cultures.
   B. Decreased white blood cell count.
   C. Pulmonary infiltrates seen on chest x-ray examination.
   D. Prolonged PT and PTT.
   E. Elevated blood urea nitrogen (BUN) and creatinine levels.
   F. Respiratory alkalosis followed by metabolic acidosis.

ASSOCIATED NURSING DIAGNOSES

I. Alteration in tissue perfusion.

II. Fluid volume deficit.

III. Decreased cardiac output.

IV. Potential for injury.

V. Alteration in comfort.

VI. Hyperthermia.

NURSING PLANNING AND IMPLEMENTATION

I. Interventions to maximize safety for the client.
   A. Assess environment for safety—bed in low position and side rails up.
   B. Orient client to time, place, and person.
   C. Maintain infection control measures—handwashing, oral care, perineal care, limitation of invasive procedures, and care of invasive equipment.

II. Interventions to decrease the severity of symptoms associated with septic shock.
   A. Report early signs and symptoms of septic shock to physician immediately.
   B. Obtain critical elements of diagnostic workup as ordered with a limited time frame.
   C. Initiate antibiotic or antifungal therapy immediately after ordered.
   D. Encourage client to turn, cough, and deep breathe to mobilize pulmonary secretions.
   E. Explain procedures, treatments, monitoring activities, and significance of changes in condition to decrease anxiety.

III. Interventions to monitor for sequelae of septic shock.
   A. Monitor vital signs (pulse, blood pressure, and respirations) at intervals dictated by clinical condition.
   B. Assess skin color, temperature, and capillary refill.
   C. Monitor intake and output.
   D. Weigh client each day.
   E. Assess potential sites of infection and obtain order for cultures of suspicious areas.
   F. Assess peripheral pulses.
   G. Monitor for signs and symptoms of complications of septic shock—DIC, adult respiratory distress syndrome.

IV. Interventions to monitor response to medical management.
   A. Monitor vital signs every 4 hours or more often as clinically indicated; report significant changes in vital signs (marked decrease in temperature, blood pressure, or pulse pressure or marked increase in pulse or respiratory rate) to physician.
   B. Monitor changes in laboratory values and report significant changes (growth in cultures, increase in white blood count) to physician.
   C. Monitor for signs and symptoms of fluid overload.

V. Interventions to enhance adaptation and rehabilitation.
   A. Maintain bedrest for acutely ill client.
   B. Organize care activities to minimize energy expenditure and oxygen consumption.
   C. Encourage range of motion and isometric exercises.
   D. Reinforce principles of infection prevention and control in preparation for discharge.

EVALUATION OF CLIENT AND FAMILY OUTCOMES
   I. Describe personal risk factors for septic shock.

   II. List critical signs and symptoms of septic shock that should be reported to a member of the health care team.

   III. Discuss strategies to decrease the risks of septic shock.

Tumor Lysis Syndrome

THEORY
   I. Pathophysiology.
   A. Tumor lysis syndrome is a metabolic imbalance that occurs with the rapid release of intracellular potassium, phosphorus, and nucleic acid into the blood as a result of tumor cell kill (Figure 9-3).
   B. The syndrome includes:
      1. Hyperkalemia.
      2. Hyperphosphatemia.
      3. Hyperuricemia—results from conversion of nucleic acid to uric acid.
      4. Hypocalcemia—results from increased phosphorus binding to calcium to form calcium phosphate salts.

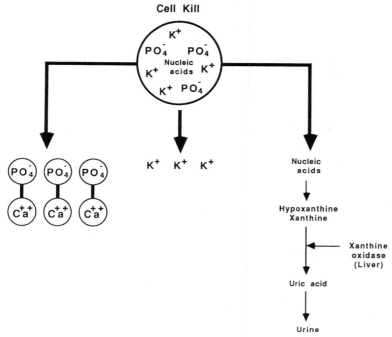

Figure 9-3 Metabolic consequences of cell death.

C. Potential effects of tumor lysis syndrome include:
  1. Renal failure—kidneys are the primary route of elimination for phosphorus, uric acid, and potassium.
  2. Cardiac arrhythmias.

II. Principles of medical management.
  A. Diagnostic tests:
    1. Serum electrolytes (potassium, phosphorus, and calcium) and uric acid.
    2. Renal function studies—BUN and creatinine.
    3. Electrocardiography (ECG).
  B. Nonpharmacological interventions:
    1. Intravenous hydration.
    2. Hemapheresis.
    3. Dialysis.
    4. Potassium and phosphorus restrictions.
  C. Pharmacological interventions:
    1. Allopurinol:
      a. Blocks xanthine oxidase to decrease uric acid production.
      b. Potential side effects—rash, fever, gastrointestinal upset, and diarrhea.
    2. Diuretics:
      a. Maintains urinary output.
      b. Potential side effects—dehydration.
      c. Usually maintained for 3 to 5 days after chemotherapy begins.
    3. Aluminum hydroxide:
      a. Binds dietary phosphate from small bowel.
      b. Potentail side effect—constipation.

4. Exchange resins such as sodium polystyrene sulfonate (Kayexalate):
   a. Decrease potassium levels.
   b. Potential side effects—hypokalemia, hypocalcemia, hypomagnesia, and constipation.
5. Sodium bicarbonate—alkalinizes urine.

DATA COLLECTION
I. Identification of clients at risk.
   A. Diagnosis of leukemia, lymphoma, or small-cell lung cancer.
   B. Diagnosis of tumors with a high growth fraction.
   C. Recent chemotherapy or radiation therapy for cancer.
   D. Concurrent renal or cardiac disease.

II. Physical examination.
   A. Early signs and symptoms:
      1. Neuromuscular—muscle weakness, twitching, paresthesia, lethargy, confusion, and fatigue.
      2. Cardiovascular—arrhythmias and bradycardia.
      3. Gastrointestinal—nausea, vomiting, and anorexia.
      4. Renal—oliguria, flank pain, hematuria, weight gain, and edema.
   B. Late signs and symptoms:
      1. Seizures.
      2. Cardiac arrest.
      3. Acute renal failure.

III. Evaluation of laboratory data.
   A. Elevated BUN and serum creatinine levels.
   B. Elevated potassium and phosphorus levels.
   C. Decreased calcium and creatinine clearance.
   D. Elevated uric acid level.

ASSOCIATED NURSING DIAGNOSES
I. Potential for injury.
II. Self-care deficit.
III. Decreased cardiac output.
IV. Fluid volume excess.
V. Altered nutrition: less than body requirements.

NURSING PLANNING AND IMPLEMENTATION
I. Interventions to maximize safety for the client.
   A. Recognize clients at risk before initiation of treatment.
   B. Institute safety measures for changes in level of consciousness:
      1. Maintain bed in low position with side rails up.
      2. Place call light within reach.
      3. Evaluate client at regular intervals.
   C. Institute seizure precautions as electrolyte levels warrant.
   D. Place emergency equipment within access if severe hyperkalemia or hypocalcemia present.

II. Interventions to decrease incidence and severity of symptoms associated with tumor lysis syndrome.

A. Teach client and family about strategies to decrease the incidence of tumor lysis syndrome:
   1. Maintain adequate oral fluid intake.
   2. Take allopurinol as ordered by physician.
   3. Report signs and symptoms of tumor lysis syndrome to health care team.
B. Notify physician if pH of urine is less than 7.0.
C. Consult with dietician to modify diet if renal dysfunction is present.

III. Interventions to monitor for sequelae of tumor lysis syndrome or treatment.
   A. Assess for symptoms of cardiac arrhythmias:
      1. Decrease in blood pressure.
      2. Increase in pulse rate.
      3. Irregular pulse.
      4. Chest pain.
      5. Shortness of breath.
   B. Assess for symptoms of renal failure:
      1. Decrease in urinary output to less than 600 ml/day.
      2. Changes in mental status.
      3. Anorexia, nausea, and vomiting.
      4. Diarrhea.
      5. Increase in weight.
   C. Assess for side effects of treatment (see section, "Pharmacological Interventions").

EVALUATION OF CLIENT AND FAMILY OUTCOMES

I. Describe personal risk factors for tumor lysis syndrome.

II. Participate in strategies to decrease the risk and severity of tumor lysis syndrome.

III. Describe signs and symptoms of tumor lysis syndrome or side effects of treatment to report to the health care team.

IV. Identify emergency resources in the community.

Anaphylaxis

THEORY

I. Pathophysiology.
   A. Anaphylaxis is an immediate hypersensitivity reaction that usually occurs within seconds to minutes.
   B. Immediate hypersensitivity reactions are mediated by immunoglobulin E (IgE), which is produced by B lymphocytes (Figure 9-4).
   C. The antigen-specific IgE binds to mast cells and sensitizes them to the antigen.
   D. On subsequent exposure of the sensitized mast cell to the antigen, a series of reactions occur that result in degranulation of the mast cell and release of mediators of the hypersensitivity reaction (Table 9-2).
   E. Signs and symptoms of the immediate hypersensitivity reaction are a result of the effects of the mediators on target organs of the skin, lung, and gastrointestinal tract.

II. Principles of medical management.
   A. Diagnostic tests:
      1. Allergy skin tests.
      2. Test dose of agents:

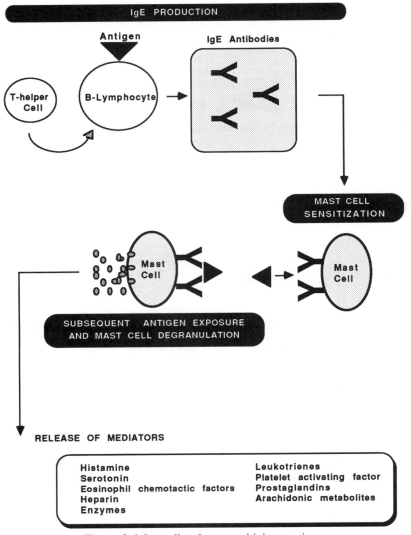

Figure 9-4 Immediate hypersensitivity reaction.

       a. Administer small dose of agent that may cause anaphylaxis.
       b. Keep line open if agent given intravenously.
       c. Monitor for signs and symptoms of anaphylaxis (see section, "Physical Examination").
       d. If no reaction occurs, administer total dose as ordered by physician.
  B. Nonpharmacological interventions:
    1. Intravenous fluid replacement.
    2. Oxygen therapy.
    3. Maintenance of patent airway:
       a. Intubation.
       b. Emergency tracheostomy if upper airway edema occurs.
    4. Hemodynamic monitoring.
  C. Pharmacological interventions:
    1. Prophylaxis—diphenhydramine, prednisone, and cimetidine.
    2. Emergency agents (Table 9-3).

Table 9-2
MEDIATORS OF THE IMMEDIATE HYPERSENSITIVITY REACTION

Mediator	Action
Histamine	Contraction of smooth muscle Increased permeability of vessels Modulation of chemotaxis and prostaglandins
Serotonin	Contraction of smooth muscle Increased permeability of vessels
Eosinophil chemotactic factors	Attraction and deactivation of eosinophils and neutrophils
Heparin	Anticoagulation
Enzymes	Proteolysis, hydrolysis, and cleavage
Leukotrienes	Contraction of smooth muscle Increased permeability of vessels Modulation of histamine, prostaglandins, and chemotaxis
Platelet activating factor	Promotion of platelet aggregation and adhesion
Prostaglandins and arachidonic metabolites	Contraction and relaxation of smooth muscle Chemotaxis

Table 9-3
PHARMACOLOGICAL AGENTS USED TO TREAT ANAPHYLAXIS

Agent	Results of Action	Nursing Implications
Epinephrine	Elevates blood pressure Dilates bronchi Constricts peripheral vessels Decreases itching	Monitor pulse rate, rhythm, and regularity.
Diphenhydramine	Decreases itching Blocks histamine actions	Monitor for sudden decrease in blood pressure. Encourage oral hygiene practices for dry mouth. Teach client about safety issues associated with drowsiness.
Hydrocortisone	Prevents delayed symptoms Inhibits synthesis of mediators of immune response	Take medication with food. Report signs and symptoms of gastrointestinal distress to physician.
Cimetidine	Decreases laryngeal edema	Monitor for marked decrease in blood pressure.
Aminophylline	Dilates bronchi	Monitor pulse rate, rhythm, and regularity.

DATA COLLECTION

I. Identification of clients at risk.
   A. Receiving antineoplastic agents such as L-asparaginase, bleomycin, or cisplatin.
   B. Risk for anaphylaxis increases when agents are:
      1. Crude preparations of the agent such as those used in phase I studies.
      2. Derived from bacteria such as L-asparaginase.
      3. Given intravenously.
      4. Given at high doses.
      5. Given in successive doses.
   C. Previous exposure to agent.
   D. Previous allergic reactions to agents such as foods, radiographic contrast media, blood products, insulin, and opiates.

II. Physical examination.
   A. Early signs and symptoms usually occur within 30 minutes:
      1. Integumentary—pruritus, urticaria, erythema, and angioedema.
      2. Cardiovascular—tightness in chest, flushing, dizziness, and warmth.
      3. Gastrointestinal—nausea, vomiting, diarrhea, and abdominal discomfort.
      4. Respiratory—dyspnea.
      5. Neurological—anxiety, feeling of doom, and agitation.
   B. Late signs and symptoms:
      1. Cardiovascular—hypotension, tachycardia, chest pain, and arrhythmias.
      2. Respiratory—laryngeal edema, bronchospasm, and stridor.

III. Evaluation of laboratory data.
   A. Arterial blood gas values.
   B. IgE antibody level.

ASSOCIATED NURSING DIAGNOSES

I. Alteration in comfort.

II. Anxiety.

III. Decreased cardiac output.

IV. Fluid volume deficit.

NURSING PLANNING AND IMPLEMENTATION

I. Interventions to maximize safety for the client.
   A. Have emergency agents and equipment within reach during administration of high-risk agents.
   B. Maintain free-flowing intravenous infusion when administering a potential allergen.
   C. Obtain baseline vital signs.
   D. Label medical record with allergy history.
   E. Remain with client for 30 minutes after administering agent.
   F. If a reaction occurs, ask client to remain in bed, put bed in low position, and raise side rails.

II. Interventions to decrease severity of symptoms associated with anaphylaxis.
   A. At first sign of reaction:
      1. Stop flow of agent.
      2. Maintain intravenous infusion according to institutional protocol.
      3. Evaluate patency of airway, pulse, respirations, and blood pressure.
      4. Notify physician of signs and symptoms observed and actions taken.

     5. Administer emergency drugs (see Table 9-3) as ordered by physician or per institutional protocol.
  B. Position client to decrease respiratory distress symptoms (elevate head of bed).
  C. Position client to maintain blood pressure (Trendelenburg) unless contraindicated by respiratory distress.

III. Interventions to monitor for sequelae of anaphylaxis or treatment.
  A. Observe for symptoms of respiratory distress:
    1. Increase in respiratory rate, rhythm, and effort.
    2. Presence of adventitious breath sounds.
    3. Changes in arterial blood gas values as ordered by physician.
  B. Observe for signs of fluid overload:
    1. Changes in weight greater than 5 pounds per day.
    2. Changes in intake and output ratio.
    3. Jugular neck vein distention.
  C. Observe for signs of anxiety:
    1. Remain with client during acute reaction.
    2. Be calm and confident while implementing emergency procedures.
    3. Explain the process and rationale for each procedure.
  D. Check for impaired skin integrity:
    1. Clip nails to decrease risk of scratching skin surfaces.
    2. Decrease pressure, friction, and sheering forces on skin surfaces.
    3. Encourage client to avoid scratching skin surfaces.

EVALUATION OF CLIENT AND FAMILY OUTCOMES

  I. Identify personal risk factors for anaphylactic reaction.

 II. Describe signs and symptoms of anaphylaxis to report to the health care team— itching, hives, difficulty breathing, and anxiety.

III. Participate in strategies to decrease risk or severity of anaphylaxis:
  A. Avoid allergen.
  B. Inform care providers of allergy.
  C. Maintain emergency kit in environment in which potential exposure to an allergen may occur.
  D. Wear medic-alert jewelry.

IV. List the location and telephone numbers of available community emergency services.

Hypercalcemia

THEORY

  I. Pathophysiology.
  A. Normal levels of calcium are regulated by the action of the parathyroid gland (production of parathyroid hormone), gastrointestinal tract (absorption of vitamin D), and the kidneys (excretion) (Figure 9-5).
    1. When calcium levels fall below normal, the parathyroid gland is stimulated to produce parathyroid hormone.
    2. Parathyroid hormone acts on the bone, a reservoir for calcium, and causes an increase in the amount of calcium released from the bone into the circulation and ultimately the extracellular fluid.
    3. When calcium levels rise above normal, the kidney increases excretion of calcium to return the level to normal.

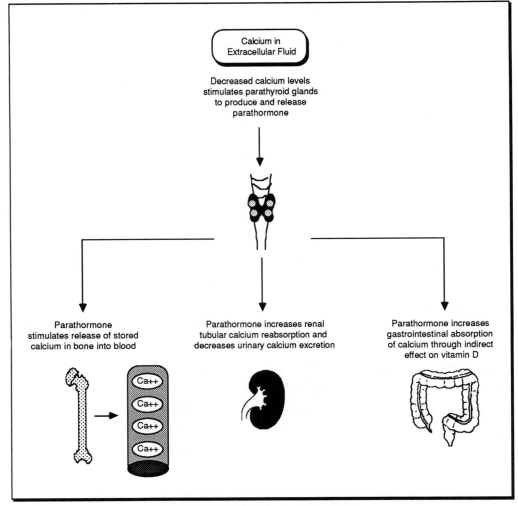

Figure 9-5 Regulation of calcium levels.

   B. Hypercalcemia is defined as a serum calcium level greater than 11 mg/dl.
   C. Potential causes of hypercalcemia among persons with cancer include:
      1. Increased bone resorption secondary to osteoclast activity stimulated by the tumor.
      2. Increased bone resorption secondary to direct tumor invasion of the bone.
      3. Decreased ability of the kidneys to clear calcium from the blood.
      4. Increased calcium absorption from the gut.
   D. Hypercalcemia occurs in 10% to 20% of persons with cancer and is the most common oncological emergency.

  II. Principles of medical management.
   A. Diagnostic tests:
      1. Serum and urine calcium.
      2. Serum potassium, sodium, and phosphorus.
      3. BUN and creatinine.
      4. ECG.

B. Nonpharmacological interventions:
  1. Administer intravenous fluids:
    a. Restore hydration.
    b. Increase the glomerular filtration rate.
    c. Treatment of choice for temporary improvement of symptoms.
  2. Maintain mobility.
  3. Provide dialysis—provides rapid, temporary relief.

Table 9-4
PHARMACOLOGICAL INTERVENTIONS FOR HYPERCALCEMIA

Agent	Action	Nursing Considerations
Furosemide	Blocks calcium reabsorption Inhibits sodium absorption	Monitor for signs of dehydration. Monitor for signs of hypokalemia. Weigh client daily.
Prednisone	Inhibits bone resorption	Assess for signs of hyperglycemia. Evaluate gastrointestinal symptoms. Weigh client daily.
Calcitonin	Inhibits bone resorption	Monitor for gastrointestinal symptoms—nausea and vomiting. Evaluate for signs and symptoms of allergic reaction.
Etidronate disodium	Inhibits bone resorption	Evaluate renal function studies as ordered by physician. Monitor for gastrointestinal symptoms.
Mithramycin	Inhibits bone resorption	Monitor for decrease in blood pressure. Assess for signs and symptoms of thrombocytopenia. Evaluate renal and hepatic function studies as ordered by physician. Use extravasation precautions with administration.
Indomethacin	Inhibits prostaglandin synthesis	Monitor for gastrointestinal symptoms—nausea, pain, bleeding, and vomiting. Evaluate renal function studies as ordered by physician. Monitor intake and output ratio. Evaluate central nervous system reactions—depression, headache, or increase in seizure activity or Parkinson's symptoms.
Phosphates	Inhibits bone resorption Limits calcium absorption from gut Promotes soft-tissue and skeletal calcification	Monitor for gastrointestinal symptoms—nausea, vomiting, and diarrhea. Evaluate for signs of hypocalcemia. Monitor for a decrease in blood pressure. Evaluate renal function studies as ordered by physician. Monitor intake and output ratio. Monitor character of urine.

C. Pharmacological interventions:
1. Administer antineoplastic therapy for primary and metastatic tumor.
2. Administer drugs to lower serum calcium (Table 9-4).
3. Discontinue agents that contribute to hypercalcemia—thiazide diuretics, estrogen therapy.

DATA COLLECTION

I. Identification of clients at risk.
A. Diagnosis of breast, lung, renal, head, or neck cancer (80%).
B. Diagnosis of multiple myeloma, lymphoma, and leukemia (20%).
C. Primary hyperparathyroidism.
D. Immobility.
E. Dehydration.
F. Renal dysfunction.
G. Skeletal fractures.
H. History of thiazide diuretic, lithium, and estrogen therapy.
I. Age.

II. Physical examination—symptomatology related to the calcium level and the rapidity of onset.
A. Early signs and symptoms:
1. Cardiovascular—bradycardia, arrhythmias, and increased digitalis sensitivity.
2. Neuromuscular—fatigue, weakness, hyporeflexia, bone pain, lethargy, confusion, apathy, and personality changes.
3. Gastrointestinal—anorexia, constipation, nausea, and vomiting.
4. Renal—weight loss, renal calculi, polydipsia, and polyuria.
B. Late signs and symptoms:
1. Cardiovascular—heart block and cardiac arrest.
2. Neuromuscular—stupor and coma.
3. Gastrointestinal—ileus.
4. Renal—renal failure.

III. Evaluation of laboratory data.
A. Elevated serum calcium level (normal range, 8.5 to 10.5 ml/dl)

Corrected serum calcium =
Measured serum calcium + (4.0 − serum albumin value) × 0.8

B. Decreased serum potassium, sodium, and phosphorus.
C. Elevated BUN and creatinine levels.
D. ECG changes:
1. Arrhythmias.
2. Shortened QT interval.
3. Broadened T wave.
4. Increased PR interval.

ASSOCIATED NURSING DIAGNOSES

I. Alteration in bowel elimination: constipation.

II. Altered thought process.

III. Potential for injury.

IV. Alteration in comfort: pain.

V. Self-care deficit.

VI. Impaired physical mobility.

NURSING PLANNING AND IMPLEMENTATION
 I. Interventions to maximize safety for the client.
   A. Maintain bed in low position with side rails up for clients with changes in mental status.
   B. Place call light within reach.
   C. Encourage client to use assistive personnel or devices with ambulation.
   D. Use transfer devices and strategies for immobile clients to decrease risk of pathological fractures.

 II. Interventions to decrease the incidence and severity of symptoms associated with hypercalcemia.
   A. Maintain level of mobility consistent with disease status and presenting symptoms:
     1. Full range of activity with assistive personnel or devices.
     2. Active range-of-motion exercises.
     3. Passive range-of-motion exercises.
     4. Weight-bearing activities such as standing at the bedside.
     5. Isometric exercises.
     6. Footboard.
   B. Implement measures to control pain (see Chapter 7).
   C. Encourage oral fluid intake.
   D. Modify diet—avoid excessive intake of calcium, vitamin D, vitamin A, and retinoids.
   E. Recommend discontinuance of multivitamin preparations and antacids.

 III. Interventions to monitor for sequelae of hypercalcemia or treatment (see Table 9-4).
   A. Evaluate changes in character of pulse—decreased rate and irregular rhythm.
   B. Assess renal function—monitor intake and output, character of urine, laboratory tests as ordered by the physician, and daily weights.
   C. Evaluate changes in the character of pain—location, severity, aggravating and alleviating factors, and affect on activities of daily living.

EVALUATION OF CLIENT AND FAMILY OUTCOMES
 I. Identify personal risk factors for hypercalcemia.

 II. Describe signs and symptoms of hypercalcemia to report to the health care team—bone pain, changes in mental status or personality, nausea, and vomiting.

 III. Participate in strategies to decrease the risk or severity of hypercalcemia.

 IV. Describe community resources available for emergency care.

Inappropriate Antidiuretic Hormone Secretion (SIADH)
THEORY
 I. Pathophysiology.
   A. Antidiuretic hormone (ADH) is released normally from the posterior pituitary in response to:
     1. Increased plasma osmolality.
     2. Decreased plasma volume.

B. ADH acts on the distal renal tubules and collecting ducts to increase permeability and thus increase water reabsorption.

C. Excess production or stimulation of ADH results in excessive water retention and dilutional hyponatremia.

II. Principles of medical management.

   A. Diagnostic tests:

     1. Decreased serum sodium.

     2. Decreased serum osmolality.

     3. Increased urinary sodium.

     4. Increased urinary osmolality.

   B. Nonpharmacological interventions:

     1. Fluid restriction (800 to 1000 ml/day):

       a. Used for mild to moderate SIADH (sodium level greater than 125 mg).

       b. Corrects elevated sodium level over 7 to 10 days.

       c. Not recommended treatment for clients with chronic SIADH or severe symptoms.

     2. Hypotonic saline solution:

       a. Used for severe SIADH.

       b. Normal saline solution (3% to 5%) infused intravenously over 2 to 3 hours.

       c. Furosemide usually is given concurrently to increase fluid excretion.

   C. Pharmacological interventions:

     1. Treat underlying pathology such as cancer or infection.

     2. Discontinue agents contributing to SIADH such as morphine, diuretics, or antidepressants.

     3. Administer other medications (Table 9-5).

DATA COLLECTION

I. Identification of clients at risk.

   A. Diagnosis of cancer of the lung, pancreas, duodenum, prostate, or brain or Hodgkin's disease.

Table 9-5
PHARMACOLOGICAL AGENTS USED TO TREAT SIADH

Agent	Action	Nursing Implications
Demeclocycline	Interferes with antidiuretic hormone (ADH) action on tubules	Avoid offering medication with meals. Assess female clients for pregnancy. Assess clients for history of liver disease. Monitor urinary output. Monitor for complaints of nausea or episodes of vomiting. Teach clients to use sun glasses, sunscreen, long-sleeved clothing, hats, and avoidance of sun to decrease risks of photosensitivity. Monitor for symptoms of diabetes insipidus.
Lithium	Interferes with ADH action	Monitor for complaints of nausea, vomiting, and anorexia. Assess neurological status—presence of tremors or weakness. Assess cardiac status—pulse rate, regularity.
Urea	Causes osmotic diuresis	Monitor for complications of nausea, vomiting, and anorexia.

    B. Presence of pulmonary infections—pneumonia, abcesses, or tuberculosis.

    C. History of trauma, infection, or lesions of the central nervous system.

    D. History of previous cancer therapy.

    E. Treatment with cyclophosphamide, vincristine, cisplatin, thiazide diuretics, morphine, or antidepressants.

    F. Concurrent cardiac, renal, or hepatic diseases.

    G. Severe pain.

    H. Stress.

    I. Fear.

II. Physical examination.

    A. Early signs and symptoms:

      1. Constitutional—weakness and fatigue.

      2. Neurological—confusion, irritability, weakness, headache, lethargy, and altered mental status.

      3. Gastrointestinal—nausea, vomiting, diarrhea, anorexia, thirst, and abdominal cramping.

      4. Renal—decreased urinary output and weight gain.

      5. Muscular—myalgias and muscle cramping.

    B. Late signs and symptoms:

      1. Progressive lethargy to coma.

      2. Seizure activity.

III. Evaluation of laboratory data.

    A. Serum sodium less than 130 mEq/L.

    B. Serum osmolality less than 280 mOsm/kg of water.

    C. Urinary sodium greater than 20 mEq/L.

    D. Urinary osmolality greater than 1400 mOsm/L.

    E. BUN and creatinine levels within normal ranges.

    F. Hypouricemia.

ASSOCIATED NURSING DIAGNOSES

  I. Fluid volume excess.

  II. Altered thought process.

  III. Potential for injury.

  IV. Altered nutrition: less than body requirements.

  V. Alteration in comfort: pain.

NURSING PLANNING AND IMPLEMENTATION

  I. Interventions to maximize safety for the client.

    A. Bed in low position and side rails up.

    B. Call light and personal items within reach.

    C. Assistance with activities of daily living as needed.

    D. Bed check device if client is confused.

    E. Use of rate regulator for intravenous infusions.

  II. Interventions to decrease the severity of symptoms associated with SIADH.

    A. Thirst:

      1. Assist client to divide amount of fluids between day, evening, and night hours.

      2. Offer sugarfree candy or gum to stimulate salivation.

Table 9-6
SEIZURE PRECAUTIONS

Remain with patient.

Alter environment to promote safety.

Loosen tight clothing.

Turn head to side.

Monitor for respiratory distress.

Monitor for another seizure before complete recovery from previous seizure.

    3. Rinse mouth with water every 2 hours.
    4. Monitor intravenous fluid intake.
  B. Neurological changes:
    1. Orient to person, time, and place as needed.
    2. Use environmental cues such as calendars and clocks.
    3. Implement seizure precautions (Table 9-6).

III. Interventions to monitor for sequelae of SIADH or treatment.
  A. Observe for fluid overload:
    1. Weigh client daily.
    2. Maintain strict intake and output records.
    3. Test urine for specific gravity.
  B. Monitor for electrolyte abnormalities:
    1. Monitor vital signs.
    2. Evaluate for changes in mental status.
    3. Assess for signs and symptoms of hypokalemia.
    4. Assess for signs and symptoms of hyponatremia.
    5. Monitor laboratory data (electrolyte values and osmolality of serum and urine) as ordered by physician.
  C. Monitor for side effects of pharmacological therapy (see Table 9-5).

EVALUATION OF CLIENT AND FAMILY OUTCOMES

  I. Discuss personal risk factors for SIADH.

  II. Participate in measures to decrease the severity of symptoms associated with SIADH.

  III. Describe signs and symptoms to report to the health care team—weight gain greater than 5 pounds in 1 day; decrease in urinary output to less than 60 ml/hour; mental status changes; nausea; or any seizure activity.

  IV. Demonstrate self-care skills related to monitoring and treatment of SIADH—measuring urinary output; administering medications; and weighing.

  V. List community resources available for emergency care.

BIBLIOGRAPHY
Bajorunas, D.R. (1990). Clinical manifestations of cancer-related hypercalcemia. *Semin Oncol 17*(2, suppl 5), 16-25.
Barry, S.A. (1989). Septic shock: special needs of patients with cancer. *Oncol Nurs Forum 16*(1), 31-35.
Bick, R.L. (1988). Disseminated intravascular coagulation and related syndromes: a clinical review. *Semin Thromb Hemost 14*(4), 299-338.

Bodey, G.P. (1986). Infection in cancer patients. A continuing association. *Am J Med 81*(1A), 11-26.

Bonner, J.R. (1988). Anaphylaxis. Part I. Etiology and pathogenesis. *Ala J Med Sci 25*(3), 283-287.

Bonner, J.R. (1988). Anaphylaxis. Part II. Prevention and treatment. *Ala J Med Sci 25*(4), 408-411.

Carr, M.E., Jr. (1987). Disseminated intravascular coagulation: pathogenesis, diagnosis, and therapy. *J Emerg Med 5*(4), 311-322.

Chernecky, C.C., Ramsey, P.W., & Kline P.M. (1984). *Critical Nursing Care of the Client With Cancer*. Norwalk, Conn: Appleton-Century-Crofts.

Coward, D.D. (1986). Cancer-induced hypercalcemia. *Cancer Nurs 9*(3), 125-132.

Coward, D.D. (1988). Hypercalcemia knowledge assessment in patients at risk of developing cancer-induced hypercalcemia. *Oncol Nurs Forum 15*(4), 471-476.

Craig, J.B. & Capizzi, R.L. (1985). The prevention and treatment of immediate hypersensitivity reactions from cancer chemotherapy. *Semin Oncol Nurs 1*(4), 285-291.

DeVita, V.T., Jr., Hellman, S., Rosenberg, S.A. (eds). (1989). *Cancer: Principles & Practice of Oncology* (3rd ed). Philadelphia: J.B. Lippincott Co.

Dickerson, M. (1988). Anaphylaxis and anaphylactic shock. *Crit Care Nurs Q 11*(1), 68-74.

Dietz, K.A. & Flaherty, A.M. (1990). Oncologic emergencies. In S.L. Groenwald, M.H. Frogge, M. Goodman & C.H. Yarbro (eds). *Cancer Nursing: Principles and Practice*. Boston: Jones & Bartlett Publishers, pp. 644-668.

Dunlay, R.W., Camp, M.A., Alion, M., Fanti, P., Malluche, H.H., & Liach, F. (1989). Calcitriol in prolonged hypocalcemia due to the tumor lysis syndrome. *Ann Intern Med 110*(2), 162-164.

Ellerhorst-Ryan, J.M. (1985). Complications of the myeloproliferative system: infection and sepsis. *Semin Oncol Nurs 1*(4), 244-250.

Gerson, S.L. & Lazarus, H.M. (1989). Hematopoietic emergencies. *Semin Oncol 16*(6), 532-542.

Hartnett, S. (1989). Septic shock in the oncology patient. *Cancer Nurs 12*(4), 191-201.

Hughes, C. (1987). Tumor lysis syndrome: a serious complication of chemotherapy. Implications for the IV nurse. *NITA 10*(2), 112-114.

Kim, M.J., McFarland, G.K., & McLane, A.M. (eds). (1989). *Pocket Guide to Nursing Diagnoses* (3rd ed). St. Louis: C.V. Mosby Co.

Kinzie, B.J. (1987). Management of the syndrome of inappropriate secretion of antidiuretic hormone. *Clin Pharm 6*(8), 625-633.

Larcan, A., Lambert, H., & Gerard, A. (1987). *Consumption Coagulopathies*. New York: Masson Publishing.

Lazarus, H.M., Creger, R.J., & Gerson, S.L. (1989). Infectious emergencies in oncology patients. *Semin Oncol 16*(6), 543-560.

Lind, J.M. (1985). Ectopic hormonal production: nursing implications. *Semin Oncol Nurs 1*(4), 251-258.

Litt, M.R., Bell W.R., & Lepor, H.A. (1987). Disseminated intravascular coagulation in prostatic carcinoma reversed by ketoconazole. *JAMA 258*(10), 1361-1362.

Littleton, M.T. (1988). Pathophysiology and assessment of sepsis and septic shock. *Crit Care Nurs 11*(1), 30-47.

Mahon, S.M. (1989). Signs and symptoms associated with malignancy-induced hypercalcemia. *Cancer Nurs 12*(3), 153-160.

Mathewson, M.K. (1986). Antidiuretic hormone. *Crit Care Nurs 6*(5), 88-93.

Meriney, D.K. (1990). Diagnosis and management of acute promyelocytic leukemia with disseminated intravascular coagulopathy: a case study. *Oncol Nurs Forum 17*(3), 379-383.

Miaskowski, C. (1991). Oncologic emergencies. In S.B. Baird, R. McCorkle, & M. Grant (eds). *Cancer Nursing: A Comprehensive Textbook*. Philadelphia: W.B. Saunders Co., pp. 885-893.

Miyagawa, C.I. (1986). The pharmacologic management of the syndrome of inappropriate secretion of antidiuretic hormone. *Drug Intell Clin Pharm 20*(7-8), 527-531.

Mundy, G.R. & Yates, A.J.P. (1989). Recent advances in pathophysiology and treatment of hypercalcemia of malignancy. *Am J Kidney Dis 14*(1), 2-12.

Nace, C.S. & Nace, G.S. (1985). Acute tumor lysis syndrome: pathophysiology and nursing management. *Crit Care Nurs 5*(3), 26-34.

Patterson, L.M. & Norolan, E.L. (1989). Diabetes insipidus versus syndrome of inappropriate antidiuretic hormone. *Dimens Crit Care Nurs 8*(4), 226-234.

Poe, C.M. & Taylor, L.M. (1989). Syndrome of inappropriate antidiuretic hormone: assessment and nursing implications. *Oncol Nurs Forum 16*(3), 373-381.

Randall, B.J. (1986). Reacting to anaphylaxis. *Nursing 16*(3), 34-40.

Ratnoff, O.D. (1989). Hemostatic emergencies in malignancy. *Semin Oncol 16*(6), 561-571.

Reinhart, K. & Eyrich, K. (eds). (1989). *Sepsis. An Interdisciplinary Challenge*. New York: Springer-Verlag.

Ritch, P.S. (1990). Treatment of cancer-related hypercalcemia. *Semin Oncol 17*(2, suppl 5), 26-33.

Sathe, S. & Weinstein, M.P. (1987). Etiology, diagnosis, and treatment of bacteremia. *Compr Ther 13*(2), 24-31.

Schneider, S.M. & Distelhorst, C.W. (1989). Chemotherapy-induced emergencies. *Semin Oncol 16*(6), 572-578.

Schulmeister, L. (1989). Developing guidelines for bleomycin test dosing. *Oncol Nurs Forum 16*(2), 205-207.

Siegrist, C.W. & Jones, J.A. (1985). Disseminated intravascular coagulopathy and nursing implications. *Semin Oncol Nurs 1*(4), 237-243.

Silverman, P. & Distelhorst, C.W. (1989). Metabolic emergencies in clinical oncology. *Semin Oncol 16*(6), 504-515.

Singer, F.R. (1990). Role of the bisphosphonate etidronate in the therapy of cancer-related hypercalcemia. *Semin Oncol 17*(2, suppl 5), 34-39.

Sparano, J., Ramirez, M., & Wiernik, P.H. (1990). Increasing recognition of corticosteroid-induced tumor lysis syndrome in non-Hodgkin's lymphoma. *Cancer 65*(5), 1072-1073.

Stafford, C.T. (1989). Life-threatening allergic reactions. Anticipating and preparing the best defenses. *Postgrad Med 86*(1), 232-242, 245.

Stuckey, P. & Waters, H. (1988). Oncology alert for the home care nurse: syndrome of inappropriate antidiuretic hormone. *Home Healthcare Nurse 6*(6), 26-30.

Suchak, B.A. & Barbon, C.B. (1989). Disseminated intravascular coagulation: a nursing challenge. *Orthop Nurs 8*(6), 61-69.

Ulrich, S.P., Canale, S.W., & Wendell S.A. (1990). *Nursing Care Planning Guides: A Nursing Diagnosis Approach* (2nd ed). Philadelphia: W.B. Saunders Co.

Waters, H.F. & Stuckey, P.A. (1988). Oncology alert for the home care nurse: hypercalcemia. *Home Healthcare Nurse 6*(1), 32-36.

Issues and Trends in Cancer Care

Sociodemographic and Attitudinal Changes Affecting Cancer Care

Jennifer S. Webster, MN, MPH, RN, OCN

I. Sociodemographic changes in incidence.
   A. Deaths caused by lung cancer continue to rise.
      1. Supportive and explanatory data:
         a. Lung cancer death is the primary cause of cancer mortality in men and women in the United States.
         b. Since 1940 age-adjusted lung cancer death rates in men have increased from 11 per 100,000 population to 73 per 100,000 in 1982; presently the trend is leveling at approximately 74 per 100,000.
         c. Since 1960 age-adjusted lung cancer death rates in women have risen from 6 per 100,000 population to 28 per 100,000 (Figure 10-1).
         d. Smoking causes 85% of lung cancer deaths in men and 75% of lung cancer deaths in women:
            (1) Men began smoking decades before women smoked and smoked more heavily, thus accounting for the difference in mortality rates.
            (2) The gap between men and women smokers has narrowed since the 1950s (Figure 10-2).
            (3) The 20-year latency period between starting to smoke and the development of lung cancer explains the steady increase in lung cancer in women since the 1970s.
         e. In 1987 lung cancer surpassed breast cancer as the leading cause of cancer mortality in women.
         f. Lung cancer is preventable; 83% of all lung cancers would be eliminated if people did not smoke.
         g. Exposure to sidestream smoke (passive smoking) increases the risk of lung cancer and other respiratory diseases in nonsmokers.
         h. Informational and legislative changes have influenced cigarette consumption (Figure 10-3).
         i. In the past 20 years the per capita cigarette consumption has gradually declined, particularly in men (Figure 10-3).
         j. Lung cancer mortality rates in men should start to decline in the 1990s because of the 20-year latency period between starting to smoke and the development of lung cancer.

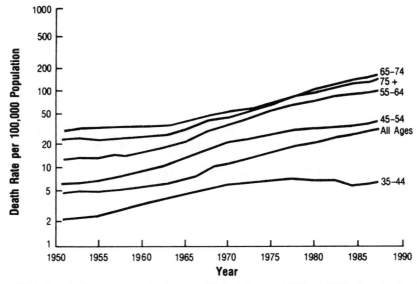

Figure 10-1 Female lung cancer death rates, United States, 1950 to 1987. Standardized on the age distribution of the population of the United States, 1970. *(From Garfinkel, L. & Silverberg, E. [1991]. Lung cancer and smoking trends in the United States over the past 25 years. CA 41,[3], 138.)*

2. Nursing implications:
   a. Target young people and nonsmokers for educational programs to decrease the initiation of tobacco use.
   b. Increase tobacco use cessation via educational and support programs targeted toward smokers.

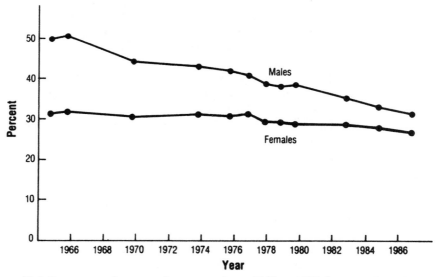

Figure 10-2 Percentage of current cigarette smokers, 1965 to 1987, by sex. *(From Department of Health and Human Services [1989]. Reducing the Health Consequences of Smoking: 25 years of progress. A report of the Surgeon General. DHHS Publication No. [CDC] 89-8411, Washington, D.C.: The Department.)*

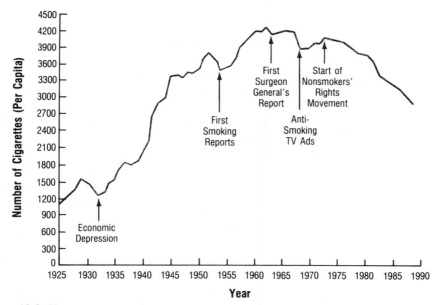

Figure 10-3 Cigarette consumption per capita, age 18 and older, United States, 1925 to 1989. *(From Garfinkel, L. & Silverberg, E. [1991]. Lung cancer and smoking trends in the United States over the past 25 years.* CA 41[3], *140.)*

    c. Support legislative changes that restrict the advertising, distribution, and use of tobacco products.

    d. Propose and support local community initiatives to restrict tobacco use in the workplace and public settings.

    e. Act as role models for clients and the public.

B. Aging U.S. population increases cancer incidence and mortality rates.

    1. Supportive and explanatory data:

        a. From 1950 to 1980 the elderly population increased more rapidly than the population as a whole, and this trend is continuing.

        b. By the year 2030 approximately 20% of the U.S. population will be 65 years or older.

        c. Age is the greatest risk factor for developing cancer; 50% of all cancers occur after age 65; 60% of all cancer deaths occur after age 65.

        d. The most common cancers in the elderly are colorectal, prostate (men), lung cancer, and breast cancer (women):

           (1) Advances in treatment have increased survival rates and decreased mortality rates for childhood cancer and low-incident malignancies (leukemia, Hodgkin's disease, testicular cancer) but have had minimal influence on the cancers most common in the elderly.

           (2) Incidence rates for breast cancer have increased 3% per year since 1980.

           (3) More than 80% of prostatic tumors occur in men over age 65.

    2. Nursing implications:

        a. Target the elderly for education and prevention services.

        b. Be well informed about particular problems and care of the elderly.

        c. Offer and encourage screening of the asymptomatic elderly for breast, colorectal, and prostate cancer to enhance early detection and treatment.

      d. Support increased funding of Medicare to cover cancer screening in the elderly.

      e. Continue to initiate and apply research about prevention, early detection, and coping behaviors of the elderly with cancer and explore factors that motivate or act as barriers to cancer screening.

      f. Create educational materials suitable for the changes in sensorium that may accompany aging.

  C. The socioeconomically disadvantaged continue to have higher cancer incidence rates and lower survival rates than the total U.S. population.

    1. Supportive and explanatory data:

      a. Overall 5-year cancer survival rate of poor Americans is an estimated 10% to 15% lower than that of non-poor Americans; at least half the difference in survival among poor people is attributed to late diagnosis.

      b. Differences in survival rates were historically based on race:

        (1) Studies conducted in the 1970s and 1980s compared cancer incidence and mortality based on racial differences.

        (2) In the late 1980s socioeconomic factors were recognized as more important determinants of cancer incidence and mortality.

      c. Members of minority groups more likely are socioeconomically disadvantaged than whites.

      d. Economic disadvantages account for the majority of cancer incidence and survival discrepancies between minorities and whites:

        (1) Poverty rate for black Americans is 34%, compared with 12% for white Americans.

        (2) Overall 5-year cancer survival rate of black Americans is 38%; survival rate of white Americans is 50%.

        (3) Hispanic Americans and black Americans have less knowledge about cancer prevention and early detection methods and are less likely to have had some form of cancer screening.

      e. Culture and life-style are important, but no known genetic basis exists to explain major racial differences in cancer incidence and outcome.

    2. Nursing implications:

      a. Target specific socioeconomic and cultural groups for cancer education, prevention, and screening.

      b. Develop educational materials that are:

        (1) Culturally sensitive.

        (2) Written/spoken in the appropriate language.

        (3) Written/spoken at the appropriate educational level.

      c. Support legislative initiatives to increase funding for cancer prevention, detection, and treatment in poor communities.

      d. Continue to initiate and apply research about prevention, early detection, and coping behaviors of the poor with cancer and explore factors that motivate or act as barriers to cancer screening.

  D. Life-style changes are being recognized as major factors in cancer prevention.

    1. Supportive and explanatory data:

      a. Approximately 80% of all diagnosed cancers have some life-style component that influences the disease:

        (1) Smoking is most important life-style factor contributing to cancer risk.

        (2) Diet, alcohol, exposure to sunlight, multiple sexual partners, and estrogen therapy are contributors to increased risks of cancer.

        (3) Occupational exposures to toxic industrial substances such as vinyl chloride, nickel, chlorine fumes, and coal dust increase risks of cancer.

        (4) Cigarette smoking has a synergistic effect when combined with exposure to asbestos, increasing the risk of lung cancer 60 times.

        (5) Smokeless tobacco increases the risk of cancer of the mouth, larynx, throat, and esophagus; smokeless tobacco is emerging again as a popular habit, especially among young males.

    b. All cancers caused by cigarette smoking and alcohol use could be prevented.

    c. An estimated 600,000 skin cancers were diagnosed in 1991; approximately 90% could have been prevented by protection from sunlight.

    d. The general public is becoming more involved and interested in health promotion and disease prevention:

        (1) The public increasingly wants to know what can be done to promote health and prevent cancer.

        (2) Smoking cessation, dietary changes, and weight loss are life-style factors of particular interest to the public.

        (3) Insurance companies and individual consumers are seeking ways to reduce health care costs by increasing self-care options and promoting educated consumerism of services.

  2. Nursing implications:

    a. Life-style changes are difficult to make when changing lifelong habits is required:

        (1) Target young people for educational programs to implement positive life-style behaviors.

        (2) Target young males for programs to prevent the use of smokeless tobacco.

        (3) Offer educational and support programs to adults making changes in life-style.

    b. Capitalize on the trend toward self-help and disease prevention with cancer prevention educational programs:

        (1) Target the general public through churches, health fairs, community centers, businesses, and schools.

        (2) Target those individuals already seeking health care at clinics, hospitals, and physician offices.

    c. Smoking cessation is the single most influential life-style change in preventing cancer that the oncology nurse can implement with clients.

    d. Educational programs that address life-style factors such as diet, alcohol consumption, sunlight exposure, sexual activity, occupational hazards, and estrogen therapy are needed.

    e. Mass media influence the health practices of the public:

        (1) Use the media to disseminate health care information to the public.

        (2) Support legislation that limits the advertising of tobacco and alcohol products.

    f. Support strict enforcement of rules that protect workers from occupational exposure to carcinogens.

E. Improvement in screening and early detection can increase cancer survival rates.

  1. Supportive and explanatory data:

    a. Despite improvement in treatment of advanced cancers, early detection provides the best chance for survival.

        (1) The use of the Papanicolaou (Pap) test to detect dysplasia has markedly reduced mortality from cervical cancer.

        (2) Mammography and physical examination by a health care professional

are proven methods of detecting early breast cancer; early-stage breast cancer has a survival rate greater than 90%.

(3) The detection and removal of premalignant colorectal lesions may reduce the incidence of colorectal cancer.

b. Lung cancer is difficult to detect early; survival rates remain at 13%.

2. Nursing implications:

a. Continue to develop and apply education and screening programs that emphasize early detection:

(1) Teach "cancer's seven warning signals" to clients and the general public.

(2) Teach and encourage self-examination practices—breast, skin, oral, vulvar, and testicular.

(3) Encourage individuals to seek cancer screening and detection services, especially individuals at high risk.

b. Identify high-risk groups and target educational and screening programs toward these groups:

(1) The elderly, even if asymptomatic, comprise a high-risk group.

(2) The poor and poorly educated are less likely to seek services and need nursing intervention.

(3) Individuals who have a history of cancer in the family or who practice risky life-style behaviors are targets for early detection programs.

II. Access to health care is an increasing problem for many Americans.

A. Supportive and explanatory data:

1. Important components of access:

a. Availability of personnel and facilities within a defined geographical location.

b. Availability of services that are affordable, appropriate, culturally sensitive, comprehensive, timely, and treat the individual with respect and dignity.

c. Availability of effective cancer prevention, education, and early detection services.

2. The poverty level is defined as a family of four living on less than $12,000 a year:

a. An estimated 36 million poor people live in the United States—5.5 million Hispanic Americans, 9.7 million black Americans, and 21.4 million white Americans are classified as poor.

b. One in five children lives in a poor family.

3. During the 1980s, as health care costs increased, the federal government introduced regulatory changes that:

a. Reduced Medicaid and Medicare expenditures.

b. Reduced state funding of health care programs.

c. Reduced funding of Women, Infants, and Children (WIC) nutrition programs.

4. In 1988 55% of the poor in the United States made too much money to be eligible for Medicaid:

a. A family may become ineligible for Medicaid if income is greater than 50% of defined poverty level.

b. Cutoff for Medicaid eligibility varies from state to state.

5. An estimated 37 million people in the United States do not have health insurance:

a. Twenty million uninsured individuals live above the official poverty line.

b. Young adults and children are most likely to be uninsured.

6. As health insurance premiums rise, employers are demanding that employees pay an increasing percentage of premiums and health care costs:
   a. Many employers have discontinued health benefits as a result of the rise in cost.
   b. Uninsured workers often do not qualify for public assistance.
7. Poor Americans and uninsured Americans combined constitute a total of approximately 55 million people deprived of health care for financial reasons.
8. The number of people with health problems who reported no health care visit during the year increased by 70% in the last 5 years; a major factor cited for the increase was inability to pay.
9. The poor and/or uninsured receive fewer preventive services (Pap smears, breast examination, or mammograms).
10. The poor and/or uninsured are more likely to receive primary care in out-patient clinics or emergency clinics than in physician offices, which results in:
    a. Symptomatic care only, with limited follow-up and diagnostic services.
    b. A delay in diagnosis and lower survival rate.
11. Other barriers to adequate health care include:
    a. The closure of many small and/or rural hospitals as a result of financial pressure.
    b. Reduced health services in rural areas and reduced funding for the National Health Service.
12. Many urban health care centers are understaffed, underfunded, and over-whelmed with demands for services; 10% of the hospitals provide care for 40% of the uninsured.
13. Other obstacles discouraging the poor or uninsured from seeking health care:
    a. Lack of transportation to and from health care facilities.
    b. Inflexible work hours and limited hours services are offered.
    c. Lack of child care services.
    d. Long waiting periods in health care facilities.
    e. Discourteous or harried staff.
    f. Language barriers.
    g. Culturally inappropriate information.
B. Nursing implications:
   1. Make respectful, affordable, and appropriate cancer prevention, early detection, treatment, and rehabilitation services a goal for all oncology nurses.
   2. Initiate an environmental surveillance of the work place with respect to criteria for accessible services and initiate changes based on the assessment:
      a. Are the educational services appropriate for the population served?
      b. Is adequate transportation available to reach the facility?
      c. Do the hours of operation facilitate use of the facility?
      d. Are users of the facility made to feel welcome and respected?
      e. Does the facility offer outreach services to the community?
   3. Develop educational materials for the socioeconomically disadvantaged:
      a. Monitor reading level of published materials and assess community appropriateness.
      b. Develop educational materials that are culturally sensitive, at the appropriate reading level, and written in the appropriate language for the community.
      c. Develop visual aids to communicate to the low-literacy population.
   4. Adapt early detection and prevention programs to needs of minority and poor populations such as:

        a. Developing a mobile screening clinic to access hard-to-reach populations.

        b. Involving lower socioeconomic community leaders in the identification of specific issues that may block use of the programs by the poor.

        c. Employing members of the community in programs to act as advocates for the population and to promote the programs within the community.

    5. Participate in political activity at the local, regional, state, or national level to develop advocacy groups/coalitions for the medically underserved or socioeconomically disadvantaged.

    6. Participate in raising public awareness of the issues.

III. Attitudes and beliefs of public are affecting cancer care.

  A. Supportive and explanatory data:

    1. Perception of cancer is based on:

        a. Individual experience.

        b. Cultural heritage.

        c. Religious beliefs.

        d. Family and societal attitudes.

        e. Education.

        f. Present circumstances.

    2. The poor, the elderly, and the poorly educated often have the least accurate information about cancer prevention, detection, and treatment.

    3. Poor people often make health a low priority when budgeting their money and efforts, thus deterring early treatment or detection of cancer.

    4. The poor often feel powerless to change life's circumstances and helpless to develop or control cancer.

    5. A fatalistic attitude toward cancer is prevalent among poor people, especially black Americans:

        a. Cancer is widely believed invariably fatal.

        b. Fatalism contributes to delays in seeking treatment and following preventive practices.

    6. Socioeconomically disadvantaged people may feel isolated from a formal health care structure:

        a. Non-English-speaking individuals feel greater isolation.

        b. Staff members who do not convey respect for the individual enhance feelings of isolation.

    7. Beliefs that cancer detection methods (mammography, x-ray examinations) may cause cancer deter participation in screening.

    8. The elderly may confuse symptoms of illness with the normal signs of aging (fatigue, poor appetite, bowel or bladder problems, changes in appearance of the skin).

    9. Young people may not seek prevention and early detection services because of feelings of invincibility, especially teenagers and young adults.

   10. Cultural practices (folk medicine) may conflict with standard medical practice:

        a. People seek help first from familiar resources such as a folk healer, midwife, relative, or home remedies.

        b. Only when these methods fail is medical attention sought.

        c. If the individual believes that personal cultural values are not respected, health services will be rejected.

        d. If local beliefs are integrated into modern treatments, acceptance may be increased.

   11. Despite increasing awareness of the curability of cancer, fear that cancer is fatal exists at all levels of society and deters early diagnosis and treatment.

12. Unproven methods often are sought if one feels alienated from the traditional medical establishment (see Chapter 25).
B. Nursing implications:
   1. Oncology nurses must be sensitive to the complexity of decisions made to seek or not seek conventional medical services:
      a. Become familiar with the practices and beliefs of the community served.
      b. Incorporate community beliefs into education programs, outreach services, and screening services.
   2. Recognize that fear of cancer is a deterrent to seeking care and educate the community about the benefits of early detection.
   3. Educate the elderly about symptoms of cancer that may be attributed to aging.
   4. Discuss unproven treatments in a nonthreatening and open manner:
      a. Outline the pros and cons of the treatment.
      b. Explore the underlying reason for seeking unproven methods and address these issues.
      c. Offer support and education to the client and family.
      d. Contact local American Cancer Society for information on specific unproven methods.
      e. Provide sources for client to seek additional information on both conventional and unproven treatment (National Cancer Institute: 1-800-4-CANCER; American Cancer Society: 1-800-ACS-2345).

BIBLIOGRAPHY

Allen, M.E. & Edwards, K. (1987). Cancer prevention: implications for ethnic and racial minorities. *Fam Community Health 10*(3), 62-66.

American Cancer Society (1991). *Cancer Facts and Figures-1991*. Atlanta: The American Cancer Society.

Barro, A.R. (1986). Women and cancer: the impact and feasibility of practicing prevention. *Health Values 10*(1), 5-15.

Bloom, J.R., Hayes, W.A., Saunders, F., & Flatt, S. (1987). Cancer awareness and secondary prevention practices in Black Americans: implications for intervention. *Fam Community Health 10*(3), 19-30.

Dellefield, M.E. (1988). Informational needs and approaches for early cancer detection in the elderly. *Semin Oncol Nurs 4*(3), 156-168.

Doty, P., Liu, K., & Wiener, J. (1985). An overview of long-term care. *Health Care Financing Rev 6*(3), 69-78.

Flynt, J.W. (1989). The poor: who and where? In *Bridging the Gaps in Health Care: Proceedings for the National Conference on Cancer in the Poor*. Atlanta: American Cancer Society, pp. 21-26.

Frank-Stromborg, M. (1988). Future projected trends in the care of the elderly individual with cancer, and implications for nursing. *Semin Oncol Nurs 4*(3), 224-231.

Freeman, H.P. (1989). Cancer in the socioeconomically disadvantaged. *CA 39*(5), 266-288.

Garfinkel, L. & Silverberg, E. (1991). Lung cancer and smoking trends in the United States over the past 25 years. *CA 41*(3), 137-145.

Given, B.A. & Kellman, L. (1990). Cancer in the elderly population: research issues. *Oncol Nurs Forum 17*(1), 121-123.

Holland, J.C. (1982). Why patients seek unproven cancer remedies: a psychological perspective. *CA 32*(1), 10-14.

Lerner, M. (1989). Access to the American health care system: consequences for cancer control. *CA 39*(5), 289-295.

Miaskowski, C. (1990). The future of oncology nursing: a historical perspective. *Nurs Clin North Am 25*(2), 461-473.

Metter, G.E. (1986). Cancer trends: measures and limitations and their relevance to cancer in women. *Health Values 10*(1), 41-44.

National Cancer Advisory Board (1989). Fighting cancer in America: achieving the "year 2000 goal." *Cancer Nurs 12*(6), 359-368.

Newell, G.R., Spitz, M.R., & Sider, J.G. (1989). Cancer and age. *Semin Oncol 16*(1), 3-9.

National Cancer Institute (1986). *Cancer Among Blacks and Other Minorities: Statistical Profiles*. Washington, D.C.: U.S. Department of Health and Human Services.

National Cancer Institute (1985). *Cancer Rates and Risks* (3rd ed). Bethesda, Md: The Institute.

Porter/Novelli (1988). *Cancer Prevention and Control Needs of Disadvantaged Americans: An Exploratory Study*. Washington, D.C.: Author.

Short, P.F. (1988). Trends in employee health benefits. *Health Affairs 7*(3), 186-196.

Stewart, J.A. & Foster, R.S., Jr. (1989). Breast cancer and aging. *Semin Oncol 16*(1), 41-50.

Ultmann, J.E. (1988). A fight worth fighting: reflections on the National Cancer Program. *Cancer Invest 6*(3), 357-360.

U.S. Office of the Assistant Secretary for Health (1980). *Promoting Health/Preventing Disease: Objectives for the Nation*. Washington, D.C.: Public Health Service.

Williams, R.D., Edwards, K., & Hane, N. (1987). Barriers to breast cancer screening in older women. *Fam Community Health 10*(3), 51-56.

Yarbro, C.H. (1990). Unproven methods of cancer treatment. In S.L. Groenwald, M.H. Frogge, M. Goodman, & C.H. Yarbro (eds). *Cancer Nursing: Principles and Practice*. Boston: Jones & Bartlett Publishers, pp. 1216-1227.

Changes in Oncology Health Care Settings

Deborah Stephens Mills, MN, RN, OCN

I. Decision making regarding care settings.
  A. Decision makers vary.
    1. Client and family have ultimate freedom of choice.
    2. Members of health care team contribute according to respective area of expertise:
      a. Physician—diagnosis, treatment, follow-up of disease; disease progression; iatrogenic responses; complications; side effects.
      b. Nurse—diagnosis and treatment of human responses to actual or potential health problems; education; resource development; coordination of care (between primary in-hospital and office or home health nurses).
      c. Social worker/case manager—evaluation of resources; discharge planning; utilization review; family support; coordination of outpatient care and equipment.
      d. Dietitian—diet education; diet enhancement.
      e. Chaplain/minister—spiritual care; community support.
    3. Client/family treated as unit of care—encouraging to remain autonomous and independent and interdependent.
  B. Decision-making process is dynamic.
    1. Collaboration facilitates comprehensive approach.
      a. Health care team is adjunctive to primary care provider.
      b. Client and family are included in care planning.
    2. Ongoing—revised as changes occur and needs arise.
    3. Proactive—includes anticipated needs of client/family; is sensitive, creative, and adapted to changing needs of clients/families within rapidly changing hospital or community health care systems.
  C. Decision-making process is systematic, involving:
    1. Data collection.
      a. Assessment of client needs:
        (1) Begins with the presenting problem of the client in any setting.
        (2) Includes (but is not limited to) physiological needs (disease state,

treatment demands, symptom management) stated in the Oncology Nursing Society (ONS) Practice Standards:
  (a) Prevention and early detection.
  (b) Current knowledge and information needs.
  (c) Coping strategies affecting health.
  (d) Comfort/discomfort and management.
  (e) Current nutritional status.
  (f) Functioning of protective mechanisms.
  (g) Level of mobility.
  (h) Elimination patterns (past/present).
  (i) Sexual patterns and current functioning.
  (j) Ventilation/current respiratory status.
  (k) Circulation (adequate tissue perfusion).
  (3) Encompasses social needs (relating to family and community—including coping with the disease and physical changes).
  (4) Includes emotional and spiritual needs (dealing with sense of self and meaning of cancer experience).
  (5) Involves determination of socioeconomic and vocational needs (work and financial responsibilities).
b. Assessment of family and/or significant other's needs:
  (1) Elicit past experiences with illness.
  (2) Assess strengths gained from past illnesses.
  (3) Assess unresolved losses or maladaptive responses to previous losses.
  (4) Determine meaning of cancer and treatment for client and family members.
  (5) Explore ways that family may participate in therapy.
  (6) Identify any sense of loss or fears family may be experiencing (e.g., client suffering, anticipated role changes, fear of unknown, difficulty getting information).
  (7) Evaluate family composition, roles, availability for care.
c. Assessment of present care setting:
  (1) Determine why the client is in the present care setting.
  (2) Evaluate adequacy in meeting the needs of the client/family.
  (3) Identify the primary care provider.
  (4) Verify availability of appropriate support persons, equipment, medications, and resources.
  (5) Determine accountability for ongoing assessment or care and follow-up.
  (6) Consider home the preferred setting whenever possible.
  (7) Begin discharge planning and/or follow-up with client/family upon diagnosis or admission.
d. Assessment of potential care settings:
  (1) Determine client/family eligibility for resources/community agencies.
  (2) Assess availability of resource people, supportive services, and health delivery agencies within the community and beyond (call local American Cancer Society [ACS] or develop catalogue of resources).
  (3) Evaluate services, criteria for admission, costs, and goals.
  (4) Assess client's/family's usual resources for skills, services, and funds.
  (5) Develop a data base for referral (National Cancer Institute ([NCI], university hospitals) when access to care is limited within home community.

    2. Evaluation of alternatives.
      a. Assessment of perceived obstacles to selecting appropriate care setting:
        (1) Change in socioeconomic status (e.g., loss of job, decreased income).
        (2) Exceeding limits of insurance coverage.
        (3) Disagreement among client/family and health care providers about choice of care setting.
      b. Weight of relative benefits among alternative settings.
  D. Consider special care issues affecting selection:
    1. Persons with human immunodeficiency virus (HIV)-related illnesses.
    2. Socioeconomically disadvantaged populations.
    3. Ethnic minorities.
    4. Persons undergoing nontraditional therapies or early phase research protocols.
    5. Treatment using radioisotopes or radioactive implants.
    6. Bone marrow transplantation—preoperative and postoperative care, insurance coverage.
    7. Terminally ill children.
    8. The following is an *example* of consideration of special care needs of the client with HIV-related illnesses:
      a. Confronting the care needs of persons with HIV-related illnesses has become a tremendous challenge to nursing today:
        (1) Reminiscent of the cancer problem 20 to 30 years ago.
        (2) Services and therapy for persons with cancer have improved over last several years, which can in turn have a positive effect on the care environments of persons with HIV-related illnesses.
      b. Caring for persons with HIV-related illnesses involves four areas of concern: occupational risks, infection control, professional competence, and re-examination of personal values/prejudices:
        (1) With appropriate education and support, all health care professionals can safely assume responsibility for care of persons with HIV-related illnesses.
        (2) Given experience with immunocompromised patients, oncology nurses are especially well prepared to care for these patients.
        (3) The oncology unit may be the setting of choice for in-hospital care of same.
      c. With incorporation of universal blood/body fluid precautions (Centers for Disease Control [CDC] recommendations and guidelines; see Chapter 37), persons with HIV-related diseases and persons immunocompromised secondary to cancer/cancer therapy can be housed safely on the same unit; in using universal precautions, all clients are treated as potentially infectious, thereby eliminating the need to differentiate HIV-infected persons from others.
      d. Persons with HIV-related disorders often have a clinical disease course of remissions interspersed with acute exacerbations, ending with a variable period of terminal illness. Factors that complicate the choice of care setting include:
        (1) Social isolation and disapproval of life-style.
        (2) Nontraditional or limited support systems.
        (3) Limited or expended financial resources.
        (4) High incidence of neuropsychiatric problems.
        (5) Poor prognosis and limited community services.
        (6) Uncertainty, leading to helplessness and hopelessness.

(7) Need for specialty care (e.g., infectious diseases).

    e. Decentralized and out-of-hospital community liaison services for persons with HIV-related illnesses enhance services available outside metropolitan acquired immunodeficiency syndrome (AIDS) centers.

    f. Persons with HIV-related illnesses receive care in varied settings—hospitals, homes, clinics (general or AIDS/HIV primary care), physicians' offices, schools, public health centers, drug treatment facilities, mental health centers, residential care facilities, nursing homes, hospices, and others:

        (1) Case management and primary care are recommended to promote continuity of care.

        (2) Sensitive, comprehensive approach is warranted for meeting many levels of needs through disease trajectory.

E. Care settings to consider in planning and implementation:

  1. In-hospital care.

  2. Ambulatory care.

  3. Home care.

  4. Nursing home or convalescent care.

  5. Hospice care.

II. Planning care in hospital settings.

A. The oncology unit.

  1. Definition: a designated hospital area that facilitates the team approach to comprehensive cancer care by bringing into close proximity personnel and facilities necessary for such care; provides not only for the physical needs of the cancer client, but also for the ongoing emotional, social, and spiritual support of the client and his or her family or significant others.

  2. An oncology unit should be organized if cancer admissions to a hospital equal 15% or more of total medical-surgical admissions.

  3. Six conditions must be met in opening an oncology unit:

    a. A physical setting with ample room for nurses to work and conference and for client/family comfort (including private space, kitchen facilities, and sleeping facilities for family).

    b. Professional nursing staff to meet the specific needs of cancer clients as determined by a client-classification system (regarding client acuity and nursing hours).

    c. Policies and procedures for unit operation using a multidisciplinary treatment approach.

    d. A philosophy of nursing that focuses on the client/family unit and incorporates the importance of service, education, and research.

    e. A nurturing work environment in which staff is actively supported through:

        (1) Specialty orientation.

        (2) Ongoing staff development.

        (3) Stress management.

        (4) Individualized reward systems.

    f. An excellence of practice that is marked by continuous evaluation of quality of care.

  4. Advantages of oncology unit:

    a. Specialized needs of persons with catastrophic and sometimes life-threatening diseases addressed by specialty nursing personnel.

    b. Technical proficiency combined with sensitivity to cancer as a disease affecting the whole family.

       c. "High touch in a high-tech environment."

       d. High degree of trust and individualization of care of clients/families and nurses well known to each other.

    5. Disadvantages of oncology unit: professional burnout—related to the continuous close contact with cancer clients; major factors are:

       a. Staffing shortages.

       b. Frustrating client/family demands.

       c. Personal psychological strains.

B. The scattered-bed unit.

    1. Definition: mixed medical-surgical or nononcology specialty unit in hospitals in which cancer admissions do not justify an organized oncology unit or in which administrative support for such a unit is lacking.

    2. Advantages of scattered-bed unit:

       a. Even with substantial cancer admissions, a scattered-bed approach may be considered more cost-effective.

       b. Cancer-specific skilled nursing care is still possible with:

         (1) An oncology clinical nursing specialist on staff.

         (2) Ongoing continuing education programs specific to the needs of clients with cancer.

         (3) Oncology transition service and case management.

         (4) Collaboration with nurses in oncology office practices.

    3. Disadvantages of scattered-bed unit:

       a. Continuity of care can suffer; families need special consideration when confronted by different nurses on every hospital admission.

       b. Family-centered nursing may not be orientation of the unit.

       c. Subtle changes in client's status may be missed or thought unimportant because of unfamiliarity with disease process or client's history.

       d. Client education may be more generic rather than individualized or specific to current status or treatment regimen.

III. Planning care in ambulatory settings.

A. Oncology office practice setting.

    1. Definition: associated office practices that may include any or all of the following oncology specialties:

       a. Surgery and gynecology.

       b. Medical oncology (including hematology).

       c. Immunology and infectious diseases.

       d. Pediatric oncology.

       e. Radiation oncology.

    2. Often affiliated with regional cancer centers and other large hospitals but also found in smaller communities.

    3. Disease- and treatment-related sequelae monitored frequently to avoid unnecessary discomfort or toxicity.

    4. The role of oncology office nurse instrumental in the success of therapy for clients in at least three areas:

       a. Direct care (e.g., chemotherapy, comfort, symptom management).

       b. Information exchange (e.g., education, interpretation of reports).

       c. Client/family support (e.g., support groups, phone follow-up, and counseling).

    5. Advantages:

       a. Expert, specialized care.

       b. Hospitalizations minimized, with problems managed in ambulatory setting whenever possible.

        c. Accessibility of research programs to enhance treatment options.

        d. Frequently, physician-nurse team assumes primary responsibility for care, adding to trust and confidence of client and family; clients and families encouraged to call office to manage symptoms or to clarify instructions.

    6. Disadvantages:

        a. Professional stress related to:

           (1) High patient volume-to-time ratios.

           (2) Time-consuming functional tasks.

           (3) Inadequate staffing ratios, long hours.

        b. Because of urgency (related to above), client and family may not feel a part of the treatment-planning process.

        c. Time required for consultation, physician visits, and treatment often frustrating for all involved.

B. General/primary practice setting.

    1. Definition: client-care system wherein all or most of the problems of the client are managed by one physician or physician group (e.g., general surgeon, family practitioner, internist).

    2. Often in rural settings with few physicians the same physician who assessed the initial symptomatology may proceed with surgery and later oversee follow-up.

    3. In more urban settings issue of primary care sometimes complicates treatment decisions; private practice physician may consult with specialists but retain primary responsibility for workup and management of presumed malignancy.

    4. Requires that office or clinic staff (physician and nurse) be both generalist and specialist.

    5. Advantages:

        a. Allows client to remain in home community to receive therapy.

        b. High level of trust and commitment already established between client/family and physician/nurse.

    6. Disadvantages:

        a. Tremendous challenge to physician and nurse to provide optimal cancer-related care, depending on resources such as:

           (1) Professional cancer journals and textbooks.

           (2) Affiliation with cancer centers and organizations.

           (3) Regional or national specialty seminars or inservices.

        b. Lack of case volume to develop expertise in managing more obscure diagnoses or complications or to participate in clinical trials.

        c. Ethical dilemma of whether client is receiving optimal care.

C. Employee health service.

    1. Definition: personnel assistance program providing routine examinations, follow-up laboratory studies, and even chemotherapy in the workplace as incentive to clients to remain actively involved in the work force.

    2. Advantages:

        a. Cost-effective and time-efficient to employer and employee.

        b. Especially important to persons who are presently cancer free but have some risk(s):

           (1) Several years after diagnosis and/or treatment.

           (2) No longer under the supervision of an oncologist.

           (3) Cancer prone—strong family history of cancer or life-style promoting cancer risk (e.g., smoking, obesity, alcoholism).

      c. Can be instrumental in enhancing health promotion activities or life-style changes because of employer support.
   3. Disadvantages:
      a. Workup may not be comprehensive.
      b. Physician-nurse team may not be current on cancer-related symptomatology or even risk factor management.
      c. Focus is returning employee to workforce; therefore, some complaints may not be evaluated thoroughly.
      d. Very dependent on the employer health belief system; varies among employers.
IV. Planning care for home settings.
  A. Home nursing agencies and home health care agencies.
   1. Definition: according to the Department of Health and Human Services, home health care is "that component of a continuum of comprehensive health care whereby health services are provided to individuals and families in their places of residence for the purpose of promoting, maintaining or restoring health, or of maximizing the level of independence, while minimizing the effects of disability and illness, including terminal illness."
   2. Home health agencies provide assistance by:
      a. Dealing with client problems such as pain, poor nutrition, elimination disturbances, sleeplessness, emotional strain.
      b. Engaging other family or community members to assist in client care, thereby extending the stay at home.
      c. Offering respite for primary care providers to support the client's choice to stay in the home.
      d. Cooperating as partners with client's primary physician-nurse team in providing comprehensive care.
   3. The client may contract with home health agency for varied services from care providers, including:
      a. Home care nurses and home health aides.
      b. Social workers and chaplains.
      c. Physical and occupational therapists.
      d. Pharmacists and medical equipment venders.
      e. Respiratory therapists.
      f. Dietitians and others.
   4. High-acuity support services available in the ambulatory setting make home care an option for clients who have an ongoing need for:
      a. Intravenous (IV) therapy and/or parenteral nutrition.
      b. Chemotherapy (IV, arterial infusion pump, intrathecal, peritoneal).
      c. Antibiotic therapy.
      d. Analgesic infusion pump therapy.
      e. Specimen sampling for laboratory studies.
   5. The commitment of family members to provide care in the home must not be disregarded or undervalued by the health care professionals involved in the care:
      a. Sensitivity toward and support of home care provider is essential.
      b. Need exists for continual assessment of options available to:
        (1) Support care in home (usually client's choice).
        (2) Build family confidence and expertise.
        (3) Allay anxieties while offering services and resources.
   6. Advantages of home care setting:
      a. High level of care in the comfort of home; all other care settings coordinate with home care.

        b. Increased self-sufficiency of client/family unit; home is client's natural social environment.

        c. Reduction in frequency and number of hospitalizations.

        d. Reduction in the incidence of infections (especially pulmonary).

        e. Prevention and/or recognition of potentially life-threatening complications and implementation of appropriate actions by home care team.

        f. Restoration and maintenance of optimal performance of activities of daily living.

        g. Promotion of compliance with medical regimen.

    7. Disadvantages of home care setting:

        a. Occasional conflicting goals among client/family members (e.g., client wants to stay in home; family prefers security of institutional care).

        b. High level of stress for home care provider:

           (1) Clients/families may choose institutional care over home if a feeling of burden or inability to provide client comfort or safety exists.

           (2) Home care provider maintains major role as first line observer of changes in client's health and comfort status, which may be anxiety provoking and difficult to continue over time.

           (3) Home care provider must contend with multiple roles, requiring new skills and the need to delegate tasks (which may be difficult).

        c. Burnout of home care provider—requires respite intervention (either institutional care or recruiting helpers).

        d. Possibly complicated reimbursement schedules or third-party payer requirements for services rendered.

V. Planning care in nursing home or residential settings.

    A. Definition: according to the Social Security Act, "posthospital extended care for continuation of necessary medical treatment in an institution that provides a level of care distinguished from the intensive care ordinarily furnished by a hospital," including either:

        1. Skilled nursing services.

        2. Intermediate care (health services for persons needing institutional care but not skilled nursing).

    B. Occasionally clients or families initiate hospitalization and/or nursing home placement in response to a home care crisis; these admissions may be painful if seen by families as a failure to meet client's needs at home.

    C. If the client and family still prefer home care, that option should be restored if at all possible; temporary or permanent nursing home placement may be considered as an alternative if other resource avenues have been exhausted.

    D. Advantages of nursing home or residential care placement:

        1. A care option for clients who no longer require hospitalization but do not have the resources needed at home or an available home care provider.

        2. An opportunity for respite for the primary caregiver at home even when home nursing support is available but not adequate at present for caregiver under stress.

        3. For elderly clients, specialty care geared toward needs and concerns of senior adults.

    E. Disadvantages of nursing home or residential care placement:

        1. Stigma attached by many clients/families and rejection of care option by same.

        2. Client-staff ratios and staffing composition that differ from hospital to nursing home (possible disruptions in care).

3. Philosophies of care (i.e., pain management protocols) may differ, thereby affecting continuity of care.
4. Complications of cancer therapies may not be familiar to nursing home staff, thus detection and intervention may differ.
5. Accountability issue (who will assume primary care responsibility).

VI. Planning for hospice care.
   A. Hospice care.
     1. Definition: a system of specialized care that provides support and assistance for the most difficult of journeys—facing one's own death; hospice nursing involves intensive caring, collaborative sharing, continuous knowing, and continuous giving.
     2. A concept of care that concentrates on rehumanizing the experience of dying and joins sophisticated methods of pain and symptom control and sensitive, respectful, noninvasive caring; with hospice support, clients who choose to die at home usually can.
     3. On November 1, 1983, legislation provided funding for certified hospices to care for Medicare-eligible clients.
     4. Hospices provide many rewards for nurses, yet the care is demanding and support services are needed to alleviate stress and prevent burnout.
   B. Types of hospice care settings and approaches.
     1. Community-based program:
       a. No facility other than an office.
       b. A multidisciplinary team.
       c. Home care is the focus; goal is to provide comfort, autonomy, and emotional and physical support to client/family.
       d. Clients may continue in cancer therapy.
       e. Hospice team collaborates with cancer treatment team to provide optimal cross-coverage and continuity of care.
     2. Hospital-based program:
       a. May be an inpatient program or a hospital-based home care program.
       b. Inpatient program allows, for example, for hospital admission for respite care or new pain management protocol.
       c. Hospital-based home care program may have partial or full hospital backing from hospice interdisciplinary team or consultants from various departments.
     3. Hospital-based hospice team:
       a. May also be called the palliative care team.
       b. Clients are received through in-hospital referral or consultation.
       c. The team physician may become the client's primary physician, or the referring physician may remain, working in concert with the hospice team.
       d. Hospital beds may be allocated for hospice care, or clients may be seen throughout the hospital.
       e. The hospice team makes rounds each day, making recommendations as needed.
     4. Freestanding hospice:
       a. A freestanding facility, usually with a home care program.
       b. If unable to maintain care in the home, the client or family may elect admission to the hospice facility.
       c. Hospice care is uninterrupted because the same team members facilitate transition between home and hospice facility.

    d. Cancer therapy usually has been discontinued, and the primary physician may have relinquished all care responsibility to the hospice physician.

C. Advantages of hospice care setting (also criteria for hospice care):
1. The client and family comprise the unit of care.
2. Care includes around-the-clock care commitment (staff available on premises or on call 24 hours per day).
3. Practitioner competence is enhanced.
4. Communication is facilitated by interdisciplinary team planning and family input.
5. Volunteers are recruited actively and used as members of care team.
6. A physician is an integral part of the team, usually as the medical director.
7. Accepting and nonjudgmental attitudes persist among members of the care team.
8. Pain or symptom control is highly emphasized, but commitment also is made to psychosocial, emotional, and spiritual needs of client and family.
9. Hospice care continues with the family after the client's death through bereavement follow-up.
10. Continuous, comprehensive care is very appealing to clients and families who may find health care costly and episodic as the disease progresses.

D. Disadvantages of hospice care setting and approach:
1. Hospice programs vary widely from community to community; client and family must assess services available to them.
2. Medicare pays only for hospice care administered through certified programs (can be confusing for clients/families when a home nursing program offers "hospice" care but is not really a hospice program).
3. Stigma is associated with hospice for some who focus on the terminal care component of program.
4. Stress level is high for staff and primary caregiver during time when client's condition deteriorates; support for both hospice staff and family is essential.

VII. Trends in cancer care related to settings.
A. Ambulatory care settings are becoming the treatment site choice of clients; care planning is more proactive than reactive, exploring creative means of delivering care to clients who prefer the comfort of home.
1. The phone is a vital link in ambulatory care, and nurses on oncology units and in office practices can optimize care through phone triage.
2. Phone conversations between client/family and nurse promote early problem solving and curtail complications.
3. Documentation of problems and nursing actions promote continuity and legal record of practice.
B. Because clients and families are voicing not only concerns but preferences in cancer care, health care providers are responding.
1. An interagency task force, including health professionals and lay community members, can provide the objectivity and creativity needed to offer new client-driven services.
2. Many of the support programs presently offered were initiated by clients who could not find needed resources (e.g., Reach to Recovery, United Ostomy Association).
C. Alliances between hospitals and home care agencies are expanding:
1. Collaboration between agencies provides continuity of care and individualized, comprehensive care that enhances accountability and reduces gaps in care.

2. In the future this same practice should be seen more frequently between nursing homes and home health care agencies.
D. Hospice care has become a model for holistic care.
   1. Hospice philosophy has influenced caregivers at stages of the life cycle other than dying.
   2. Models for multidisciplinary care that support a continuum of physical, psychosocial, and spiritual need have been developed.
E. Primary nursing has become a model of care that:
   1. Promotes continuity and quality of care through 24-hour accountability.
   2. May be implemented best through nurse-physician teams.
   3. In oncology nursing, allows the primary nurse to be a clinician, teacher, care manager, consultant, and/or researcher.
F. Qualified nurses are practicing independently:
   1. In fee-for-service bereavement therapy through a local hospital of funeral home referral system.
   2. In a joint or collaborative practice in which the care of a client population is shared with a physician and other health care professionals.
   3. In a direct contract with clients and families.
      a. The client or family may request education or a specific service.
      b. The nurse may provide a wide range of services as defined by the nurse practice act of the respective state; services may include:
         (1) Physical assessment.
         (2) Family and client education.
         (3) Family and client counseling and psychotherapy.
         (4) Coordination of contracted services (social services, nutritional counseling, physical therapy, and home nursing services).

VIII. Cancer rehabilitation—an approach to care across settings.
   A. Definition: preventive, restorative, supportive, and palliative activities engaged to improve the quality of life for maximal productivity with minimal dependence, regardless of life expectancy and within the limits imposed by disease and treatment.
   B. More than 50% of clients diagnosed with cancer today will be alive in 5 years.
      1. Cancer rehabilitation begins at the time of diagnosis.
         a. From diagnosis, cancer clients should be considered survivors, not victims.
         b. This perception and commitment to wellness and healing influence quality of life.
      2. Cancer can create dependency, and the goal of cancer rehabilitation is to promote independence through the coordinated efforts of the rehabilitation team, including:
         a. Nurses and physicians.
         b. Occupation, physical, and recreational therapists.
         c. Art and music therapists.
         d. Chaplains, counselors, and social workers.
         e. Appliance fitters.
         f. Speech therapists.
         g. Community liaisons.
   C. Rehabilitation is a process that need not be confined to a facility (Table 11-1).
      1. Prescriptions for rehabilitation can be completed through a hospital, a freestanding cancer facility, or office practice(s).
      2. The ambulatory care setting is the most natural and least disruptive for clients and families engaging in a rehabilitation program.

Table 11-1
REHABILITATION ISSUES ASSOCIATED WITH SPECIFIC CANCER SITES

Cancer Site	Rehabilitation Issues
Head and neck cancers	Maintenance of optimal nutrition and deglutition Shoulder dysfunction rehabilitation Neck dysfunction rehabilitation Self-care considerations Speech/communication Restoring acceptable appearance and function
Breast cancer	Physical restoration of affected arm Psychosocial rehabilitation regarding loss, body image alterations, and sexuality Cosmetic rehabilitation with form, prosthesis, or reconstruction
Bone and soft-tissue malignancies	Restore near-normal function through prostheses, appliances, and aids to ambulation Restore acceptable appearance Vocational rehabilitation Psychosocial restoration
Lung cancer	Preoperative rehabilitation emphasizes breathing retraining Pulmonary disability prevention after radiation or surgery
Colorectal and bladder malignancies resulting in ostomies	Self-concept adjustment Elimination control and ostomy adjustment Self-care considerations Psychosocial rehabilitation Effective skin care
Central nervous system	Preventing unnecessary loss of function and diminished quality of life Cognitive function evaluation Mobility modifications Retraining for activities of daily living Bowel and bladder management

Modified from DeLisa, J.A., Miller, R.M., Melnick, R.R., Gerber, L.H., & Hillel, A.B. (1989). Rehabilitation of the cancer patient. In V.T. DeVita, S. Hellman, & S.A. Rosenberg (eds). *Cancer: Principles and Practice*. Philadelphia: J.B. Lippincott Co.

    D. Clients and families also seek rehabilitation services through self-help and other support services:
        1. I Can Cope—support group and educational program sponsored by the ACS.
        2. We Can Weekend—a guided family experience with individual and group activities geared toward enhancing family communication and coping with cancer.
        3. WIN—a unique physical conditioning and rehabilitation program for women cancer survivors (similar to Outward Bound).
        4. National Coalition for Cancer Survivorship—a network of independent organizations and individuals working in cancer survivorship and support to generate a nationwide awareness of survivorship as a vibrant productive life after the diagnosis of cancer:
           a. Cancer survivors speak on their own behalf to address educational, employment, and social needs.

   b. The focus is health promotion, risk preventions, and promotion of care settings committed to careful follow-up and support of health-protective activities.
 E. In some communities comprehensive cancer rehabilitation services may be minimal; reasons for the deficit may include:
   1. A persistent and common view that cancer is a terminal rather than a curable or chronic illness.
   2. Lack of third-party reimbursement for such services.
   3. Perceived hierarchy of needs for limited services in which resources are concentrated on acute care versus rehabilitation.
   4. Lack of awareness of rehabilitative needs and demands by the public for services.
 F. Improved diagnostic and treatment regimens have resulted in longer and healthier lives among individuals with cancer and have made cancer rehabilitation an integral part of the treatment plan.

IX. Evaluation of desired outcomes.
 A. Clients and families report the availability of professional assistance needed to:
   1. Seek a health restorative process.
   2. Maintain an adapted health status.
   3. Cope with end-stage or terminal phase of cancer.
 B. Nurses actively assess services available in the community and identify areas that need enhancement.
 C. Nursing research supports changes in care delivery.
   1. Nurses collaborate with physicians and other colleagues to identify gaps in care.
   2. Nurses use research to validate clinical assumptions about nursing needs of clients with cancer: (As illustrated by Hull who identified 4 needs with respect to cancer nursing):
     a. Twenty-four–hour accessibility and availability.
     b. Effective communication skills.
     c. Accepting and nonjudgmental attitudes.
     d. Practitioner competence.
   3. Nurses secure financial support for research through pharmaceutical companies, the ACS, and cancer nursing organizations.
 D. Initial treatment services support continuity of care through:
   1. Interdisciplinary communication between the client, family, and treatment team and involvement in decision making related to therapeutic modalities.
   2. Early discharge planning and follow-up care.
 E. Transition services are available to coordinate care between inpatient and outpatient settings to enhance ease of setting change and accessibility.
   1. Types of available assistance include hospital services under titles such as "Continuity of Care" or "Managed Care," nursing agencies, physicians' offices, employee health departments, and liaison personnel.
   2. The nurse in transition services:
     a. Supports the client and family as educator and advocate.
     b. Provides a communication link between client/family and the community health care system.
     c. Facilitates personalized, cost-effective care planning and comfort for the client, family, and public.
 F. Support services are available for the dying client and primary caregiver.
   1. Respite care, support groups, use of volunteers, and appropriate staffing and coverage are facilitated in community oncology care services.

2. An option for home death within personal surroundings with family members present is valued and supported in the community.

G. Oncology nurses manifest active involvement in the challenge of maintaining quality care to increasing numbers of ill clients in all health care settings.

BIBLIOGRAPHY

Amenta, M. (1991). Hospice services. In S.B. Baird, R. McCorkle, & M. Grant (eds). *Cancer Nursing: A Comprehensive Textbook*. Philadelphia: W.B. Saunders Co., pp. 1033-1043.

Amenta, M.O. (1984). Hospice USA 1984—steady and holding. *Oncol Nurs Forum 11*(5), 68-74.

American Nurses' Association and Oncology Nursing Society (1987). *Standards of oncology nursing practice*. Kansas City, Mo: American Nurses' Association.

Anderson, J.L. (1989). The nurse's role in cancer rehabilitation. Review of the literature. *Cancer Nurs 12*(2), 85-94.

Aydelotte, M.K. (1987). Nursing's preferred future. *Nurs Outlook 35*(3), 114-120.

Baird, S.B. (ed) (1988). *The Role of the Oncology Nurse in the Office Setting*. Columbus, Ohio: Adria Laboratories.

Barhamand, B.A. (1991). A survey of the role, benefits, and realities of the office-based oncology nurse. *Oncol Nurs Forum 18*(1), 31-37.

Bennett, J.A. (1987). Nurses talk about the challenge of AIDS. *Am J Nurs 87*(9), 1150-1155.

Blank, J.J., Clark, L., Longman, A.J., & Atwood, J.R. (1989). Perceived home care needs of cancer patients and their caregivers. *Cancer Nurs 12*(2), 78-84.

Brown, J.K. (1985). Ambulatory services: the mainstay of cancer nursing care. *Oncol Nurs Forum 12*(1), 57-59.

Burdman, G.D.M., Benoliel, J.Q., Dohner, C.W., Schaad, D., & Strand, D. (1987). A focus on cancer: development of a course on prevention and early detection. *J Contin Educ Nurs 18*(3), 93-96.

Chang, P.N. (1991). Psychosocial needs of long-term childhood cancer survivors: a review of literature. *Pediatrician 18*(1), 20-24.

De Muth, J.S. (1989). Patient teaching in the ambulatory setting. *Nurs Clin North Am 24*(3), 645-654.

Dobratz, M.C. (1990). Hospice nursing: present perspectives and future directives. *Cancer Nurs 13*(2), 116-122.

Dudas, S. & Carlson, C.E. (1988). Cancer rehabilitation. *Oncol Nurs Forum 15*(2), 183-188.

Dufour, D.F. (1989). Home or hospital care for the child with end-stage cancer: effects on the family. *Issues Compr Pediatr Nurs 12*(5), 371-383.

Elpern, E.H., Rodts, M.F., DeWald, R.L., & West, J.W. (1983). Associated practice: a case for professional collaboration. *J Nurs Adm 13*(11), 27-31.

Esparza, D.M., Young, N., & Luongo, J.A. (1989). Effective planning for office and outpatient chemotherapy administration. *Semin Oncol Nurs 5*(2, suppl 1), 8-14.

Farley, B.A. (1991). Ambulatory care settings. In S.B. Baird, R. McCorkle, & M. Grant (eds). *Cancer Nursing: A Comprehensive Textbook*. Philadelphia: W.B. Saunders Co., pp. 1011-1022.

Ferrell, B.A., Ferrell, B.R., & Osterweil, D. (1990). Pain in the nursing home. *J Am Geriatr Soc 38*(4), 409-414.

Gambosi, J.R. & Ulreich, S. (1990). Recovering from cancer: a nursing intervention program recognizing survivorship. *Oncol Nurs Forum 17*(2), 215-219.

Grady, C. (1989). Acquired immunodeficiency syndrome: the impact on professional nursing practice. *Cancer Nurs 12*(1), 1-9.

Greenwald, H.P., Dirks, S.J., Borgatta, E.F., McCorkle, R., Nevitt, M.C., & Yelin, E.H. (1989). Work disability among cancer patients. *Soc Sci Med 29*(11), 1253-1259.

Habeck, R.V., Romsaas, E.P., & Olsen, S.J. (1984). Cancer rehabilitation and continuing care: a case study. *Cancer Nurs 7*(4), 315-319.

Halloran, J., Hughes, A., & Mayer, D.K. (1988). Oncology Nursing Society position paper on HIV-related issues. *Oncol Nurs Forum 15*(2), 206-217.

Harris, M.D. & Parente, C.A. (1991). Home care services. In S.B. Baird, R. McCorkle, & M. Grant (eds). *Cancer Nursing: A Comprehensive Textbook*. Philadelphia: W.B. Saunders Co., pp. 1023-1032.

Harris, M.G. & Bean, C.A. (1991). Changing the role of the nurse in the hematology-oncology outpatient setting. *Oncol Nurs Forum 18*(1), 43-46.

Hilderley, L.J. (1991). Nurse-physician collaborative practice: the clinical nurse specialist in a radiation oncology private practice. *Oncol Nurs Forum 18*(3), 585-591.

Holmes, B.C. (1985). Private practice in oncology nursing. *Oncol Nurs Forum 12*(3), 65-67.

Hull, M.M. (1991). Hospice nurses: caring support for caregiving families. *Cancer Nurs 14*(2), 63-70.

Johnson, J.B. & Kelly, A.W. (1990). Multifaceted rehabilitation program for women with cancer. *Oncol Nurs Forum 17*(5), 691-695.

Lewis, F.M. (1990). Strengthening family supports. Cancer and the family. *Cancer, 65*(3), 752-759.

Lone, P. (1989). A place to call home. *Am J N 89*(4), 490-492.

Mayer, D. & O'Connor, L. (1989). Rehabilitation of persons with cancer: an ONS position statement. *Oncol Nurs Forum 16*(3), 433.

McCorkle, R. (1979). A new beginning: the opening of a multidisciplinary cancer unit. Part I. *Cancer Nurs 2*(3), 201-209.

McCorkle, R. (1979). A new beginning: the opening of a multidisciplinary cancer unit. Part II. *Cancer Nurs 2*(4), 269-278.

McCorkle, R. (1988). The four essentials. *J Palliative Care 4*(1-2), 59-61.

McCorkle, R., Benoliel, J.Q., Donaldson, G., Georgiadou, F., Moinpour, C. & Goodell, B. (1989). A randomized clinical trial of home nursing care for lung cancer patients. *Cancer 64*(6), 1375-1382.

McCorkle, R. & Germino, B. (1984). What nurses need to know about home care. *Oncol Nurs Forum 11*(6), 63-69.

McMahon, K.M. & Coyne, N. (1989). Symptom management in patients with AIDS. *Semin Oncol Nurs 5*(4), 289-301.

Miaskowski, C. (1990). The future of oncology nursing: a historical perspective. *Nurs Clin North Am 25*(2), 461-473.

Mills, D.S. & Pennoni, M. (1986). A nurturing work environment: In philosophy and practice. *Cancer Nurs 9*(3), 117-124.

Moinpour, C.M. & Polissar, L. (1989). Factors affecting place of death of hospice and non-hospice cancer patients. *Am J Public Health 79*(11), 1549-1551.

Moseley, J.R. & Brown, J.S. (1985). The organization and operation of oncology units. *Oncol Nurs Forum 12*(5), 17-24.

Nail, L.M., Greene, D., Jones, L.S., & Flannery, M. (1989). Nursing care by telephone: describing practice in an ambulatory oncology center. *Oncol Nurs Forum 16*(3), 387-395.

NCCS News briefs. (1991). *Coping 4*(3), 21.

Neal, M.C. (1982). *Nurses in Business*. Pacific Palisades, Calif.: Nurseco.

Padella, G. & Kirshner, T. (1991). Continuity of care and discharge planning. In S.B. Baird, R. McCorkle, & M. Grant (eds). *Cancer Nursing: A Comprehensive Textbook*. Philadelphia: W.B. Saunders Co., pp. 1000-1007.

Pappas, C.A. & Van Scoy-Mosher, C. (1988). Establishing a profitable outpatient community nursing center. *J Nurs Adm 18*(5), 31-33.

Parkes, C.M. (1985). Terminal care: home, hospital, or hospice? Lancet *1*(8421), 155-157.

Parkes C.M. (1988). Not always! *J Palliative Care 4*(1-2), 50-52.

Pasacreta, J.V. & Jacobsen, P.B. (1989). Addressing the need for staff support among nurses caring for the AIDS population. *Oncol Nurs Forum 16*(5), 659-663.

Paulen, A. (1984). High touch in a high tech environment. *Cancer Nurs 7*(3), 201.

Rodek, C.F. & Jacob, S. (1984). Hospice legislation: a new trial. *Cancer Nurs 7*(5), 385-389.

Romsaas, E.P. & McCormick J.M. (1986). Assessment and resource utilization for cancer patients. *Arch Phys Med Rehabil 67*(7), 459-462.

Rose, M.A. (1989). Health promotion and risk prevention: applications for cancer survivors. *Oncol Nurs Forum 16*(3), 335-340.

Rowland, H.S. & Rowland, B.L. (1984). *The Nurse's Almanac* (2nd ed). Rockville, Md: Aspen Systems Corp.

Satterwhite, B.E., Settle, J.T., Cushnie, P.B., & Kaplowitz, L.G. (1991). Ambulatory care for patients with HIV/AIDS: creating a specialty clinic. *Oncol Nurs Forum 18*(3), 555-558.

Smith, S.N. & Bohnet, N. (1983). Organization and administration of hospice care. *J Nurs Adm 13*(11), 10-16.

Stein, S., Linn, M.W., & Stein, E.M. (1989). Psychological correlates of survival in nursing home cancer patients. *Gerontologist 29*(2), 224-228.

Tehan, C. (1982). Hospice in an existing home care agency. *Fam Community Health 5*(3), 11-20.

Tighe, M.G., Fisher, S.G., Hastings, C., & Heller, B. (1985). A study of the oncology nurse role in ambulatory care. *Oncol Nurs Forum 12*(6), 23-27.

Tornberg, M.J., McGrath, B.B., & Benoliel, J.Q. (1984). Oncology transition services: partnerships of nurses and families. *Cancer Nurs 7*(2), 131-137.

Vinciguerra, V. (1988). How it can be done: a pilot project in comprehensive home cancer treatment. *J Palliative Care 4*(1-2), 53-55.

Vinciguerra, V., Degnan, T.J., Sciortino, A., O'Connell, M., Moore, T., Brody, R., Budman, D., Eng, M., & Carlton, D. (1986). A comparative assessment of home versus hospital comprehensive treatment for advanced cancer patients. *J Clin Oncol 4*(10), 1521-1528.

Watson, P.G. (1990). Cancer rehabilitation: the evolution of a concept. *Cancer Nurs 13*(1), 2-12.

Weinstein, S.M. (1984). Specialty teams in home care. *Am J Nurs 84*(3), 342-345.

Wells, R.J. (1990). Rehabilitation: making the most of time. *Oncol Nurs Forum 17*(4), 503-507.

Williams, H.A. (1988). Social support and social networks: a review of the literature. *J Assoc Pediatr Oncol Nurs 5*(3), 6-10.

Wright, K. & Dyck, S. (1984). Expressed concerns of adult cancer patients' family members. *Cancer Nurs 7*(5), 371-374.

Yates, J.H. & Lyons, C. (1991). The organization of cancer service settings. In S.B. Baird, R. McCorkle, & M. Grant (eds). *Cancer Nursing: A Comprehensive Textbook*. Philadelphia: W.B. Saunders Co., pp. 993-999.

12

Professional Issues in Cancer Care

Mary Cunningham, MS, RN

Professional Development

I. Professional mandates related to professional development.
   A. American Nurses' Association (ANA)/Oncology Nursing Society (ONS) Standards of Oncology Nursing Practice, Standard VII: professional development—the oncology nurse assumes responsibility for professional development and continuing education and contributes to the professional growth of others.
   B. ONS Standards of Oncology Nursing Education: Generalist and Advanced Practice Levels.
      1. Standard V: learner-oncology nurse generalist—the oncology nurse generalist:
         a. Assumes responsibility for personal/professional development in oncology nursing.
         b. Contributes to the professional growth of others.
      2. Standard V: learner-advanced level oncology nurse—the advanced level oncology nurse assumes responsibility for personal professional development in oncology practice, education, consultation, administration, and research.
   C. Joint Commission of Accreditation of Healthcare Organizations.
      1. Nursing care chapter from the 1991 *Accreditation Manual for Hospitals,* Standard NC 2: all members of the nursing staff are competent to fulfill their assigned responsibilities.
         a. Required characteristic NC 2.1: each member of the nursing staff is assigned clinical and/or managerial responsibilities based on educational preparation, applicable licensing laws and regulations, and assessment of current competence.
         b. Required characteristic NC 2.3: nursing staff members participate in orientation, regularly scheduled staff meetings, and ongoing education designed to improve their competence.

II. Professional development strategies.
   A. Identification of professional development needs.
      1. Conduct self-assessment of learning needs.
      2. Develop plan for meeting learning needs.
      3. Initiate independent learning activities (e.g., reading professional literature, participating in professional organizations, identifying resource staff, participating in professional support groups).

4. Participate in continuing education activities.
5. Maintain an awareness of personal beliefs, values, biases, and traditions that influence patient care.

B. Professional certification.

1. Rationale for certification: enables a profession to define and articulate for its members the new knowledge required for practice.
2. Definition: one measure of continued competency of individuals and as the means of documenting, to some extent, continued professional development.
3. Rationale for recertification: competency changes over time as knowledge and technology changes.

C. Continued professional competency: National Council of State Boards of Nursing, Inc., identified six methods to assure continued competency:

1. Peer review.
2. Continuing education.
3. Client review.
4. Periodic refresher courses.
5. Competency examinations.
6. Minimal practice requirements.

III. Outcomes of professional development.

A. Enhancement of the development of the profession.
B. Beneficial to individual professional.
C. Beneficial to recipients of care.
D. Fulfillment of the characteristics of a profession:

1. Specialized knowledge—profession is based on specialized knowledge that is passed to new practitioners through education and demonstration.
2. Commitment—implies career orientation; concerned not only with present work performance but also with improving standards and the status of the profession.
3. Vital service—provides a service of critical importance to society.
4. Autonomy—self-regulating or self-governing; responsible for developing standards that govern practice and performance; accountable.
5. Authority—the power to act independently because of competency.

Multidisciplinary Collaboration

I. Professional mandates related to multidisciplinary collaboration.

A. ANA/ONS Standards of Oncology Nursing Practice, Standard VIII: multidisciplinary collaboration—the oncology nurse collaborates with the multidisciplinary team in assessing, planning, implementing and evaluating care.

1. Rationale: the complexity of cancer care delivery necessitates a multidisciplinary approach for the provision of services to clients.
2. Collaboration among professionals is essential to promote efficient and effective care and to help the client achieve optimal health.

B. ONS Standards of Oncology Nursing Education: Generalist and Advanced Practice Levels.

1. Standard V: learner-oncology nurse generalist—the oncology nurse generalist collaborates with the multidisciplinary team to access, plan, implement, and evaluate primary, secondary, and tertiary care.
2. Standard V: learner-advanced level oncology nurse—the advanced level oncology nurse collaborates with clients to minimize cancer risks and to promote health.

   C. Joint Commission of Accreditation of Health Care Organizations: nursing staff members collaborate, as appropriate, with physicians and other clinical disciplines in making decisions regarding each patient's need for nursing care.

   D. Five essential factors of National Joint Practice Commission Model for collaborative practice between nurses and physicians:
1. Communication.
2. Competence.
3. Accountability.
4. Trust.
5. Administrative support.

   E. Association of Community Cancer Centers (ACCC), Standard 1: there is a multidisciplinary team approach to planning, implementing, and evaluating the care of cancer patients and families.

   F. ANA Nursing, Social Policy Statement: the nursing profession is particularly concerned with the working relationships essential to the carrying out its health orientated mission.

   G. Society: society's emphasis on health care requires health care planning as opposed to fragmentation into disciplines such as medical care, nursing care, physical therapy services; the very nature of health care mandates involvement of more than a single health care provider.

II. Types of working relationships.

   A. Slave-master relationships—person with power gives a command that another individual obeys; assumes that the responding individual has little knowledge, few skills, and little or no judgment or initiative.

   B. Detente—recognized power among individuals; a recognition and acceptance of separate spheres of activity and responsibility; mutuality of interests and commonality of goals.

   C. Collaboration—a true partnership in which the power on both sides is valued by both, with recognition and acceptance of separate and combined spheres of activity and responsibility, mutual safeguarding of the legitimate interests of each party, commonality of goals that is recognized by both parties; individuals in a true partnership believe that collaboration provides synergism of talents and efforts.

III. Barriers to the development of collaborative relationships.

   A. Lack of identification with one's own profession.

   B. Tendency to regard professional expertise as bias.

   C. Discomfort with responsibility.

   D. Felt discrimination in relationships.

   E. Failure of others to value one's profession.

   F. Competency inconsistencies within one's profession because of lack of uniform preparation.

   G. Lack of clearly defined, distinct domain of influence.

   H. Lack of understanding for another's perception.

   I. Overlapping and changing domains of practice that produce competition.

   J. Perceived threats to autonomy.

   K. Lack of administrative support for collaborative relationships.

   L. Lack of recognition for knowledge and expertise.

   M. Role confusion (role extension versus role expansion) within or among professions.

IV. Opportunities for collaboration.
   A. Potential for collaboration among healthcare providers/agencies exists wherever and with whomever the client and family have contact. Although emphasis is often placed on physician-nurse collaboration, nurses have the potential of collaborative relationships with any member of the multidisciplinary health care team.
   B. Nurse-to-nurse collaboration may be influenced by the following:
      1. Role—clinician, educator, researcher, administrator (clinician-researcher collaboration in the identification of a clinical problem and evaluation of applicable research findings to address the problem; educator-administrator-clinician collaboration in the development, implementation, and evaluation of staff nurse orientation; clinician-administrator-researcher collaboration in the development and testing of a client acuity classification system).
      2. Domain of responsibility such as shift and performance standards (day, evening, and night shift nurses collaborate on developing change of shift report guidelines; primary nurse and associate nurse collaborate on the nursing process).
      3. Specialization (collaboration among nurses with a specialty [oncology, critical care, intraoperative care] in planning for continuity of care for the client diagnosed with lung cancer undergoing a thoracotomy).
      4. Subspecialization (collaboration among nurses with a subspecialty [medical oncology, surgical oncology, radiation oncology, biotherapy] in the development of a cancer care orientation packet for clients and families).
      5. Practice setting—acute care, outpatient, ambulatory treatment center, office practice, home care, hospice care, comprehensive cancer treatment center, community hospital, rural community (collaboration among nurses from a variety of practice settings to develop a chronic pain protocol).
   C. Collaborative relationships may extend beyond direct care health care providers to members of voluntary agencies and organizations (nurse, Leukemia Society volunteer, and patient collaborate in the development and implementation of a client/family support group).

V. Benefits of collaborative relationships.
   A. Maximizes the unique skills of each person.
   B. Assumes shared responsibility.
   C. Delineates shared and individual responsibilities and accountability.
   D. Reduces duplication of efforts.
   E. Expedites planned action.
   F. Enhances communication.
   G. Creates and modifies norms.
   H. Facilitates role clarification by revealing the uniqueness of each professional domain.
   I. Benefits recipients of service.

Research

I. Professional mandates related to research.
   A. ANA/ONS Standards of Oncology Nursing Practice, Standard XI: research—the oncology nurse contributes to the scientific base of nursing practice and the field of oncology through the review and application of research.
   B. ONS Standards of Oncology Nursing Education: Generalist and Advanced Practice Levels.

    1. Oncology Nurse Generalist Standard III: curriculum; the curriculum includes:
      a. Application of research findings to oncology nursing practice.
      b. Delineation of the role of the nurse in cancer care, education, and research.
    2. Oncology Nurse Generalist Standard V: learner; oncology nurse generalist participates in oncology nursing research problem identification, implementation, and/or application to cancer care.
    3. Advanced Practice Standard III: curriculum; the curriculum includes:
      a. Opportunities to develop skills as a consumer of research as a beginning researcher.
      b. Application of nursing process, theories, and research to the practice of oncology nursing at the advanced level.
    4. Advanced Practice Standard V: learner; the advanced level oncology nurse:
      a. Applies the scientific method to initiate, evaluate, and apply oncology nursing research within the scope of advanced practice.
      b. Contributes to the development of nursing theory, research, and practice.
      c. Assumes responsibility for personal and professional development in oncology practice, education, consultation, administration, and research.

II. Research roles of nurses by level of education.
  A. ANA Cabinet on Nursing Research developed a hierarchy of research roles based on research preparation by level of education.
  B. Research roles of nurses for the five levels of research preparation include:
    1. Associate degree:
      a. Identify clinical problems.
      b. Assist in data collection.
      c. Collaborate in using research in clinical practice.
    2. Baccalaureate degree:
      a. Evaluate research reports.
      b. Understand ethical principles in research.
      c. Assist investigators in accessing research subjects.
      d. Provide input about data collection methods.
      e. Use research findings in clinical practice.
    3. Master's degree:
      a. Provide clinical expertise for the research process.
      b. Evaluate clinical relevance of research findings.
      c. Ensure integration of research into practice.
      d. Generate a clinical practice environment supportive to conducting research.
    4. Doctorate degree:
      a. Conduct independent investigations in collaboration with other scientists and clinicians.
      b. Acquire external research funding.
      c. Disseminate research findings.
    5. Postdoctoral education—develop research programs.

III. Implementation of research role of oncology nurse generalist.
  A. Research role of the oncology nurse generalist includes:
    1. Identification of practice problems through observation of client populations and quality assurance activities; focus of practice problem may include:
      a. Developing and testing interventions designed to improve client outcomes such as the ability to perform central venous catheter care after one-to-one teaching compared to effect of group teaching or the impact of oral care protocol after the administration of mucosa toxic chemotherapy.

      b. Identifying variables associated with specific client problems or needs such as pattern of diarrhea and perineal skin breakdown after the administration of high-dose Ara-C (cytosine arabinoside).

      c. Describing the characteristics of a given situation such as non-nursing tasks assigned to nurses in the outpatient clinic or content of change-of-shift reports.

      d. Testing methods of delivering nursing care such as time and motion studies of nursing activities to determine whether to administer intravenous intermittent antibiotic therapy via intravenous piggyback or multichannelled pumps.

2. Participation in evaluation of existing research.

3. Collaboration in identifying solution to clinical problem.

    a. Incorporate applicable research into clinical practice.

    b. Identify need for research study.

4. Participation in research activities under the guidance of a qualified researcher.

    a. Conceptualization and design of a research study:

      (1) Establish the clinical significance of the problem.

      (2) Identify important clinical variables and client eligibility criteria.

      (3) Assess the feasibility of the methods and procedures proposed for the study.

    b. Implementation of research protocol:

      (1) Deliver prescribed interventions.

      (2) Identify potential research subjects.

      (3) Collect data.

      (4) Serve as research subject.

    c. Interpretation of results.

B. Characteristics of employer support of research role of oncology nurse generalist:

1. Values nursing research as evidenced by:

    a. Inclusion of research role in job description and performance standards.

    b. Maintenance of nursing research committee.

2. Supports research activities with time, money, resources, and recognition.

3. Provides opportunities for nurse to participate in research activities.

4. Values expertise of nurse generalist in identifying research problem.

5. Provides resource staff to assist the nurse in:

    a. Research critique.

    b. Incorporation of research findings into practice.

    c. Evaluation of outcomes of incorporating research findings into practice.

IV. Guidelines for evaluating research reports.

A. Areas fundamental to research reports include:

1. Problem and purpose.

    a. Statement of the research problem includes:

      (1) Generalized discussion of the problem.

      (2) Introduction to the area of study.

      (3) Statement of the importance of the subject.

      (4) Summarization of the related facts and theories.

    b. Statement of the purpose includes:

      (1) Focus of the study.

      (2) Specific variables.

      (3) Data collection methods.

      (4) Setting.

      (5) Nature of the sample.

   c. Statement of the purpose can be written as:
     (1) Question.
     (2) Statement.
     (3) Hypothesis.
2. Theoretical framework—support of hypothesis, research statement, or question by a clear and concise review of relevant research, literature, and conceptual framework or scientific theory.
3. Methodology.
   a. Description of how the investigator plans to seek answer to the research question.
   b. Types of research designs—qualitative and quantitative:
     (1) Qualitative research.
       (a) Purpose—to describe and explore phenomena or to gain understanding.
       (b) Characteristics—process focused, subjective, and not generalizable.
       (c) Types—descriptive, surveys, phenomenology, and content analysis.
     (2) Quantitative research.
       (a) Purpose—to describe relationships and cause and effect and to identify facts.
       (b) Characteristics—outcome focused, objective, generalizable.
       (c) Types—quasi-experimental, experimental, and correlational.
   c. Research design selection depends on:
     (1) Current knowledge about the problem.
     (2) Setting.
     (3) Ethics.
     (4) Skills of the researcher.
     (5) Time.
     (6) Resources (Table 12-1).
     (7) Funding (Table 12-1).
   d. Description of the sample.
     (1) Method of sample selection.
     (2) Representiveness of sample to larger population.
   e. Methods to collect data.
     (1) Discussion of the instrument(s).
     (2) Rationale of instrument(s) selection.
   f. Instrument(s) development.
     (1) Instrument(s) reliability.
     (2) Instrument(s) validity.
   g. Analysis of the data.
     (1) Description of the sample.
     (2) Description of statistics applied to the data.
     (3) Statistical procedures determined by research question/design and the level of measurement of the variables.
       (a) Research question.
         i. Description of phenomena—descriptive statistics such as the frequencies, means, and standard deviation.
         ii. Prediction of differences and relationships—inferential statistics such as t-test, analysis of variance (ANOVA), or chi square (χ^2).
       (b) Level of measurement.

Table 12-1
RESEARCH FUNDING RESOURCES AND AGENCIES

Bauer, D. (1988). The Complete Grants Sourcebook for Nursing and Health. New York: American Council on Education and MacMillan Publishing.

Provides profiles on federal, corporate, and foundation support of nursing research activities. For each funding source, author details the following: program title and address, purpose, areas of interest, types of assistance, examples of funding recipients, funding restrictions, financial profile, application process, and review process/selection criteria. Explains preparation of grant applications and provides examples.

Catalogue of Federal Domestic Assistance (CFDA)

Provides extensive information of federal programs and sources of research funding.

c/o Superintendent of Documents
U.S. Government Printing Office
Washington, DC 20402

Foundation centers

Publications provide regional details of the philanthropic industry and support of research.

Northeast	*Midwest*	*South*	*West*
Foundation Center	Foundation Center	Foundation Center	Foundation Center
79 Fifth Ave	Kent H. Smith Library	1001 Connecticut Ave. NW	312 Sutter Street
New York, NY 10003	1442 Hana Building	Washington, DC 20036	San Francisco, CA 94108
	1422 Euclid Ave.		
	Cleveland, Ohio 44115		

National Institutes of Health Guide for Grants and Contracts

Contains program announcements and requests for applications detailing specific research areas of interest to NIH institutes, centers and divisions and information on types of award mechanisms and updates on existing programs and policies.

NIH Guide Distribution Center
NIH
Building 31
Room B4-BN08
Bethesda, MD 20892

Office of Information and Legislative Affairs. National Center of Nursing Research. National Institute of Health (1990). Facts About Funding. (NIH Pub. No. 90-3112). Bethesda, Md: NCNR.

Explains the types of research and research training supported by the National Center for Nursing Research (NCNR) and the National Institutes of Health (NIH) mechanisms available to provide this support.

Office of Information and Legislative Affairs
National Center for Nursing Research
National Institutes of Health
Building 31, Room 5B03
Bethesda, MD 20892

NCNR within the NIH was created in 1986. With the creation of NCNR, many new opportunities exist to obtain funding for nursing research, research training, and career development. Ada Sue Hinshaw, RN, PhD, FAAN, is the director of NCNR.

National Center for Nursing Research
National Institutes of Health/Public Health Service
Building 38A/Room B2E17
Bethesda, MD 20894

Table 12-1
RESEARCH FUNDING RESOURCES AND AGENCIES *Continued*

Sigma Theta Tau International Honor Society of Nursing

Information and grant applications can be obtained from the following address:

Sigma Theta Tau
Attention: Program Department
550 West North Street
Indianapolis, IN 46202
317-634-8171

American Nurses' Foundation

The American Nurses' Foundation of the American Nurses' Association underwrites 25 grants each year. Information and grant applications can be obtained from the following address:

American Nurses' Foundation
1101 14th Street NW
Suite 200
Washington, DC 20005
202-789-1800

Oncology Nursing Society and the Oncology Nursing Foundation Research Grants

Information and grant applications can be obtained from the following address:

Oncology Nursing Society
501 Holiday Drive
Pittsburgh, PA 15220
412-921-7373

---

       i. Application of descriptive or inferential statistics applied depends on the types of variables measured—nominal, ordinal, interval, or ratio.

      ii. The higher the level of measurement, the more powerful the statistical test applied and the greater the degree of certainty the results are factual rather than chance occurrence.

  4. Interpretation and conclusions.

    a. Presentation of the findings—discussion of statistically significant findings and probable explanation for both significant and nonsignificant findings.

    b. Conclusion.

      (1) Integration of the research findings with previous literature, research, and theory.

      (2) Identification of practical and statistical significance.

      (3) Application of findings to nursing practice.

      (4) Suggestions for further research.

B. Questions asked before implementation of research findings into nursing practice:

  1. Are the resources and institutional support adequate to implement the findings?

  2. Are the results clinically significant?

  3. Can the results be generalized?

  4. Are the implementation strategies discussed by the researcher desirable and feasible in practice?

  5. Can the outcome of implementing the findings be measured?

V. Research priorities.
   A. National Center for Nursing research (1990):
      1. Low birth weight—mothers and infants.
      2. Human immunodeficiency virus (HIV) infection—prevention and care.
      3. Long-term care for older adults.
      4. Symptom management.
      5. Information systems.
      6. Health promotion for children and adolescents.
      7. Technology dependency across the life span.
   B. Oncology Nursing Society survey (1988):
      1. Prevention and early detection.
      2. Symptom management.
      3. Pain control and management.
      4. Patient or health education.
      5. Coping and stress management.

Work-Related Stress

I. Professional mandates related to work-related stress.
   A. ANA/ONS Standards for Oncology Nursing Practice, Standard VII: professional development—the oncology nurse assumes responsibility for professional development and continuing education and contributes to the professional growth of others.
      1. Structure criteria—a mechanism is in place to provide staff development and continuing education opportunities informing staff about legal aspects of oncology nursing, stress management for oncology nursing, and occupational hazards.
      2. Outcome criteria—the oncology nurse maintains his or her physical, mental, and emotional health.
   B. ONS Standards of Oncology Nursing Education: Generalist and Advanced Practice Levels, Standard V: learner-generalist and advanced level oncology nurse—oncology nurse generalist and advanced level oncology nurse practice health behaviors consistent with health promotion as a role model for the public.

II. Stress and burnout concepts.
   A. Definitions of stress:
      1. Stress is necessary for life.
      2. Stress demands adaptational change—physical, emotional, and intellectual.
      3. Stress involves a transaction between an individual and the environment.
      4. The individual is the focal mediator between the stress stimulus and the response.
      5. Individual judgment and evaluation of the stimulus influence perception of the stimulus and the nature of the response.
   B. Stress becomes problematic when the level of stress exceeds one's ability to respond effectively and when the adaptation becomes growth inhibiting rather than growth promoting.
   C. Professional stress demands adaptation in the performance of one's professional role.
   D. The impact of stress is intensified by:
      1. Suddenness of onset.
      2. Chronicity of stressor(s).

3. High degree of intensity.
4. Significance of the stressor to the individual.
5. Vulnerability of the individual.
6. Occurrence of multiple stressors.
E. Definition of burnout:
  1. Burnout is exhaustion caused by excessive demands on energy, strength, or resources.
  2. Burnout is insidious, cumulative, and progressive.
F. Professional burnout is the deterioration of professional performance that is directly related to the demand for adaptational change brought on by perceived stressors in the work environment.
G. Chronic stress is implicated in contributing to job dissatisfaction, turnover, impaired job performance, and lack of productivity.

III. Stressors affecting oncology nurses—work-related stress in oncology nursing is multidimensional, involving:
  A. Characteristics of the individual nurse.
    1. Overly dedicated and committed.
    2. High need to control.
    3. Over identification with clients and families.
    4. Strong dependency needs.
    5. Perfectionism.
    6. Unrealistic goals and self-expectations.
    7. Diffuse personal boundaries.
    8. Idealistic.
  B. Characteristics of cancer client population and nature of care.
    1. Elusive cause.
    2. Heterogeneity of malignancies.
    3. Variability of prognosis.
    4. Unpredictability of health-illness trajectory.
    5. Confrontation with disfigurements, disability, pain, and death.
    6. Social stigma of working with people diagnosed with cancer.
    7. Knowledge base constantly in a state of flux.
    8. Confrontation with labile emotions of clients families, and staff.
    9. Inability to restore health.
    10. Repeated sense of failure if cure orientated.
  C. Characteristics within the work setting.
    1. Inadequate nurse-client ratio.
    2. Limited opportunity to participate in decision making.
    3. Limited recognition and rewards for work performance.
    4. Limited autonomy.
    5. Unclear role expectations.
    6. Conflicts between professional goals and organizational goals.
    7. Inadequate psychological support from peers.
    8. Deficient administrative support.
    9. Competitive rather than collaborative relationships.
    10. Limited upward mobility.
    11. Limited open and honest communications with peers, nurse managers, and physicians.
    12. Inappropriate discharges.
    13. Work overload.

IV. Stress responses.
  A. Physical responses.
    1. Constant state of fatigue.
    2. Sleep disturbances.
    3. Change in food, alcohol, drug, and/or cigarette consumption.
    4. Changes in physical appearance.
    5. Repetitive accidents.
    6. Change in sexual behavior.
    7. Exacerbation of physical illness.
    8. Muscular pain (e.g., neck and lower back).
  B. Emotional responses.
    1. Angry outbursts.
    2. Irritability.
    3. Feelings of worthlessness.
    4. Feelings of helplessness.
    5. Depression.
    6. Isolation of self from others.
    7. Self-criticism.
    8. Feelings of guilt.
    9. Inability to identify and express feelings.
    10. Difficulty forming and maintaining intimate relationships.
    11. Martyrdom.
    12. Numbing feelings through addictions.
    13. Cynical and negative feelings toward clients, families, and coworkers.
    14. Whining.
  C. Intellectual responses.
    1. Forgetfulness.
    2. Preoccupations.
    3. Mathematical and grammatical errors.
    4. Lack of concentration.
    5. Lack of attention to details.
    6. Denial.
    7. Assuming responsibility for behavior or feelings of others.
    8. Indecisiveness.
    9. Difficulty setting limits.
    10. Lying when telling the truth would be easier.
    11. Past, rather than present or future orientation.
    12. Diminished productivity.
    13. Impaired problem solving.
    14. Resistance to change.
    15. Change to abstract and analytical thinking.
    16. Feelings of powerlessness.
    17. Breakdown in effective communication.
    18. Strict adherence to rules rather than consideration of the uniqueness of others.
    19. Objectifying clients (e.g., "the new leukemic").
    20. Pessimism.
    21. Uncooperativeness.
    22. Tardiness or absenteeism.

V. Stress management strategies.
  A. Goals of stress management strategies include:
    1. Eliminating those stressors that can be eliminated.

    2. Mastering stress that cannot be eliminated.

    3. Developing techniques for recognition and modification of stress responses.

B. Stress management strategies include:

    1. Legitimizing one's own needs by commitment to self-care.

    2. Conducting a self-assessment, which might entail the following:

        a. Needs.

        b. Motivations.

        c. Goals.

        d. Support systems—work and social.

        e. Stress responses:

            (1) Physical.

            (2) Emotional.

            (3) Intellectual.

        f. Communication style.

        g. Time management ability.

        h. Conflict resolution skills.

        i. Sources of stress.

C. Based on self-evaluation, strategies for self-care and stress management may include:

    1. Increasing physical activity.

    2. Engaging in social activity.

    3. Becoming open to emotionally intimate relationships.

    4. Establishing realistic goals and expectations.

    5. Identifying and working to eliminate irrational beliefs.

    6. Seeking professional counseling.

    7. Practicing relaxation techniques.

    8. Maintaining a personal journal to record and analyze feelings and thoughts.

    9. Taking responsibility when appropriate; delegating when appropriate.

  10. Acquiring new skills through continuing education courses (time management, dealing with difficult people, conflict-resolution techniques).

  11. Advocating the following in the work setting:

        a. Development of support groups.

        b. Balanced nurse-client ratios that support the provision of quality care.

        c. Employee benefit packages that provide for vacations, mental health days, and reimbursement for professional counseling.

        d. Recognition and financial incentives that reward quality performance.

        e. Establishment of ethics committee.

        f. Participation in decision making.

        g. Agency philosophy that supports multidisciplinary collaboration.

        h. Acquisition of the "Ten Basic Rights for . . . Health Care Professionals": the right to be treated with respect; to a reasonable workload; to an equitable wage; to determine your own priorities; to ask for what you want; to refuse without making excuses or feeling guilty; to make mistakes and be responsible for them; to give and receive information as a professional; to act in the best interest of the client; to be human.

Quality Assurance

I. Professional mandates related to quality assurance.

  A. ANA/ONS Standards of Oncology Nursing Practice, Standard IX: quality assurance—the oncology nurse participates in peer review and interdisciplinary program evaluation to assure that high quality nursing care is provided to clients.

    1. Rationale: evaluation of the quality of nursing care through examination of the nursing process is one way to fulfill the profession's obligation to ensure adherence to professional practice standards.

    2. Peer review, interdisciplinary program evaluation, management, nursing quality assurance programs, and nursing research are used in this endeavor.

B. ANA Nursing, A Social Policy Statement: each nurse remains accountable for the quality of her or his practice within the full scope of nursing practice. Nursing practice demands professional intention and commitment carried out in accordance with the ANA *Standards of Nursing Practice* and its ethical code. All nurses are ethically and legally accountable for actions taken in the course of nursing practice as well as for actions delegated by the nurse to others assisting in the delivery of nursing care. Such accountability may be accomplished through the regulatory mechanisms of licensure, through criminal and civil laws, through the code of ethics of the profession, and through peer evaluation.

C. ANA Code for Nurses:

    1. The nurse acts to safeguard the patient when his care and safety are affected by incompetent, unethical or illegal conduct of any person.

    2. The nurse participates in efforts of the profession to define and upgrade standards of nursing practice and education.

    3. The nurse maintains individual competence in nursing practice, recognizing and accepting responsibility for individual actions and judgments.

II. General statements about quality assurance.

A. Society gives professional bodies the privilege to govern their concerns, empowering professions to manage their own functions; in return, professions are accountable to society for their actions.

B. Self-regulation to assure quality in performance and products is a hallmark of a profession.

C. Nurses have a professional responsibility to assure quality control.

D. Nursing has the right and professional responsibility to define and control its own practice.

E. In that nursing is a major component of health care, quality assurance in nursing is essential to guarantee the overall quality of health care.

F. Professional and practice standards provide a mechanism to assure and evaluate quality care.

    1. Practice standards pertain to theory, data collection, diagnosis, planning, intervention, and evaluation.

    2. Professional standards pertain to professional behavior—professional development, interdisciplinary collaboration, quality assurance, ethics, and research.

G. Professional and practice standards may be found in the following:

    1. State nurse practice acts.

    2. Published standards of professional organizations such as:

        a. *ANA Standards of Nursing Practice.*

        b. *ANA/ONS Standards of Oncology Nursing Practice.*

        c. *ONS Standards of Oncology Nursing Education: Generalist and Advanced Practice Levels.*

        d. *ONS Standards of Oncology Education—Patient/Family and Public.*

        e. *ONS Standards of Advanced Practice in Oncology Nursing.*

    3. Federal agencies guidelines and regulations (Joint Commission on Accreditation of Health Care Organization [JCAHO], Social Security Administration).

    4. Hospital or agency policy and procedure manuals.

     5. Job description and performance evaluation criteria.
     6. Professional organizations publications (*ANA Nursing: A Social Policy Statement; ANA: A Code for Nurses*).
     7. Professional literature.
  H. No one source is sufficient to describe quality of care or performance.
   I. Professional quality assurance strategies may include:
     1. Mandatory licensure.
     2. Peer review.
     3. Development and implementation of quality assurance programs.
     4. Professional certification.
     5. Certification of education programs and continuing education programs.
     6. Risk management.

III. Peer review.
  A. Peer review is a process in which professional nurses appraise the quality of care provided by professional nurse(s) in accordance with established standards.
  B. Peer review process includes both appraisal of nursing care delivered by a group of nurses and the appraisal of an individual nurse.
     1. Nursing Professional Standards Review: review of nursing care provided by a group of nurses; purposes of Nursing Professional Standards Review include:
       a. Evaluation of the quality of nursing care to identify the extent of consistency to established standard.
       b. Identification of strengths and weaknesses in nursing care.
       c. Justification for recommendations for new or revised policies, procedures, and standards to improve nursing care.
       d. Identification of practice areas in which knowledge is needed.
     2. Nursing Performance Review: review of nursing care provided by an individual nurse; purposes of Nursing Performance Review include:
       a. Provision of assistance for the nurse in improving the quality of practice.
       b. Provision of commendation and/or constructive criticism of an individual nurse's performance when applicable.
       c. Protection of the nurse from ill-founded and unjust accusations.
       d. Appraisal of how the practice of the nurse maintains or deviates from accepted practice and professional standards.
     3. Data collected from Nursing Performance Review may be used to make recommendations to a certification board and/or provide input into the performance evaluation that qualifies the nurse for clinical advancement or salary increases.

IV. Ten-step model for quality assurance: the 10-step model developed by the Joint Commission on Accreditation of Healthcare Organizations can serve as a framework for unit-based to organization-wide quality assurance activities; the steps in the model are as follows:
  A. Assign responsibility for monitoring and evaluation activities.
  B. Delineate the scope of care provided, including a description of the following:
     1. Types of clients served.
     2. Treatments or activities performed.
     3. Basic clinical activities required.
     4. Types of practitioners providing care.
  C. Identify important aspects of care—essential elements of activities that constitute nursing care.
  D. Identify indicators for monitoring the important aspects of care that are measurable variables relating to the structure, process, or outcomes of care.

1. Structure criteria describe organizational, financial, and physical attributes of the agency and provider characteristics (agency philosophy, nurse-patient ratio, qualifications of staff, equipment, environment, educational preparation of professional staff [annual continuing education requirements, certification], client classification system used to determine staffing needs).
2. Process criteria describe actions and behaviors that focus on the nature of activities, interventions, and sequence of events in the delivery of nursing care (job descriptions, performance standards, procedures, protocols, implementation strategies of nursing care plans).
3. Outcome criteria describe expected end results of nursing care such as measurable changes in the health status of the client (health knowledge, improved health status [physiological, psychological, and/or functional], satisfaction).

E. Establish the thresholds for evaluation for the indicators—a threshold for evaluation is an established level or point in the cumulative data that will trigger an intensive evaluation of care (aspect of care—vesicant extravasation; indicator—number of clients who experience a vesicant extravasation; threshold for evaluation—0%; intensive evaluation—any vesicant extravasation).

F. Monitor the important aspects of care by collecting and organizing measurements needed to determine whether or not standards are attained—data collection methods may include concurrent and retrospective audit, direct observation of nurse or client performance, questionnaire, interview, knowledge testing.

G. Evaluate care when thresholds for the indicators are reached to identify problems or opportunities for improvement.

H. Develop and implement a plan of action to correct identified problems or improve care; the plan may include:
   1. Description of the problem.
   2. Who or what is expected to change or improve.
   3. What resources are needed.
   4. Who is responsible for implementing action.
   5. What action is appropriate in view of cause (insufficient knowledge, defects in systems, deficient behavior or performance), scope, and severity.
   6. When change is expected to occur.
   7. When reevaluation will occur.
   8. Who is responsible for evaluation of the plan.

I. Evaluate the effectiveness of the actions and document the improvement in care.

J. Communicate the results of the monitoring and evaluation process to relevant individuals, departments, and to the organization-wide quality assurance program.

V. Practice acts.
   A. The nurse practice act is the state law that governs the practice of nursing.
   B. The board of nursing is the administrative agency that implements the statutes, with power granted by the state legislature.
   C. Basic components of nurse practice acts include:
      1. Definition of professional nursing.
      2. Requirements for licensure.
      3. Provisions for endorsements or sanctioning for persons licensed in another state.
      4. Specifications of exemptions from licensure.
      5. Grounds for disciplinary actions, which may include:
         a. Improper procurement of a license.
         b. Conviction for a felony.

    c. Physical or mental incapacity.

    d. Unprofessional conduct.

    e. Incompetence, negligence, and malpractice.

    f. Substance abuse.

  6. Provisions for the board of nursing with an outline of their responsibilities.

  7. Penalties for practicing without a license or substance abuse.

VI. Certification.

  A. Certification is a process by which a nongovernmental agency or association certifies that an individual licensed to practice a profession has met certain predetermined standards specified by that profession for specialty practice; its application to nursing means that a nurse has achieved competence in a field of specialty within the profession.

  B. Certification enables a profession to define and articulate for its members the new knowledge required to practice.

  C. Purposes of certification include:

    1. Protection of the public.

    2. Recognition of expert practitioner.

Occupational Health Hazards: Infections (Human Immunodeficiency Virus and Hepatitis) (Table 12-2)

I. Professional mandates related to occupational health hazards: HIV and hepatitis B virus (HBV) infections.

  A. ANA/ONS Standards of Oncology Nursing Practice, Standard VII: professional development—the oncology nurse assumes responsibility for professional development and continuing education and contributes to the professional growth of others.

    1. Structure criteria—a mechanism is in place to provide staff development and continuing education opportunities informing staff about legal aspects of oncology nursing, stress management for oncology nurses, and occupational hazards.

    2. Outcome criteria—the oncology nurse maintains his or her physical, mental, and emotional health.

  B. Centers for Disease Control:

    1. 1985—development of strategies for universal blood and body fluid precautions, stressing that all clients should be assumed infectious for HIV and other blood-borne pathogens.

    2. 1987—development of recommendations for prevention of transmission of HIV.

    3. 1988—recommendation for universal precautions to include protection against transmission of HIV and HBV.

  C. Department of Health and Human Services and Department of Labor: 1987—recommendation of HBV vaccination for workers exposed to blood and body fluids.

  D. Occupational Safety and Health Administration (OSHA): 1991—Occupational Exposure to Bloodborne Pathogens Standard—requires that Hepatitis B vaccination be made available by the employing agency after the employee has received information regarding HBV infections and transmission and HBV vaccination and within 10 working days of initial assignment to all employees who have occupational exposure.

Table 12-2
OCCUPATIONAL HEALTH HAZARDS: RESOURCES

AIDS Action Council

The purpose of the AIDS council is to lobby for fast, sensible action on AIDS research, education, and policy issues.

2033 "M" Street, NW No. 802
Washington, DC 20036
202-293-2886

AIDS Information

U. S. Public Health Service
Hubert Humphrey Building
Room 721-H
200 Independence Ave., SW
Washington, DC 20201
202-245-6866 (English)
202-245-SIDA (Spanish)

AIDS Hotline

1-800-342-AIDS

AZT Information Hotline

1-800-843-9388

American Hospital Association

Provides information about workplace safety, including transmission of infection.

840 N. Lake Shore Drive
Chicago, IL 60611-2431
312-280-6000
Order Processing Department
1-800-AHA-2626

American Hospital Association (1985). Patient Educator's Resource Guide: Organizational and Print Resources for Program Development. Chicago: Author.

This publication includes names of national organizations and their available publications and client education resources.

Centers for Disease Control

Mail Stop C06
1600 Clifton Rd. NE
Atlanta, GA 30333
404-639-3311

National AIDS Information Clearinghouse

Centralized resource for information on HIV/AIDS programs, services, and materials. A service of the U.S. Department of Health and Human Services, Public Health Service, and Centers for Disease Control.

P.O. Box 6003
Rockville, MD 20850
1-800-458-5231
FAX 1-301-738-6616

Table 12-2
OCCUPATIONAL HEALTH HAZARDS: RESOURCES *Continued*

National Directory of AIDS-Related Services

Provides information about national, regional, and local AIDS-related services.

The Fund for Human Dignity
80 Fifth Ave., Suite 1601
New York, NY 10011

National Health Information Center

Free service produces directories, resource guides, and bibliographies and distributes publications from the Office of Disease Prevention and Health Promotion.

c/o ONHIC
P.O. Box 133
Washington, DC 20013-1133
1-800-336-4797 (in Virginia, 703-522-2590)

National Hospice Organization

A nonprofit organization that provides literature and information about hospice care and referral to local, regional, and national resources.

1901 North Moore Street, Suite 901
Arlington, VA 22209
703-243-5900

National Institute of Mental Health

Provides booklet, *Coping with AIDS,* for health care professionals.

Public inquiries:
Park Lawn Building
Room 15C-15
5600 Fishers Lane
Rockville, MD 20857

The Shanti Project

Provides list of training materials for professional and public education.

890 Hayes Street
San Francisco, CA 94117
415-777-2273

U.S. Department of Occupational Safety and Health

The directorate of technical support provides information about work-related hazards and occupational injuries and illnesses.

Administration (OSHA)
Directorate of Technical Support
200 Constitution Ave. NW
Washington, DC 20210
202-523-7047

U.S. Department of Health and Human Services

Information Office
Washington, DC 20210
(202) 245-8705

E. Joint Commission of Accreditation for Healthcare Organizations, infection control chapter: 1991 *Accreditation Manual for Hospitals*.
   1. Standard 1C.1: there is an effective organization-wide program for the surveillance, prevention, and control of infection.
   2. Standard IC.1.3.2—activities are conducted to prevent and control infections in clients and personnel.
F. ANA: 1985—statement urging nurses to develop and promote effective education programs for the public and health care community with AIDS.
G. ONS:
   1. 1987—ONS Twelfth Annual Congress: adopted resolutions recognizing the role of oncology nurses in caring for HIV-infected persons and in educating professionals and public about AIDS.
   2. 1987—established ONS AIDS Task Force.
   3. 1988—published a position paper on HIV-related issues.
      a. Education—oncology nurses have a responsibility to be involved in HIV-related education at all levels.
      b. Clinical management of HIV-related illnesses—all nurses have a professional responsibility to care for individuals with HIV-related illnesses; the oncology nurse is particularly well prepared to care for these individuals.
      c. Safety issues:
         (1) ONS endorses the AIDS recommendations and guidelines proposed by the CDC; these guidelines include universal employment of blood and body fluid precautions for all clients in all health care settings.
         (2) ONS endorses the Centers for Disease Control (CDC) guidelines for the employment of health care workers who are HIV antibody positive.
      d. Public policy—oncology nurses should participate in addressing the complex health policy issues related to HIV illnesses; this participation may occur in the work place, in the community, through professional organizations or at the governmental level.
      e. Ethics—the ONS endorses the ANA Code for Nurses as the appropriate framework for dealing with HIV-associated ethical issues.
      f. Research—the oncology nurse fulfills a variety of roles in HIV-related research activities.
H. National Center for Nursing Research at the National Institutes of Health.
   1. 1988—set the National Nursing Research Agenda (NNRA); identified HIV infection as a high-priority area.
   2. 1989—appointed an HIV expert panel to identify priority areas for HIV nursing research:
      a. Prevention of HIV transmission.
      b. Physiological aspects of nursing care.
      c. Psychological aspects of nursing care.
      d. Delivery of nursing care.
      e. Applied ethics.

II. Infectious hazards in the workplace.
   A. HIV infection and acquired immunodeficiency syndrome (AIDS).
      1. HIV infection.
         a. CDC estimates that 1 to 2 million Americans are infected with HIV but are asymptomatic.
         b. A member of the retrovirus family.
         c. Infects human T cells, particularly the CD4 lymphocyte, which is essential to normal functioning of the immune system.

   d. Transmission:
      (1) Sexual contact.
      (2) Needle sharing.
      (3) Exposure to blood or blood products.
      (4) Through breast milk.
      (5) Perinatal.
   e. Diagnostic tests for HIV infection:
      (1) Enzyme-linked immunosorbent assay (ELISA).
      (2) Immunofluorescence assay, followed by a confirmatory Western blot.
2. AIDS.
   a. CDC reports that 150,000 Americans have been diagnosed with AIDS; of them, 70,000 have died as of 1990.
   b. AIDS is caused by the HIV.
   c. AIDS is a profound impairment of cellular immunity that results in the development of opportunistic infections and/or secondary cancers.
   d. Criteria for AIDS diagnosis:
      (1) Development of opportunistic infection or neoplasm.
      (2) Depletion of CD4 + cells (<200 cells/mm^3).
3. CDC classification of HIV disease:
   a. Group 1—acute symptomatic viral infection (myalgia, fever, headache, lymphadenopathy, rash, peripheral neuropathy) that appears 2 to 8 weeks after exposure to HIV.
   b. Group 2—laboratory evidence of HIV infection.
      (1) Person is asymptomatic.
      (2) HIV antibodies generally develop 2 to 8 weeks after the start of viral replications.
      (3) The cells predominantly infected are CD4 + lymphocytes.
   c. Group 3—persistent generalized lymphadenopathy.
   d. Group 4—patients with diverse HIV-related disease:
      (1) Subgroup A—constitutional symptoms, including fever, night sweats, weight loss, and diarrhea.
      (2) Subgroup B—neurological symptoms such as dementia, myelopathy, or peripheral neuropathy.
      (3) Subgroup C—secondary infection such as herpes zoster, thrush, pneumococcal infection, tuberculosis, or low CD4 + -lymphocyte counts.
      (4) Subgroup D—secondary cancer such as Kaposi's sarcoma or non-Hodgkin's lymphoma (see Chapter 37).
4. Treatment.
   a. Zidovudine (Retrovir) or azidothymidine (AZT).
      (1) Antiviral agent—reverse-transcriptase inhibitor.
      (2) Usual dose—100 to 250 mg orally every 4 hours.
      (3) Recommended for all HIV-infected individuals with T$_4$ count less than 500/mm^3.
      (4) Efficacy—increased survival, reduced incidence of opportunistic infections, no significant improvement in immunological status.
      (5) Side effects:
         (a) Hematological—anemia, neutropenia, and fever.
         (b) Gastrointestinal—nausea and vomiting.
         (c) Neurological—insomnia, confusion, and agitation.
         (d) Integumentary—rashes, pruritus, and nail pigmentation.
   b. Investigational agents.
      (1) Reverse-transcriptase inhibitors.

          (a) Dideoxycytidine (DDC).

          (b) Dideoxyinosine (DDI).

          (c) Dideoxydidehydrothymidine (D4T).

          (d) AzdU.

          (e) Foscarnet.

          (f) Carbovir.

        (2) Immunomodulators.

          (a) α-Interferon.

          (b) Interleukin-2.

          (c) HIV vaccines.

    5. Postexposure management.

      a. Counsel exposed employee about risk of infection.

      b. Provide exposed employee with a clinical evaluation and serological testing.

      c. Advise exposed employee to report any acute febrile illness within 12 weeks of exposure.

      d. Advise exposed employee to follow U.S. Public Health Services recommendations about prevention of HIV transmission such as no blood or organ donations, no breast-feeding, or no unprotected sexual intercourse.

      e. Seronegative exposed employee should be retested at 6 weeks, 12 weeks, and 6 months after exposure.

      f. Postexposure use of zidovudine is inconclusive.

B. Hepatitis.

    1. Hepatitis A (HAV)—infectious hepatitis.

      a. Onset—acute.

      b. Incubation—14 to 45 days.

      c. Transmission—feces.

      d. Symptomatology:

        (1) Fever usually precedes jaundice.

        (2) Jaundice.

        (3) Elevated serum glutamic-oxaloacetic transaminase (SGOT) or serum glutamic pyruvate transaminase (SGPT) levels for 1 to 3 weeks.

      e. Pre-exposure immune globulin (IG) prophylaxis for hospital personnel not recommended unless HAV outbreak; inoculate persons exposed to feces with IG.

      f. Postexposure IG prophylaxis recommended.

    2. HBV—serum hepatitis.

      a. Onset—gradual.

      b. Incubation—6 weeks to 6 months.

      c. Transmission—blood, blood products, saliva, and semen.

      d. Risk of HBV after parenteral exposure is directly proportional to the following:

        (1) Presence of HB surface antigen (HBsAg).

        (2) Immunity status of recipient.

        (3) Efficiency of transmission.

      e. Symptomatology:

        (1) Fever uncommon.

        (2) Jaundice.

        (3) Elevated SGOT or SGPT for 1 to greater than 8 months.

        (4) HBsAg (Australia antigen) present in incubation period and acute phase and may persist.

(5) Rash.

(6) Joint pain.

   f. HBV infection is a principal cause of acute and chronic hepatitis, cirrhosis, and primary hepatocellular carcinoma.

   g. CDC estimates that 12,000 health care workers whose jobs entail exposure to blood become infected with HBV annually; of the infected health care workers, approximately 250 will die—12 to 15 from fulminant hepatitis, 170 to 200 from cirrhosis, and 40 to 50 from liver cancer.

   h. Pre-exposure HBV vaccine recommended.

   i. Postexposure HBV vaccine recommended; hepatitis B immune globulin also may be recommended.

   j. Types of HBV vaccines:

     (1) Plasma-derived—Heptavax-B.

     (2) Recombinant HBV vaccine (yeast)—Recombivax-HB and Engerix-B.

       (a) Administration guidelines for recombinant vaccine—deltoid intramuscular injections.

       (b) Schedule—day 0, 1 month, and 6 months.

  3. Hepatitis C—non-A, non-B hepatitis.

   a. Onset—gradual.

   b. Incubation—15 to 180 days.

   c. Transmission—blood and feces.

   d. Symptomatology:

     (1) Fever—uncommon.

     (2) Jaundice.

     (3) Elevated SGOT or SGPT.

   e. Postexposure IG recommended.

  4. Delta hepatitis (HDV).

   a. Coinfection of HBV or superinfection in HBV carriers.

   b. Prevention of HDV by prevention of HBV.

III. Protective practices.

  A. All clients should be assumed infectious for HIV and other blood-borne pathogens.

  B. The development of protective practices programs should include the following steps:

   1. Classification of work activity.

   2. Development of standard operating policies and procedures.

   3. Provision of training and education.

   4. Development of procedures to ensure and monitor compliance.

   5. Workplace design.

  C. Universal precautions guidelines advise to take precautions when the possibility of exposure to blood or body fluids exists; the type of anticipated exposure prescribes the type of protective barriers worn.

   1. Use gloves when touching blood and body fluids, mucous membranes, non-intact skin, and surfaces soiled with blood and/or body fluids.

   2. Use gloves to perform invasive procedures.

   3. Use masks and eyewear during procedures likely to generate droplets of blood or body fluids.

   4. Wear gowns or aprons during procedures likely to generate splashes of blood or body fluids.

   5. Wash hands and skin and mucous membrane surfaces immediately after exposure.

6. Wash hands after glove removal.
7. Place used needles and sharps in a puncture-resistant disposable container that is labeled as infectious waste; used needles should not be bent, broken, sheared, or recapped by hand.
8. Health care workers with exudative lesions or weeping dermatitis should refrain from direct client care contact or handling of soiled equipment until skin condition resolves.
9. Pregnant health care workers are at no higher risk and should adhere strictly to protective practices.

BIBLIOGRAPHY

Professional Development

American Nurses' Association and Oncology Nursing Society (1987). *Standards of Oncology Nursing Practice*. Kansas City, Mo.: American Nurses' Association.
Gunning, C. (1983). The profession itself as a source of stress. In S.F. Jacobson & H. McGrath (eds). *Nurses Under Stress*. New York: John Wiley & Sons, pp. 113-126.
Itano, J. & Miller, C.A. (1990). Learning needs of oncology nursing society members. *Oncol Nurs Forum* 17(5), 697-703.
Joint Commission on Accreditation of Healthcare Organizations (1990). *Accreditation Manual for Hospitals*. Chicago: Author.
Oncology Nursing Society (1989). *Standards of Oncology Nursing Education: Generalist and Advanced Practice Levels*. Pittsburgh: Author.
Scofield, R. (1986). Why a generalist exam in a specialty area? *Oncol Nurs Forum* 13(1), 89.
Sheets, J. (1990). Director of Public Policy, Nursing Practice, and Education. National Council of State Boards of Nursing, Inc. Personal communication.
Steel, J.E. (1985). Getting our "C's" in order. *Oncol Nurs Forum* 12(3), 88-89.
Sullivan, S. (1985). The impact of certification on specialty associations. *Oncol Nurs Forum* 12(4), 145-146.
Volker, D.L. (1987). Learning needs assessment. *Oncol Nurs Forum* 14(5), 60-62.

Research

American Nurses' Association (1989). *Education for Participation in Nursing Research*. Kansas City, Mo.: Author.
American Nurses' Association and Oncology Nursing Society (1987). *Standards of Oncology Nursing Practice*. Kansas City, Mo.: American Nurses' Association.
Brown, M.L. (1983). The use of theory and conceptual frameworks in nursing research and practice. *Oncol Nurs Forum* 10(2), 111-112.
Ferrell, B.R., Grant, M., & Rhiner, M. (1990). Bridging the gap between research and practice. *Oncol Nurs Forum* 17(3), 447-448.
Foltz, A. & Stromborg, M. (1982). Research questions and answers. *Oncol Nurs Forum* 9(4), 86-88.
Frank-Stromborg, M. (ed) (1988). *Instruments for clinical nursing research*. Norwalk, Conn.: Appleton & Lange.
Funkhouser, S.N. & Grant, M.M. (1989). 1988 ONS survey of research priorities. *Oncol Nurs Forum* 16(3), 413-416.
Hinshaw, A.S. (1988). The National Center for Nursing Research: challenges and initiatives. *Nurs Outlook* 36(2), 54, 56.
Lindsey, A.M. (1983). Research: the problem and the purpose. *Oncol Nurs Forum* 10(3), 97-98.
McGuire, D. & Grant, M. (1983). Study designs: definitions and examples. *Oncol Nurs Forum* 10(4), 98-102.
Nail, L.M. (1990). Involving clinicians in nursing research. *Oncol Nurs Forum* 17(4), 621-623.
Office of Information and Legislative Affairs. National Center for Nursing Research. National Institutes of Health (1990). *Facts About Funding* (NIH Pub. No. 90-3112). Bethesda, Md: NCNR.
Oncology Nursing Society (1989). *Standards of Oncology Nursing Education: Generalist and Advanced Practice Levels*. Pittsburgh: Author.
Polit, D.F. & Hungler, B.P. (1991). *Nursing research: Principles and methods* (4th ed) Philadelphia: J.B. Lippincott Co., pp. 624-654.
Ropka, M.E. (1983). Utilization of research in nursing practice. *Oncol Nurs Forum* 10(1), 92-94.
Schmitt, M.H. (1986). Defining a clinical research problem and identifying a specific research question. *Oncol Nurs Forum* 13(5), 111-112, 118-119.
Schmitt, M.H. (1986). The research process versus related processes. *Oncol Nurs Forum* 13(4), 125-126, 131.

Schreier, A. (1984). Research questions and answers. *Oncol Nurs Forum 11*(1), 116-117.

Tornquist E.M. & Funk, S.G. (1990). How to write a research grant proposal. *Image 22*(1), 44-51.

Quality Assurance

American Nurses' Association (1975). *A Plan for Implementation of the Standards of Nursing Practice.* Kansas City, Mo.: Author.

American Nurses' Association (1976). *Code for Nurses With Interpretive Statements.* Kansas City, Mo.: Author.

American Nurses' Association (1976). *Guidelines for Review of Nursing Care at the Local Level.* Kansas City, Mo.: Author.

American Nurses' Association (1980). *Nursing, A Social Policy Statement.* Kansas City, Mo.: Author.

American Nurses' Association and Oncology Nursing Society (1987). *Standards of Oncology Nursing Practice.* Kansas City, Mo.: American Nurses' Association.

Beckman, J.S. (1987). What is a standard of practice? *J Nurs Quality Assurance 1*(2), 1-6.

Hegyvary, S.T. & Dieter-Haussmann, R.K. (1976). The relationship of nursing process and patient outcomes. *J Nurs Administration 6*(9), 18-21.

Joint Commission on Accreditation of Healthcare Organizations (1989). Characteristics of clinical indicators. *Quality Rev Bull 15*(11), 330-339.

Joint Commission on Accreditation of Healthcare Organizations (1991). *Accreditation Manual for Hospitals—1991.* Chicago: Author.

Lovett, R.B. (1989). Clinical practice evaluation in an oncology setting. *J Nurs Quality Assurance 3*(3), 24-35.

Lower, M.S. & Burton, S. (1989). Measuring the impact of nursing interventions on patient outcomes—the challenges of the 1990s. *J Nurs Quality Assurance 4*(1), 27-34.

Marker, C. (1987). The marker model: a hierarchy for nursing standards. *J Nurs Quality Assurance 1*(2), 7-20.

Miaskowski, C. & Rostad, M. (1990). Implementing the ANA/ONS standards of oncology nursing practice. *J Nurs Quality Assurance 4*(3), 15-23.

Steel, J.E. (1985). Getting our "C's" in order. *Oncol Nurs Forum 12*(3), 88-89.

Multidisciplinary Collaboration

American Nurses' Association (1980). *Nursing, A Social Policy Statement.* Kansas City, Mo.: Author.

American Nurses' Association and Oncology Nursing Society (1987). *Standards of Oncology Nursing Practice.* Kansas City, Mo.: American Nurses' Association.

Baggs, J.G. & Schmitt, M.H. (1988). Collaboration between nurses and physicians. *Image 20*(3), 145-149.

Devereux, P.M. (1981). Essential elements of nurse-physician collaboration. *J Nurs Administration 11*(5), 19-23.

Enrk, R. (1987). ACCC standards: Past, present, and future. *J Cancer Prog Management 2*(1), 11-21.

Joint Commission on Accreditation of Healthcare Organizations (1991). *Accreditation manual for hospitals.* Chicago: Author.

Kerstetter, N.C. (1990). A stepwise approach to developing and maintaining an oncology multidisciplinary conference. *Cancer Nurs 13*(4), 216-220.

Lewis, F.M. (1991). Consultation and collaboration among health care providers. In S.B. Baird, R. McCorkle, & M. Grant (eds). *Cancer Nursing: A Comprehensive Textbook.* Philadelphia: W.B. Saunders Co., pp. 957-964.

Makadon, H.J. & Gibbons, M.P. (1985). Nurses and physicians: prospects for collaboration. *Annals of Internal Medicine 103*(1), 134-136.

National Joint Practice Commission (1981). *Guidelines for establishing joint or collaborative practice in hospitals.* Chicago: Author.

Oncology Nursing Society. (1989). *Standards of Oncology Nursing Education. Generalist and Advanced Practice.* Pittsburgh: Author.

Prescott, P.A. & Bowen, S.A. (1985). Physician-nurse relationships. *Ann Intern Med 103*(1), 127-133.

Richardson, A.T. (1986). Nurses interfacing with other members of the health care team. In D.A. England (ed). *Collaboration in Nursing.* Rockville, Md.: Aspen, pp. 163-185.

Infectious Hazards

American Nurses' Association. (1985). Nursing profession urges health care community to step up efforts on AIDS. Press release. Kansas City, Mo.

American Nurses' Association and Oncology Nursing Society. (1987). *Standards of Oncology Nursing Practice.* Kansas City, Mo.

Bartlett, J. (1990). Current and future treatment of HIV infection. *Oncology 4*(11), 19-26, 29.

Benedict, S. (1990). Nursing research priorities related to HIV/AIDS. *Oncol Nurs Forum 17*(4), 571-573.

Department of Labor. (1987). Joint advisory notice; Department of Labor/Department of Health and Human Services; HBV/HIV. *Federal Register* 52(210), 41818-41824.

Department of Labor: Occupational Safety and Health Administration (1989). Occupational exposure to blood-borne pathogens. *Federal Register 54*(102), 23042-23139.

(1989). Guidelines for prevention of transmission of human immunodeficiency virus and hepatitis B virus to health-care and public-safety workers. *MMWR 38*(suppl 6), 1-37.

Halloran, J., Hughes, A., & Mayer, D.K. (1988). Oncology nursing society position paper on HIV-related issues. *Oncol Nurs Forum 15*(2), 206-217.

Joint Commission on Accreditation of Healthcare Organizations (1991). *Accreditation Manual for Hospitals— 1991*. Chicago: Author.

Larson, E. & Ropka, M.E. (1991). An update on nursing research and HIV infection. *Image 23*(1), 4-12.

Pasacreta, J.V. & Jacobsen, P.B. (1989). Addressing the need for staff support among nurses caring for the AIDS population. *Oncol Nurs Forum 16*(5), 659-663.

(1990). Protection against viral hepatisis. Recommendations of the immunization practices advisory committee. *MMWR 39*(RR-2), 1-26.

(1990). Public Health Service statement on management of occupational exposure to human immunodeficiency virus, including considerations regarding zidovudine postexposure use. *MMWR 39*(RR-1), 1-14.

(1985). Recommendations for preventing transmission of infection with human T-lymphotropic virus type III/ lymphadenopathy-associated virus in the workplace. *MMWR 34*(45), 681-686, 692-695.

(1987). Recommendations for prevention of HIV transmission in health-care settings. *MMWR 36*(suppl 2), 1S-18S.

Weber, D. & Rutala, W.A. (1989). Hepatitis B immunization update. *Infect Control Hosp Epidemiol 10*(12), 541-546.

Williamson, K.M., Selleck, C.S., Turner, J.G., Brown, K.C., Newman, K.D., & Sirles, A.T. (1988). Occupational health hazards for nurses: infection. *Image 20*(1), 48-53.

Stress

American Nurses' Association and Oncology Nursing Society (1987). *Standards of Oncology Nursing Practice*. Kansas City, Mo.: American Nurses' Association.

Benoliel, J.Q., McCorkle, R., Georgiadou, F., Denton, T., & Spitzger, A. (1990). Measurement of stress in clinical nursing. *Cancer Nurs 13*(4), 221-228.

Bram, P.J. & Katz, L.F. (1989). A study of burnout in nurses working in hospice and hospital oncology settings. *Oncol Nurs Forum 16*(4), 555-560.

Calhoun, G.L. & Calhoun, J.G. (1984). Occupational stress: implications for hospitals. In H. Selye (ed). *Selye's Guide to Stress Research* (vol 3). New York: Van Nostrand Reinhold, pp. 99-110.

Charlesworth, E.A. & Nathan, R.G. (1984). *Stress Management: a Comprehensive Guide to Wellness*. New York: Antheneum.

Chenevert, M. (1985). *Pro-Nurse Handbook*. St. Louis: C.V. Mosby.

Clark, C.C. (1980). Burnout: assessment and intervention. *J Nurs Adm 10*(9), 39-43.

Cox, A. & Andrews, P. (1981). The development of support systems on oncology units. *Oncol Nurs Forum 8*(3), 31-35.

Donovan, M.I. (1981). Stress at work: cancer nurses report. *Oncol Nurs Forum 8*(2), 22-25.

Ellis, A. & Harper, R.A. (1975). *A New Guide to Rational Living*. Englewood Cliff, N.J.: Prentice-Hall.

Haber, J., Leach, A.M. Schudy, S.M., & Sideleau, B.F. (eds) (1982). *Comprehensive Psychiatric Nursing* (2nd ed). New York: McGraw-Hill.

Hall, S.F. & Wray, L.M. (1989). Codependency: nurses who give too much. *Am J Nurs 89*(11), 1456-1460.

Jacobson, S. & McGrath, H. (1983). *Nurses Under Stress*. New York: John Wiley & Sons.

Lazarus, R.S. (1966). *Psychological Stress and the Coping Process*. New York: McGraw-Hill.

McElroy, A.M. (1982). Burnout—a review of the literature with application to cancer nursing. *Cancer Nurs 5*(3), 211-217.

Newlin, N.J. & Wellisch, D.K. (1978). The oncology nurse: life on an emotional roller coaster. *Cancer Nurs 1*(6), 447-449.

Ogle, M.E. (1983). Stages of burnout among oncology nurses in the hospital setting. *Oncol Nurs Forum 10*(1), 31-34.

Oncology Nursing Society (1989). *Standards of Oncology Nursing Education: Generalist and Advanced Practice Levels*. Pittsburgh: Author.

Patrick, P.K.S. (1981). Burnout: antecedents, manifestations, and self-care strategies for the nurse. In L.B. Marino (ed). *Cancer Nursing*. St. Louis: C.V. Mosby, pp. 87-104.

Storlie, F.J. (1979). Burnout: the elaboration of a concept. *Am J Nurs 79*(12), 2108-2111.

Vachon, M.S. (1979). Staff stress in care of the terminally ill. *Quality Rev Bull 5*(5), 13-17.

Selected Ethical Issues in Cancer Care

Robin Renee Gwin, MN, RN, OCN
Joan Exparza Richters, MN, RN, OCN

I. Informed consent.
  A. Definition: a decision made freely by the client or a legally authorized representative after full knowledge and understanding of risks, benefits, and available options about various treatment alternatives are obtained.
  B. Purpose
    1. Enable autonomous choice.
    2. Protect client against harm.
    3. Ensure responsible medical professional actions.
    4. Avoid exploitation.
  C. Situations requiring consent.
    1. Intrusive procedure.
    2. Treatment with significant risks.
    3. Clinical trials.
    4. Research.
  D. Components of informed consent.
    1. Disclosure—explanation of the purpose, expected duration, and description of the procedure that includes known risks, discomforts, benefits, and alternative treatment.
    2. Understanding—ability to comprehend and apply judgment.
    3. Voluntariness—ability to act freely without constraint or coercion.
    4. Competence—mental, physical, and legal capacity to identify appropriate means to a desired goal.
      a. Mental capacity—ability to reason without psychological or cognitive deficits.
      b. Physical capacity—ability to reason despite psychomotor deficits.
      c. Legal capacity—ability of a person of legal age to make decisions independent of others.
    5. Consent—approval or acceptance of an act done or proposed by another.
  E. Factors inappropriate in obtaining informed consent.
    1. Coercion—influencing a person to act against his or her will.
    2. Captivity—restraint of a person without consent.
    3. Deception—misrepresentation of information.

      4. Paternalism—assumption of decision-making responsibilities for another person.

      5. Unvalidated understanding—no proof of comprehension of knowledge by the person receiving treatment.

      6. Language barriers—incongruent languages, illiteracy, and incomprehensible language without an interpreter or intermediary.

      7. Sensory impairment—sight, hearing, and speech deficits.

      8. Confusion/disorientation—altered level of consciousness.

      9. Medication influences—altered thought processes resulting from effects of medication.

    10. Vulnerability/powerlessness—feelings of loss of control, loss of power, and helplessness related to disease process and treatment.

    11. Quackery—unproven treatment modalities.

F. Guidelines for the consent process.

      1. Medical explanation of the condition warranting treatment.

      2. Explanation of the purpose of the treatment or procedure.

      3. Description of the treatment or procedure.

      4. Explanation of known risks, benefits, alternatives, or consequences of not accepting treatment.

      5. Explanation of right to refuse consent or withdraw consent at any time.

G. Situations in which complete disclosure is not required.

      1. Therapeutic privilege:

        a. The individual may elect not to be informed.

        b. The individual may have prior knowledge of the treatment or procedure.

        c. The physician may anticipate that harm could come to the individual if information is disclosed.

        d. In emergency situations consent is inferred.

      2. Therapeutic use of placebos when used for the welfare of the client.

      3. Incomplete disclosure with research subjects when full knowledge would affect results (randomization, double-blind experiments, and other methods used to compensate for bias).

H. The role of the nurse in informed consent.

      1. Disclosure.

        a. Physicians are responsible for explaining medical treatments or procedures.

        b. Nurses are responsible for explaining human responses to treatments or procedures.

          (1) Reinforce information presented and provide supplemental explanations and educational materials.

          (2) Notify physician if ascertained that comprehension is poor.

          (3) Inform physician of possible medication administration that may interfere with comprehension.

          (4) Ascertain documentation of informed consent on the medical record.

      2. Client advocacy.

        a. Notify physician if client seems ambivalent.

        b. Respect the right of the client to choose.

        c. Encourage the client to ask questions and participate actively in decision making.

        d. Assess and report anxiety associated with the treatment.

II. Clinical trials.

A. Definition: method consisting of four phases used in research or evaluation of investigational drugs that may have therapeutic implications for clients.

1. Phase I—determination of safe *drug levels* and/or *schedules* of a new drug using human subjects.
2. Phase II—determination of therapeutic *efficacy* when performed on clients with different diagnoses.
3. Phase III—once efficacy is established, *comparison* of the drug to an existing, effective, *standard therapy* for the same diagnosis.
4. Phase IV—use as standard therapy to determine *optimal use* of the drug with large client populations.
B. Ethical principles.
   1. Justice—the investigator treats the client fairly.
   2. Autonomy—the right of a person to make independent decisions about personal affairs.
   3. Beneficence—obligation of health care workers to do good for clients.
   4. Nonmaleficence—obligation of health care workers to do no harm to clients.
C. Obligations of the researcher.
   1. Obtain Investigational Review Board approval for most educational and health care agencies and all institutions receiving Department of Health and Human Services funds.
   2. Maintain separation between practice and research.
   3. Obtain informed consent (see first section).
   4. Ensure confidentiality.
   5. Ensure anonymity when appropriate to the research design.
   6. Be sure client selection is congruent with phase criteria.
D. Role of the nurse in clinical trials.
   1. Ensure that informed consent is obtained and documented.
   2. Assess the response to treatment.
   3. Manage symptoms related to treatment.
   4. Provide physical and psychosocial care.
   5. Collaborate with research team.
   6. Document response to treatment.
   7. Maintain current knowledge of the drugs and other procedures and treatments used.
   8. Encourage client autonomy throughout the research period through reiteration of client rights.

III. No codes.
   A. Definition: a decision made by the client or his or her legal representative not to perform cardiopulmonary resuscitation in the event that heartbeat and respiration cease.
   B. Purpose: to validate agreement between the client, family, and health care team about right to die without resuscitation.
      1. Potential indications—brain death; poor prognosis; in accordance with client wishes.
      2. Contraindications—any client/family ambiguity about code status.
   C. Role of the nurse.
      1. Ensure a clear understanding exists between the physician and the client/family members about no-code orders.
      2. Promote independent decision making throughout hospitalization by encouraging client/family members to communicate openly with health care team.
      3. Ensure proper documentation and appropriate renewal procedures of no-code orders according to institutional policy.
      4. Examine cultural values regarding death and dying.

5. Validate emotional responses of the client and family to the no-code orders.
6. Respect right of client/family to choose or deny no-code orders.
7. Refer the client and family to other appropriate resources (support groups, pastoral care, clinical nurse specialist) if deemed necessary.

D. Legal issues.
1. If client is not able to speak for himself or herself, power of attorney is respected.
2. If a no-code order is not present or current on the chart, the health care team is responsible for resuscitation.

BIBLIOGRAPHY

Creighton, H. (1986). *Law Every Nurse Should Know* (5th ed). Philadelphia: W.B. Saunders Co.

Davis, A.J. (1987). The boundaries of intervention: issues in the noninfliction of harm. In M.D.M. Fowler & J. Levine-Ariff (eds). *Ethics at the Bedside: a Source Book for the Critical Care Nurse*. Philadelphia: J.B. Lippincott Co., pp. 50-61.

Donovan, C.T. (1990). Ethics in cancer nursing practice. In S.L. Groenwald, M.H. Frogge, M. Goodman, & C.H. Yarbro (eds). *Cancer Nursing: Principles and Practice* (2nd ed). Boston: Jones & Bartlett, pp. 1201-1215.

Eisenberg L. (1989). The social imperatives of medical research. In T.L. Beauchamp & L. Walters (eds). *Contemporary Issues in Bioethics* (3rd ed). Belmont, Calif: Wadsworth Publishing Co., pp. 425-432.

Fisher, B. (1984). Clinical trials for the evaluation of cancer therapy. *Cancer 54* (11, suppl), 2609-2617.

Fowler, M.D.M. & Levine-Ariff, J. (eds) (1987). *Ethics at the Bedside: A Source Book for the Critical Care Nurse*. Philadelphia: J.B. Lippincott Co.

Fry, S.T. (1991). Ethics and cancer care. In S.B. Baird, R. McCorkle, & M. Grant (eds). *Cancer Nursing: A Comprehensive Textbook*. Philadelphia: W.B. Saunders Co., pp. 31-37.

Johnson, J.M. (1986). Clinical trials: new responsibilities and roles for nurses. *Nursing Outlook 34*(3), 149-153.

Jonas, H. (1989). Philosophical reflections on experimenting with human subjects. In T.L. Beauchamp & L. Walters (eds). *Contemporary Issues in Bioethics* (3rd ed). Belmont, Calif: Wadsworth Publishing Co., pp. 432-440.

Schafer A. (1989). The ethics of the randomized clinical trial. In T.L. Beauchamp & L. Walters (eds). *Contemporary Issues in Bioethics* (3rd ed). Belmont, Calif: Wadsworth Publishing Co., pp. 441-447.

Varricchio, C.G. & Jassak, P.F. (1989). Informed consent: an overview. *Semin Oncol Nurs 5*(2), 95-98.

Legal Issues Influencing Cancer Care

Mary Magee Gullatte, MN, RN

I. Definition: pertaining to a law, conformity with a given law, or statute.

II. Primary sources of law affecting health-related issues include:
   A. Statutes—written laws enacted by legislatures that encompass the rules of society and are signed by a president or governor.
   B. Common law—court-made law that serves as the basis for most malpractice litigation.
   C. Administrative law—law made by administrative agencies appointed by the executive branch of government.

III. Purposes—concern over legal issues in the area of health care result from a need to:
   A. Protect the rights of citizens, both the public and professionals.
   B. Delineate the responsibilities of recipients and providers of health care.
   C. Delineate the scope of practice for health care professionals and institutions.
   D. Ensure the provision of reasonable and customary health care.

IV. Sources used in legal decision making relevant to oncology nursing practice.
   A. Professional documents used to establish minimal acceptable standards of practice and health care:
      1. Nurse practice acts:
         a. Provide definition and role of nursing by state.
         b. Regulate the practice of nursing.
         c. Delineate requirements and specifications of licensure.
         d. Establish a board of nursing.
         e. Provide a mechanism for due process and penalties.
      2. Professional standards of practice.
         a. *ANA Standards of Nursing Practice*.
         b. *ONS/ANA Standards of Oncology Nursing Practice*.
         c. *ONS Standards for Oncology Education: Patient/Family and the Public*.
         d. *ONS Standards of Oncology Nursing Education: Generalist and Advanced Practice Levels*.
   B. Agency or institutional policies and procedures:
      1. Regulations override institutional policies.
      2. Statutes override regulations.

Table 14-1
PATIENT RIGHTS ORGANIZATIONS

Organization	Goals/Objectives	National Office
American Civil Liberties Union (ACLU)	Actively protects the Constitutional rights of citizens Rights to privacy, equal protection, confidentiality, access to records, and equal access to care	ACLU 132 W. 43rd Street New York, NY 10036
American Society of Law and Medicine	Professional continuing education related to current trends in health law Journals: *Law, Medicine and Health Care American Journal of Law and Medicine*	American Society of Law and Medicine 765 Commonwealth Avenue Boston, MA 02215
Children in Hospitals, Inc.	Helps parents stay with and support their children during hospitalization Publishes a newsletter	Children in Hospitals, Inc. 31 Wilshire Park Needham, MA 02192
Concern for Dying and Society for the Right to Die (formerly the Euthanasia Educational Council)	Provides information and support for those interested in exercising their rights as patients, especially the right to refuse medical treatment Developed the living will *Right to Die:* an annual updated collection of all state living will laws	Concern for Dying 250 W. 57th Street New York, NY 10107 Society for the Right to Die (same address)
The Hemlock Society	Promotes legislation to legalize physician-assisted suicide and distributes literature on the subject	The Hemlock Society P.O. Box 11830 Eugene, OR 97440

Modified from Dorsen, N. and Annas, G. (eds)(1989). *The Basic ACLU Guide to Patient Rights*. (2nd ed). Carbondale, Ill: Southern Illinois University Press, pp. 275-279.

C. Requirements of accrediting or governing agencies:
1. Joint Commission on Accreditation of Health Care Organizations (JCAHO).
2. American College of Surgeons.
3. Occupational Safety and Health Administration (OSHA)—safety standards.
4. Centers for Disease Control—infection control standards.
5. Department of Health and Human Services.
D. Client rights (Table 14-1):
1. American Hospital Association (AHA)—Patient's Bill of Rights.
2. JCAHO—standards of care related to client rights.
3. Right of self-determination.
4. Informed consent documents.
E. Client and proxy agreements:
1. Living wills.

Table 14-1
PATIENT RIGHTS ORGANIZATIONS *Continued*

Organization	Goals/Objectives	National Office
Law, Medicine and Ethics Program	Education, research, and advocacy in health law, with emphasis on patient rights, health care regulation, and medical ethics	Law, Medicine and Ethics Program Boston University Schools of Medicine and Public Health 80 E. Concord Street Boston, MA 02118
The National Hospice Organization	Information center about hospices Publishes a national directory and provides information	The National Hospice Organization 1901 North Fort Myer Drive Suite 902 Arlington, VA 22209
National Health Law Program	Legal services and back-up center, specializing in health law, Medicaid, and access issues for the poor Publishes a newsletter	National Health Law Program 26396 South LaCienega Blvd. Los Angeles, CA 90034
People's Medical Society	Provides information on issues regarding patient rights Membership organization for consumers of medical services	People's Medical Society 14 East Minor Street Emmaus, PA 18049
Public Citizen Health Research Group	Ralph Nader–affiliated consumer advocacy group Concerned with issues of medical care, drug safety, medical device safety, physician competence, and consumer health care issues	Public Citizen Health Research Group 2000 P Street N.W. Suite 708 Washington, DC 20036

      2. Directives for organ and tissue donation.
      3. Directives for withholding or withdrawing life-support measures.

  V. Individual and professional nurse accountability.
     A. Individual nurse is responsible for professional nursing practice.
     B. "Respondent superior" renders employer liable and responsible for the actions of the employee.

 VI. Liability.
     A. Negligence—deviation from the acceptable standard of care that a reasonable person would use in a specific situation.
     B. Malpractice—deviation from a professional standard of care.
     C. Duty—care relationship between client and provider.
     D. Breach of duty—failure to meet an acceptable standard of care.

VII. Litigations involving oncology nurses include:
     A. Medication errors.
     B. Failure to follow acceptable standard of care, resulting in client harm.

      C. Incomplete or absence of documentation in medical record.

      D. Inadequate referral or follow-up.

      E. Lack of teaching.

      F. Insufficient discharge planning.

VIII. Potential actions resulting from legal allegations.

      A. Out-of-court settlement, which may include monetary or other restitution.

      B. Trial by jury resulting in monetary restitution, imprisonment, public service payback, or loss of licensure if found guilty; admissible evidence includes medical records, sworn testimony, and expert witnesses.

      C. Agency or institutional sanctions.

      D. Professional sanctions by state board of nursing.

IX. Prudent actions by nurses to ensure "reasonable or customary care" is rendered to the client and is documented in the medical record.

      A. Demonstrate knowledge of and adherence to professional standards and procedures as determined by self-evaluation and peer review.

      B. Participate in policy review and revisions within the agency, private practice, and professional organizations.

      C. Maintain current knowledge of personal and institutional liability.

      D. Maintain adequate individual and agency liability insurance coverage.

      E. Keep diligent records with respect to:

        1. Accuracy of entries.

        2. Timeliness of charting.

        3. Accurate and timely filing of incident reports according to agency policy.

        4. Referrals and follow-up care.

X. Cancer legislation—current legislative issues related to cancer care focus on:

      A. Prevention and early detection of disease.

      B. Research and clinical trials.

      C. Evaluation of alternative treatments.

      D. Investigation using human subjects.

      E. Minority health issues.

      F. Treatment of socioeconomically disadvantaged clients, including the poor, elderly, homeless, and refugees of all races and ethnic groups.

      G. Health issues of women.

      H. Environmental hazards.

      I. Occupational hazards.

      J. Access to health care.

      K. Economics of cancer care.

      L. Research ethics.

      M. Research funding.

XI. Issues pertinent to oncology nursing practice.

      A. Ownership of human cells and tissues.

      B. Right to self-determination and autonomy.

      C. Withholding care to terminally ill clients.

      D. Withdrawing medical treatment.

      E. Occupational and environmental hazards.

      F. Smoking among oncology nurses.

      G. Human subject research.

      H. Alternative treatments.

      I. Chemical dependency among health care workers.

      J. Informed consent—explicit versus implied.

K. Quality of life and survivorship.

L. Political reform related to access to health care for all.

XII. Nurse managers—a wide range of legal issues confront the nurse manager, including:

A. The nursing shortage and the issue of liability; recommendations to reduce liability include the following responsibilities:

1. Communicate staffing shortages.

2. Define system to measure acuity objectively.

3. Define the number and types of staff needed to provide safe client care.

4. Identify equipment and supply needs.

5. Initiate client care standards.

6. Document impact of inadequate staffing on client care.

7. Assure that "reasonable" efforts have been taken to address the staffing problem.

B. Temporary staff and agency nurse liability—ostensible agency or apparent authority (client believes a health care worker is an employee of the hospital); recommendations to reduce liability of hospital with respect to acts of independent contractors include the following responsibilities:

1. Verify credentials such as nursing licensure, malpractice insurance, and cardiopulmonary resuscitation.

2. Orient to hospital and care unit.

3. Review hospital policies and procedures.

4. Validate psychomotor skills.

5. Identify professional as agency nurse.

6. Evaluate care given.

7. Contract with a limited number of agencies.

C. Labor relations—collective bargaining is becoming more pervasive in the health care system.

1. Taft-Hartley Act exempted nonprofit hospitals from jurisdiction of the National Labor Relations Board (NLRB).

2. Hospitals became subject to the NLRB after 1974.

3. Solicitation for union member—a "no solicitation" rule is often in effect to inhibit union solicitation within the hospital.

4. Recommendations for maintaining a "union-free" workplace include:

a. Fair labor practices.

b. Wide range of benefits.

c. Avoidance of discrimination on basis of sex, color, creed, or national origin.

d. Equitable hiring and promotion practices.

e. Fair and competitive wages.

f. Open lines of communications between management and labor.

D. Impaired health care professionals (chemical dependency).

1. State boards of nursing report chemical dependency as the leading cause of disciplinary action; the number of addicted nurses is reported at 10% to 12%.

2. Factors contributing to chemical dependency among nurses—job-related stress, easy access to controlled substances, inadequate narcotic control on nursing unit, financial concerns, home situations, failure of colleagues to report suspicious behaviors.

3. Management responsibilities:

a. Establish hospital policy on impaired professionals.

b. Investigate suspected abuse promptly.

c. Protect client and hospital from harm and liability.

d. Notify board of nursing and document actions.

e. Offer support through peer or employee assistance programs.

f. Provide reentry support.

BIBLIOGRAPHY

Annas, G.J. (1989). *The Rights of Patients: The Basic ACLU Guide to Patient Rights* (2nd ed). Carbondale, Ill.: Southern Illinois University Press.

Bartholome, W.G. (1989). A new understanding of consent in pediatric practice: consent, parental permission, and child assent. *Pediatr Ann 18*(4), 262-265.

Billue, J.S. (1989). Who owns the patient? *Heart Lung 18*(5), 530-532.

Burris, D.S. (1969). *The Right to Treatment; a Symposium.* New York: Springer Publishing Co.

Cassel, C.K. (1989). Care of the dying: the limits of law, the limits of ethics. *Law Med Health Care 17*(3), 232-233.

Chamorro, T. (1991). Legal responsibilities of the nurse. In S.B. Baird, R. McCorkle, & M. Grant (eds). *Cancer Nursing: A Comprehensive Textbook.* Philadelphia: W.B. Saunders Co., pp. 1139-1448.

Childress, J.F. (1989). Dying patients: who's in control? *Law Med Health Care 17*(3), 227-231.

Cohen, A. (1989). The management rights clause in collective bargaining. *Nurs Management 20*(11), 24-26, 28-30, 34.

Dimond, M. (1989). Health care and the aging population. *Nurs Outlook 37*(2), 76-77.

Fiesta, J. (1983). *The Law and Liability: a Guide for Nurses.* New York: John Wiley & Sons.

Fiesta, J.; (1990). Agency nurses—whose liability? *Nurs Management 21*(3),16-17.

Fiesta, J. (1990). The impaired nurse—who is liable. *Nurs Management 21*(10), 20, 22.

Fiesta, J. (1990). The nursing shortage: whose liability problem? Part II. *Nurs Management 21*(2), 22-23.

Fiesta, J. (1991). Law for the nurse manager. QA and risk management: reducing liability exposure. *Nurs Management 22*(2), 14-15.

Fowler, M.D. (1989). Slow code, partial code, limited code. *Heart Lung 18*(5), 533-534.

Goldsmith, M.F. (1988). Health decisions for the American people subject of new national bioethical policy group. *JAMA 260*(17), 2478.

Hurt, R.D., Berge, K.G., Offord, K.P., Leonard, D.A., Gerlach, D.K., Renquist, C.L. & O'Hara, M.R. (1989). The making of a smoke-free medical center. *JAMA 261*(1), 95-97.

Leikin, S. (1989). When parents demand treatment. *Pediatr Ann 18*(4), 266-68.

McCabe, M.S., Piemme, J.A., & Donoghue, M. (1991). Cancer legislation. In S.B. Baird, R. McCorkle, & M. Grant (eds). *Cancer Nursing: A Comprehensive Textbook.* Philadelphia: W.B. Saunders Co., pp. 1149-1161.

Miaskowski, C. & Nielson, B. (1991). Documentation of the nursing process in cancer nursing. In S.B. Baird, R. McCorkle, & M. Grant (eds). *Cancer Nursing: A Comprehensive Textbook.* Philadelphia: W.B. Saunders Co., pp. 1126-1131.

Meisel, A. (1989). Refusing treatment, refusing to talk, and refusing to let go: on whose terms will death occur? *Law Med Health Care 17*(3), 221-226.

Reynolds, J.J. (1989). Love, medicine, and money: issues of access, use, and advocacy. *Health Soc Work 14*(1), 6-7.

Rizzo, R.F. (1989). The living will: does it protect the rights of the terminally ill? *NY State J Med 89*(2), 72-79.

Taylor, I. (1988). Patients' rights and clinical research. *Lancet 2*(8624), 1370.

Salladay, S.A. & McDonnell, M.M. (1989). Spiritual care, ethical choices, and patient advocacy. *Nurs Clin North Am 24*(2), 543-549.

Scanlon, C. & Fleming, C. (1989). Ethical issues in caring for the patient with advanced cancer. *Nurs Clin North Am 24*(4), 977-986.

Schulmeister, L. (1987). Litigation involving oncology nurses. *Oncol Nurs Forum 14*(2), 25-28.

Wachter, R.M., Luce, J.M., Lo, B., & Raffin, T.A. (1989). Life-sustaining treatment for patients with AIDS. *Chest 95*(3), 647-652.

White, G.B., & O'Connor, K.W. (1990). Rights, duties, and commercial interests: John Moore versus the regents of the University of California. *Cancer Invest 8*(1), 65-70.

Zweibel, N.R. & Cassel, C.K. (1989). Treatment choices at the end of life: a comparison of decisions by older patients and their physician-selected proxies. *Gerontologist 29*(5), 615-621.

15

Cancer Survivorship Issues

Susan Leigh, BSN, RN

THEORY

I. Definition of survivorship.
  A. Cancer survivors have been defined historically as individuals who live either 5 years after a cancer diagnosis or remain free of disease 5 years after completion of therapy.
  B. Cancer survivors have also been defined as family members or significant others who live after the death of an individual with cancer.
  C. A broader definition of cancer survivor ("people with histories of cancer") has been proposed by the National Coalition for Cancer Survivorship (NCCS).
    1. Implications of the NCCS definition for health care providers and the public:
      a. Cancer survival begins at the moment of diagnosis and proceeds along a continuum through and beyond treatment to remissions, recurrences, cure, and the final stages of life, regardless of cause.
      b. Survivorship is the concept of living through and beyond a diagnosis of cancer.
    2. Survivors also encompass persons affected by the disease other than the diagnosed client—family members, significant others, friends, coworkers, health care professionals, and social support networks.

II. Seasons of survival—a dynamic model of life after a cancer diagnosis consisting of three "seasons"—acute stage of survival, extended stage of survival, and permanent stage of survival.
  A. Acute stage:
    1. Begins at the moment of diagnosis and extends through the initial treatment.
    2. Individuals may be dealing with:
      a. Actual or potential losses.
      b. Fear of dying or impending death.
      c. Acute side effects of treatment.
      d. Disruption of family and social roles.
  B. Extended stage:
    1. Follows the completion of the initial treatment.
    2. Individuals may be in remission, on maintenance therapy, or terminal.
    3. Individuals may be dealing with:

        a. Severing of treatment-based support systems.

        b. Feeling ambiguous about the joy of being alive, fear of recurrence, or fear of death.

        c. Adjusting to physical or psychosocial compromise.

        d. Reintegrating and reorganizing individual and family concerns.

        e. Isolating the individual because of external or self-imposed forces.

        f. Seeking community-based support systems.

C. Permanent stage:

  1. Gradual evolution to a time of diminished probability for disease recurrence.

  2. If cancer is arrested permanently, some survivors may be considered "cured."

  3. Individuals may be dealing with:

        a. Discrimination in the workplace.

        b. Procurement or maintenance of adequate insurance coverage.

        c. Adaptation to the physical and psychosocial changes resulting from disease.

        d. Treatment for long-term or late effects of disease and treatment.

           (1) Long-term effects are chronic sequelae that may develop during or result from treatment and may persist for months to years after the cancer is eradicated and treatment is complete (amputations, hair loss, and scarring).

           (2) Late effects are subclinical sequelae that may become apparent months to years after completion of treatment (pulmonary fibrosis, second malignancies, and disease recurrence).

        e. Maintenance of adequate follow-up care.

III. Impact of survival.

A. The impact of cancer survival may be long-term or delayed.

B. Multiple factors determine the occurrence, frequency, and severity of actual or potential effects:

  1. Type of cancer.

  2. Location of disease.

  3. Size and extent of the primary tumor.

  4. Type and aggressiveness of therapy.

  5. Age of the individual at diagnosis.

  6. State of general physical and mental health of the individual at diagnosis.

  7. Quantity and quality of psychosocial support available.

C. Four primary categories of effects are recognized—biomedical, psychosocial, economic/legal, and spiritual/existential.

  1. Biomedical effects:

        a. Recurrence of disease.

        b. Second malignancies.

           (1) Overall risk is low but remains a serious problem for those affected.

           (2) Risk of second malignancies does not contraindicate therapy.

        c. Structural changes or losses such as amputations or scars.

        d. Decreased physical stamina.

        e. System-related effects with examples:

           (1) Neurological—neuropathies, delayed radiation necrosis, and neuralgias.

           (2) Cardiovascular—cardiomyopathy, pericardial effusion, and arterial and venous obstruction or occlusion.

           (3) Pulmonary—fibrosis, pleural effusions, and spontaneous pneumothorax.

           (4) Urological—nephritis, tubular atrophy, cystitis, and urinary diversions.

    (5) Gastrointestinal—transient liver enzyme elevations, bowel diversions, adhesions, obstruction, and hepatic veno-occlusive disease.

    (6) Sexual/reproductive—sterility, impotence, testicular atrophy, premature menopause, and changes in sexual response times.

    (7) Musculoskeletal—fractures and muscle atrophy.

2. Psychosocial effects:

  a. Fear of recurrence (Damocles syndrome).

  b. Heightened sense of vulnerability.

  c. Recurrent episodes of anxiety during routine health care follow-up or cancer-related anniversaries.

  d. Ambivalence about health care follow-up, ranging from hypochondriacal obsession to complete avoidance.

  e. Changes in body image or self-concept that result in less-than-satisfactory expression of self and sexuality.

  f. Social stigma associated with external sources (shunning by others) or internal sources (isolationism).

  g. Transition from sick role to return to previous roles or development of new roles and responsibilities.

  h. Inconsistent perceptions of the state of health of the survivor among the individual, family, and social acquaintances.

  i. Continued need for psychosocial support after therapy.

3. Economic/legal effects—employment discrimination based on common misconceptions that anyone with cancer will die; that cancer is contagious; and that people with cancer will be less productive because of continued illness:

  a. Employment-related problems may include avoidance by coworkers; demotion or lack of promotion; job-lock for fear of losing benefits; and dismissal from the job.

    (1) Legal protection is provided through the Federal Rehabilitation Act of 1973 that prohibits discrimination against the handicapped or those perceived as handicapped by employers who receive federal funding (federal agencies, hospitals, and universities).

    (2) Additional protection is provided for workers not protected by the Federal Rehabilitation Act under the Americans with Disabilities Act (ADA) of 1990.

    (3) Federal and state laws specifically prohibit cancer-related employment discrimination; contain information on how to file a complaint and with whom; prohibit employers from requiring pre-employment examinations; and allow medical questions only after one is offered a job and only if the questions are related specifically to the job.

  b. Insurance-related problems may include refusal of new applications, waiver or exclusion of preexisting conditions, extended waiting periods, an increase in premiums and reduction of benefits for the employee and employer, or cancellation of health and life insurance policies.

    (1) Legal protection includes Consolidated Omnibus Budget Reconciliation Act (COBRA) of 1986, which mandates that employers of more than 20 workers offer group medical coverage to employees (18 months) and their dependents (36 months) if they lose a job or need to work fewer hours.

    (2) High-risk insurance pools in some states for the medically uninsurable—insurers share both the risks and expenses with the high-risk population.

(3) Social Security Disability Insurance Program is available to individuals who have paid into the program previously; eligibility begins 6 months after being declared medically or mentally impaired.
4. Spiritual/existential issues:
   a. Changes in life priorities and values after critical evaluation and a search for meaning.
   b. Deepening sense of spirituality that may or may not be associated with organized religion.
   c. Expressed concerns about the quality of one's life.
   d. Increased self-love or self-acceptance.
   e. Increased passion or zest for life.
   f. Ambivalent feelings about occasional periods of depression.
   g. Survivor's guilt, especially during follow-up examinations when confronted with others who are not doing well, are more debilitated, or are terminal.

ASSOCIATED NURSING DIAGNOSES

I. Disturbances in self-concept.

II. Spiritual distress.

III. Ineffective individual coping.

IV. Ineffective family coping.

V. Sexual dysfunction.

VI. Anxiety.

NURSING PLANNING AND IMPLEMENTATION

I. Nursing planning and interventions are guided by two beliefs and values.
   A. Each person diagnosed with cancer and his or her family are cancer survivors.
   B. Cancer survivors are entitled to certain rights (Table 15-1):
      1. Assurance of lifelong medical care, as needed.
      2. Pursuit of happiness.
      3. Equal job opportunities.
      4. Assurance of adequate public or private health insurance.

II. Acute stage interventions.
   A. Begin to incorporate rehabilitation models of care at the time of diagnosis.
   B. Encourage client and family involvement in treatment decisions and planning for transitions in level of care and services.
   C. Introduce survivorship potential and support with factual information and available resources.
   D. Assess changes in individual and family coping demands and resources throughout the seasons of survivorship.
   E. Establish exit interviews as clients complete initial treatment to assist in the transition to the extended stage.

III. Extended stage interventions.
   A. Encourage periodic follow-up examinations and continued access to health care.
   B. Make referrals to appropriate supportive services within the treatment center and the community such as the American Cancer Society, United Ostomy Association, and vocational rehabilitation.

Table 15-1

AMERICAN CANCER SOCIETY: THE CANCER SURVIVORS' BILL OF RIGHTS

1. Survivors have the right to assurance of lifelong medical care as needed. The physicians and other professionals involved in their care should continue their constant efforts to be:

- Sensitive to the cancer survivors' life-style choices and their need for self-esteem and dignity
- Careful, no matter how long they have survived, to have symptoms taken seriously and not have aches and pains dismissed for fear of recurrence is a normal part of survivorship
- Informative and open, providing survivors with as much or as little candid medical information as they wish and encouraging their informed participation in their own care
- Knowledgeable about counseling resources and willing to refer survivors and their families, as appropriate, for emotional support and therapy that will improve the quality of individual lives

2. In their personal lives, survivors, like other Americans, have the right of the pursuit of happiness. This means they have the right:

- To talk with their families and friends about their cancer experience if they wish but to refuse to discuss it if that is their choice and not to be expected to be more upbeat or less blue than anyone else
- To be free of the stigma of cancer as a "dread disease" in all social relations
- To be free of blame for having gotten the disease and of guilt for having survived it

3. In the workplace, survivors have the right to equal job opportunities. This means they have the right:

- To aspire to jobs worthy of their skills and for which they are trained and experienced and thus not to have to accept jobs they would not have considered before the cancer experience
- To be hired, promoted, and accepted on return to work, according to their individual abilities and qualifications and not according to "cancer" or "disability" stereotypes
- To privacy about their medical histories

4. Since health insurance coverage is an overriding survivorship concern, every effort should be made to assure all survivors adequate health insurance, whether public or private. This means:

- For employers, that survivors have the right to be included in group health coverage, which is usually less expensive, provides better benefits, and covers the employee regardless of health history
- For physicians, counselors, and other professionals concerned, that they keep themselves and their survivor-clients informed and up-to-date on available group or individual health policy options, noting, for example, what major expenses like hospital costs and medical tests outside the hospital are covered and what amount must be paid before coverage (deductibles)

From Silverberg, E. & Lubera, J.A. (1988). Cancer survivor's bill of rights: *CA* 3:32.

    C. Keep client, family, and children updated and informed of changes in the status of the client.

IV. Permanent stage interventions.

    A. Encourage the development of systematic follow-up programs for long-term survivors.

    B. Encourage participation in activities related to changes in public and private policies affecting cancer survivors.

BIBLIOGRAPHY

Baez, S.B., Dodd, M.J. & DiJuleo, J.E. (1991). Nursing management of persons treated for cure: prototype-Hodgkin's Disease. In S.B. Baird, R. McCorkle, & M. Grant (eds). *Cancer Nursing: A Comprehensive Textbook*. Philadelphia: W.B. Saunders Co., pp. 673-688.

Carter, B.J. (1989). Cancer survivorship: a topic for nursing research. *Oncol Nurs Forum 16*(3), 435-437.

Cella, D.F. (1987). Cancer survival: psychosocial and public issues. *Cancer Invest 5*(1), 59-67.

Christ, G.H. (1987). Social consequences of the cancer experience. *Am J Pediatr Hematol Oncol 9*(1), 84-88.

Dudas, S. & Carlson, C.E. (1988). Cancer rehabilitation. *Oncol Nurs Forum 15*(2), 183-188.

Hoffman, B. (1989). Current issues of cancer survivorship. *Oncology 3*, 85-94.

Kudsk, E.G. & Hoffmann, G.S. (1987). Rehabilitation of the cancer patient. *Primary Care 14*(2), 381-390.

Loescher, L.J., Clark, L., Atwood, J.R., Leigh, S., & Lamb, G. (1990). The impact of the cancer experience on long-term survivors. *Oncol Nurs Forum 17*(2), 223-229.

Loescher, L.J., Welch-McCaffrey, D., Leigh, S.A., Hoffman, B., & Meyskens, F.L., Jr. (1989). Surviving adult cancers. Part I. Physiologic effects. *Ann Intern Med 111*(5), 411-432.

Mellette, S.J. (1989). Rehabilitation issues for cancer survivors: psychosocial challenges. *J Psychosoc Oncol 7*(4), 93-109.

Mullan, F. (1984). Re-entry: the educational needs of the cancer survivor. *Health Educ Q 10*(special suppl), 88-94.

Mullan, F. (1985). Seasons of survival: reflections of a physician with cancer. *N Engl J Med 313*(4), 270-273.

Quigley, K.M. (1989). The adult cancer survivor: psychosocial consequences of cure. *Semin Oncol Nurs 5*(1), 63-69.

Rose, M.A. (1989). Health promotion and risk prevention: applications for cancer survivors. *Oncol Nurs Forum 16*(3), 335-340.

Welch-McCaffrey, D., Hoffman, B., Leigh, S.A., Loescher, L.J., & Meyskens F.L., Jr. (1989). Surviving adult cancer. Part II. Psychosocial implications. *Ann Intern Med 111*(6), 517-524.

Pathophysiology of Cancer

16

Pathophysiology of Cancer

Deborah L. Volker, MA, RN, OCN

I. What is cancer?
- A. Definition: a single transformed cell that does not conform to regulation of cellular differentiation and proliferation; forms a clone; and continues to grow without respect to body needs.
- B. Pathology—mutations (deoxyribonucleic acid [DNA] changes) that affect either or both types of oncogenes (oncogene—a gene whose expression plays a causative role in carcinogenesis):
   1. Proto-oncogenes—the genetic portion of the DNA that regulates normal cell growth and repair; mutation may allow cells to proliferate beyond normal body needs.
   2. Antioncogenes—the genetic portion of the DNA that stops cell division; mutation may allow cells to proliferate beyond normal body needs.
- C. Cause—the three-stage theory of causation (carcinogenesis) is the most widely used explanation of the process by which a normal cell is transformed into a cancer cell:
   1. Initiation—a carcinogen (cancer-causing agent) damages the DNA by changing a specific gene; this gene then may:
      - a. Undergo repair, and no cancer results.
      - b. Become permanently changed but not cause cancer unless subsequently exposed to threshold levels of cancer promoters.
      - c. Become transformed and produce a cancer cell line if the initiator is a complete carcinogen (acts as both an initiator and promoter).
   2. Promotion.
      - a. Definition of promotion: process by which carcinogens are subsequently introduced, resulting in one of the following changes:
         (1) Reversible damage to the proliferation mechanism of the cell; the effects of promoting factors may be inhibited by:
            (a) Cancer-reversing agents—present studies include agents such as retinoids, vitamin C, and indoles (found in cruciferous vegetables).
            (b) Host characteristics such as an effective immune system.
            (c) Time or dose limits on the exposure to the promoter (Figure 16-1).

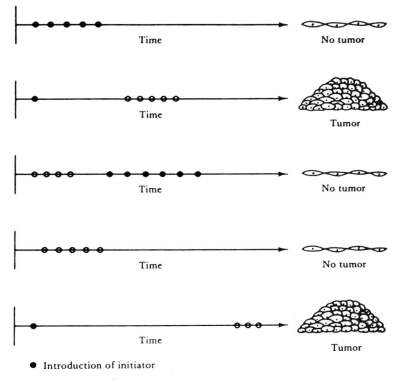

● Introduction of initiator

O Introduction of promoter

Figure 16-1 Initiation *(closed circles)* and promotion *(open circles).* Initiation must precede promotion for a tumor to develop; promotion alone will not produce a tumor. *(From Yarbro, J. [1990].* Carcinogenesis. In S.L. Groenwald, M.H. Frogge, M. Goodman, & C.H. Yarbro [eds]. Cancer Nursing: Principles and Practice [2nd ed]. Boston: Jones & Bartlett Publishers, p. 33.)

        (2) Irreversible damage to the proliferation mechanism, resulting in cancer cell transformation.
    b. Characteristics of promoting factors:
        (1) Can induce tumors in initiated cells.
        (2) Will not cause tumors when applied *before* the initiating factor.
        (3) Have a threshold level—if a subthreshold dose or widely spaced doses are given, no effect occurs.
        (4) May also be initiators (cigarette smoke, asbestos, alcohol).
  3. Progression.
    a. Invasion—cells continue to divide; increased bulk and pressure result in local spread and invasion of surrounding structures (exception: *carcinoma in situ*—malignancy limited to the epithelium; has not yet invaded the basement membrane [underlying tissue]).
    b. Metastasis—the production of secondary tumors at distant sites.
        (1) Routes of metastasis (Figure 16-2)—cells may spread by:
           (a) Seeding throughout a body cavity such as the peritoneal cavity.
           (b) Dissemination via the lymphatic system—entrapment may occur in the first lymph node encountered, or cells may bypass the first node and reach more distant sites ("skip metastasis").
           (c) Dissemination via blood capillaries and veins; most metastases form by this method; proposed mechanism:

Formation of a Metastasis

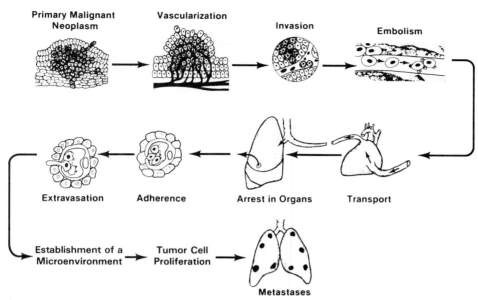

Figure 16-2 Process of metastasis consists of multiple sequential and highly selective steps. *(From Fidler, I.J. & Nicolson, G.L. [1987]. The process of cancer invasion and metastasis.* Cancer Bull 39,[3] 127.)

      i. Migration of metastatic cells to the periphery of the primary tumor.
     ii. Penetration of the extracellular matrix of the tumor by enzymes and other factors.
   iii. Penetration of surrounding blood vessel walls.
   iv. Dissemination into the bloodstream.
    v. Interaction with host factors (platelets, lymphocytes).
   vi. Formation of clusters or emboli.
  vii. Adherence to blood vessel walls in distant organ.
 viii. Extravasation out of blood vessel into adjacent tissue.
   ix. Proliferation of the metastatic deposit of cells.
    x. Formation of a supporting vascular system via secretion of tumor-angiogenesis factor (TAF).

(2) Sites:
  (a) Most common—bone, lung, liver, and central nervous system.
  (b) Predilection for specific sites may be influenced by:
     i. Patterns of blood flow.
    ii. Cell receptors and genes that direct the cell to travel to specific sites.
   iii. Necessary growth factors, which can be elicited only in selected organs.

(3) Clinical implications:
  (a) Metastasis is the major cause of death from cancer.
  (b) Most tumors have begun to metastasize at the time of detection.

c. Heterogeneity—refers to differences among individual cells within a tumor; degree of heterogeneity increases as the tumor grows (Figure 16-3).

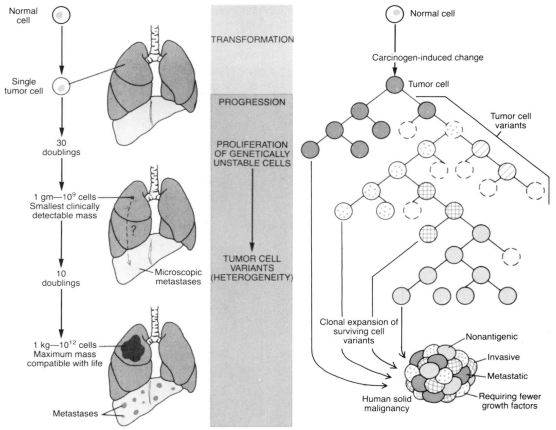

Figure 16-3 Biology of tumor growth. The left panel depicts minimal estimates of tumor cell doublings that precede the formation of clinically detectable tumor mass. It is evident that by the time a solid tumor is detected, it has already completed a major portion of its life cycle as measured by cell doublings. The right panel illustrates clonal evolution of tumors and generation of tumor cell heterogeneity. New subclones arise from the descendants of the original transformed cell, and with progressive growth the tumor mass becomes enriched for those variants that are more adept at evading host defenses and are likely to be more aggressive. *(Modified from Tannock, I.F. [1983]. Biology of tumor growth. Hosp Pract 18:81.)*

(1) Differences include:
  (a) Genetic composition.
  (b) Invasiveness.
  (c) Growth rate.
  (d) Hormonal responsiveness.
  (e) Metastatic potential.
  (f) Susceptibility to antineoplastic therapy.
(2) Heterogeneity is caused by random mutations during tumor progression.
(3) Clinical implications—can cause tumors to be highly resistant to any one specific therapy.
II. What causes cancer (carcinogenesis)?
  A. Exposure to carcinogens.
    1. Exposure to radiation—cellular DNA damaged by a physical release of energy.
      a. Ionizing radiation.

(1) Damage to the cell by this source:
   (a) Is usually repaired and no mutation results.
   (b) May give rise to a malignancy when damage affects proto-onco-genes or antioncogenes.
   (c) Depends on numerous factors:
      i. Level of tissue oxygenation—well-oxygenated cells are more radiosensitive.
      ii. Genetic composition—certain genetic disorders, particularly those associated with inefficient DNA repair mechanisms, increase risk.
      iii. Age—children, fetuses, and elderly are at higher risk.
      iv. Cell-cycle phase (Figure 16-4)—G2 more sensitive than S or G1.
      v. Degree of differentiation—immature cells most vulnerable.
      vi. Cell proliferation rate—cells with high mitotic index most vulnerable.
      vii. Tissue type—hematopoietic and gastrointestinal tissue very sensitive.
      viii. Total dose and rate of dose—the higher the cumulative dose and dose rate, the greater is the likelihood of mutation.
(2) Most exposure is from natural, unavoidable sources.
(3) Examples of ionizing radiation:
   (a) Diagnostic or therapeutic sources—diagnostic x-rays, radiation therapy, radioisotopes used in diagnostic imaging.
   (b) Cosmic rays.
   (c) Radioactive ground minerals and gases—radon gas, radium, uranium.
(4) Cancers linked to exposure to ionizing radiation include:
   (a) Skin cancer.
   (b) Leukemia (particularly acute myelogenous leukemia [AML] and chronic myelogenous leukemia [CML]).
   (c) Lung cancer.
   (d) Thyroid cancer.
   (e) Breast cancer.
   (f) Osteosarcoma.

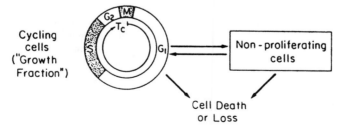

Figure 16-4 Model of a tumor cell population. The tumor contains proliferating cells (referred to as the growth fraction) and nonproliferating cells. The latter population may include cells that have lost the ability to proliferate (e.g., by differentiaton) or cells that can revert to proliferation if factors such as cellular nutrition improve. Most tumors contain a high rate of cell death or loss from the tumor. *(From Tannock, I.F. [1989]. Principles of cell proliferation: cell kinetics. In V.T. DeVita, Jr., S. Hellman, & S.A. Rosenberg [eds]. Cancer: Principles & Practice of Oncology [3rd ed]. Philadelphia: J.B. Lippincott Co., p. 5.)*

   b. Ultraviolet radiation (UVR).
      (1) Sources of UVR:
         (a) Sunlight.
         (b) Tanning booths.
         (c) Industrial sources—welding arcs and germicidal lights.
      (2) Risk of carcinogenesis by UVR is increased by:
         (a) Prolonged exposure as a result of occupational or recreational activities.
         (b) Hereditary diseases characterized by inefficient DNA repair mechanisms (examples—xeroderma pigmentosum, ataxia-telangiectasia).
         (c) Skin pigmentation—the greater the amount of melanin, the greater is the protection against UVR.
      (3) Cancers most commonly associated with UVR include:
         (a) Melanoma.
         (b) Basal cell carcinoma.
         (c) Squamous cell carcinoma.

Table 16-1
CHEMICALS AND MIXTURES CARCINOGENIC OR PROBABLY CARCINOGENIC IN HUMANS

Agent	Site
Life-Style/Personal-Choice Exposure	
Tobacco	Lung, pancreas, oral cavity and pharynx, larynx, urinary tract
Tobacco quids and betel nut	Oral mucosa
Ethanol with smoking	Esophagus
Industrial Exposure	
Arsenic compounds	Skin, lungs
p-Biphenylamine and o-nitrobiphenyl	Urinary bladder
Asbestos	Pleura, peritoneum, lung
Asbestos with cigarette smoking	Synergistic increase in lung
Benzidine (4,4′-diaminobiphenyl)	Urinary bladder
Bis(chloromethyl) ether	Lung
Bis(2-chloroethyl) sulfide	Respiratory tract
Chromium compounds	Lung
2(or β)-Naphthylamine	Urinary bladder
Nickel compounds	Lungs, nasal sinuses
Soots, tars, oils	Skin, lungs
Vinyl chloride	Liver mesenchyme
Radon gas (radiation)	Lung
Radon gas with cigarette smoking	Synergistic increase in lung
Drugs and Therapeutic Exposure	
N,N-Bis(2-chloroethyl)-2-naphthylamine (Chlornaphazine)	Urinary bladder
Cancer chemotherapy regimens (alkylating agents)	Leukemias, lymphomas, solid tumors
Diethylstilbestrol	Vagina
Estrogen	Breast, uterus
Phenacetin	Renal pelvis
Psoralen with ultraviolet radiation	Skin

From Lieberman, M.W. & Lebovitz, R.M. (1990). Neoplasia. In J.M. Kissane (ed). *Anderson's Pathology* (9th ed). St. Louis: C.V. Mosby Co., p. 596.

2. Chemical carcinogens—chemical substances that alter DNA (Table 16-1); examples include:
    a. Alkylating antineoplastic agents—cyclophosphamide, nitrogen mustard, melphalan, busulfan, nitrosoureas.
    b. Aromatic hydrocarbons—soot, pitch, coal tar, benzene.
    c. Organic compounds—vinyl chloride, isopropyl oil.
    d. Tobacco products—cigarette smoke, chewing tobacco, snuff.
    e. Inorganic compounds—chromates, asbestos, nickel.
    f. Plant and microbial products—*Senecio* alkaloids in herbal teas and medicines, aflatoxin B, betel nuts, griseofulvin, cycasin, safrol.
    g. Hormones—estrogens and diethylstilbestrol.
    h. Others—chromium, polychlorinated biphenyls (PCBs), some insecticides and fungicides.
3. Viruses (Table 16-2):
    a. Infect DNA, resulting in proto-oncogene changes and cell mutation.

Table 16-2
ONCOGENIC VIRUSES

Family	Virus	Associated Tumors	Other Risk Factors
DNA Viruses			
Hepadenovirus	Hepatitis B group (HBV)	Liver cancer	Alcohol Smoking Fungal toxins Other viruses
Papovavirus	Human papilloma virus (HPV)	Genital, laryngeal, and skin warts	
		Skin cancers in clients with epidermodysplasia verruciformis	Sunlight Genetic disorders possibly affecting immunity
		In situ and invasive cancers of the vulva and uterine cervix	
Herpesvirus	Epstein-Barr virus (EBV)	Burkitt's lymphoma Immunoblastic lymphoma Nasopharyngeal carcinoma	Malaria Immune deficiency Histocompatibility antigen genotype
	Herpes simplex type 2 (HSV-2)	Cancer of uterine cervix	
	Cytomegalovirus (CMV)	Kaposi's sarcoma	Immune deficiency Histocompatibility antigen genotype
RNA Viruses			
Type D	Human T-cell leukemia virus-1 (HTLV-1)	Adult T-cell leukemia/ lymphoma	

From Fernoglio-Preiser, C.M., et al. (1986). *New Concepts in Neoplasia as Applied to Diagnostic Pathology.* Baltimore, Md: Williams & Wilkins, p. 133.

b. Effects modified by:
(1) Age—the very young and elderly are more susceptible.
(2) Immunocompetence—many viruses are oncogenic only if the host is immunocompromised.
B. Compromised immune system.
1. Immune surveillance against cancer—theory that proposes recognition and destruction of cancer cells by the immune system.
2. Surveillance occurs via recognition of tumor-associated antigens (TAAs) that mark cancer cells as foreign.
3. Immune response may fail because of:
a. Constitutional factors:
(1) Age—an immature or senescent immune system.
(2) Tumor burden:
(a) Too little—insufficient to stimulate response.
(b) Too much—overwhelms the immune system.
(3) Cancer cells may:
(a) Shed substances that:
i. Suppress immune activity.
ii. Shield the cell from recognition.
iii. Resemble normal cells and thus escape detection.
(b) Invade the bone marrow, resulting in decreased production of lymphocytes.
(c) Become coated with fibrin and escape detection.
b. Iatrogenic factors:
(1) Immunosuppressive drug therapy—incidence of malignancy increases with use of glucocorticosteroids, alkylating agents, azathioprine, cyclosporine.
(2) Radiation-induced suppression of immune response.
C. Genetic predisposition—predisposition to certain cancers may be inherited; mechanism is unclear in most cases, although some are linked to inheritance of dominant antioncogenes; examples:
1. Familial polyposis coli.
2. Multiple endocrine neoplasia.
3. Dysplastic nevus syndrome.
4. Neurofibromatosis.
5. Wilms' tumor.
6. Retinoblastoma.
7. Xeroderma pigmentosum.
8. Ataxia-telangiectasia.
9. Fanconi's anemia.
III. How is cancer diagnosed?
A. Microscopic studies show structural changes in cancer cells that are described in pathological terms (Figure 16-5) such as:
1. Pleomorphism—cells are variable in size and shape:
a. Some are unusually large; others are too small.
b. Multiple nuclei can be present.
2. Hyperchromatism—nuclear chromatin more pronounced upon staining.
3. Polymorphism—nucleus enlarged and variable in shape.
4. Aneuploidy—unusual numbers of chromosomes present.
5. Abnormal chromosome arrangements:
a. Translocations—exchange of material between chromosomes.

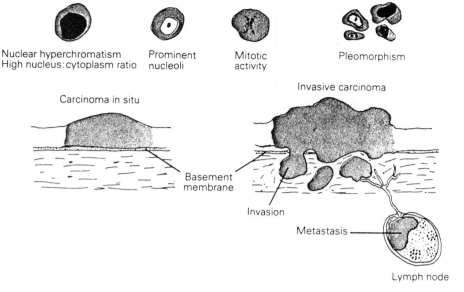

Nuclear hyperchromatism   Prominent   Mitotic   Pleomorphism
High nucleus:cytoplasm ratio   nucleoli   activity

Carcinoma in situ   Invasive carcinoma

Basement
membrane

Invasion

Metastasis

Lymph node

Figure 16-5 Features of malignant neoplasms. *(From Lefkowitch, J.H. [1989]. Histopathology of Disease. New York: Churchill Livingstone, p. 17.)*

    b. Deletions—loss of chromosome segments.
    c. Additions—extra chromosome sites.
    d. Fragile sites—weak points on chromosomes; more sensitive to carcinogens; can facilitate chromosome rearrangement.
  B. Biochemical studies show differences in cell metabolism and products such as:
    1. Cell membrane changes:
      a. Production of surface enzymes that may aid in invasion and metastasis.
      b. Loss of glycoproteins that normally aid in cell-to-cell adhesion and organization.
      c. Loss of antigens that otherwise label the cell as "self;"
      d. Production of new "tumor-associated antigens" that mark the cell as "non-self;" examples:
        (1) Oncofetal antigens—antigens that are expressed by certain normal cells during fetal development but are subsequently repressed; may reappear when cell becomes malignant; examples:
          (a) Carcinoembryonic antigen (CEA)—may be elevated in colorectal, breast, lung, liver, pancreatic, and gynecological cancers.
          (b) α-Fetoprotein (AFP)—may be elevated in hepatocellular, testicular, lung, pancreatic, and ovarian cancers.
        (2) Placental antigens—antigens normally produced by the placenta.
          (a) Examples—human chorionic gonadotropin (HCG) and human placental lactogen (HPL).
          (b) Usually are associated with gynecological cancers.
        (3) Differentiation antigens—found in normal differentiating tissue; associated with acute lymphocytic leukemia (ALL), chronic lymphocytic leukemia (CLL), and lymphoblastic lymphoma.
        (4) Lineage-associated determination antigens:
          (a) Example—CA-125.
          (b) Associated with ovarian cancer.
        (5) Viral antigens—appear in certain cancers associated with viral origins.

e. Clinical usefulness—certain tumor antigens may be used as tumor markers (biochemical substances synthesized and released by tumor cells; may be used as indicators of tumor presence but may also be present in a variety of benign conditions); most tumor markers lack specificity to cancer.

2. Abnormal glycolysis—higher rate of anaerobic glycolysis, making the cell less dependent on oxygen.

3. Abnormal production of substances that give rise to the paraneoplastic syndromes (signs or symptoms that occur in a cancer client but are not due directly to the local effects of the tumor) (Table 16-3).

   a. Hormone or hormonelike substances, especially from nonendocrine cells.

   b. Procoagulant materials that affect the clotting mechanism.

C. Cell kinetic (growth and division) studies show:

1. Loss of contact inhibition (the normal inhibition of cell movement and division once in contact with other cells) (Figure 16-6).

2. Defect in cell-to-cell recognition and adhesion—cancer cells do not recognize and adhere to each other as well as normal cells do.

3. Increased mitotic index (the proportion of cells in a tissue that are in mitosis at any given time).

Table 16-3
PARANEOPLASTIC SYNDROMES

Clinical Syndrome	Underlying Cancers	Causal Substance
Cushing's syndrome	Bronchogenic (small cell) carcinoma Pancreatic carcinoma Neural tumors	Adrenocorticotropic hormone (ACTH) or ACTH-like substance
Hyponatremia	Bronchogenic carcinoma Intracranial neoplasms	Antidiuretic hormone (ADH) or ADH-like substance
Hypercalcemia	Bronchogenic squamous cell carcinoma Breast carcinoma Renal carcinoma Adult T-cell lymphoma	(?) Parathyroid hormone-like substance Transforming growth factor (TGF)-α
Hyperthyroidism	Blood dyscrasias Bronchogenic carcinoma Prostatic carcinoma	Thyroid-stimulating hormone (TSH) or TSH-like substance
Hypoglycemia	Fibrosarcoma Other mesenchymal sarcomas Hepatocellular carcinoma	Insulin or insulin-like substance
Carcinoid syndrome	Bronchial adenoma (carcinoid) Pancreatic carcinoma Gastric carcinoma	Serotonin, bradykinin, (?) histamine
Polycythemia	Renal carcinoma Cerebellar hemangioma Hepatocellular carcinoma	Erythropoietin
Venous thrombosis	Pancreatic carcinoma Bronchogenic carcinoma Other cancers	(?) Hypercoagulability

Modified from Cotran, R.S., Kumar, V., & Robbins, S.L. (1989). *Robbins Pathologic Basis of Disease* (4th ed). Philadelphia: W.B. Saunders Co., p. 295.

A Cancer cells or normal cells

B Cancer cells or normal cells
    in culture (early)

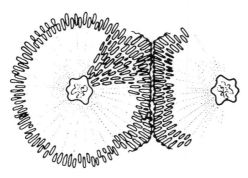

C Normal cell

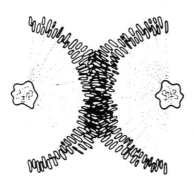

D Cancer cells

Figure 16-6 Impaired contact inhibition of cancer cells. *(From Kupchella, C.E. [1990]. Cellular biology of cancer. In S.L. Groenwald, M.H. Frogge, M. Goodman, & C.H. Yarbro [eds]. Cancer Nursing: Principles and Practice [2nd ed]. Boston: Jones & Bartlett Publishers, p. 48.)*

    a. Large numbers of mitotic cells reflect the higher proliferative activity of the tumor.

    b. A high mitotic index is not unique to cancer; however, normal cells in, for example, the gastrointestinal system, bone marrow, and hair follicles have a rapid rate of cell turnover and thus a high mitotic index.

  4. Abnormal cell differentiation.

    a. Differentiation—refers to the extent to which tumor cells resemble comparable normal cells, both morphologically and functionally.

      (1) Grade—an evaluation of the degree of differentiation of the tumor.

(a) Often characterized as grade I, II, III, or IV.

(b) Grade I—well differentiated; also termed *low grade*.

(c) Grade IV—poorly differentiated; also termed *high grade*.

(2) Benign tumors—composed of well-differentiated cells; tend to resemble the mature, functionally normal cells of the tissue of origin.

(3) Malignant tumors—may be composed of cells that range from well differentiated to undifferentiated, primitive cells.

(4) Anaplasia, or lack of differentiation, is:

(a) A hallmark of malignancy.

(b) The result of proliferation of transformed cells that do not mature.

(c) Not a result of "dedifferentiation" (a reversion of the maturational process).

b. Functional changes:

(1) The greater the degree of differentiation of a cell, the more likely it will have some of the functional capabilities of its normal counterpart.

(2) The more anaplastic the tumor, the less likely any specialized function will be present.

5. Growth characteristics—the length of time required for a tumor to become clinically detectable is influenced by:

a. Growth fraction—the ratio of the total number of cells to the number of proliferating cells (cells that will subsequently divide).

(1) Normal tissue.

(a) Growth fraction is variable, depending on type of tissue.

(b) Example—intestinal epithelium contains approximately 16% actively proliferating cells; central nervous system cells are nonproliferating.

(2) Type of malignancy.

(a) Growth fraction also is variable, depending on type of cancer.

(b) Examples:

i. Many solid tumors—2% to 8% of cells are actively proliferating.

ii. Very aggressive, rapidly growing tumors—20% to 30% of cells are actively proliferating.

b. Tumor volume-doubling time.

(1) The time within which the total cancer cell population doubles.

(2) Average volume-doubling time of most primary solid tumors—2 to 3 months, with a range of 11 to 90 weeks.

(3) Influencing variables:

(a) Tumor type—most tumors have a high proportion of nonproliferating cells.

(b) Vascularity:

i. Supplies necessary nutrients and removes wastes.

ii. Varies within tumor (Figure 16-7).

(i) Center is poorly vascular; hence, slower growing.

(ii) Periphery is more vascular; hence, increased growth.

(c) Cell loss by:

i. Continuous shedding from the primary tumor.

ii. Death caused by toxic products released from other necrotic cells within the tumor.

(d) Hormone levels.

i. Certain cancers (that arise in hormone-dependent tissue) require hormones for growth.

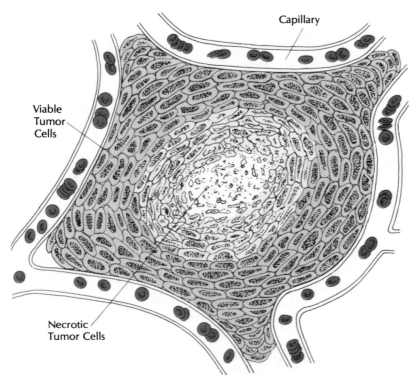

Capillary

Viable
Tumor
Cells

Necrotic
Tumor Cells

Figure 16-7 A, In many tumors, viable tissue and necrotic tissue are arranged in one of two patterns: cylindrical or nodular. Both patterns appear to reflect the presence or absence of proximate vascular support. The nodular pattern is depicted here. Viable tissue lies around the outer margins of the nodule, near surrounding vessels, whereas the center is necrotic. *(Reproduced with permission. Tannock, I.F. [1983]. Biology of tumor growth.* Hosp Pract 18[4], 86. *Illustration by Nancy Lou Makris.)*

          ii. Reduction in hormone levels reduces tumor growth.
          iii. Increased hormone levels promote growth.
     c. Clinical conclusions (Figure 16-3):
        (1) Tumor growth rates vary widely.
        (2) Growth increases exponentially at first (tumor growth doubles constantly over time).
        (3) Growth then slows.
        (4) Smallest clinically detectable mass equals:
          (a) One gram in weight.
          (b) One cubic centimeter in diameter.
          (c) Ten billion to 100 billion cells.
          (d) Approximately 30 tumor volume-doubling times.
        (5) Growth from 1 g to 1 kg (potentially lethal size) requires only 10 more doublings.
        (6) Tumors increase in size because rate of cell production exceeds rate of cell death.
  D. Tumor growth patterns (Figure 16-8).
    1. Noncancerous and precancerous growth changes.
     a. Hypertrophy:
       (1) An increase in the size of cells.

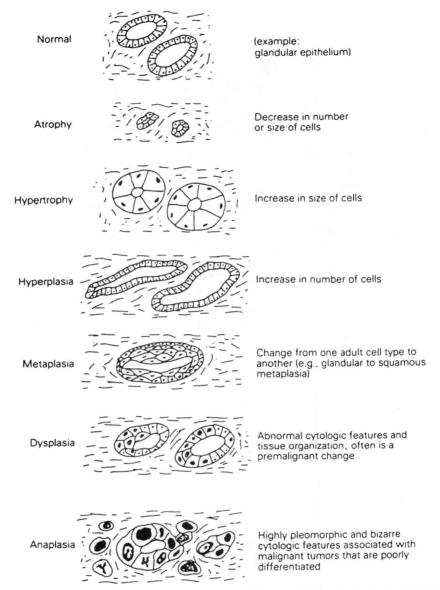

Normal — (example: glandular epithelium)

Atrophy — Decrease in number or size of cells

Hypertrophy — Increase in size of cells

Hyperplasia — Increase in number of cells

Metaplasia — Change from one adult cell type to another (e.g., glandular to squamous metaplasia)

Dysplasia — Abnormal cytologic features and tissue organization; often is a premalignant change

Anaplasia — Highly pleomorphic and bizarre cytologic features associated with malignant tumors that are poorly differentiated

Figure 16-8 Features of reactive and neoplastic growth processes. *(From Lefkowitch, J.H. [1989]. Histopathology of Disease. New York: Churchill Livingstone, p. 160.)*

       (2) Can result from hormonal stimulation, increased workload, or compensation secondary to functional loss of other tissue.
   b. Hyperplasia:
       (1) A reversible increase in the number of cells in a tissue.
       (2) Can result from hormonal stimulation (during pregnancy).
       (3) Abnormal hyperplastic changes such as those associated with chronic irritation can lead to increased risk of malignancy.
   c. Metaplasia:
       (1) Reversible process involving replacement of one mature cell type by another mature cell type not usually found in the involved tissue.

(2) Initiated by chronic irritation, inflammation, vitamin deficiency, or other pathological process.

(3) Example—replacement of columnar epithelial cells in respiratory passages of smokers with squamous cell epithelium.

  d. Dysplasia:

(1) Alteration in normal adult cells.

(2) Characterized by variations in size, shape, and organization.

(3) Can result from chronic irritation or inflammation.

(4) Smokers may exhibit dysplastic changes in respiratory tissues and oral mucosa.

(5) Possibly reversible if stimulant is removed.

(6) Strongly associated with subsequent neoplastic changes.

2. Hyperplasia, metaplasia, and dysplasia are not neoplastic per se but may precede the development of cancer.

3. Cancerous conditions.

  a. Anaplasia:

(1) The cytological and positional disorganization of cells.

(2) Degree of anaplastic changes may vary.

(3) Most often used to describe malignancy.

  b. *Neoplasm* versus *tumor*.

(1) Interchangeable terms.

(2) Refers to abnormal growth of tissue that serves no function and continues to grow unchecked once a stimulus is removed.

(3) Can be benign or malignant.

  c. *Cancer*—common term for all malignancies.

E. Tumor nomenclature (Table 16-4).

1. Usually named according to tissue of origin (numerous exceptions exist).

2. Benign tumors:

  a. Labeled by adding the suffix *oma* to the tissue of origin.

  b. Examples:

(1) Lipoma—benign tumor composed of lipid cells.

(2) Adenoma—benign tumor composed of glandular cells.

3. Malignant tumors (Table 16-4):

  a. Classified according to:

(1) Tissue of origin.

(2) Biological behavior.

(3) Anatomical site.

(4) Degree of cell differentiation.

  b. Carcinomas:

(1) Arise in epithelial tissue.

(2) Prefixes describe specific type of epithelial tissue.

    (a) *Adeno:*

      i. Describes tumors arising from glandular epithelium (columnar).

      ii. Organ of origin also included.

      iii. Example—pancreatic adenocarcinoma (a malignant epithelial neoplasm located in the pancreas).

    (b) *Squamous:*

      i. Describes tumors arising from squamous epithelium.

      ii. Organ of origin is included.

      iii. Example—squamous cell carcinoma of the skin.

Table 16-4
NOMENCLATURE OF TUMORS

Tissue of Origin	Benign	Malignant
Composed of One Parenchymal Cell Type		
Tumors of mesenchymal origin		*Sarcomas*
Connective tissue and derivatives	Fibroma	Fibrosarcoma
	Myxoma	Myxosarcoma
	Lipoma	Liposarcoma
	Chondroma	Chondrosarcoma
	Osteoma	Osteogenic sarcoma
Endothelial and related tissues		
Blood vessels	Hemangioma	Angiosarcoma
	Capillary	
	Cavernous	
Lymph vessels	Lymphangioma	Lymphangiosarcoma
Synovia		Synovioma (synoviosarcomae)
Mesothelium (lining cells of body cavities)		Mesothelioma
Brain coverings	Meningioma	Invasive meningioma
Glomus	Glomus tumor	
Blood cells and related cells		
Hematopoietic cells		Myelogenous leukemia
		Monocytic leukemia
Lymphoid tissue		Malignant lymphomas
		Lymphocytic leukemia
		Plasmacytoma (multiple myeloma)
Langerhans' cells		Histiocytosis X
Monocyte-macrophage		(?) Histiocytic lymphoma
		(?) Hodgkin's disease
Muscle		
Smooth muscle	Leiomyoma	Leiomyosarcoma
Striated	Rhabdomyoma	Rhabdomyosarcoma
Tumors of epithelial origin		*Carcinomas*
Stratified squamous	Squamous cell papilloma	Squamous cell or epidermoid carcinoma
Basal cells of skin or adnexa		Basal cell carcinoma
Skin adnexal glands		
Sweat glands	Sweat gland adenoma	Sweat gland carcinoma
Sebaceous glands	Sebaceous gland adenoma	Sebaceous gland carcinoma

From Cotran, R.S., Kumar, V., & Robbins, S.L. (1989). *Robbins Pathologic Basis of Disease* (4th ed). Philadelphia: W.B. Saunders Co., p. 242.

    c. Sarcomas:
       (1) Originate in connective tissue.
       (2) Prefixes for specific connective tissue sarcomas include:
          (a) *Osteo*—arising from bone.
          (b) *Chondro*—arising from cartilage.

Table 16-4
NOMENCLATURE OF TUMORS *Continued*

Tissue of Origin	Benign	Malignant
Epithelial lining		
Glands or ducts—well-differentiated group	Adenoma Papilloma Papillary adenoma Cystadenoma	Adenocarcinoma Papillary carcinoma Papillary adenocarcinoma Cystadenocarcinoma
Poorly differentiated group		Medullary carcinoma Undifferentiated carcinoma (simplex)
Respiratory passages		Bronchogenic carcinoma Bronchial "adenoma"
Neuroectoderm	Nevus	Melanoma (melanocarcinoma)
Renal epithelium	Renal tubular adenoma	Renal cell carcinoma (hypernephroma)
Liver cells	Liver cell adenoma	Hepatoma (hepatocellular carcinoma)
Bile duct	Bile duct adenoma	Bile duct carcinoma (cholangiocarcinoma)
Urinary tract epithelium (transitional)	Transitional cell papilloma	Papillary carcinoma Transitional cell carcinoma Squamous cell carcinoma
Placental epithelium	Hydatidiform mole	Choriocarcinoma
Testicular epithelium (germ cells)		Seminoma Embryonal carcinoma
More Than One Neoplastic Cell Type—Mixed Tumors—Usually Derived From One Germ Layer		
Salivary glands	Pleomorphic adenoma (mixed tumor of salivary gland origin)	Malignant mixed tumor of salivary gland origin
Renal anlage		Wilms' tumor
More Than One Neoplastic Cell Type Derived From More Than One Germ Layer—Teratogenous		
Totipotential cells in gonads or in embryonic rests	Mature teratoma, dermoid cyst	Immature teratoma

        (c) *Lipo*—arising from fat.
        (d) *Rhabdo*—arising from skeletal muscle.
        (e) *Leiomyo*—arising from smooth muscle.
     d. Hematological malignancies:
       (1) Leukemias:
          (a) Arise from hematopoietic stem cells.
          (b) Classified according to cell type and maturity.
          (c) *Lympho* denotes leukemia of lymphoid origin.
          (d) *Myelo* denotes leukemia of myeloid origin.

(2) Lymphomas:
   (a) Malignancies of the lymphocyte.
   (b) Subclassified as:
      i. Hodgkin's disease.
      ii. Non-Hodgkin's lymphoma.
(3) Multiple myeloma—arises from the plasma cell (B lymphocyte) line.

IV. How do these concepts relate to nursing care?
   A. Form the basis for client teaching about prevention and health promotion:
      1. Avoidance of known carcinogens at:
         a. Home—see Table 16-1 for specific substances.
         b. Occupational sites, especially:
            (1) Asbestos.
            (2) Carcinogenic chemicals.
            (3) Sun.
            (4) Tobacco (smokefree work environment).
         c. Recreational activities—sun, tanning booths.
      2. Emphasis on health promotion and life-style choices:
         a. Smoking cessation.
         b. Dietary choices.
         c. Methods to avoid sexually transmitted viral carcinogens.
         d. Screening and follow-up when at risk for familial carcinogenesis.
         e. Self-examination for early cancer detection:
            (1) Breast.
            (2) Testes.
            (3) Skin.
            (4) Oral.
            (5) Vulvar.
         f. Other screening activities (per American Cancer Society guidelines).
      3. Investigative potential of reversing agents (retinoids, vitamin C, indoles).
      4. Emphasis on reversibility of cellular changes (as appropriate)—behavior or life-style changes *can* make a difference.
      5. Clarification of misconceptions about carcinogenic potential of screening and diagnostic radiological examinations:
         a. Average yearly exposure to natural, background radiation—0.7 to 1.5 mGy.
         b. Biological effects not apparent until 1000 mGy (1 Gy) incurred.
         c. Approximate doses for common radiographic procedures:
            (1) Chest x-ray—0.05 mGy.
            (2) Abdominal computed tomography—5.0 mGy.
            (3) Mammography—0.8 mGy.
         d. Carcinogenic risk from diagnostic procedures is extremely minimal.
      6. Emphasis on risk of *not* undergoing screening radiography (i.e., undetected cancer).
   B. Form the basis of client teaching about cancer diagnoses:
      1. Pathology necessary for cancer diagnosis.
      2. Cytological examinations (Papanicolaou smear):
         a. Detection before palpable lesion is present.
         b. Promotion of chance for early cure.
      3. Tumor-associated antigens are used as tumor markers:
         a. At the time of diagnosis.

      b. During treatment.

      c. After treatment to monitor recurrence or progression.

    4. Radiologic examinations are necessary for detection of micrometastases.

C. Form the basis of client teaching about treatment:

    1. High mitotic index of certain cancer cells renders them more susceptible to cytotoxic effects of chemotherapeutic agents.

    2. Stable cells (bone, neural tissue) are less sensitive to effects of chemotherapy because of lower mitotic index.

    3. Use of hyperoxygenation procedures are based on principles of cell sensitivity to radiation effects.

    4. Tumor heterogeneity explains the necessity for:

      a. Intense initial treatment.

      b. Subsequent, repeated treatments with a variety of drugs.

      c. Failures in treatment of metastases.

    5. Adjuvant therapy is used for presumed micrometastases to kill the last remaining cancer cells.

    6. Use of hormonal manipulation for tumors is effective only in hormone-dependent tissues.

    7. Use of fractionated radiation therapy is to minimize damage to healthy tissue while achieving lethal effect to malignant cells.

    8. Carcinogenic potential of alkylating chemotherapeutic agents and radiation therapy necessitates long-term client follow-up to detect iatrogenic malignancies.

D. Form the basis for understanding treatment side effects:

    1. Chemotherapy and radiation therapy are nonselective between malignant and normal cells.

    2. Effect on normal cells (especially rapidly dividing cells) accounts for treatment-related side effects (myelosuppression, alopecia, mucositis, nausea and vomiting, diarrhea, dysphagia).

E. Explain paraneoplastic syndromes:

    1. Related clinical problems are based on ectopic production of hormones and other substances by the malignant cells.

    2. Hormones are atypical of the tissue that gives rise to the tumor, resulting in clinical syndromes (endocrine, coagulant).

F. Form the basis for client teaching and follow-up to detect metastasis:

    1. Likelihood of metastasis at time of diagnosis may necessitate:

      a. Extensive diagnostic workup.

      b. Systemic approach to therapy.

      c. Adjuvant therapy.

    2. Potential for disease recurrence via metastasis necessitates frequent and long-term follow-up.

V. What are the implications for the professional development of the nurse?

A. Promotes understanding of terminology and nomenclature necessary for client teaching and interdisciplinary communication or collaboration.

B. Promotes understanding of cancer prevention and early detection.

C. Forms basis for understanding rationale for treatment protocols, timing of treatment, and diagnostic follow-up.

D. Enhances understanding of reasons for intensity of initial treatment protocols.

E. Forms basis for understanding current research and trends in care.

F. Forms basis for understanding and initiating cancer nursing research.

G. Promotes understanding of prognostic implications of disease.

H. Enhances participation in identification and discussion of ethical issues related to disease and treatment.

BIBLIOGRAPHY

Adelstein, S.J. (1987). Uncertainty and relative risks of radiation exposure. *JAMA 258*(5), 655-657.

Alkire, K. & Groenwald, S.L. (1990). Relation of the immune system to cancer. In S.L. Groenwald, M.H. Frogge, M. Goodman, & C.H. Yarbro (eds). *Cancer Nursing: Principles and Practice* (2nd ed). Boston: Jones & Bartlett Publishers, pp. 72-88.

Bates, S.E. & Longo, D.L. (1987). Use of serum tumor markers in cancer diagnosis and management. *Semin Oncol 14*(2), 102-138.

Bunn, P.A., Jr. & Ridgway, E.C. (1989). Paraneoplastic syndrome. In V.T. DeVita, Jr., S. Hellman, & S.A. Rosenberg (eds). *Cancer: Principles & Practice of Oncology* (3rd ed). Philadelphia: J.B. Lippincott Co., pp. 1896-1940.

Cotran, R.S., Kumar, V., & Robbins, S.L. (1989). *Robbins Pathologic Basis of Disease* (4th ed). Philadelphia: W.B. Saunders Co.

Eddy, D.M., Hasselblad, V., McGivney, W., & Hendee, W. (1988). The value of mammography screening in women under age 50 years. *JAMA 259*(10), 1512-1519.

Fidler, I.J. & Balch, C.M. (1987). The biology of cancer metastasis and implications for therapy. *Curr Probl Surg 24*(3), 129-209.

Fidler, I.J. & Nicolson, G.L. (1987). The process of cancer invasion and metastasis. *Cancer Bull 39*(3), 126-131.

Fitzpatrick, T.B. (1986). Ultraviolet-induced pigmentary changes: benefits and hazards. *Curr Probl Dermatol 15*, 25-38.

Friedberg, E.C. (1985). *DNA Repair*. New York: W.H. Freeman and Co.

Fry, R.J.M. (1989). Principles of carcinogenesis: physical. In V.T. DeVita, Jr., S. Hellman, & S.A. Rosenberg (eds). *Cancer: Principles & Practice of Oncology* (3rd ed). Philadelphia: J.B. Lippincott Co., pp. 136-148.

Gallucci, B.B. (1987). The immune system and cancer. *Oncol Nurs Forum 14*(6 suppl), 3-12.

Gallucci, B.B. (1991). Cancer biology: molecular and cellular aspects. In S.B. Baird, R. McCorkle, & M. Grant (eds). *Cancer Nursing: A Comprehensive Textbook*. Philadelphia: W.B. Saunders Co., pp. 115-129.

Gohagan, J.K., Darby, W.P., & Spitznagel, E.L. (1986). Radiogenic breast cancer effects of mammographic screening. *J Natl Cancer Inst 77*(1), 71-76.

Hansen, M.F. & Cavenee, W.K. (1987). Genetics of cancer predisposition. *Cancer Res 47*(21), 5518-5527.

Harley, N.H. & Harley, J.H. (1990). Potential lung cancer risk from indoor radon exposure. *Ca 40*(5), 265-275.

Hecht, F., Hecht, B.K., & Sandberg, A.A. (1989). Cytogenetics and human neoplasia. In A.E. Sirica (ed). *The Pathobiology of Neoplasia*. New York: Plenum Press, pp. 231-246.

Henderson, B.E. (1989). Establishment of an association between a virus and a human cancer. *J Nat Cancer Inst 81*(5), 320-321.

Heppner, G.H. & Miller, B.E. (1989). Therapeutic implications of tumor heterogeneity. *Semin Oncol 16*(2), 91-105.

Hubbard, S.M. & Liotta, L.A. (1991). The biology of metastases. In S.B. Baird, R. McCorkle, & M. Grant (eds). *Cancer Nursing: A Comprehensive Textbook*. Philadelphia: W.B. Saunders Co., pp. 130-142.

Killion, J.J. & Fidler, I.J. (1989). The biology of tumor metastasis. *Semin Oncol 16*(2), 106-115.

Kupchella, C.E. (1990). Cellular biology of cancer. In S.L. Groenwald, M.H. Frogge, M. Goodman, & C.H. Yarbro (eds). *Cancer Nursing: Principles and Practice* (2nd ed). Boston: Jones & Bartlett Publishers, pp. 43-57.

Kupchella, C.E. (1990). The spread of cancer: invasion and metastasis. In S.L. Groenwald, M.H. Frogge, M. Goodman, & C.H. Yarbro (eds). *Cancer Nursing: Principles and Practice* (2nd ed). Boston: Jones & Bartlett Publishers, pp. 58-71.

Lieberman, M.W. & Lebovitz, R.M. (1990). Neoplasia. In J.M. Kissane (ed). *Anderson's Pathology* (9th ed). St. Louis: C.V. Mosby Co., pp. 566-613.

Lilley, L.L. & Schaffer, S. (1990). Human papillomavirus: a sexually transmitted disease with carcinogenic potential. *Cancer Nurs 13*(6), 366-372.

Liotta, L.A., Stracke, M.L., Wewer, U.M., & Schiffmann, E. (1989). Tumor invasion and metastases: biochemical mechanisms. In A.E. Sirica (ed). *The Pathobiology of Neoplasia*. New York: Plenum Press.

Loken, M.K. (1987). Physicians' obligations in radiation issues. *JAMA 258*(5), 673-676.

Lovejoy, N.C., Thomas, M.L. Halliburton, P., & Mimnaugh, L. (1987). Tumor markers: relevance to clinical practice. *Oncol Nurs Forum 14*(5), 75-82.

Mettlin, C. & Mirand, A.L. (1991). The causes of cancer. In S.B. Baird, R. McCorkle, & M. Grant (eds). *Cancer Nursing: A Comprehensive Textbook*. Philadelphia: W.B. Saunders Co., pp. 104-114.

Nicolson, G.L. (1988). Organ specificity of tumor metastasis: role of preferential adhesion, invasion and growth of malignant cells at specific secondary sites. *Cancer Metastasis Rev 7*(2), 143-188.

Nonaka, S., Kaidbey, K.H., & Kligman, A.M. (1983). The influence of UVA and visible radiation on acute damage by short-wave UVR (lambda less than 320 nm). *J Invest Dermatol 81*(6), 524-527.

Pitot, H.C. (1989). Principles of carcinogenesis: chemical. In V.T. DeVita, Jr., S. Hellman, & S.A. Rosenberg (eds). *Cancer: Principles & Practice of Oncology* (3rd ed). Philadelphia: J.B. Lippincott Co., pp. 116-135.

Ruddon, R.W. (1987). *Cancer Biology* (2nd ed). New York: Oxford University Press.

Schnipper, L. (1986). Clinical implications of tumor-cell heterogeneity. *N Engl J Med 314*(22), 1423-1431.

Sell, S. (1987). *Immunology, Immunopathology, and Immunity* (4th ed). New York: Elsevier Science Publishing Co.

Sirica, A.E. (1989). Classification of neoplasms. In A.E. Sirica (ed). *The Pathobiology of Neoplasia*. New York: Plenum Press, pp. 25-38.

Stewart, D.S. (1987). Indoor tanning: the nurse's role in preventing skin damage. *Cancer Nurs 10*(2), 93-99.

Stites, D.P., Stobo, J.D., & Wells, J.V. (1987). *Basic and Clinical Immunology* (6th ed). Los Altos, Calif: Lange Medical Publications.

Sulitzeanu, D. (1985). Human cancer-associated antigens: present status and implications for immunodiagnosis. *Adv Cancer Res 44*, 1-42.

Tannock, I.F. (1987). Tumor growth and cell kinetics. In I.F. Tannock & R.P. Hill (eds). *The Basic Science of Oncology*. New York: Pergamon Press, pp. 140-159.

Tannock, I.F. (1989). Principles of cell proliferation: cell kinetics. In V.T. DeVita, Jr., S. Hellman, & S.A. Rosenberg (eds). *Cancer: Principles & Practice of Oncology* (3rd ed). Philadelphia: J.B. Lippincott Co., pp. 3-13.

Virji, M.A., Mercer, D.W., & Herberman, R.B. (1988). Tumor markers in cancer diagnosis and prognosis. *CA 38*(2), 104-126.

Woodruff, M. (1990). *Cellular Variation and Adaptation in Cancer: Biological Basis and Therapeutic Consequences*. New York: Oxford University Press.

Yarbro, J.W. (1990). Carcinogenesis. In S.L. Groenwald, M.H. Frogge, M. Goodman, & C.H. Yarbro (eds). *Cancer Nursing: Principles and Practice* (2nd ed). Boston: Jones & Bartlett Publishers, pp. 31-42.

Yunis, J.J. & Hoffman, W.R. (1989). Fragile sites as a mechanism in carcinogenesis. *Cancer Bull 41*(5), 283-292.

Section Four

Cancer Epidemiology

17

Cancer Epidemiology

Ruth Bope Dangel, MN, RN

I. Epidemiological purposes, methods, and principles.
   A. Definition: the scientific study of factors that influence the frequency and distribution of cancer in humans.
   B. Goals—to:
      1. Discover causes of cancer.
      2. Detect and quantify risk factors.
      3. Increase understanding of carcinogenesis.
      4. Evaluate preventive measures.
   C. Methods—research methods include descriptive, analytic, and molecular studies.
      1. Descriptive studies.
         a. Purposes:
            (1) Measure the occurrence of cancer within groups of people.
            (2) Use demographic characteristics such as age, sex, race, marital status, residence, and occupation to delineate the groups.
            (3) Provide data about frequency and distribution of cancer in populations and high-risk groups.
            (4) Identify geographical areas of frequent occurrence.
            (5) Evaluate the effectiveness of preventive measures.
            (6) Identify changes in patterns of occurrence.
            (7) Generate hypotheses about causal relationships.
         b. Example—cancer rates of migrant populations demonstrated that Japanese who migrated to Hawaii and California experienced an increased risk of large bowel cancer within a few decades of migration.
      2. Analytical studies.
         a. Purposes:
            (1) Test hypotheses regarding the causal relationships between variables and cancer.
            (2) Provide data about causative agents or causal models.
            (3) Generate new hypotheses regarding causation.
            (4) Suggest further need for descriptive studies.
         b. Types of analytical studies:
            (1) Prospective analytical studies:

(a) Test hypotheses regarding disease causation by quantifying factors thought related to cancer in populations who do not have cancer; the proportion that develops the disease is studied over a designated period of time.

(b) Example—study of smokers followed over time suggested the positive association between level of smoking (package years) and lung cancer.

(c) Advantages:

    i. Can generalize from the sample to the reference population with some certainty.

    ii. Can quantify the risk of developing cancer.

    iii. Can establish that the variable preceded the cancer.

    iv. Can decrease bias in reporting since the variable is described before the outcome is measured.

(d) Disadvantages:

    i. Costly in time and personnel.

    ii. Follow-up can be difficult.

    iii. Provide limited data when condition is rare.

    iv. Attrition occurs in both the sample and among investigators.

    v. Changes occur that affect data but are not studied.

(2) Retrospective analytical studies:

(a) Comparison of characteristics of groups who have cancer with groups who do not.

(b) Example—endometrial cancer among women who used estrogen and non-users.

(c) Advantages:

    i. Require less time and expense than prospective studies.

    ii. Useful for studying cancers that rarely occur.

    iii. Attrition is less than in prospective studies.

    iv. Conclusions can be supported by retrospective studies conducted by different investigators on different populations.

(d) Disadvantages:

    i. Generalization is difficult because of lack of information about the reference population.

    ii. Making estimates of risks is difficult because of uncertainty as to whether the characteristic preceded or was consequent to the disease.

    iii. The possibility of bias exists if the population has selective recall.

    iv. Can study only those who survived the disease.

3. Cross-sectional studies.

  a. Method—identify a reference population, select a sample of that population, and ascertain and study characteristics and conditions simultaneously.

  b. Advantages:

    (1) Generalization to a reference group makes it possible to make prevalence and risk estimates.

    (2) Require less time and less expense than prospective studies.

    (3) Bias and attrition can be minimized by research design.

  c. Disadvantage—cannot always distinguish between antecedent and consequent relationships.

    4. Biochemical or molecular epidemiological studies.
       a. Method—new approach using analytical methods and laboratory studies of biological markers to determine molecular or biochemical changes caused by exposure to carcinogens.
       b. Advantages:
          (1) Laboratory study permits the study of exposure to oncogenic viruses, chemical and physical agents, dietary, or genetic factors.
          (2) Assist to clarify early preneoplastic events, host factors, and mechanism of action.
       c. Disadvantages—cannot extrapolate from animal species to humans.
  D. Epidemiological indicators—incidence, mortality, and lost life expectancy.
    1. Incidence—the number of new cases of cancer occurring during a certain time period among a given population.
       a. Measure of the probability of developing cancer.
       b. Useful in comparing rates of cancer between different populations.

$$\textbf{Incidence rate} = \frac{\textbf{Number of persons developing cancer in a unit of time}}{\textbf{Total population living at that time}}$$

    2. Prevalence—the number of cases of cancer in existence in a given population at a certain time.
       a. A measure of the burden of cancer in a population.
       b. Useful in planning health services.

$$\textbf{Prevalence rate} = \frac{\textbf{Number of persons with cancer at a given point in time}}{\textbf{Total population living at that time}}$$

    3. Mortality—number of deaths from cancer during a certain period of time.
       a. Reflects the occurrence of cancer sites with the worst prognosis.
       b. Useful in evaluating trends and geographical variations.
       c. Helpful in clarifying incidence rate, which may be misleading because of increased case reporting.

$$\textbf{Mortality rate} = \frac{\textbf{Number of persons dying from cancer in a unit of time}}{\textbf{Total population living at that time}}$$

    4. Lost life expectancy—a functional measure of the frequency of cancer and the socioeconomic impact; useful as a measure of the public health significance of cancer.

      Lost life expectancy: a death *n* years before a specified age contributes *n* years of lost life expectancy.

 E. Focus of epidemiological study—interaction of agent-host-environment (Table 17-1).
    1. Agent.
       a. Definition: a factor that must be present for disease to occur.
       b. Examples:
          (1) Tobacco is directly related to approximately 30% of all cancers and is the most important carcinogenic factor identified to date.
          (2) Alcohol accounts for approximately 3% of all cancer deaths.
          (3) Medications may account for 2% of all cancers (estrogens, alkylating agents, immunosuppressive agents).
    2. Host.
       a. Definition: a person susceptible to disease.

Table 17-1
ENVIRONMENTAL CAUSES OF HUMAN CANCER

Agent	Type of Exposure	Site of Cancer
Alcoholic beverages	Drinking	Mouth, pharynx, esophagus, larynx, liver
Alkylating agents (melphalan, cyclophosphamide, chlorambucil, semustine)	Medication	Leukemia
Androgen-anabolic steroids	Medication	Liver
Aromatic amines (benzidine, 2-naphthylamine, 4-aminobiphenyl)	Manufacturing of dyes and other chemicals	Bladder
Arsenic (inorganic)	Mining and smelting of certain ores, pesticide manufacturing and use, medications, drinking water	Lung, skin, liver (angiosarcoma)
Asbestos	Manufacturing and use	Lung, pleura, peritoneum
Benzene	Leather, petroleum, and other industries	Leukemia
Bis(chloromethyl) ether	Manufacturing	Lung (small cell)
Chlornaphazine	Medication	Bladder
Chromium compounds	Manufacturing	Lung
Estrogens Synthetic (DES)	Medication	Cervix, vagina (adenocarcinoma)
Conjugated (Premarin)		Endometrium
Steroid contraceptives		Liver (benign)
Immunosuppressants (azathoprine, cyclosporin)	Medication	Non-Hodgkin's lymphoma, skin (squamous carcinoma and melanoma), soft tissue tumors (including Kaposi's sarcoma)
Ionizing radiation	Atomic bomb explosives, treatment, and diagnosis, radium dial painting, uranium and metal mining	Most sites

From Fraumeni, J.F., Jr., Hoover, R.N., Devesa, S.S., & Kinlen, L.J. (1989). Epidemiology of cancer. In V.T. DeVita, Jr., S. Hellman, & S.A. Rosenberg (eds). *Cancer: Principles & Practice of Oncology* (3rd ed). Philadelphia: J.B. Lippincott Co. p. 217.

b. Examples:
  (1) Diet is suspected as a cancer risk by direct influence on or by modulation of the immune system.
  (2) Genetic susceptibility may contribute to a small percent of cancer occurrence (retinoblastoma, nevoid basal cell carcinoma, polyposis coli, dysplastic nevus syndrome); some families have an aggregation of site-specific cancers that appear consistent with autosomal dominant inheritance.
  (3) Data on the influence of psychological characteristics on the incidence of cancer are inconclusive.

Table 17-1
ENVIRONMENTAL CAUSES OF HUMAN CANCER *Continued*

Agent	Type of Exposure	Site of Cancer
Isopropyl alcohol	Manufacturing by strong acid process	Nasal sinuses
Leather industry	Manufacturing and repair (boot and shoe)	Nasal sinuses, bladder
Mustard gas	Manufacturing	Lung, larynx, nasal sinuses
Nickel dust	Refining	Lung, nasal sinuses
Parasites	Infection	
Schistosoma haematobium		Bladder (squamous carcinoma)
Clonorchis sinensis		Liver (cholangiocarcinoma)
Phenacetin-containing analgesics	Medication	Renal pelvis
Polycyclic hydrocarbons	Cool carbonization products and some mineral oils	Lung, skin (squamous carcinoma)
Tobacco chews, including betel nut	Snuff dipping and chewing of tobacco, betel, lime	Mouth
Tobacco smoke	Smoking, especially cigarettes	Lung, larynx, mouth, pharynx, esophagus, bladder, pancreas, kidney
Ultraviolet radiation	Sunlight	Skin (including melanoma), lip
Viruses	Infection	
Epstein-Barr virus		Burkitt's lymphoma; nasopharyngeal carcinoma (?)
Hepatitis-B virus		Hepatocellular carcinoma
Human T-lymphotrophic virus, Type I		T-cell leukemia/lymphoma
Vinyl chloride	Manufacturing of polyvinyl chloride	Liver (angiosarcoma)
Wood dust	Furniture manufacturing (hardwood)	Nasal sinuses (adenocarcinoma)

    (4) Viral infections in the host may account for approximately 5% of cancers in the United States (Epstein-Barr virus [EBV] causing Burkitt's lymphoma and possibly hepatocellular carcinoma; hepatitis B virus [HBV] causing hepatocellular carcinoma; infection with human T-lymphotrophic virus type I [HTLV-I] linked with adult T-cell leukemia; and human immunodeficiency virus [HIV] causing Kaposi's sarcoma and lymphoma).
 3. Environment.
   a. Definition: factors to which the host is exposed.
   b. Examples:
    (1) Epidemiological studies indicate that an estimated 75% to 80% of cancers in the United States are caused by environmental and life-style factors.

(2) Occupational exposures may account for approximately 5% of all cancer deaths (asbestos, benzene).

(3) Environmental pollutants account for an estimated 2% of cancer deaths (Table 17-1).

(4) Ionizing radiation accounts for an estimated 3% of all cancer deaths.

    a. All body sites are vulnerable to the carcinogenic effects of radiation, but the most radiosensitive sites are the bone marrow, breast, and thyroid.

    b. Recent concerns include risk of lung cancer from indoor radon.

(5) Solar radiation is the major risk factor for skin cancer (squamous, basal cell, melanoma).

II. Historical development of cancer epidemiology.

  A. Epidemiological observations.

    1. 1700—Bernardino Ramazzini, an occupational physician, reported breast cancer occurred more in nuns than other women and suggested celibacy as a factor.

    2. 1775—Sir Percivall Pott, a surgeon, linked adult scrotal cancer to childhood experiences as chimney sweeps.

    3. 1761—Hill reported a risk of nasal cancer among snuff users.

    4. 1795—von Soemmering reported a link between pipe smoking and lip cancer.

    5. 1879—Harting and Hesse reported lung cancer in metal miners.

    6. 1888—Hutchinson reported skin cancer in clients treated with arsenic-containing solutions.

    7. 1895—Rehm reported bladder cancer among aniline dye workers.

  B. First epidemiological study—Rigoni-Stern (1842) attempted to quantify the risks of uterine cancer among nuns and other women in Verona and reported that uterine cancer was significantly less common in nuns.

  C. Largest epidemiological studies.

    1. Cancer Prevention Study I (CPS I) conducted by the American Cancer Society from 1959 through 1972:

      a. Approximately 68,000 volunteers enrolled 1,078,000 men and women from 25 states into the study.

      b. Subjects completed questionnaires annually during 1960 to 1965 and twice during 1971 and 1972.

      c. Supplemental questionnaires were completed in alternate years, and a further evaluation occurred in 1972.

      d. Through 1971 98.4% of the follow-up was complete.

      e. In 1976 a decision was made to continue tracking long-term survivors.

      f. The relationship between smoking and death was established using these data.

    2. Cancer Prevention Study II (CPS II) begun in 1982 by the American Cancer Society:

      a. A long-term prospective study of habits and exposures of more than 1 million Americans to study life-style and environmental factors related to cancer development.

      b. CPS II is modeled after CPS I but is larger in scope and in number of participants.

      c. Questions involve current concerns such as risks of drug, food, and occupational exposures, low-tar nicotine cigarette use, consumer products, low-level radiation exposure, and health effects of air and water pollution.

d. By comparing mortality rates of groups with different exposure, factors that increase risks of developing cancer, carry little or no risk, and may prevent cancer may be identified.

e. Preliminary data indicate a drastic decrease in the percentage of men who smoke.

III. Current data sources.

A. Surveillance, Epidemiology, and End Results (SEER)—begun in 1973 by the National Cancer Institute to gather data from population-based registries and to evaluate long-term trends in cancer incidence and survival.

B. CPS II—discussed above; data analyses in progress.

C. International Agency for Research on Cancer—compiles data from registries of countries in five continents; useful for proposing etiological hypotheses.

D. National Cancer Data Base (NCDB)—created in 1989 by the American Cancer Society and the American College of Surgeons to gather data from existing tumor registries and to combine regional data about cancer diagnosis, treatment, and survival into one national data base; provides the first data resource based on clinical treatment and outcome rather than the traditional population-based incidence, mortality, and survival data.

IV. Current cancer statistics.

A. Incidence (Figure 17-1):

CANCER INCIDENCE BY SITE AND SEX*

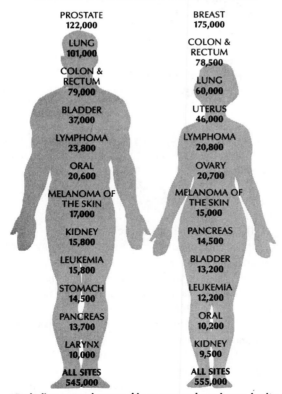

*Excluding nonmelanoma skin cancer and carcinoma in situ.

Figure 17-1 Cancer incidence by site and sex—1991 estimates. *(From American Cancer Society [1991]. Cancer Facts and Figures—1991. Atlanta: Author.)*

1. Approximately 1,100,000 people were diagnosed with cancer in 1991, excluding nonmelanoma skin cancer and carcinoma in situ.
2. For males and females combined, the highest incidence rates are for lung cancer, followed by cancer of the colon and rectum.
3. For males, the highest incidence rates are for prostate, lung, and colon and rectal cancer.
4. For females, the highest incidence rates are for breast, colon and rectum, and lung.
5. Breast cancer will develop in approximately one of every nine women.
6. Prostate cancer will develop in approximately one of every 11 men.
7. Incidence rate of cancer increases with advancing age.
8. Cancer in children is rare, but an estimated 7800 new cases occurred in 1991 (leukemia; osteogenic sarcoma and Ewing's sarcoma; neuroblastoma, rhabdomyosarcoma; brain cancers; lymphomas and Hodgkin's disease; retinoblastoma; and Wilms' tumor).
9. Incidence rates of cancer for black Americans are higher than for white Americans.
   a. In 1987 6% difference existed—incidence rates were 402.5 per 100,000 for blacks and 379.1 per 100,000 for whites.
   b. Cancer sites with significantly higher incidence rates for blacks include esophagus, uterine cervix, stomach, liver, prostate, larynx, and multiple myeloma.
   c. The incidence rate for esophageal cancer is three times higher among blacks than among whites.
   d. Black males have the highest rate of prostate cancer in the world.
   e. Black females have an incidence rate of invasive cancer of the cervix twice that of white females.
   f. The incidence rate for endometrial cancer for white females is almost double that of black females.
   g. Socioeconomic disadvantage is a greater contributor than race in explaining black-white differences.
B. Prevalence:
   1. Approximately 76 million Americans now living will develop cancer.
   2. Over 7 million living Americans have a history of cancer, and 3 million of the 7 million were diagnosed 5 or more years ago (most can be considered cured).
   3. Cancer will occur in three out of four families.
C. Mortality (Figure 17-2):
   1. Over 500,000 people died of cancer in 1991.
   2. Cancer is the second leading cause of death among adults and children ages 1 to 4 in the United States.
   3. In the United States one of every five deaths from all causes is from cancer.
   4. For males and females combined, lung cancer is the leading cause of cancer death, and colon and rectal cancer is the second leading cause.
   5. For men, the three leading causes of death from cancer are lung, prostate, and colon and rectal cancer.
   6. For women, the three leading causes of death from cancer are lung, breast, and colon and rectal cancer.
   7. Smoking is the most preventable cause of death in the United States; tobacco use causes more than one in six deaths in the United States.
   8. Cancer is the leading cause of death in children between the ages of 1 and 14 years.

CANCER DEATHS BY SITE AND SEX

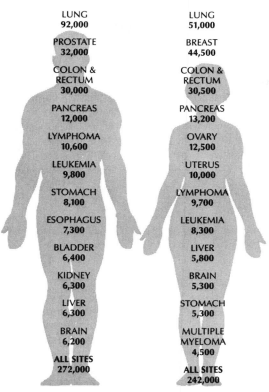

Figure 17-2 Cancer deaths by site and sex—1991 estimates. *(From American Cancer Society [1991]. Cancer Facts and Figures—1991. Atlanta: Author.)*

    9. In 1991, approximately 1500 cancer deaths in children occurred (one third were from leukemia).
   10. Mortality rates are higher for black Americans than for white Americans.
 D. Survival (Table 17-2):
    1. Approximately 4 of 10 people (440,000 Americans) diagnosed with cancer in 1991 will be alive 5 years after diagnosis.
      a. The observed survival rate is 40%.
      b. The survival rate adjusted for normal life expectancy is 50%.
    2. Five-year survival rates vary according to site.
      a. Lung cancer—the 5-year relative survival rate is 13% for all stages combined; the 5-year survival rate for lung cancers detected while localized is 37%, but only 20% are discovered while localized.
      b. Colon and rectal cancer—the 5-year survival rate for early localized stage is 85%; for regional spread to adjacent organs or lymph nodes, 55%; for distant metastases, approximately 6%.
      c. Breast cancer—the 5-year survival rate for localized disease is 91%; for cancer in situ, almost 100%; for regional spread, 69%; and for distance metastases, 18%.
      d. Cancer of the prostate—the 5-year relative survival rate for localized cancer is 85%; for all stages combined, 71%.
      e. Childhood cancer—the 5-year survival rate for all sites is 67%; for bone cancer, 54%; for neuroblastoma, 56%; for brain and central nervous

Table 17-2
FIVE-YEAR SURVIVAL RATES FOR SELECTED SITES*

Selected Site	All Stages (%)	Local (%)	Regional (%)	Distant (%)
Oral	52	75	41	18
Colon-Rectum	53	85	55	6
Pancreas	3	6	4	1
Lung	13	37	13	1
Melanoma	81	90	55	14
Female Breast	75	91	69	18
Cervix Uteri	67	88	51	13
Corpus Uteri	85	93	68	26
Ovary	38	85	44	18
Prostate	71	85	74	29
Testis	88	96	91	54
Bladder	76	88	44	9

*Adjusted for normal life expectancy. This chart is based on cases diagnosed in 1974-1986.
From American Cancer Society (1991). *Cancer Facts and Figures-1991*. Atlanta: Author.

system, 59%; for Wilms' tumor, 83%; and for Hodgkin's disease, 85% (data are for white children; data for other ethnic groups are not available).

  E. Morbidity:
    1. Definition: the condition of being diseased.
    2. Advances:
      a. Pain control—pain medication on a regular schedule, analgesics by infusion or injections, and procedures to interrupt pain pathways.
      b. Noninvasive diagnostic procedures—magnetic resonance imaging and computerized tomography often can replace exploratory surgery and define the location of tumors more precisely.
      c. Less mutilative treatment (limb-salvage techniques are sometimes used to treat primary bone cancer of the arm and leg by replacing a section of bone rather than amputation of the limb; the larynx can be conserved in early cancers; lumpectomy for early breast cancer minimizes disfigurement).
      d. Less toxicity of treatment—the use of growth factors to stimulate normal bone marrow cells allows use of higher doses of chemotherapeutic drugs with less toxicity.
      e. Greater awareness of psychosocial needs and knowledge of interventive strategies for clients and families have facilitated coping with cancer.

BIBLIOGRAPHY

American Cancer Society (1991). *Cancer Facts and Figures—1991*. Atlanta: Author.
Boring C.C., Squires, T.S., & Tong T. (1991). Cancer statistics, 1991. *CA 41*(1), 19-36.
Fraumeni, J.F., Jr., Hoover, R.V., Devesa, S.S., & Kinlen, L.J. (1989). Epidemiology of cancer. In V.T. DeVita, Jr., S. Hellman, & S.A. Rosenberg (eds). *Cancer: Principles & Practice of Oncology* (3rd ed). Philadelphia: J.B. Lippincott Co., pp. 196-235.

Lew, E.A. & Garfinkel, L. (1990). Mortality at ages 75 and older in the cancer prevention study (CPS I). *CA 40*(4), 210-224.

McGrath, B.B. (1987). Terminology. In C.R. Ziegfeld (ed). *Core Curriculum for Oncology Nursing.* Philadelphia: W.B. Saunders Co., pp. 31-33.

Menck, H.R., Garfinkel, L., & Dodd, G.D. (1991). Preliminary report of the National Cancer Data Base. *CA 41*(1), 7-18.

Mettlin, C. (1988). Descriptive and analytic epidemiology. Bridges to cancer control. *Cancer 62* (suppl 8), 1680-1687.

Murphy, G.P. (1991). The national cancer data base (editorial). *CA 41*(1), 5-6.

National Cancer Institute (undated). *Cancer Statistics Review.* Washington, D.C.: National Cancer Advisory Board.

Oleske, D.M. (1991). Epidemiologic principles for nursing practice: assessing the cancer problem and planning its control. In S.B. Baird, R. McCorkle, & M. Grant (eds). *Cancer Nursing: A Comprehensive Textbook.* Philadelphia: W.B. Saunders Co., pp. 91-103.

Oleske, D.M. & Groenwald, S.L. (1990). Epidemiology of cancer. In S.L. Groenwald, M.H. Frogge, M. Goodman, & C.H. Yarbro (eds.) *Cancer Nursing: Principles and Practices.* Boston: Jones & Bartlett, pp. 3-30.

Perera, F.P. (1990). Molecular epidemiology: a new tool in assessing risks of environmental carcinogens. *CA 40*(5), 277-288.

Peters, P.S. (1987). Cancer incidence and trends. In C.R. Ziegfeld (ed). *Core Curriculum for Oncology Nursing.* Philadelphia: W.B. Saunders Co., pp. 35-39.

Woods, N.F. & Woods, J.S. (1981). Epidemiology and the study of cancer. In L.B. Marino (ed). *Cancer Nursing.* St. Louis: C.V. Mosby Co., pp. 139-175.

Treatment of Cancer

18

Implications of Diagnosis and Staging on Treatment Goals and Strategies

Roberta Anne Strohl, MN, RN

THEORY

I. Decisions related to the treatment of cancer are made after review of the clinical, pathological, laboratory, and diagnostic data by a multidisciplinary team of cancer specialists.

II. Key factors to evaluate before making a treatment decision:
  A. Site of cancer.
     1. Review of client history.
     2. Physical examination.
     3. Radiological examination.
     4. Laboratory data.
  B. Histological type and grade of cancer.
     1. Diagnosis of cancer is determined by tissue biopsy.
        a. Incisional biopsy:
           (1) Aspiration.
           (2) Fine needle biopsy—removal of a core of tissue.
           (3) Punch biopsy—removal of tissue from the core of the tumor.
        b. Excisional biopsy—removal of tissue with client under general or local anesthesia:
           (1) Provides an opportunity to remove the entire lesion.
           (2) Serves as mechanism for removal of an adequate sample of tissue for diagnosis.
        c. Cytology—examination of fluid containing cells that have been shed:
           (1) A positive result from cytology may be adequate for diagnosis.
           (2) A negative result from cytology is inconclusive, and additional attempts to obtain tissue for diagnosis are indicated.
     2. Biopsy confirmation is important in that proof of a diagnosis is mandated by insurance companies for coverage.
     3. Tissue biopsy allows for histopathological grading of the tumor:
        a. Grade—a qualitative assessment of the degree of differentiation of the tumor; resemblance to the normal tissue origin is the primary criterion used for evaluation.

b. Classification for grading according to American Joint Committee on Cancer (AJCC):
   (1) G_x—grade cannot be assessed.
   (2) G_1—well differentiated.
   (3) G_2—moderately well differentiated.
   (4) G_3—poorly differentiated.
   (5) G_4—undifferentiated.
      (a) Well-differentiated tumors more closely resemble normal tissues and reproduce slowly.
      (b) Well-differentiated tumors generally have a more favorable prognosis.
C. Extent of disease or stage of cancer.
   1. Knowledge of the usual pattern of spread of specific cancers provides guidelines for the staging workup.
   2. Obtaining an extensive history and physical examination is the initial step of the staging procedure.
   3. Tests selected for the staging procedure are designed to evaluate the extent of local disease and potential sites of metastatic disease:
      a. Noninvasive procedures such as x-ray examinations, computed tomographic (CT) scans, magnetic resonance imaging (MRI), and ultrasound.
      b. Invasive procedures such as exploratory laparotomy.
   4. Staging systems.
      a. A uniform system for staging:
         (1) Allows comparisons of treatment results across client populations.
         (2) Serves as an aid to indicate appropriate and standard therapy.
      b. TNM—most widely accepted system for staging (Figure 18-1):
         (1) T—extent of primary *tumor.*
         (2) N—absence or presence and extent of regional lymph *node* metastasis.
         (3) M—absence or presence of distant *metastases.*
         (4) Addition of numbers after each letter indicate the extent of disease; the higher the number, the more advanced is the disease.
         (5) Addition of prefixes to the TNM indicate the timing of the staging (Table 18-1).
D. General health status of the client.
   1. Physical examination.

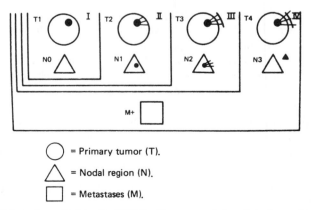

Figure 18-1 TNM staging. (*Rubin, P. [1983]. Statement of the clinical oncologic problem. In P. Rubin, R.F. Bakemeier, & S.K. Krackov [eds]. Clinical oncology: A multidisciplinary approach. [6th ed]. New York: American Cancer Society, p. 12.*)

Table 18-1
CLASSIFICATIONS OF TNM STAGING SYSTEM

Type of Classification	Symbol	Data Sources
Clinical classification	cTNM	Based on data available before treatment
Pathological classification	pTNM	Based on data available before treatment and on pathological examination of the resected specimen.
Retreatment classification	rTNM	Based on data available before definitive treatment after a disease-free interval Tissue confirmation required
Autopsy classification	aTNM	Based on data available at the time of autopsy

    2. Additional radiological and laboratory tests are conducted to determine the ability of the client to withstand the demands of and potential consequences of the proposed therapies.

    3. Evaluation of pulmonary, renal, liver, gastrointestinal, and cardiac function are often obtained.

    4. Host performance scales (Table 18-2).

E. Types of therapy.

    1. Primary treatment—major modality used to treat the cancer.

    2. Adjuvant treatment—therapy given *after* the primary treatment to control potential or known sites of metastasis.

    3. Neoadjuvant treatment—adjuvant therapy given *before* the primary treatment to control potential or known sites of metastasis.

    4. Prophylactic treatment—treatment directed to a sanctuary site when the risk for developing cancer at the site is high.

F. Goals of therapy.

    1. Cure—eradication of cancer cells in the body.

        a. Maximal risk of recurrence of disease usually occurs within the first 2 years after primary treatment.

        b. Clients who have been diagnosed with one cancer may be at higher risk for the development of another cancer that shares similar causative factors, such as breast and endometrial cancers; lung, head, neck, and esophageal cancers.

        c. Continued annual follow-up is required for evaluation of the presence of recurrence and late effects of treatment.

    2. Control—containment of the growth of cancer cells without complete eradication.

    3. Palliation—comfort and relief of symptoms when the possibility of cure is hopeless.

        a. Treatment may include any of the therapeutic modalities.

        b. Treatment course generally is shorter than treatment given with curative intent.

III. Treatment may include single and multimodal approaches.

A. Single-modality approach.

    1. Reserved for clients with small local disease and without evidence of predilection for metastasis.

    2. Examples of cancers for which single-modality treatment is appropriate—early skin cancer, colon cancer, head and neck cancers, and leukemia.

Table 18-2
HOST PERFORMANCE SCALES

American Joint Committee on Cancer

H   The physical state (performance scale) of the client, considering all cofactors determined at the time of stage classification and subsequent follow-up examinations

H0   Normal activity

H1   Symptomatic and ambulatory; cares for self

H2   Ambulatory more than 50% of time; occasionally needs assistance

H3   Ambulatory 50% or less of the time; nursing care needed

H4   Bedridden; hospitalization may be needed

Karnofsky Scale: Criteria of Performance Status (PS)

Able to perform normal activity; requires no care.	100	Normal; no complaints or evidence of disease
	90	Able to perform normal activity; minor signs and symptoms of disease
	80	Able to perform normal activity with effort; some signs and symptoms of disease
Unable to work; able to live at home and care for most personal needs; requires varying amount of assistance	70	Cares for self; unable to perform normal activity or to do active work
	60	Requires occasional assistance but is able to care for most of own needs
	50	Requires considerable and frequent medical care
Unable to care for self; requires equivalent of institutional or hospital care; disease may be progressing rapidly	40	Requires special care and assistance; disabled
	30	Hospitalization indicated, although death not imminent; severely disabled
	20	Hospitalization necessary; active supportive treatment required; very sick
	10	Fatal processes progressing rapidly; moribund
	0	Dead

Eastern Cooperative Oncology Group Scale (ECOG)

0   Fully active; able to perform all predisease activities without restriction

1   Restricted in physically strenuous activity but ambulatory and able to perform work of a light or a sedentary nature

2   Ambulatory and capable of all self-care but unable to perform any work activities; up and about more than 50% of waking hours

3   Capable of only limited self-care; confined to bed or chair 50% or more of waking hours

4   Completely disabled; cannot carry on any self-care; totally confined to bed or chair.

    B. Multimodal approach.
       1. Reserved for clients with bulky tumors or high likelihood of or actual metastatic disease.
       2. Surgery, radiation therapy, chemotherapy, and biotherapy may be combined sequentially or given concurrently.
       3. Examples of cancers for which multimodal treatment is appropriate—breast cancer, lymphoma, lung cancer, and endometrial cancer.

IV. Evaluation of the response to treatment.
  A. Complete response—absence of signs and symptoms of cancer for at least 1 month.
  B. Partial response:
    1. A 50% or more reduction in the sum of the products of the greater and lesser diameters of all measured lesions,
    2. Lasts at least 1 month, and
    3. Without the development of any new lesions during therapy.
  C. Progression:
    1. A 25% or more increase in the sum of the products of the greater and lesser diameters of all measured lesions or
    2. Development of any new lesions.

DATA COLLECTION

I. Pertinent personal history.
  A. Personal experiences with others with a diagnosis of cancer.
  B. Educational level.
  C. Concurrent diseases of the heart, liver, kidneys, lungs, and gastrointestinal tract.

II. Physical examination (see Chapter 5).

III. Psychosocial examination (see Chapter 3).
  A. Psychosocial factors that may affect the ability to participate in decision making.
  B. Factors that may affect the motivation or commitment to complete recommended workup or therapy.

ASSOCIATED NURSING DIAGNOSES

I. Knowledge deficit.

II. Decisional conflict.

III. Hopelessness.

NURSING PLANNING AND IMPLEMENTATION

I. Interventions to prepare the client and family for diagnostic and metastatic workup.
  A. Coordinate scheduling for laboratory and radiological procedures.
  B. Describe the rationale for and demands of the procedure:
    1. Temporal aspects expected.
    2. Sensations likely to be experienced.
  C. Describe the steps of the procedure.
  D. Discuss potential side effects or complications that may occur.
  E. Identify measures that can be used to prevent or minimize sequelae of the procedure.
  F. Describe the time frame for receiving results of the procedure.

II. Interventions to help the client and family understand the implications of staging procedures and type of tumor on treatment recommendations.
  A. Seek consensual validation of the perceptions of the client and family about information provided about the diagnosis, treatment, and prognosis.
  B. Clarify misconceptions about efficacy of selected treatment modalities.
  C. Provide information about the relative risks and benefits of selected treatments.

III. Interventions to assist the client and family understand the goals of and responses to therapy.

   A. Encourage the client and family to express concerns about the treatment or follow-up plan.

   B. Describe the demands of continued follow-up for the site-specific cancer.

   C. Teach the client and family signs and symptoms of long-term consequences of treatment modalities used in care.

EVALUATION OF CLIENT AND FAMILY OUTCOMES

   I. Describe the rationale for and findings of pretreatment and metastatic workup.

  II. Discuss the rationale for treatment selection based on the site, type, and stage of tumor and the general health status of the client.

 III. Identify the demands of treatment and follow-up care.

 IV. List community resources to assist with demands of treatment and follow-up care.

BIBLIOGRAPHY

Beahrs, O.H., Henson, D.E., Hutter, R.V. & Myers, M.H. (eds) (1987). *Manual for Staging of Cancer* (3rd ed). Philadelphia: J.B. Lippincott Co., pp. 1-25.

Davis, M. (1987). Assessing and diagnosing cancer. In C.R. Ziegfeld (ed). *Core Curriculum for Oncology Nursing*. Philadelphia: W.B. Saunders Co., pp. 71-87.

Ford, R. (ed) (1987). *Patient Teaching Manual* (vol 2). Pennsylvania: Springhouse Corp., pp. 118-168.

Gordon, D. (1987). Staging: a classification system for cancer. In C.R. Ziegfeld (ed). *Core Curriculum for Oncology Nursing*. Philadelphia: W.B. Saunders Co., pp. 87-94.

Griffiths, M.J., Murray K.H., & Russo, P.C. (1984). *Oncology Nursing: Pathophysiology, Assessment, and Intervention*. New York: MacMillan Publishing Co., pp. 64-89.

Mood, D.W. (1991). The diagnosis of cancer: a life transition. In S.B. Baird, R. McCorkle, & M. Grant. (eds). *Cancer Nursing: A Comprehensive Textbook*. Philadelphia: W.B. Saunders Co., pp. 219-235.

O'Mary, S.S. (1990). Diagnostic evaluation, classification, and staging. In S.L. Groenwald, M.H. Frogge, M. Goodman, & C.H. Yarbro (eds). *Cancer Nursing: Principles and Practice* (2nd ed). Boston: Jones & Bartlett Publishers, pp. 161-174.

Implications of Surgical Treatment for Nursing

Thomas J. Szopa, MS, RN, OCN, CETN

THEORY

I. Principles of surgery.
  A. Surgery is the treatment of choice for malignant tumors that:
    1. Have low growth fractions and long cell-cycle times.
    2. Are confined locally and/or regionally.
  B. Surgery is planned to:
    1. Remove the malignant tumor and a margin of adjacent normal tissue.
    2. Remove the malignant tumor with attention to resulting structural, functional, and cosmetic changes.
  C. Surgical procedures include strategies to decrease the local and systemic spread of cancer.
    1. Ligation of local blood vessels and local and regional draining lymphatics.
    2. Irrigation of wounds with cytotoxic agents.
    3. Changing surgical gloves frequently.
    4. Cleaning surgical instruments with cytotoxic solutions.
    5. Using a "no-touch" technique with tumor tissue.

II. Role of surgery in cancer care.
  A. Establish a tissue diagnosis.
    1. Incisional biopsy (Table 19-1).
    2. Excisional biopsy (Table 19-1).
    3. Needle biopsy (Table 19-1).
  B. Determine the stage of disease.
    1. Obtain multiple biopsies to identify and determine the extent of disease.
    2. Remove tumor along with affected organs or tissues.
    3. Mark residual tumor on affected organs to assist in subsequent cancer treatment planning and delivery.
  C. Treat disease.
    1. Primary treatment—removal of the malignant tumor and a margin of adjacent normal tissue.
    2. Adjuvant treatment—removal of tissues to decrease the risk of cancer incidence, progression, or recurrence.

Table 19-1
SURGICAL PROCEDURES

Type of Procedure	Uses in Cancer Care	Advantages	Disadvantages
Incisional biopsy	Obtain tissue for pathological examination	Simple method to obtain diagnosis	Additional, more extensive surgical procedure generally performed to remove tumor
Excisional biopsy	Establish tissue diagnosis and tumor removal	Quick, simple removal of tumor at biopsy time; may not require hospitalization; decreased cost; minimal cosmetic effects	Tumor cells may be implanted along surgical path and incision, resulting in local recurrence
Needle biopsy	Obtain tissue for pathological examination	Simple to perform, reliable, inexpensive, performed with client under local anesthesia on outpatient basis	Risk of injury to adjacent structures; risk of tumor cell implantation along needle tract and recurrence
Diagnostic laparotomy	Determine stage and extent of disease	Provides more accurate diagnostic information for treatment planning	Major surgical procedure with risk for postoperative complications; requires hospital stay, costly, multiple life-style disruptions
Local excision	Primary treatment Cytoreductive surgery Removal of solitary metastasis Palliative treatment	Minimal tissue removal with little effect on functional status and appearance; may not require hospital stay or short hospital stay	Risk of microscopic residual disease left in tissue, resulting in local recurrence
Wide excision	Primary treatment Cytoreductive surgery Prophylactic surgery	Eliminates visible and microscopic disease locally and in adjacent tissue that has increased risk for disease spread	Longer, more involved rehabilitation required; may cause major changes in functional ability and appearance; may require reconstructive procedures

     a. Cytoreductive surgery—reduction of the tumor volume to improve the effect of other cancer treatment modalities.

     b. Prophylactic surgery—removal of nonvital organs that have an extremely high risk of subsequent cancer (Table 19-2).

  3. Salvage treatment—use of an extensive surgical approach to treat local disease recurrence after the use of a less extensive primary approach (Table 19-3).

  4. Palliative treatment—use of procedures to promote client comfort and quality of life without the goal of cure of disease.

     a. Examples—bone stabilization, relief of obstruction, removal of solitary metastasis, therapy for oncologic emergencies, ablative surgery, and management of cancer pain.

     b. Benefit of palliative treatment depends on the biological pace of the cancer, projected life expectancy, and expected primary treatment outcome.

Table 19-1
SURGICAL PROCEDURES *Continued*

Type of Procedure	Uses in Cancer Care	Advantages	Disadvantages
Laser	Primary treatment Cytoreductive surgery Palliation	Can be used in all body systems; decreased blood loss and need for blood products; decreased local recurrence rates; minimal side effects, including minimal pain during and after surgery, decreased wound drainage, earlier return of functional ability, reduced incidence of functional disabilities; minimal preparation time and easy to deliver treatment; decreased procedure time; decreased or eliminated hospital stay; may be repeated on recurrent tumor; may perform immediate graft; may be performed when traditional surgery is contraindicated (e.g., because of location of tumor; client is a poor surgical risk as a result of health status)	None noted
Photodynamic therapy	Primary treatment	More precise in locating cancer cells, particularly when all sites of disease are unknown; decreased risks and variety of side effects as compared to traditional surgery	Photosensitivity for 4-6 weeks, causing possible lifestyle disruptions

5. Combination treatment—use of surgery with other treatment modalities to improve tumor resectability; decrease the extent of tissue removed; limit the change in physical appearance and functional ability; and improve treatment outcomes.
   a. Examples—preoperative chemotherapy, radiation therapy, or immunotherapy; intraoperative chemotherapy or radiation therapy; and postoperative chemotherapy, radiation therapy, or immunotherapy.

Table 19-2
SURGERY THAT CAN PREVENT CANCER

Underlying Condition	Associated Cancer	Prophylactic Surgery
Cryptorchidism	Testicular	Orchiopexy
Polyposis coli	Colon	Colectomy
Familial colon cancer	Colon	Colectomy
Ulcerative colitis	Colon	Colectomy
Multiple endocrine neo-plasia types II and III	Medullary cancer of the thyroid	Thyroidectomy
Familial breast cancer	Breast	Mastectomy
Familial ovarian cancer	Ovary	Oophorectomy

From DeVita, V.T., Jr., Hellman, S., & Rosenberg, S.A. (eds). *Cancer: Principles & Practice of Oncology* (3rd ed). Philadelphia: J.B. Lippincott, Co., p. 241.

    b. Risk of type and severity of side effects experienced increases with each additional treatment modality used.
      (1) Chemotherapy may affect wound healing (methotrexate); renal function (cisplatin); cardiac function (doxorubicin); or pulmonary function (bleomycin).
      (2) Radiation therapy may affect wound healing in the treatment field or function of organs within the treatment field (pulmonary fibrosis).
    c. Current research issues.
      (1) Timing of combination therapies.
      (2) Sequencing of combination therapies.
      (3) Identifying combination therapies most effective in controlling cancer with minimal untoward effects.
  D. Place therapeutic and supportive hardware such as a gastrostomy tube, hyper-alimentation lines, ventricular reservoir, external or implantable vascular access catheters, ports, and pumps, and radioactive implants.
  E. Assess response to treatment by "second-look" procedures.
    1. Procedure performed within a predetermined time frame after initial therapy.
    2. Sites and volume of residual tumor are identified and resected if possible.

Table 19-3
EXAMPLES OF SALVAGE THERAPY

Cancer Site	Primary Conservative Approach	Salvage Approach
Breast	Lumpectomy and radiation therapy	Mastectomy
Bladder	Primary radiation therapy	Radical cystectomy
Early glottic carcinoma	Primary radiation therapy	Hemilaryngectomy
Prostate	Primary radiation therapy	Radical prostatectomy

F. Reconstruct affected body parts.
  1. Repair or reduce anatomical defects from cancer surgery to improve function and/or cosmetic appearance.
  2. Examples—fecal or urinary diversion, breast reconstruction, fistula excision, skin flap development, and prosthesis placement.

III. Types and classifications of surgery (see Table 19-1).
  A. Surgical blades.
    1. Local excision—removal of cancer with a small margin of normal tissue.
    2. Wide excision—removal of cancer, tissue containing primary lymph nodes, contiguous structures involved, and contiguous structures at high risk for tumor spread.
  B. Electrosurgery—use of electrical current for cell destruction.
  C. Cryosurgery—use of liquid nitrogen to freeze tissue to result in cell destruction.
  D. Chemosurgery—use of combined topical chemotherapy and layer-by-layer surgical removal of abnormal tissue.
  E. Laser (*Light Amplification by Stimulated Emission of Radiation*) surgery (see Table 19-1).
    1. Contact tip or "laser scalpel" provides a focused form of energy within a precise location and depth of tissue.
    2. Photodynamic therapy—intravenous injection of a light-sensitizing agent (hematoporphyrin derivative [HPD]) with uptake by cancer cells, followed by exposure to laser light within 24 to 48 hours of injection (see Table 19-1).
      a. Results in fluorescence of cancer cells and cell death.
      b. Used for determining extent of disease and response to treatment.

IV. Safety measures in the delivery of surgery.
  A. Aseptic techniques are used to reduce the risks of infection:
    1. Skin preparation to specific surgical site.
    2. Sterile techniques during procedures.
    3. Wound dressings.
  B. Type of anesthesia is selected based on client preference, previous response to anesthesia, physical and mental history, type and duration of procedure, surgical site, and positioning during the surgical procedure.
  C. Electrical hazards are prevented by proper grounding plate placement within the operating room and by checking electrical cords, plugs, and outlets.
  D. Client is prepared for the surgery:
    1. Delivery of specific operative site or system preparations such as bowel preparations, medications, or nutritional interventions.
    2. Positioning during the surgical procedure to prevent joint damage, muscle stretch or strain, and pressure ulcers.
  E. Informed consent is obtained:
    1. The nature of and reason for surgery is explained.
    2. All available options and risks associated with each option are discussed.
    3. Risks of the surgical procedure and administration of anesthesia are described.
    4. Potential benefits and outcomes of the treatment are explained.

DATA COLLECTION

I. Pertinent personal history.
  A. Factors that may increase the incidence of complications of surgery:
    1. Presence of preexisting cardiovascular, pulmonary, renal, neurological, musculoskeletal, gastrointestinal, or liver disease.

     2. Previous surgical history—type of surgery, experience with anesthetic agents, blood transfusions, and surgical complications.

     3. Life-style activities such as tobacco use, alcohol ingestion, use of illegal medications, or abuse of over-the-counter medications.

     4. Previous cancer therapy and the length of time since therapy completed.

     5. Present medications.

     6. Allergies.

     7. Physiological changes of aging (Table 19-4).

  B. Factors that may assist with discharge planning:

     1. Home environment.

     2. Financial status.

     3. Self-care capabilities.

     4. Anticipated changes in self-care capabilities resulting from surgery.

     5. Support personnel or services available and patterns of use.

     6. Employment status and type of work.

II. Physical examination.

  A. Cardiovascular—heart rate and rhythm, blood pressure, presence and quality of regional pulses, color and temperature of regional extremities.

  B. Pulmonary—respiratory rate, depth, and rhythm; lung expansion; posture.

  C. Renal—color and odor of urine; urinary elimination patterns; previous urinary output.

  D. Gastrointestinal—color, consistency, and caliber of stool; bowel elimination patterns.

  E. Mobility—muscle strength and endurance; range of motion; gait; activity level.

  F. Nutrition—weight; skin turgor; amount, content, and patterns of nutritional intake.

  G. Comfort level.

III. Psychosocial examination.

  A. Explore client/family concerns.

     1. Meaning attached to the loss of body part and/or functioning.

     2. Expectations related to the procedure, such as pain, disability, or survival.

     3. Perceived impact of surgery on life-style and relationships.

  B. Assess client's/family's current level of coping.

     1. Coping strategies used in previous illnesses or times of stress.

     2. Support systems available and patterns of use.

     3. Community resources available and patterns of use.

IV. Critical laboratory and diagnostic data unique to surgery.

  A. Cardiovascular—electrocardiogram (ECG).

  B. Hematological—complete blood count, prothrombin time, and partial thromboplastin time.

  C. Hepatic—liver function studies.

  D. Renal—urinalysis, blood urea nitrogen, creatinine, and electrolytes.

  E. Pulmonary—chest x-ray examination.

  F. Nutritional—serum albumin.

ASSOCIATED NURSING DIAGNOSES

  I. Alteration in comfort.

 II. Impaired skin integrity.

III. Knowledge deficit.

Table 19-4
PHYSIOLOGICAL CHANGES RELATED TO THE AGING PROCESS THAT CAN AFFECT SURGERY

Physiological Changes	Effects	Potential Postoperative Complications
Cardiovascular		
Decreased elasticity of blood vessels	Decreased circulation to vital organs	Shock (hypotension), thrombosis with pulmonary emboli, delayed wound healing, postoperative confusion, hypervolemia, decreased response to stress
Decreased cardiac output	Slower blood flow	
Decreased peripheral circulation		
Respiratory		
Decreased elasticity of lungs and chest wall	Decreased vital capacity	Atelectasis, pneumonia, postoperative confusion
Increased residual lung volume	Decreased alveolar volume	
Decreased forced expiratory volume	Decreased gas exchange	
Decreased ciliary action	Decreased cough reflex	
Fewer alveolar capillaries		
Urinary		
Decreased glomerular filtration rate	Decreased kidney function	Prolonged response to anesthesia and drugs, overhydration with intravenous fluids, hyperkalemia, urinary tract infection, urinary incontinence
Decreased bladder muscle tone	Stasis of urine in bladder	
Weakened perineal muscles	Loss of urinary control	
Musculoskeletal		
Decreased muscle strength	Decreased activity	Atelectasis, pneumonia, thrombophlebitis, constipation, or fecal impaction
Limitation of motion		
Gastrointestinal		
Decreased intestinal motility	Retention of feces	Constipation or fecal impaction
Metabolic		
Decreased gamma globulin level	Decreased inflammatory response	Delayed wound healing, wound dehiscence, or evisceration
Decreased plasma proteins		
Immune System		
Fewer killer T cells	Decreased ability to protect against invasion by pathogenic microorganisms	Wound infection, wound dehiscence, pneumonia, urinary tract infection
Decreased response to foreign antigens		

From Phipps, W.J., Long, B.C., Woods N.F., & Cassmeyer V.L. (eds) (1991). *Medical-Surgical Nursing: Concepts and Clinical Practice* (4th ed). St. Louis: Mosby–Year Book.

IV. Alteration in nutrition.

V. Ineffective airway clearance.

VI. Anxiety.

NURSING PLANNING AND IMPLEMENTATION

I. Interventions to maximize safety for the client/family.
  A. Implement preoperative medical preparation regimen as ordered.
    1. Dietary restrictions.
    2. Bowel preparation.
    3. Skin preparation.
  B. Use aseptic or clean technique, as indicated, for invasive procedures such as insertion of tubes, drains, or intravenous lines.

II. Interventions to decrease incidence and severity of complications unique to surgery.
  A. Ineffective airway clearance:
    1. Teach turning, coughing, and deep breathing (TCDB) techniques to client/family and schedule activities postoperatively.
    2. Demonstrate use of incentive spirometry.
    3. Use suction devices to assist client to remove mucus or sputum.
  B. Impaired skin integrity:
    1. Assist client to turn and shift positions in bed every 2 hours.
    2. Massage uninjured areas gently.
    3. Use mattress overlays such as therapeutic foam mattress, alternating air mattress, or water mattress or specialty beds such as low-airflow, air-fluidized, or kinetic therapy for high-risk clients.
    4. Establish a schedule for changing the surgical dressing.
    5. Use protective film, hydrocolloid barriers, and/or collection devices around drains or tubes with copious drainage.
    6. Encourage early ambulation.
  C. Alteration in comfort:
    1. Teach splinting of incision during TCBD or with movement.
    2. Use nonpharmacological methods for pain control:
      a. Progressive muscle relaxation.
      b. Guided imagery.
      c. Music.
      d. Massage.
      e. Diversional activities.
    3. Administer analgesic and antiemetic medications as ordered by physician.
  D. Anxiety:
    1. Allow client and family to discuss feelings, fears, and concerns.
    2. Provide client and family teaching:
      a. Plan of care and rationale for procedures.
      b. Anticipated care settings, equipment, and experiences related to surgery.
      c. Self-care strategies to prevent or minimize complications of surgery.
    3. Encourage use of coping strategies that have been effective in the past during times of stress.
    4. Allow for adequate rest periods between care activities.

III. Interventions to monitor for unique complications of surgery.
  A. Ineffective airway clearance:
    1. Assess client on a routine basis for changes in respiratory effort, rate, rhythm, and subjective responses to breathing.
    2. Inspect chest wall for symmetrical movement, use of accessory muscles, diaphragmatic breathing, and sternal retraction.

  3. Auscultate lungs for adventitious or absent breath sounds.
  B. Impaired skin integrity:
      1. Assess incision site for redness, swelling, increased drainage, discomfort, and approximation of surgical margins.
      2. Assess bony prominences for areas remaining red 30 minutes or longer after pressure relieved.
  C. Alteration in nutrition:
      1. Assess for return of bowel sounds.
      2. Assess for physical signs of dehydration—color and moisture of mucous membranes; skin turgor.
      3. Assess fluid loss via incisional or fistular wounds, urinary output, and tube or drain drainage.
      4. Assess intake and output ratio.
      5. Weigh client daily.
      6. Evaluate tolerance to progressive diet—appetite, amount and type of foods eaten, and responses to eating.
      7. Monitor laboratory parameters of nutritional status.

IV. Interventions to enhance adaptation and rehabilitation.
  A. Implement postoperative teaching plan that includes changes in self-care activities and activities resulting from surgery, progressive return to maximal activity level, anticipated discharge medications, wound management, proper use of assistive or prosthetic devices, community resources available for home care, plans for follow-up care, contact should questions arise, and changes in condition to report to the health care team.
  B. Involve client and family in assessment, planning, and evaluation of care through transition periods.
  C. Instruct client/family about rehabilitation programs available such as physical and occupational therapy, speech therapy, ostomy outpatient clinics, and prosthetic fitting services.
  D. Refer client/family to support programs available such as Reach to Recovery, Re-Con Group, Voicemasters, Make Today Count, International Association of Laryngectomees, and United Ostomy Association chapters.
  E. Refer client/family to professional counselors as indicated.

EVALUATION OF CLIENT AND FAMILY OUTCOMES

  I. Describe the type of and rationale for surgery.

  II. List potential immediate and long-term complications of the surgery.

  III. Describe self-care measures to decrease the incidence and severity of complications of surgery.

  IV. Demonstrate new self-care skills demanded by structural or functional effects of surgery.

  V. Describe schedule and procedures for routine follow-up care.

  VI. List changes in condition that should be reported to the health care team.
  A. Signs and symptoms of infection.
  B. Persistent nausea, vomiting, or a decrease in appetite.
  C. Poor wound healing.
  D. Changes in bowel or bladder patterns.
  E. Changes in location or increased severity of pain or intolerance to discomfort.
  F. Inability to resume functional ability within anticipated time frame.

  VII. Identify potential community resources to meet unique demands of therapy and rehabilitation.

BIBLIOGRAPHY

Arbeit, J. (1990). Molecules, cancer, and the surgeon. *Ann Surg 212*(1), 3-13.

Aronoff, B. (1986). The state of the art in general surgery and surgical oncology. *Laser Surg Med 6*(4), 376-382.

Baird, R.M. & Rebbeck, P.A. (1986). Impact of preoperative chemotherapy for the surgeon. *Recent Results Cancer Res 103*, 79-84.

Balch, C. (1990). The surgeon's expanded role in cancer care. *Cancer 65*(3,suppl), 604-609.

Brown, J. (1989). Peripherally inserted central catheters—use in home care. *J Intravenous Nurs 12*(3), 144-150.

Cole, W.H. & Humphrey L. (1985). Need for immunologic stimulators during immunosuppression produced by major cancer surgery. *Ann Surg 202*(1), 9-20.

Daly, J.M. & DeCosse, J.J. (1984). Horizons in surgical oncology. *Adv Surg 18*, 117-143.

DeVita, V.T., Jr., Hellman, S., & Rosenberg, S.A. (eds) (1989). *Cancer: Principles & Practice of Oncology* (3rd ed). Philadelphia: J.B. Lippincott Co.

Dixon, J. (1988). Current laser applications in general surgery. *Ann Surg 207*(4), 355-372.

Elias, G. (1989). *Handbook of Surgical Oncology*. Boca Raton, Florida: CRC Press, Inc.

Forbes, J. (1988). Principles and potential of palliative surgery in patients with advanced cancer. *Recent Results Cancer Res 108*, 134-142.

Groenwald, S.L., Frogge, M.H., Goodman, M., Yarbro, C.H. (eds) (1990). *Cancer Nursing: Principles and Practice* (2nd ed). Boston: Jones & Bartlett Publishers.

Haibeck, S. (1988). Intraoperative radiation therapy. *Oncol Nurs Forum 15*(2), 143-147.

Harvard, C.P. & Topping, A.E. (1991). Surgical oncology. In S.B. Baird, R. McCorkle, & M. Grant (eds). *Cancer Nursing: A Comprehensive Textbook*. Philadelphia: W.B. Saunders Co., pp. 235-245.

Herfarth, C. (ed). (1987). Progress symposium—advances in surgical oncology. *World J Surg 11*(4), 405-540.

Hoff, S. (1987). Concepts in intraperitoneal chemotherapy. *Semin Oncol Nurs 3*(2), 112-117.

Jako, G. (1987). The road toward 21st century surgery: new strategies and initiatives in cancer treatment. *Lasers Surg Med 7*(3), 217-218.

Lehr, P. (1989). Surgical lasers: how they work, current applications. *AORN J 50*(5), 972-977.

Minton, J. (1986). The laser in surgery: A 23 year perspective. *Ann J Surg 151*(6), 725-729.

Rosenberg, S. (1987). *Surgical Treatment of Metastatic Cancer*. Philadelphia: J.B. Lippincott Co.

Schirrmacher, V. (1985). Cancer metastasis: experimental approaches, theoretical concepts, and impacts for treatment strategies. *Adv Canc Res 43*, 1-73.

Shamberger, R. (1985). Effect of chemotherapy and radiotherapy on wound healing: experimental studies. *Recent Results Cancer Res 98*, 17-34.

Tootla, J. & Easterling, A. (1989). PDT: destroying malignant cells with laser beams . . . photodynamic therapy. *Nurs 19*(11), 48-9.

Viall, C. (1990). Your complete guide to central venous catheters. *Nurs 20*(2), 34-42.

Wickman, R. (1990). Advances in venous access devices and nursing management strategies. *Nurs Clin North Am 25*(2), 345-364.

Wong, R.J. & DeCosse, J.J. (1990). Cytoreductive surgery. *Surg Gynecol Obstet*. Mar: 170 (3), 276-281.

20

Implications of Radiation Therapy for Nursing

Jennifer Dunn Bucholtz, MS, RN

THEORY

I. Principles of radiation therapy.
  A. Radiation therapy is the use of high-energy particles or waves to treat disease.
  B. Effects of radiation on cellular structure and function.
    1. Molecules within the cell become agitated and excited.
    2. Agitated molecules break into stable molecules and chemically active substances.
    3. Chemical reactions take place inside the cell, resulting in changes to deoxyribonucleic acid (DNA) in the nucleus.
    4. Changes in DNA are expressed as a single or double chromosomal-strand break.
      a. Degree of DNA damage or cell radiosensitivity depends on:
        (1) Rate of cell division—rapidly dividing cells are more radiosensitive.
        (2) Phase of cell cycle—cells in mitosis and between G_1 and G_2 are more radiosensitive.
        (3) Oxygenation level of cell—well-oxygenated cells are more radiosensitive.
        (4) Degree of cell differentiation—poorly differentiated cells are more radiosensitive.
      b. Relationship of radiosensitivity to treatment planning.
        (1) Cancers with rapidly dividing, well-oxygenated, and poorly differentiated cells are the most radiosensitive (Table 20-1).
        (2) Normal cells and tissues can tolerate only a specified dose of radiation before complications result (Table 20-2).
        (3) Treatment is planned to deliver a tumoricidal dose of radiation within the limits imposed by the radiation tolerance of surrounding normal tissues.
      c. Cell death caused by DNA damage may occur:
        (1) Immediately—DNA altered and cannot be repaired.
        (2) During cell division—DNA damaged, but cell continues to function until cell division.

319

Table 20-1
RELATIVE RADIOSENSITIVITY OF VARIOUS TUMORS AND TISSUES

Tumors / Tissues	Relative Radiosensitivity
Lymphoma	High
Leukemia	
Seminoma	
Dysgerminoma	
Squamous cell cancer of the oropharyngeal, glottic, bladder, skin, and cervical epithelia; adenocarcinomas of the alimentary tract	Fairly high
Vascular and connective tissue elements of all tumors; secondary neurovascularization, astrocytomas	Medium
Salivary gland tumors, hepatoma, renal cancer, pancreatic cancer, chondrosarcoma, osteogenic sarcoma	Fairly low
Rhabdomyosarcoma, leiomyosarcoma, and ganglioneurofibrosarcoma	Low

From Rubin, P. (ed) (1983). Principles of radiation oncology and cancer radiotherapy. In *Clinical Oncology for Medical Students and Physicians*. New York: American Cancer Society.

   (3) With cell degeneration—cells become sterile, cannot divide, and die a natural death.
C. Normal cell and tissue response versus neoplastic cell and tissue response.
   1. Radiation damages both normal cells and neoplastic cells.
   2. Single chromosomal-strand breaks in DNA of normal cells are repaired more easily than those in DNA of neoplastic cells.
   3. Sequelae of radiation therapy result from radiation damage to normal cells within the treatment field.

II. Role of radiation therapy in cancer care.
A. Cure—eradication of disease with the expectation that the individual will live a normal life span.
   1. Examples of cancers often cured with radiation therapy—Hodgkin's disease, early-stage breast cancer, seminoma of the testes, cervical cancer, skin cancer, laryngeal cancer, Wilms' tumor (combined with chemotherapy), thyroid cancer, early-stage medulloblastoma and rhabdomyosarcoma.
   2. With cure of disease, systematic follow-up and evaluation for long-term complications of radiation therapy are required.
B. Control—limitation of the growth and spread of disease with the expectation that the individual will live for a period of time symptom free.
   1. Examples of cancers often controlled with radiation therapy—cancer of the bladder, late-stage breast cancer, large head and neck cancers, brain tumors, ovarian cancer, lung cancer.
   2. Radiation therapy may be used prophylactically to control disease that may be microscopic but not detectable (cranial irradiation for lung cancer).
C. Palliation—relief or reduction of distressing symptoms or impending complications with no expectation of extension of life span.
   1. Examples of problems often palliated with radiation therapy—pain from bony metastasis; obstructive processes of the superior vena cava, gastrointestinal tract, ureters, and trachea; spinal cord compression; brain metastases; bleeding.

Table 20-2
MAXIMAL TOLERANCE DOSE OF ORGANS BY RADIATION*

Organ	Injury	Dose (rads)	Amount of Organ Treated (or Field Size)
Bone marrow	Aplasia	450	Whole
	Pancytopenia	4000	Segment
Liver	Acute hepatitis	4000	Whole
	Chronic hepatitis	2000	Whole (strip)
Stomach	Perforation, ulcer, hemorrhage	5500	100 cm
Intestine	Ulcer, perforation, hemorrhage	5500	400 cm
		6500	100 cm
Brain	Infarction, necrosis	6000	Whole
Spinal cord	Infarction, necrosis	5500	10 cm
Heart	Pericarditis	5500	60%
	Pancarditis	8000	25%
Lung	Acute pneumonitis	3500	100 cm
	Chronic pneumonitis	2500	Whole
Kidney	Acute nephrosclerosis	2000	Whole (strip)
	Chronic nephrosclerosis	2500	Whole
Fetus	Death	400	Whole

*Maximal tolerance dose is defined as the dose to which a given population of clients is exposed under a standard set of treatment conditions resulting in a 50% severe complication rate within 5 years of treatment.
From Rubin, P. (ed) (1983). Principles of radiation oncology and cancer radiotherapy. In *Clinical Oncology for Medical Students and Physicians*. New York: American Cancer Society.

III. Types of radiation therapy.
  A. Classified according to the form of radiation used and the method of delivery.
    1. Form of radiation.
       a. Electromagnetic—radiation in the form of waves.
          (1) X-rays delivered by linear accelerators, kilovoltage machines, and betatrons.
          (2) Gamma rays delivered by machines that house radioactive sources.
       b. Particulate—radiation in the form of particles; examples of particle radiation include:
          (1) Alpha particles—positively charged particles with poor penetrating ability.
          (2) Beta particles—high-speed electrons with greater penetrating ability than alpha particles.
          (3) Electrons—particles similar to beta particles that are produced by machines and are used to treat superficial malignancies.
          (4) Neutrons—uncharged, heavy particles produced by a cyclotron used in experimental treatments.
          (5) Pions—small, negatively charged particles used in experimental treatments.
    2. Method of delivery.
       a. External beam (teletherapy)—therapy in which the source of ionizing radiation is outside the body.

(1) Machines deliver electron energy in precise beams with little radiation scatter (linear accelerator) or deliver gamma rays from radioactive cobalt or cesium sources.

(2) Process of treatment planning.

    (a) Consultation with physician, radiation oncologist, and radiation therapy nurse.

    (b) Simulation to tailor the treatment plan to the volume and location of tumor.

        i. Tumor is localized with fluoroscope and pretreatment x-ray examinations.

        ii. Immobilization devices are created as needed.

        iii. Temporary or permanent marks are placed on skin to outline treatment field.

        iv. Diagnostic studies may be done to locate vital structures within the treatment field.

    (c) Construction of blocks to shield vital structures or radiosensitive tissues from total dose of radiation.

    (d) Generation of computerized treatment plans based on tumor volume and the body contour of the client.

    (e) Calculation of total dose of radiation to give over time; fractionated dose, number of fields, and time schedule are based on:

        i. Relationship of radiosensitivity of tumor cells and normal cells and tissues.

        ii. Tumor volume and location.

        iii. Relationship of total dose and time of treatment.

        iv. Goal of treatment.

b. Internal radiation (brachytherapy)—therapy in which the radioactive source is placed into a body cavity or directly on the body.

(1) Method for delivery of high, concentrated dose of radiation to a specific part of the body and for minimizing the radiation dose to normal tissues.

(2) Cure or control is goal of care.

(3) Types of internal radiation.

    (a) Mechanically positioned—radioactive source is positioned in a specific body site.

        i. Types of sealed radioactive sources—seeds, threads, needles, and ribbons.

        ii. Position of sources may be intracavitary (cesium implant in vagina), interstitial (iridium implants in breast), or on the surface (strontium to a superficial tumor of the eye).

        iii. Implanted sources may be temporary (cesium implant for cancer of cervix) or permanent (iodine seeds into a bronchial tumor).

    (b) Metabolized or absorbed—nonsealed sources of radiation are administered orally, intravenously, or within a body cavity (Table 20-3).

B. Selection of type and method used depends on client and disease factors.

IV. Potential side effects of radiation therapy.

  A. Side effects occur when normal cells within the radiation treatment field are temporarily or permanently damaged.

  B. Types of side effects.

    1. Acute side effects occur during or within 6 months after the radiation treatment:

Table 20-3
TYPES OF METABOLIZED OR ABSORBED RADIATION

Route of Administration	Examples of Nonsealed Sources	Diseases Treated
Oral	Iodine 131	Hyperthyroidism
Intravenous	Phosphorus 32	Metastatic bone lesions
Intrapleural	Phosphorus 32	Mesothelioma
Intraperitoneal	Phosphorus	Intraperitoneal metastases from ovarian cancer

      a. Occur in cells that divide rapidly such as those cells of the skin, mucous membranes, hair follicles, and bone marrow.
      b. Damage is usually repairable.
   2. Chronic side effects occur from 6 months to years after the radiation treatment:
      a. Occur in cells that divide slowly such as those cells in muscle or vessels.
      b. Damage is usually permanent.
  C. Factors that influence the occurrence and severity of side effects.
   1. Treatment field.
      a. Only cells and tissues within the radiation field are at risk for damage.
      b. The larger the treatment field, the greater is the risk of side effects.
   2. Dose—as the fractionated and total doses increase, the incidence of acute and chronic side effects increases (Table 20-4).
   3. Method of delivery—the less penetrating the radiation, the greater is the risk for skin reactions.
   4. Individual factors.

V. Safety measures in delivery of radiation therapy.
  A. Purpose of safety measures is to protect personnel against low-level radiation believed to result in undesirable effects:
   1. Somatic effects—actual alterations in cells and tissues.
      a. Development of solid tumor—example includes increased incidence of breast cancer among women in Nova Scotia who received chest fluoroscopy frequently for follow-up of tuberculosis.
      b. Development of hematological malignancies—example includes increased incidence of leukemia among survivors of the atomic bomb in Japan.
   2. Genetic effects—potential damage to future generations of individuals exposed to radiation.
      a. Development of genetic mutations in offspring of animals (fruit flies and mice) exposed to radiation.
      b. Development of genetic mutations in offspring of survivors of the atomic bomb in Japan.
      c. Most human studies on genetic effects of radiation are based on high-dose radiation exposure; data about risks of low-dose exposure are not conclusive.
  B. Factors that determine the type and amount of radiation safety measures:
   1. Type of radiation—alpha, beta, and gamma radiation differ in penetrating ability and therefore the type of material needed to shield from exposure (Figure 20-1).

Table 20-4
COMPLICATIONS OF RADIATION THERAPY

Organ	Response	Dose (rads)	Time to Onset	Nursing Considerations
Skin	Erythema	3000-4000	2-3 wk	Assess skin at regular intervals during treatment.
	Moist desquamation	4500-6000	5-6 wk or within 6 wk from end of therapy	Instruct client to wash skin with only water. Decrease exposure to irritating substances—fabrics, sun, soap, and trauma.
	Telangiectasis	4500-6000	Months to years	
Hair	Loss within treatment area	300-400	Few weeks	Instruct client to avoid excessive shampooing, hair dryers, hot rollers. or curling irons. Encourage planning for hair loss by purchasing wig, scarf, turban, or hat before loss.
Teeth	Caries	4000	Months to years	Encourage pretreatment dental evaluation. Instruct on prophylactic oral care measures.
Mouth/tongue	Mucositis	3000	2-3 wk	Encourage to avoid alcohol, tobacco, and other irritating agents.
	Xerostomia	3000-4000	2-3 wk	
	Taste changes	3000-4000	2-3 wk	
Larynx	Edema	5000-6000	Late in treatment	Monitor for changes in quality of voice.
	Necrosis of cartilage	6500+	Months or years	Assess difficulty in breathing or talking.
Thyroid	Hypothyroidism	3500-4000	Years	Monitor for signs and symptoms of hypothyroidism.
Lung	Pneumonitis	2500-3000	6-8 wk after treatment	Evaluate pulmonary function before treatment. Monitor respiratory rate, rhythm, and effort.
	Fibrosis	4000	Months to years	Monitor for signs and symptoms of infection.
Gastrointestinal (GI) tract	Nausea Vomiting	125+	1-2 hr after treatment	Instruct in use of antiemetic agents during treatment.
Small intestines	Cramping	2000-3000	2-3 wk	Begin client on low-residue diet.
	Diarrhea	2000-3000	2-3 wk	Avoid ingestion of food or beverages that increase GI motility.
	Malabsorption	3000-4000	Months to years	Maintain adequate fluid intake.
	Necrosis	6000-7000	Months to years	Monitor stool for signs and symptoms of bleeding.
	Ulceration	6000-7000	Months to years	Evaluate changes in bowel patterns.
	Strictures	6000-7000	Months to years	
Urinary bladder	Cystitis	3000	Few weeks	Monitor for signs and symptoms of bladder irritation or bleeding.

Table 20-4
COMPLICATIONS OF RADIATION THERAPY *Continued*

Organ	Response	Dose (rads)	Time to Onset	Nursing Considerations
	Fibrosis	6500-7000	Months to years	Evaluate changes in bladder patterns. Assess character of urine.
Ovary	Sterility	500-1000	Days to weeks	Assess ovarian function before initiation of therapy. Evaluate impact of sterility on client/partner.
Uterus	Necrosis	20000+	Months to years	Monitor for signs of infection or necrosis—discharge, odor, bleeding, or pain.
Brain/spinal cord	Neurological deficits Necrosis	5000, whole brain 6500-7000, smaller areas	Months to 1 yr	Assess neurological and sensory function. Evaluate changes over time.
Bone (child)	Arrested growth	2000-3000	Depends on area	Evaluate growth pattern before initiation of therapy. Instruct parents about potential risks of arrested growth. Monitor growth and development patterns after therapy.

2. Half-life of isotope—amount of time needed to reduce the radioisotope to half of the original radioactivity (Table 20-5).
3. Dose of radioisotope—the higher the dose, the more radiation protection needed.
4. Method of isotope delivery.
    a. When radioisotopes are positioned mechanically, implant is radioactive; the individual is not.
    b. When radioisotopes are given orally or systemically, the individual and body secretions may be radioactive.
C. Principles of radiation protection based on time, distance, and shielding:
    1. Minimize time in contact with the radioactive source or individual.
    2. Maximize distance from the radioactive source or individual.

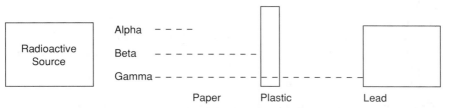

Figure 20-1 Range and penetration of alpha, beta and gamma radiation. (*Redrawn from Yasko, J. [1982]. Care of the Client Receiving External Radiation Therapy. Reston, Va: Reston Publishing Co.*)

Table 20-5
HALF-LIFE OF COMMONLY USED RADIOISOTOPES

Radioisotope	Half-Life
Cesium 137	30.00 yr
Cobalt 60	5.26 yr
Gold 198	2.70 days
Iodine 125	60.20 days
Iodine 131	8.05 days
Iridium 192	74.20 days
Radium 226	1602.0 yr
Yttrium 90	64.00 hr
Phosphorus 32	14.28 days

3. Use required shielding based on source and penetration to decrease exposure.
4. Monitor radiation exposure by use of a film badge or other monitoring device.
5. For a client with a mechanically positioned radiation source:
   a. Avoid caring for client if you are attempting to conceive or are pregnant.
   b. Never touch a dislodged sealed source of radiation.
   c. Limit time spent with client each day.
6. For a client receiving metabolized or absorbed radiation:
   a. Avoid caring for client if you are attempting to conceive or are pregnant.
   b. Limit time spent with client each day.
   c. Wear waterproof gloves when handling body secretions.
   d. Provide disposable eating trays and utensils.
   e. Keep all linens and trash in room and scan them before removal.
   f. Scan client before discharge.

DATA COLLECTION

I. Pertinent personal history.
   A. Age.
   B. History of previous cancer therapy.
   C. History of concurrent disease involving organs and tissues within the treatment field.

II. Physical examination—condition of tissues and organs within the proposed treatment field.

III. Psychosocial examination.
   A. Perceptions of client and family about radiation treatment.
   B. Ability of client to meet transportation, hospitalization, and financial demands of radiation treatment and follow-up.
   C. Expression of fear or anxiety.

IV. Critical laboratory and diagnostic data unique to radiation therapy.
   A. Hemoglobin and hematocrit levels.
   B. Additional data based on tissues and organs within the proposed treatment field.

ASSOCIATED NURSING DIAGNOSES

I. Potential impaired skin integrity.

II. Knowledge deficit related to radiation therapy.

III. Additional diagnoses are related to the location of the treatment field (see Table 20-4).

NURSING PLANNING AND IMPLEMENTATION

I. Interventions to maximize safety for the client and family. If client is receiving metabolized or absorbed radiation or mechanically positioned radiation.
  A. Label medical record and client room with radioactivity precautions.
  B. Restrict visits of pregnant women and children under 10 years of age.
  C. Limit the amount of time visitors spend in the room each day.
  D. Instruct visitors in principles of time, distance, and shielding.
  E. Monitor positioning of mechanically placed devices.
  F. Assign client to private room.

II. Interventions to decrease the incidence and severity of complications unique to radiation therapy.
  A. Note incidence and severity of complications, which depend on the location of tumor, size of the treatment field, therapeutic dose, and radiosensitivity of surrounding cells or tissues.
  B. Perform nursing assessments related to site-specific areas (Table 20-4).
  C. Refer to Chapter 7 for nursing management of specific side effects.

EVALUATION OF CLIENT AND FAMILY OUTCOMES

I. Discuss the rationale and demands of radiation therapy.

II. Participate in self-care strategies to decrease the risks and severity of predictable side effects of radiation therapy.

III. Describe recommended changes in self-care and life-style to minimize effects of radiation therapy on health.

IV. Discuss strategies to maintain valued roles and relationships during and after radiation therapy.

V. List community resources available for assistance and support.

VI. Describe the rationale and schedule for continued follow-up after radiation therapy.

VII. Identify signs and symptoms of short-term and long-term complications of radiation therapy to report to the health care team.

BIBLIOGRAPHY

Brandt, B. & Havey, J. (1989). An overview of interstitial brachytherapy and hyperthermia. *Oncol Nurs Forum 16*(6), 833-841.

Bucholtz, J. (1987). Radiation therapy. In C. Ziegfeld (ed). *Core Curriculum for Oncology Nursing*. Philadelphia: W.B. Saunders Co., pp. 207-224.

Bucholtz, J. (1987). Radiolabelled antibody therapy. *Semin Oncol Nurs 3*(1), 67-73.

Glicksman, A. (1987). Radiobiologic basis of brachytherapy. *Semin Oncol Nurs 3*(1), 15-22.

Griffiths, M.J., Murray, K.H., & Russo, P.C. (1984). Radiotherapy as a treatment modality. In M.J. Griffiths, K.H. Murray, & P.C. Russo. *Oncology Nursing: Pathophysiology, Assessment, and Intervention*. New York: Macmillan Publishing Co., pp. 137-149.

Hilderley, L. (1990). Radiotherapy. In S.L. Groenwald, M.H. Frogge, M. Goodman, & C.H. Yarbro (eds). *Cancer Nursing: Principles and Practice* (2nd ed). Boston: Jones & Bartlett Publishers, pp. 199-229.

Hilderley, L.J. & Dow, K.H. (1991). Radiation oncology. In S.B. Baird, R. McCorkle, & M. Grant (eds). *Cancer Nursing: A Comprehensive Textbook.* Philadelphia: W.B. Saunders Co., pp. 246-265.

Strohl, R. (1988). The nursing role in radiation oncology: Symptom management of acute and chronic reactions. *Oncol Nurs Forum 15*(4), 429-434.

Yasko, J.M. (1982). *Care of the Client Receiving External Radiation Therapy.* Reston, Va: Reston Publishing Co.

21

Implications of Antineoplastic Therapy for Nursing

Catherine Bender, MN, RN

THEORY

I. Principles of cancer chemotherapy.
  A. Cancer chemotherapy is the treatment of choice for malignancies of the hematopoietic system and for solid tumors that have metastasized regionally or distally.
  B. The application of antineoplastic agents to the treatment of cancer is based on concepts of cellular kinetics, which include the cell life cycle, cell cycle time, growth fraction, and tumor burden.
    1. Cell life cycle—a five-stage process of reproduction that occurs in both normal and malignant cells (Figure 21-1).
      a. Gap 0 (G_0) or resting phase.
        (1) Cells are not dividing and are temporarily out of the cell cycle.
        (2) Length of time in G_0 phase is highly variable.
      b. Gap 1 (G_1) or interphase.
        (1) As cells are activated, they enter the cell cycle at the G_1 phase.
        (2) Enzymes necessary for deoxyribonucleic acid (DNA) synthesis are produced.
        (3) Protein and ribonucleic acid (RNA) synthesis also occur.
        (4) Length of time in G_1 is approximately 18 hours.
      c. Synthesis (S).
        (1) Cellular DNA is duplicated in preparation for cell division.
        (2) Length of time in the S phase is approximately 20 hours.
      d. Gap 2 (G_2) or premitotic phase.
        (1) Protein and RNA synthesis occur.
        (2) Precursors of the mitotic spindle apparatus are produced.
        (3) Length of time in G_2 is short.
      e. M (mitosis).
        (1) Cellular division occurs in four phases—prophase, metaphase, anaphase, and telophase.
          (a) Prophase—nuclear membrane breaks down and chromosomes clump.
          (b) Metaphase—chromosomes align in the middle of the cell.

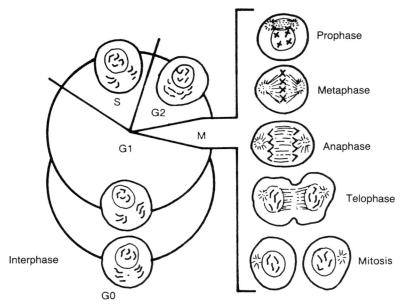

Figure 21-1 Cell life cycle. (*Redrawn from Marino, L. (1981). Cancer Nursing. St. Louis, C.V Mosby Co.*)

          (c) Anaphase—chromosomes segregate to centriole.
          (d) Telophase—cellular division occurs with the production of two daughter cells.
      (2) Length of time in M phase is approximately 1 hour.
  2. Cell cycle time—the amount of time required for a cell to move from one mitosis to another mitosis.
    a. The length of the total cell cycle varies with the specific type of cell; however, the length of the G_0 phase is the major determinant of the cell cycle time.
    b. A shorter cell cycle time results in a higher cell kill with exposure to cell cycle–specific agents.
    c. Continuous infusion of cell cycle–specific agents results in exposure of a greater number of cells and in a higher cell kill in tumors with short cell-cycle times.
  3. Growth fraction of tumor—the percentage of cells actively dividing at a given point of time.
    a. A higher growth fraction results in a higher cell kill with exposure to cycle- or phase-specific agents.
    b. Tumors with a greater fraction of cells in G_0 will be more sensitive to cell cycle–nonspecific agents.
  4. Tumor burden—the number of cells present in the tumor.
    a. Cancers with a small tumor burden are usually more responsive to antineoplastic therapy.
    b. As the tumor burden increases, the growth rate slows, and the number of cells actively dividing decreases.
    c. The higher the tumor cell burden, the higher is the probability of drug-resistant sublines.
  C. Two or more antineoplastic agents often are combined to effect a better response than can be achieved by one agent alone.

1. Combining agents with actions in different phases of the cell cycle increases the number of cells exposed to cytotoxic effects during a given treatment cycle.
2. Combining agents, one of which serves to reverse the toxic effects of the other agent, decreases the incidence and severity of side effects of therapy.
3. Criteria for selection of antineoplastic agents for combination therapy:
   a. Demonstrate cytotoxic activity when used alone to treat a specific cancer.
   b. Possess different dose-limiting toxicities.
   c. Exhibit toxicities that occur at different points of time from the treatment.
   d. Exhibit biological effects that result in enhanced cytotoxicity.
D. Factors influencing the success of treatment with antineoplastic agents.
   1. Characteristics of the tumor—location, size, growth rate, presence of resistant cells, and ratio of sensitivity of malignant cells and normal target cells.
   2. Physical status of the client.
   3. Psychosocial status of the client.

II. Roles of chemotherapy in cancer care.
   A. Cure.
      1. Single treatment modality—acute lymphocytic leukemia in children, Hodgkin's disease, lymphosarcoma, Burkitt's lymphoma, testicular carcinoma, and Ewing's sarcoma.
      2. Combined treatment modality.
   B. Control.
      1. Goal is to extend the length and quality of life when the hope of cure is not realistic.
      2. Breast cancer, chronic lymphocytic leukemia, chronic and acute myelogenous leukemia, small cell carcinoma of the lung, prostatic cancer, multiple myeloma, gastric carcinoma, endometrial carcinoma, and soft-tissue sarcomas.
   C. Palliation.
      1. Goal is to improve comfort when neither cure nor control are possible.
      2. Relief of pressure on nerves, lymphatics, and vasculature and reduction of organ obstruction.

III. Types/classifications of chemotherapy—antineoplastic agents are classified according to phase of action during the cell cycle, mechanism of action, biochemical structure, or physiological action.
   A. Phase of action during the cell cycle.
      1. Phase cycle–specific agents.
         a. Major cytotoxic effects are exerted on cells in a particular phase of the cell cycle.
         b. Only cells in the specific phase of action for the agent will be affected.
         c. Greater cytotoxic effect can be achieved if these agents are administered in divided doses or continuous infusion.
         d. Agents are most effective against tumors in which a large number of cells are dividing.
      2. Cell cycle–specific agents.
         a. Major cytotoxic effects are exerted on cells actively dividing throughout the cell cycle.
         b. Agents are not active against cells in the resting phase (G_0).
         c. Agents are most effective if administered in divided doses or continuous infusion.
         d. Cytotoxic effects occur during the cell cycle and are expressed when cell repair or division is attempted.

3. Cell cycle–nonspecific agents.
   a. Major cytotoxic effects are exerted on cells at any phase, including G_0, in the cell cycle.
   b. Agents are most effective if administered by bolus doses since the number of cells affected is proportional to the amount of drug given.
   c. Cytotoxic effects occur during the cell cycle and are expressed when cell division is attempted.
B. Biochemical structure, mechanism of action, or physiological action (Table 21-1).
   1. Alkylating agents.
      a. Mechanisms of action—interfere with DNA replication through cross-linking of DNA strands, DNA strand breaking, and abnormal base pairing of proteins.
      b. Most agents are cell cycle nonspecific.

Table 21-1
CLASSIFICATIONS OF ANTINEOPLASTIC AGENTS

Antimetabolites	Alkylating Agents	Antitumor Antibiotics	Nitrosoureas
Methotrexate	Mechlorethamine	Doxorubicin	Carmustine
Cytosine arabinoside	Cyclophosphamide	Bleomycin	Lomustine
5-fluorouracil	Chlorambucil	Mitomycin	Semustine
6-mercaptopurine	Melphalan	Daunorubicin	Streptozotocin
6-thioguanine	Triethylenethiophosphoramide	Dactinomycin (Actinomycin D)	Chlorozotozin
Floxuridine	Thiophosphoramide		
Vidarabine	Busulfan		
Hexamethylmelamine	Dacarbazine		
5-azacytidine	Cisplatin		
	Carboplatin		

Hormones	Vinca Alkaloids	Miscellaneous Agents
Testosterone	Vinblastine	Hydroxyurea
Fluoxymesterone (Halotestin)	Vincristine	Procarbazine
	Vindesine	Aminoglutethimide
Diethylstilbestrol	Teniposide (VM-26)	Amascarine
Medroxyprogesterone acetate (Provera)	Etoposide (VP-16)	
Hydroxyprogesterone caproate (Delalutin)		
Megestrol acetate (Megace)		
Tamoxifen citrate (Nolvadex)		

Table 21-2
POTENTIAL SIDE EFFECTS OF CANCER CHEMOTHERAPY

System	Side Effects	System	Side Effects
Hematopoietic	Anemia Leukopenia Thrombocytopenia	Genitourinary	Cystitis Renal toxicity
Gastrointestinal	Anorexia Nausea Vomiting Stomatitis Constipation Diarrhea Ulceration Hepatic toxicity	Cardiovascular	Cardiac toxicity Venous fibrosis Phlebitis Extravasation
		Neurological	Neurotoxicity Ototoxicity
		Pulmonary	Fibrosis
Integumentary	Dermatitis Alopecia	Reproductive	Infertility Changes in libido Erectile dysfunction

Additional Effects

Latent effects	Learning disabilities Changes in memory Second malignancies	Metabolic alterations	Hypocalcemia Hypercalcemia Hypoglycemia Hyperglycemia Hyperuricemia Hypokalemia Hyperkalemia
Mood alterations	Anxiety Depression		

    c. Major toxicities occur in the hematopoietic, gastrointestinal, and reproductive systems (Table 21-2).
  2. Nitrosoureas.
    a. Mechanisms of action—interfere with DNA replication and repair.
    b. Nitrosoureas are noncross-resistant to alkylating agents.
    c. Most agents are cell cycle nonspecific.
    d. Most agents cross the blood-brain barrier.
    e. Major toxicities occur in the hematopoietic and gastrointestinal systems.
  3. Antimetabolites.
    a. Mechanisms of action—inhibit protein synthesis, substitute erroneous metabolites or structural analogues during DNA synthesis, and inhibit DNA synthesis.
    b. Most agents are phase cycle specific (S).
    c. Major toxicities occur in the hematopoietic and gastrointestinal systems.
  4. Antitumor antibiotics.
    a. Mechanisms of action—interfere with nucleic acid synthesis and function, inhibit RNA synthesis, and inhibit DNA synthesis.
    b. Most agents are cell cycle nonspecific.
    c. Major toxicities occur in the hematopoietic, gastrointestinal, reproductive, and cardiac systems (cumulative doses) (Table 21-2).

Table 21-3
ROUTES OF ADMINISTRATION OF ANTINEOPLASTIC AGENTS

Route	Advantages	Disadvantages	Potential Complications	Nursing Implications
Oral	Ease of administration	Inconsistency of absorption	Drug-specific complications	Evaluate compliance with medication schedule.
Subcutaneous/ intramuscular	Ease of administration Decreased side effects	Adequate muscle mass and tissue required for absorption	Infection Bleeding	Evaluate platelet count (>50,000). Use smallest gauge needle possible. Prepare injection site with an antiseptic solution. Assess injection site for signs and symptoms of infection.
Intravenous	Consistent absorption Required for vesicants	Sclerosing of veins over time	Infection Phlebitis	Check for blood return before and after administration of drugs.
Intra-arterial	Increased doses to tumor with decreased systemic toxic effects	Requires surgical procedure for equipment placement	Bleeding Embolism	
Intrathecal/ intraventricular	More consistent drug levels in cerebrospinal fluid	Requires lumbar puncture or surgical placement of reservoir or implanted pump for drug delivery	Headaches Confusion Lethargy Nausea and vomiting Seizures	Observe site for signs of infection. Monitor reservoir or pump functioning.

5. *Vinca* alkaloids.
   a. Mechanisms of action—bind with microtubular proteins that crystallize the mitotic spindle, resulting in metaphase arrest, and inhibit RNA and protein synthesis.
   b. Most agents are phase specific.
   c. Major toxicities occur in the hematopoietic, integumentary, neurological, and reproductive systems (Table 21-2).
6. Hormonal agents.
   a. Androgens—alter pituitary function and directly affect the malignant cell.
   b. Corticosteroids—lyse lymphoid malignancies and have indirect effects on malignant cells.
   c. Estrogens—suppress testosterone production in males and alter the response of breast cancers to prolactin.
   d. Progestins—promote differentiation of malignant cells.
   e. Estrogen antagonists—compete with estrogens for binding with estrogen receptor sites on malignant cells.

Table 21-3
ROUTES OF ADMINISTRATION OF ANTINEOPLASTIC AGENTS *Continued*

Route	Advantages	Disadvantages	Potential Complications	Nursing Implications
Intraperitoneal	Direct exposure of intra-abdominal metastases to drug	Requires placement of Tenckhoff catheter or intraperitoneal port	Abdominal pain Abdominal distention Bleeding Ileus Intestinal perforation Infection	Warm chemotherapy solution to body temperature. Check patency of catheter or port. Instill solution according to protocol—infuse, dwell, and drain or continuous infusion.
Intravesicular	Direct exposure of bladder surfaces to drug	Requires insertion of Foley catheter	Urinary tract infections Cystitis Bladder contracture Urinary urgency Allergic drug reactions	Maintain sterile technique when inserting Foley catheter. Instill solution, clamp catheter for 1 hour, and unclamp to drain.
Intrapleural	Sclerosing of pleural lining to prevent recurrence of effusions.	Requires insertion of a thoracotomy tube	Pain Infection	Monitor for complete drainage from pleural cavity before instillation of drug. Following instillation, clamp tubing and reposition client every 10-15 min × 2 hr. Attach tubing to suction × 18 hr.

      7. Miscellaneous agents.
          a. Mechanisms of action—poorly understood.
          b. Variety of toxic effects.
  IV. Routes of administration—advantages of each route, potential complications, and nursing implications are presented in Table 21-3.

DATA COLLECTION
   I. Pertinent personal history.
     A. Type of cancer and phase of cancer trajectory.
     B. Previous cancer therapy and time interval since last therapy.
        1. Attitudes of client/family toward previous therapy.
        2. Side effects experienced.
        3. Self-care measures used to minimize side effects.
        4. Effectiveness of measures in reducing the incidence and severity of side effects.

    C. Dietary intake.

    D. Knowledge of rationale for and goals of treatment, agents to be given, potential side effects, and relative risks and benefits of treatment.

  II. Physical examination.

    A. Renal—amount and color of urinary output and patterns of urinary elimination.

    B. Gastrointestinal system:

      1. Oral cavity—cleanliness, moisture, and integrity of lips, gums, teeth, oral mucosa, and tongue.

      2. Bowel—presence of bowel sounds; consistency, color, and caliber of stool; patterns of bowel elimination.

      3. Rectum—integrity of perirectal and perineal tissue; presence of hemorrhoids, redness, or pain.

    C. Hematological system:

      1. Color of skin and mucous membranes; presence of bruising or petechiae.

      2. Activity tolerance.

      3. Presence of signs and symptoms of infection.

 III. Psychosocial examination.

    A. Previous responses to stressors and effective coping mechanisms used.

    B. Level of independence and responsibility, desire, and ability for self-care.

    C. Support systems and personnel available to client/family.

 IV. Laboratory data.

    A. Hemoglobin, hematocrit, platelet count, white blood cell count, and differential results.

    B. Blood urea nitrogen (BUN) levels.

    C. Electrolyte levels.

ASSOCIATED NURSING DIAGNOSES

  I. Knowledge deficit.

 II. Altered nutrition: less than body requirements.

III. Potential for infection.

IV. Altered oral mucous membrane.

 V. Sexual dysfunction.

VI. Activity intolerance.

VII. Body image disturbances.

NURSING PLANNING AND IMPLEMENTATION

  I. Interventions to maximize safety for the client/family.

    A. Obtain appropriate materials and agents for management of extravasation as indicated (Table 21-4).

      1. Extravasation—infiltration or leakage of an intravenous (IV) antineoplastic agent into the local tissues.

        a. Irritants—agents that may produce pain and inflammation at the administration site or along the path of a vein if leakage into subcutaneous tissue occurs (Table 21-4).

        b. Vesicants—agents that have the potential to cause cellular damage or tissue destruction if leakage into subcutaneous tissue occurs (Table 21-4).

          (1) Instruct client to report pain or burning with the infusion.

Table 21-4
VESICANT AND IRRITANT CHEMOTHERAPEUTIC MEDICATIONS

Medication	Description	Local Antidote
Carmustine (BiCNU, BCNU)	Irritant	Sodium bicarbonate (T)*
Dacarbazine (DTIC-Dome)	Irritant	Sodium thiosulfate (T)
Dactinomycin (Actinomycin D)	Vesicant	Sodium thiosulfate (T)
Daunomycin Daunorubicin (Cerubidine)	Vesicant	Hydrocortisone (T)
Doxorubicin (Adriamycin)	Vesicant	Application of cold to site (M)† NOTE: Local infiltration of site with an injectible corticosteroid and flooding of the site with normal saline solution has been known to lessen the local reaction.
Mitoxantrone (Novantrone)	Irritant	None
Streptozocin (Zanosar)	Irritant	Hydrocortisone
Vinblastine (Velban)	Vesicant	Hyaluronidase
Vincristine (Oncovin)	Vesicant	Hyaluronidase

* T, theoretical antidote.
† M, manufacturer-recommended antidote.
From Tenenbaum, L. (1989). *Cancer Chemotherapy: A Reference Guide.* Philadelphia: W.B. Saunders Co., p. 190.

    (2) Administer vesicants in larger veins of the arm, midway between the wrist and elbow.
    (3) Assess blood return after each 1 to 2 ml of the agent is infused.
  c. If extravasation occurs or is suspected:
    (1) Discontinue infusion, leaving needle or IV catheter in place.
    (2) Aspirate residual medication and blood from the IV tubing.
    (3) If recommended (Table 21-4), instill IV antidote and then remove needle.
    (4) If no IV antidote is recommended, remove needle.
      (a) Inject the subcutaneous antidote in a clockwise fashion into the infiltrated area using a 25-gauge needle for each injection.
      (b) Avoid applying pressure to the area to decrease spread of drug infiltrate.
      (c) Apply a sterile, occlusive dressing, heat, or cold as indicated (Table 21-4).
      (d) Elevate the affected extremity to decrease swelling.
    (5) Notify physician of extravasation.
    (6) Document extravasation in medical record to include—date, time, needle size and type, site, medication(s) administered, sequence of antineoplastic agents, approximate amount of agent extravasated, subjective symptoms reported by client, nursing assessment of site, nursing interventions, notification of physician and interventions, instructions given to client, follow-up measures, and signature.
B. Obtain appropriate emergency equipment and agents for management of anaphylaxis as indicated.
C. Select site for venipuncture.

Table 21-5
CHEMOTHERAPEUTIC AGENTS WITH ATYPICAL TOXICITIES AND APPROPRIATE NURSING INTERVENTIONS

Chemotherapeutic Agents	Toxicity	Nursing Interventions
Asparaginase	Hypersensitivity	Identify clients at risk—clients with previous allergic reactions to this or other medications. Assess for early signs of hypersensitivity—urticaria, pruritus. Assess for signs of anaphylactic-type reaction—local or generalized urticaria; angioedema of the face, eyelids, hands, feet; respiratory stridor; hypotension; cyanosis. Administer epinephrine in dose of 0.5-0.75 ml (solution strength, 1:1000) per physician order.
Bleomycin (Blenoxane)	Pulmonary toxicity presented as pneumonitis, which may result in pulmonary fibrosis	Monitor cumulative dose, which should not exceed 400 units; doses above this limit significantly increase the risk of pulmonary toxicity. Assess for signs of pulmonary toxicity—dry persistent cough, dyspnea, tachypnea, cyanosis, basilar rales. Prevent infection by promoting exercise, coughing and deep breathing, and humidification of air.
Cisplatin	Renal toxicity	Monitor blood urea nitrogen and creatinine levels, urinary output. Provide adequate hydration and diuresis with furosemide or mannitol as ordered by physician.
	Ototoxicity	Teach client to report tinnitus. Monitor dose levels; risk increases with doses exceeding 60-75 mg/m²; hearing loss may be cumulative with additional doses and may or may not be reversible. Refer client for regular audiograms.
Cyclophosphamide (Cytoxan)	Hemorrhagic cystitis	Ensure adequate fluid intake of 3000 ml/day unless contraindicated. Avoid urinary retention by having client void every 2 hours when possible. Assess for signs of cystitis, including urinary frequency, pain on urination, cloudy urine, hematuria, low back pain. Teach client to report signs of cystitis.

1. Select distal sites before proximal sites.
2. Evaluate general condition of veins.
3. Note type of medication(s) to be infused.
4. Avoid sites where damage to underlying tendons or nerves is more likely to occur—antecubital region, wrist, dorsal surface of the hand, areas with recent venipuncture sites, sclerosed veins, or areas of previous surgery such as skin grafts, mastectomy, or partial amputation.
D. Assess IV for blood return.
E. Infuse 5 to 10 ml normal saline solution to assess patency of vein.

Table 21-5
CHEMOTHERAPEUTIC AGENTS WITH ATYPICAL TOXICITIES AND APPROPRIATE NURSING
INTERVENTIONS *Continued*

Chemotherapeutic Agents	Toxicity	Nursing Interventions
Daunorubicin (Cerubidine) Doxorubicin (Adriamycin)	Cardiotoxicity manifested by electrocardiographic (ECG) changes, congestive heart failure, cardiomyopathy	Monitor cumulative dose of agents; maximal cumulative dose is 550 mg/m^2; doses above this limit significantly increase the risk of cardiotoxicity; maximal cumulative dose is reduced to 400 mg/m^2 in the presence of concurrent radiation therapy to the mediastinum or concurrent cyclophosphamide therapy. Assess for signs of cardiotoxicity, including ECG changes, signs of congestive heart failure (shortness of breath, hypertension, edema).
Etoposide (VePesid)	Hypotension resulting from rapid administration	Administer over 30 to 60 minutes. Monitor blood pressure every 15 minutes during administration.
5-Fluorouracil (5-FU)	Photosensitivity manifested by increased skin pigmentation or erythema	Teach client to avoid prolonged sun exposure or to use sunscreen when exposed to the sun. Assess for changes in pigmentation and/or erythema of skin.
Vincristine	Neurotoxicity	Assess for numbness of hands and feet, foot drop, constipation, tingling of fingertips and toes, decreased fine and gross motor abilities, and slapping gait. Teach client to report symptoms of neurotoxicity..

    F. Administer antineoplastic agents according to agency policy according to the five rights:
      1. Right medication.
      2. Right time.
      3. Right route.
      4. Right dose.
      5. Right client.
    G. Assess client for signs of infiltration (burning, pain, swelling, redness).
    H. Flush IV with 3 to 10 ml of normal saline solution after administering each agent and at completion of the infusion.
    I. Remove needle or venous catheter or inject heparin into central line or device.
      1. Apply adhesive bandage to site.
      2. Have client elevate extremity for 3 to 5 minutes after needle is withdrawn.
      3. Apply gentle pressure to the site to reduce local bleeding.
    J. Document medication administration and client response according to agency policy.

II. Interventions to decrease the incidence and severity of complications of chemotherapy.
    A. Interventions for common complications of chemotherapy are presented in Chapter 7.
    B. Interventions for unique complications of specific antineoplastic agents are presented in Table 21-5.

EVALUATION OF CLIENT AND FAMILY OUTCOMES

I. Describe the chemotherapy protocol—name of agent(s), route, method, schedule of administration, and schedule for routine laboratory and physical examination follow-up.

II. List potential immediate and long-term side effects of the antineoplastic agents.

III. Describe self-care measures to decrease the incidence and severity of complications of therapy.

IV. List changes that should be reported immediately to the health care team.
   A. Signs and symptoms of infection—fever greater than 101° F, pain, swelling, redness, or pus.
   B. Nausea or vomiting that persists and is unrelieved by usual control methods.
   C. Unusual bleeding or bruising.
   D. Acute changes in mental or emotional status.
   E. Diarrhea or constipation unrelieved by usual control methods.

V. Identify potential community resources to meet demands of treatment and rehabilitation.

VI. Demonstrate competence in self-care skills demanded by the treatment plan—care of venous access devices, implanted ports, or intracavitary catheters.

BIBLIOGRAPHY

Brager, B.L. & Yasko, J.M. (1984). *Care of the Client Receiving Chemotherapy*. Reston, Va: Reston Publishing Co.

Brown, J.K. & Hogan, C.M. (1990). Chemotherapy. In S.L. Groenwald, M.H. Frogge, M. Goodman, & C.H. Yarbro (eds). *Cancer Nursing: Principles and Practice* (2nd ed). Boston: Jones & Bartlett Publishers, pp. 230-283.

DeVita, V.T., Jr., Hellman, S., & Rosenberg, S.A. (eds) (1989). *Cancer: Principles & Practice of Oncology* (3rd ed). Philadelphia: J.B. Lippincott Co.

Esparza, D.M. & Weyland, J.B. (1982). Nursing care for the patient with an Ommaya reservoir. *Oncol Nurs Forum 9*(4), 17-20.

Fischer, D.S. & Tish-Knobf, M.K. (1989). *The Cancer Chemotherapy Handbook* (3rd ed). Chicago: Year Book Medical Publishers.

Fraser, M.C. & Tucker, M.A. (1988). Late effects of cancer therapy: Chemotherapy-related malignancies. *Oncol Nurs Forum 15*(1), 67-77.

Guy, J.L. (1991). Medical oncology—the agents. In S.B. Baird, R. McCorkle, & M. Grant (eds). *Cancer Nursing: A Comprehensive Textbook*. Philadelphia: W.B. Saunders Co., pp. 266-290.

Hoff, S.T. (1987). Concepts in intraperitoneal chemotherapy. *Semin Oncol Nurs 3*(2), 112-117.

Skeel, R.T. (ed) (1982). *Manual of Cancer Chemotherapy*. Boston: Little, Brown & Co.

Von Hoff, D.D., Rozencweig, M., & Piccart, M. (1982). The cardiotoxicity of anticancer agents. *Semin Oncol 9*(1), 23-33.

Principles of Preparation, Administration, and Disposal of Antineoplastic Agents

Linda Tenenbaum, MSN, RN, OCN

THEORY

I. Exposure to antineoplastic agents poses a potential health risk to personnel who prepare, handle, administer, and dispose of these drugs.
   A. Potential routes of exposure.
      1. Direct contact—skin and mucous membrane contact or inhalation.
      2. Indirect contact—body fluids and excreta of clients who have received antineoplastic agents within the past 72 hours.
   B. Potential effects of exposure to antineoplastic agents.
      1. Short-term—occur within hours or days after exposure.
         a. Dermatitis.
         b. Hyperpigmentation of skin.
         c. Other reported symptoms not linked conclusively to antineoplastic agent exposure—sores in nasal mucosa, burning of eyes, dizziness, headache, and nausea.
      2. Long-term—occur within months or years after exposure.
         a. Partial alopecia.
         b. Chromosomal abnormalities.
         c. Increased risk of cancer.

II. Institutional responsibilities with respect to antineoplastic agents.
   A. Define agency policies and procedures about use of antineoplastic agents consistent with professional and federal recommendations to minimize risks to personnel.
   B. Orient all agency personnel who may come in contact with antineoplastic agents about the potential risks of antineoplastic agents and agency policies and procedures.
   C. Review agency policies and procedures about antineoplastic agents at periodic intervals.
   D. Include compliance to policies and procedures as a component of agency quality assurance program.

E. Develop a monitoring system for reviewing incident reports involving antineoplastic agents.

DATA COLLECTION

I. Previous health history of personnel.
   A. Personal history of cancer.
   B. Family history of cancer.
   C. Personal risk factors for cancer.
   D. Presence of signs and symptoms of site-specific cancers.

II. Physical and psychosocial examination—examination as defined by agency policy.

NURSING PLANNING AND IMPLEMENTATION

I. Interventions to minimize risk of exposure during preparation.
   A. Determine a dedicated environment for drug preparation.
      1. Prepare antineoplastic agents in a centralized area.
      2. Prohibit eating, drinking, smoking, and applying cosmetics in the work area.
   B. Obtain and maintain special equipment for drug preparation.
      1. Prepare antineoplastic agents in a class II, type B biological safety cabinet for maximal protection.
         a. Hood should be vented outside if feasible.
         b. Blower should be operated 24 hours a day, 7 days a week.
         c. Hood should be serviced at regular intervals according to manufacturer recommendations.
      2. Use a disposable, plastic-backed, absorbent pad underneath work area to minimize contamination by droplets or spills.
         a. Pads are changed at a minimum at the completion of drug preparation or at the end of the shift.
         b. Pads are changed immediately after a contamination.
      3. Wear protective clothing during preparation of antineoplastic agents:
         a. Disposable, long-sleeved gown made of lint-free fabric with knitted cuffs and a closed front.
         b. Disposable, surgical latex (0.007 to 0.009 inches), non-powdered gloves with cuffs long enough to tuck over the knit cuffs of the gown.
            (1) Gloves should be discarded after each use.
            (2) Gloves should be discarded after a puncture, tear, or medication spill.
   C. Follow special procedures when preparing drugs.
      1. Wash hands thoroughly before and after preparation of antineoplastic agents.
      2. Use needles, syringes, tubing, and connectors with Luer-Lok attachments.
      3. Use special care when preparing agents packaged in ampules.
         a. Clear all fluid from the neck of the ampule.
         b. Tilt tip of the ampule away from preparer.
         c. Wrap a sterile gauze pad around the neck of the ampule.
         d. Break neck of the ampule away from preparer.
         e. Discard excess solution from ampule into a sealed waste vial or according to agency policy.
      4. Use special care when reconstituting agents packaged in vials.
         a. Use a 18- or 19-gauge needle and a 0.2 μm hydrophobic filter or dispensing pin.
         b. Create negative pressure in the vial when adding diluent by aspirating a volume of air slightly larger than the volume of diluent added.
         c. Add diluent slowly.

      d. Allow diluent to run slowly down the side of the vial.

      e. Withdraw dose of agent into syringe.

      f. Allow air pressure to equalize between the vial and syringe before removing the needle.

   5. Expel air from a syringe or tubing containing antineoplastic agents slowly onto a sterile gauze pad contained in a sealable 4 ml polyethylene bag.

   6. Prime all tubing with intravenous (IV) solution before adding antineoplastic agent(s) if possible.

II. Interventions to minimize exposure to antineoplastic agents during administration.

  A. Wear protective clothing (gloves, gown, mask, and goggles) as indicated by institutional policy when administering antineoplastic agents.

  B. Prepare agents for infusion over an absorbent, plastic-backed pad:

    1. Expulsion of air from syringe or tubing.

    2. Injection into the side arm of a running IV infusion.

    3. Spiking of a bag.

    4. Making Luer-Lok connections from tubing to venous access devices.

  C. Wash hands thoroughly after administering antineoplastic agents.

III. Interventions to minimize exposure to antineoplastic agents during disposal.

  A. Dispose of sharp objects in a puncture-resistant, leak-proof container.

  B. Dispose of filled containers and contaminated equipment in a sealable 4 ml polyethylene or 2 ml polypropylene bag.

  C. Label all waste containers "Caution: Chemotherapy."

  D. Wash hands thoroughly after disposing of antineoplastic agents and equipment.

IV. Interventions to minimize the incidence and severity of exposure to antineoplastic agents.

  A. Direct contact.

    1. Wash exposed areas with copious amounts of water or special solution.

      a. Wash exposed skin thoroughly with soap (nongermicidal) and water.

      b. Flood involved eye while holding the eyelid open with water or an isotonic eye wash for at least 5 minutes.

    2. Seek medical evaluation as soon as possible after an accidental exposure.

    3. Complete an incident report according to institutional policies and procedures.

  B. Accidental spill.

    1. Obtain a "spill kit" as recommended by the American Society of Hospital Pharmacists for spills greater than 150 ml in volume.

      a. Protective clothing—disposable dust and mist respirator, splash goggles or safety goggles, two pairs of disposable gloves (inner latex gloves and outer utility gloves), disposable low-permeability coveralls or gown and shoe covers.

      b. Special equipment—two sealable thick plastic, hazardous waste disposal bags; absorbent, plastic-backed sheets or spill pads; small scoop to collect broken glass fragments; disposable toweling; puncture-resistant container.

    2. Wear protective clothing.

    3. Absorb liquids with a spill pad or sheet.

    4. Remove powdered agents with a damp, disposable gauze pad or soft toweling.

    5. Collect glass fragments in scoop.

    6. Dispose of all contaminated materials in a sealed, thick, plastic bag labeled with a chemotherapy warning label.

V. Interventions to minimize risk of indirect exposure from body fluids of clients who have received antineoplastic agents.

A. Wear protective clothing (gloves minimum) when handling urine, stool, blood, or emesis.

B. Avoid splattering body fluids during disposal.

C. Label all laboratory specimens "Caution: Chemotherapy" or "Biohazard."

D. Place linen contaminated with body fluids in specially marked laundry bag placed inside an impervious bag labeled "Caution: Chemotherapy" or "Biohazard."

EVALUATION OF HEALTH CARE PERSONNEL OUTCOMES

I. Discuss potential risks related to handling antineoplastic agents.

II. Describe procedures designed to minimize exposure to antineoplastic agents.

III. Document accidental exposure to antineoplastic agents according to agency policy.

IV. Recognize professional and federal resources for monitoring changes in potential risks from and recommendations regarding exposure to antineoplastic agents.

BIBLIOGRAPHY

(1990) ASHP technical assistance bulletin on handling cytotoxic and hazardous drugs. *Am J Hosp Pharm* 47(15), 1033-1049.

Barstow, J. (1985). Safe handling of cytotoxic agents in the home. *Home Healthcare Nurs* 3(5), 46-47.

(1988). *Cancer Chemotherapy Guidelines Module I: Recommendations for Cancer Chemotherapy Course Content and Clinical Practicum.* Pittsburgh: Oncology Nursing Society.

(1988). *Cancer Chemotherapy Guidelines Module II: Recommendations for Nursing Practice in the Acute Care Setting.* Pittsburgh: Oncology Nursing Society.

(1988). *Cancer Chemotherapy Guidelines Module III: Recommendations for Nursing Practice in the Outpatient Setting.* Pittsburgh: Oncology Nursing Society.

(1988). *Cancer Chemotherapy Guidelines Module IV: Recommendations for Nursing Practice in the Home Care Setting.* Pittsburgh: Oncology Nursing Society.

(1988). *Cancer Chemotherapy Guidelines Module V: Recommendations for the Management of Extravasation and Anaphylaxis.* Pittsburgh: Oncology Nursing Society.

Cloak, M.M., Connor, T.H., Stevens, K.R., Theiss, J.C., Alt, J.M., Matney, T.S., & Anderson, R.N. (1985). Occupational exposure of nursing personnel to antineoplastic agents. *Oncol Nurs Forum* 12(5), 33-39.

Dunne, C.F. (1989). Safe handling of antineoplastic agents: self-learning module. *Cancer Nurs* 12(2), 120-127.

Esparza, D.M., Young, N., & Luongo, J. (1989). Effective planning for office and outpatient chemotherapy administration. *Semin Oncol Nurs* 5(2, suppl 1), 8-14.

Fiscus, J.A., Hayes, N.A., Rostad, M.A., & Whedon, M.A. (1989). *Safe Handling of Cytotoxic Drugs.* Pittsburgh: Oncology Nursing Society.

Frogge, M.H. (1982). Issues in chemotherapy administration III—sequence of administering vesicant cytotoxic drugs. B. Give the vesicants last. *Oncol Nurs Forum* 9(1), 54.

(1986). *Guidelines for Cytotoxic (Antineoplastic) Drugs.* Washington, D.C.: U.S. Department of Labor.

Goodman, M. (1991). Delivery of cancer chemotherapy. In S.B. Baird, R. McCorkle, & M. Grant (eds). *Cancer Nursing: A Comprehensive Textbook.* Philadelphia: W.B. Saunders Co., pp. 291-320.

Gullo, S.M. (1988). Safe handling of antineoplastic drugs: translating the recommendations into practice. *Oncol Nurs Forum* 15(5), 595-601.

Johnson, E.G. & Janosik, J.E. (1989). Manufacturers' recommendations for handling spilled antineoplastic agents. *Am J Hosp Pharm* 46(2), 318-319.

Laidlaw, J.L., Cannor, T.H., Theiss, J.C., Anderson, R.W., & Matney, T.S. (1984). Permeability of latex and polyvinyl chloride gloves to 20 antineoplastic drugs. *Am J Hosp Pharm* 41(12), 2618-2623.

Miller, S.A. (1987). Issues in cytotoxic drug handling safety. *Semin Oncol Nurs* 3(2), 133-141.

National Study Commission on Cytotoxic Exposure (1987). *Recommendations for Handling Cytotoxic Agents.* Boston: Author.

(1986). OSHA work-practice guidelines for personnel dealing with cytotoxic (antineoplastic) drugs. *Am J Hosp Pharm* 43(5), 1193-1204.

(1983). *Recommendations for the Safe Handling of Parenteral Antineoplastic Drugs.* Washington, D.C.: National Institutes of Health.

Sansivero, G.E. & Murray, S.A. (1989). Safe management of chemotherapy at home. *Oncol Nurs Forum* 16(5), 711-713.

Stellman, J.M. & Zoloth, S.R. (1986). Cancer chemotherapeutic agents as occupational hazards: a literature review. *Cancer Invest 4*(2), 127-135.

Tenenbaum, L. (1989). *Cancer Chemotherapy: A Reference Guide*. Philadelphia: W.B. Saunders Co.

Tish-Knobf, M.K. (1982). Intravenous therapy guidelines for oncology practice. *Oncol Nurs Forum 9*(2), 30-34.

Tobin, B.K. (1985). Hidden hazards on the job. II. Parenteral antineoplastic drugs. *Nurs Life 5*(5), 45-49.

Valanis, B. & Shortridge, L. (1987). Self-protective practices of nurses handling antineoplastic drugs. *Oncol Nurs Forum 14*(3), 23-27.

(1986). *Work Practice Guidelines for Personnel Dealing With Cytotoxic (Antineoplastic) Drugs*. Washington, D.C.: Occupational Safety and Health Administration.

23

Implications of Biological Response Modifier Therapy for Nursing

Lynne Brophy, BSN, RN, OCN
Paula Trahan Rieger, MSN, RN, OCN

THEORY

I. Principles of biotherapy.
  A. The components of immune system function to provide homeostasis, surveillance, and defense (Figure 23-1).
  B. Types of immunity.
    1. Innate immunity—mechanical barriers, chemical barriers, and the inflammatory response.
    2. Acquired immunity—recognition of self versus non-self.
      a. Cell-mediated immunity.
        (1) T lymphocyte is primary effector cell.
        (2) Provides for protection against fungi, viruses, intracellular bacteria, and initiates transplantation rejection.
      b. Humoral immunity.
        (1) Sensitized B lymphocytes produce antibodies.
        (2) Provides for protection against foreign antigens such as bacteria, viruses, and toxins.
      c. Interactions.
        (1) Initiation of immune response requires interaction between cellular and humoral immune factors.
        (2) Interactions are mediated by macrophages and protein messengers—cytokines, lymphokines, and monokines.
  C. Definition of biotherapy: treatment with agents derived from biological sources and/or able to affect biological responses.
  D. Definition of biological response modifiers—agents or approaches that change the relationship between the tumor and the host by modifying the biological response of the host to tumor cells with a resultant therapeutic effect (Table 23-1).

II. Role of biotherapy in cancer care.
  A. Diagnosis of cancer.

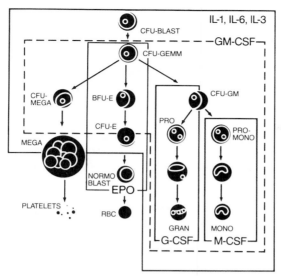

Figure 23-1 Regulation of hematopoietic cell development. *(From Gabrilove, J.L. [1989]. Introduction and overview of hematopoietic growth factors.* Semin Hematol 26[suppl 2], 2.)

    1. Monoclonal antibodies are used in differential diagnosis of cancer.
    2. Radiolabeled monoclonal antibody scans are used to detect tumors (investigational).
  B. Treatment of cancer.
    1. Primary treatment.
      a. Alpha-interferon (α-IFN) for treatment of hairy cell leukemia.
      b. High-dose α-IFN for treatment of acquired immunodeficiency syndrome (AIDS)-related Kaposi's sarcoma.
    2. Supportive treatment.
      a. Granulocyte-macrophage colony stimulating factor (GM-CSF) for treatment of neutropenia in clients after bone marrow transplant.
      b. Granulocyte colony stimulating factor (G-CSF) for treatment of neutropenia associated with antineoplastic therapy.

III. Classification of biotherapeutic agents.
  A. Agents that initiate, modify, or restore the immune response of the host.
  B. Agents that have direct antitumor activity (cytotoxic or antiproliferative mechanisms of action).
  C. Agents that have other biological effects such as affecting the differentiation or maturation of cells or the ability of the tumor cell to metastasize or survive.

IV. Safety measures in delivery of biotherapy.
  A. Aseptic techniques should be used when preparing and administering biological response modifiers.
  B. Most biological response modifiers are natural body proteins and no specific recommendations exist about handling.
  C. When biological response modifiers are attached to antineoplastic agents, cytotoxic handling procedures should be followed (see Chapter 22).
  D. When biological response modifiers are attached to radioisotopes, radiation safety precautions should be followed (see Chapter 20).

Text continued on page 354

Table 23-1
BIOLOGICAL RESPONSE MODIFIERS

Actions	Clinical Uses	Routes of Administration

Alpha (α)-Interferon (IFN)
Beta (β)-Interferon
Gamma (γ)-Interferon
Antiviral activity
Antiproliferative activities
Immunomodulatory activities
  Stimulation of interferons
  (e.g., alpha can stimulate pro-
  duction of gamma), interleu-
  kins, and tumor necrosis fac-
  tors
  Activation of T cells
  Increased phagocytic activity
  of macrophages and natural
  killer (NK) cells
	Alpha-interferon (Roferon-A, Intron A) is Food and Drug Administration (FDA) approved for hairy-cell leukemia, acquired immunodeficiency syndrome (AIDS)-related Kaposi's sarcoma, and condyloma acuminata and remains investigational for other diseases.
	In clinical trials the interferons have shown clinical activity in hematological malignancies, renal cell carcinoma, melanoma, and superficial bladder cancers.
		Subcutaneous (SQ)
		Intramuscular (IM)
		Intravenous (IV)
		Intracavitary

Interleukin-2 (IL-2) Supports growth and maturation of subpopulations of T cells Stimulates activity of NK and cytotoxic T cells Induces production of other lymphokines (i.e., γ-IFN, granulocyte-macrophage colony stimulating factor)	Investigational Clinical activity in clients with renal and melanoma cancers	IV SQ Intra-arterial Intraperitoneal

Common Side Effects	Nursing Considerations

Side effect incidence and severity increase with dose
Acute
Flulike syndrome (headaches, fever, chills, arthralgia and myalgia)
Nausea and vomiting
Chronic
Fatigue
Neurological
  Decreased short-term memory
  Decreased concentration/attention span
  Decreased ability to perform mathematical calculations.
Gastrointestinal
  Taste changes
  Anorexia
  Weight loss
Integument
  Dry skin
  Pruritus
  Partial alopecia
Hematological
  Neutropenia
  Thrombocytopenia
	Cardiopulmonary side effects are more common in clients with underlying cardiopulmonary disease.
	Thrombocytopenia, anorexia, fatigue and malaise are dose limiting.
	Neurotoxicity may necessitate discontinuance of drug.
	Chills usually occur 3-6 hr after administration.
	Premedicate with diphenhydramine before IFN administration to prevent chills; if chills occur after premedication, repeat dose of antihistamine and increase amount of premedication with subsequent doses.
	Fever occurs 30-90 min after onset of chills and may peak at 104° F (40° C) for as long as 24 hr. Admininster acetaminophen as a premedication and every 4 hr as needed after IFN dosing.
	Fever and chills may decrease or vary in severity and incidence as treatment cycle progresses.
	Maintain fluid balance.
	Store agents in refrigerator.
	Do not shake vial during preparation because foaming will occur.
	Consult pharmacy about reconstitution guidelines, available vial strengths (produced by several companies).
	Teach client injection technique.

Consitutional symptoms
Capillary leak syndrome
Nausea and vomiting
Anorexia
Central nervous system (CNS) changes
Skin changes
  Erythema
  Dry desquamation
  Pruritus
  Rash
Altered laboratory values
  Hepatic
  Hematological
  Hypocalcemia
  Hypomagnesemia
	Medicate with acetaminophen and nonsteroidal anti-inflammatory drug (NSAID) to control temperature.
	Obtain and monitor:
	  Orthostatic blood pressures/pulse
	  Daily weights
	  Input and output
	Perform skin care (see Chapter 7).
	IL-2 is produced by several companies—consult pharmacy about stability, filterability, and compatibility issues.

Table continued on following page

Table 23-1
BIOLOGICAL RESPONSE MODIFIERS *Continued*

Actions	Clinical Use	Routes of Administration
Granulocyte-Macrophage Colony Stimulating Factor (GM-CSF)		
Mediates proliferation and differentiation and enhances function of the granulocyte and macrophage lineages Stimulates production of tumor necrosis factor and interleukin-1	GM-CSF (Sargramostim) is FDA approved for neutropenia associated with bone marrow transplantation.	SQ IV
Erythropoietin		
Stimulates production and differentiation of red blood cells	Erythropoietin is FDA approved for anemia associated with dialysis-dependent end-stage renal disease. Erythropoietin is investigational for treatment of anemia in cancer clients.	IV SQ
Granulocyte Colony Stimulating Factor (G-CSF)		
Mediates primarily proliferation, differentiation, and function of neutrophils	G-CSF (Filgrastim) is FDA approved for chemotherapy-associated febrile neutropenia in clients with non-myeloid malignancies.	SQ IV
Interleukin-3 (IL-3) (also known as multi-CSF)		
Stimulates growth of multipotential stem cell	Investigational Early phase I trials	IV SQ
Macrophage Colony Stimulating Factor (M-CSF)		
Supports the proliferation and differentiation of macrophages Enhances cellular function of monocytes and macrophages	Investigational	IV
Interleukin-1 (IL-1)		
Induces release of lymphokines from activated T cells, fibroblasts Mediates inflammatory response	Investigational Early phase 1 trials	IV

Common Side Effects	Nursing Considerations
Severity is dependent on dose and route. *Low dose* Bone pain Local skin reaction Flulike syndrome (see "Interferon" for description of syndrome and management guidelines) *High dose* Third spacing at doses of 16-32 μg/kg	Agent may cause phlebitis with peripheral administration. Maximal tolerated dose is 16-32 μg/kg. Teach client SQ injection techniques. Treat bone pain with acetaminophen as needed. Monitor blood counts, including white blood cell (WBC) differential as ordered. Verify with physician WBC levels at which drug should be held. Consult pharmacy resource personnel about differences in products that may affect administration.
Hypertension Diarrhea	Teach client SQ injection techniques. Monitor blood pressure during therapy.
Bone pain	Teach client SQ injection techniques. Treat bone pain with acetaminophen as needed. Monitor clients with preexisting skin conditions such as psoriasis or eczema for signs of dermatitis (erythema, papules, fever, lesions).
Constitutional symptoms Bone pain	Monitor temperature closely for spikes unrelated to normal response to drug. Administer acetaminophen for bone pain.
Thrombocytopenia	Institute thrombocytopenic precautions for platelet count less than 50,000/mm³.
Constitutional symptoms Hypotension Phlebitis with peripheral administration	Monitor orthostatic blood pressures. Administer drug through central venous catheter (CVC). Dilute with human serum albumin (HSA) after initial reconstitution.

Table continued on following page

Table 23-1
BIOLOGICAL RESPONSE MODIFIERS *Continued*

Actions	Clinical Uses	Routes of Administration
Interleukin-4 (IL-4)		
Stimulates growth of resting B cells	Investigational	IV SQ
Tumor Necrosis Factor (TNF)		
Causes cell death by arrest at G_2 phase Damages vascular epithelium in tumor capillaries, resulting in hemorrhage and necrosis of tumor cells Enhances coagulation and depresses anticoagulation Mediates septic shock reaction	TNF is not approved by the FDA.	IV SQ IM Intracavitary Intra-arterial
Monoclonal Antibodies		

Cause cell death through interaction with immune responses
Recognize tumor-associated antigens
	Investigational
	    Diagnostic
	    Therapeutic
	    Bone marrow transplant
	Differential diagnosis of tumors by pathologist
		IV
		Intralymphatic

Common Side Effects	Nursing Considerations
Constitutional symptoms Nasal congestion ***High doses*** Capillary leak-type syndrome Rare—skin rashes	Premedicate for chills and fever. Monitor vital signs and orthostatic blood pressure. Administer drug with special tubing or prerinse tubing system with HSA or normal saline solution. Obtain daily weights.

Flulike syndrome (see "Interferon" for description and management)
Chills occur 1-6 hr after administration of agent; can progress to rigors
Fever occurs 30-60 min after onset of chills and usually peaks 1-2 hr after administration
Cardiopulmonary
  Orthostatic hypotension
Gastrointestinal
  Nausea
  Vomiting
  Anorexia
Hepatic (doses >50 μg/m^2)
  Elevated transaminases
  Hypertrigliceriedemia
  Transient increases in coagulation factors
  Decreased cholesterol
  Hyperbilirubinemia
Hematological (doses >100 μg/m^2)
  Reversible neutropenia
  Reversible thrombocytopenia
  Reversible monocytosis
Other
  Pain at tumor site
  Erythema at SQ injection site
  Weight loss
Rare
Neurological
  Seizures
  Confusion
  Aphasia
  Dyspnea
	Treat chills immediately, at onset, with meperidine sulfate intravenously as ordered by physician.
	Offer meperidine or morphine as a premedication with ensuing doses of TNF (if allergic or refractory to meperidine, use diphenhydramine or morphine sulfate as an alternative as ordered by physician).
	Offer non-pharmocological measures such as blankets or heating pads.
	Administer acetaminophen as a premedication and every 4 hr as needed.
	Monitor vital signs frequently in clients receiving doses greater than 100 μg/m^2.
	Treat significant decreases in systolic blood pressure with normal saline solution (250 ml boluses) as ordered by physician.
	Monitor changes in coagulation parameters and signs of bleeding.
	Monitor blood gases as ordered by physician.
	Apply warm soaks or dry heat to TNF injection sites.

Potential allergic reactions Consitutional symptoms	Keep emergency drugs at bedside. Monitor vital signs frequently during first hour of infusion. Administer drug by infusion pumps. Consult pharmacy about stability, compatibility, filterability of drug.

Table continued on following page

Table 23-1
BIOLOGICAL RESPONSE MODIFIERS *Continued*

Actions	Clinical Uses	Routes of Administration
Effector Cells (e.g., lymphokine-activated killer [LAK] cells or tumor-infiltrating lymphocytes [TIL] cells)		
Target tumor cells	Investigational Primarily in combination with IL-2	IV

DATA COLLECTION

I. Pertinent personal history.
   A. Assess current medications, especially those that may be contraindicated with biological response modifiers.
      1. Aspirin.
      2. Steroids.
      3. Nonsteroidal anti-inflammatory drugs (NSAIDs).
      4. Medications that may alter mentation or coagulation.
      5. Immunosuppressants.
   B. Assess for chronic illnesses that may be exacerbated by biological response modifiers therapy—heart disease, diabetes, neurological or psychiatric disorders, hypertension, and psoriasis.
   C. Assess history of prior cancer therapies—chemotherapy, radiation therapy, surgery, and biotherapy.
   D. History of smoking, oxygen therapy, anorexia, nausea, vomiting, diarrhea, and taste changes.

II. Physical examination.
   A. Cardiovascular—heart rate and rhythm, abnormal heart sounds, and orthostatic blood pressure.
   B. Pulmonary—respiratory rate, adventitious breath sounds, shortness of breath, cyanosis, and clubbing.
   C. Gastrointestinal—weight, abdominal girth, mucositis, and xerostomia.
   D. Musculoskeletal—range of motion, functional status, and presence and patterns of arthritis.
   E. Neurological—affect, orientation, memory, attention span, social engagement, and sensory perception.
   F. Integument—erythema, rash, lesions, dryness, decreased turgor, and alopecia.

III. Psychosocial examination.
   A. Assess baseline mental status.
   B. Assess current social structure, including support systems, primary caretaker, financial status, and housing and living arrangements.
   C. Assess type, number, and effectiveness of previous coping strategies used by client and family.

Common Side Effects	Nursing Considerations
Chills Fever	Medicate client for chills with intravenous meperidine. Administer acetaminophen for fevers. Do not filter cell preparations during administration. Agitate drug gently and at intervals to reduce clumping.

IV. Evaluation of laboratory data.
   A. White blood count, differential, hemoglobin, and hematocrit levels, and platelet count.
   B. Renal function—blood urea nitrogen (BUN) and creatinine levels.
   C. Liver function—lactate dehydrogenase (LDH), alkaline phosphatase, serum glutamic-oxaloacetic transaminase (SGOT), serum glutamate pyruvic transaminase (SGPT), and bilirubin levels.
   D. Nutritional parameters—electrolytes, protein, and albumin levels.

V. Client/family perceptions of treatment goals and demands.
   A. Treatment goals.
   B. Obligations of treatment such as length of hospitalization, follow-up clinic visits, laboratory and diagnostic test requirements, and financial obligations.
   C. Expected side effects of biotherapy.
   D. Ability to perform self-care skills.

ASSOCIATED NURSING DIAGNOSES

  I. Alteration in comfort.

 II. Fatigue.

III. Knowledge deficit regarding self-care skills.

IV. Potential impaired skin integrity.

 V. Alteration in nutrition: less than body requirements.

NURSING PLANNING AND IMPLEMENTATION

  I. Interventions to maximize safety for client and family.
   A. Use aseptic procedures for mixing and administering biological agents.
   B. Identify location of emergency equipment and supplies.
   C. Obtain pulse, respirations, blood pressure, and temperature before administration of biotherapy.
   D. Administer premedications (acetaminophen and diphenhydramine) as ordered by the physician.
   E. Teach client and family signs and symptoms of untoward reactions to biological response modifier therapy to report to a member of the health care team.

       1. Fever greater than 103° F.

       2. Weight gain greater than 10 pounds in 1 week.

       3. Shortness of breath.

II. Interventions to monitor for unique complications of biological response modifier therapy.

  A. Monitor orthostatic blood pressure and pulse rate.

  B. Monitor fever patterns to differentiate normal responses to treatment from septic spikes.

  C. Evaluate symptoms for frequency, severity, duration, and effects on activities of daily living.

    1. Excessive fatigue.

    2. Weight loss or gain of 10 pounds or more in 1 week.

    3. Marked mental status changes such as excessive somnolence, psychosis, or confusion.

    4. Cardiac symptoms such as chest pain, arrhythmias, and symptomatic hypotension.

    5. Other symptoms—increased dyspnea, oliguria, edema, and severe allergic or local inflammatory reactions.

  D. Follow client for adherence to outpatient regimen.

  E. Monitor critical changes in laboratory values as ordered by the physician.

III. Interventions to decrease the incidence and severity of complications unique to biological response modifier therapy.

  A. Impaired skin integrity.

    1. Bathe in shower or bath with tepid water and avoid scrubbing skin.

    2. Apply lubricants (water-based lotions or creams) to skin after bathing.

    3. Encourage measures to maintain integrity such as position changes, weight shifts, getting out of bed, and ambulation.

  B. Mental status changes.

    1. Assess, at regular intervals, risk to fall.

    2. Teach family to monitor for subtle behavioral changes and report to a member of the health care team.

    3. Maintain a safe physical environment.

    4. Evaluate impact of mental status changes on functional status, judgment, and independence in activities of daily living.

  C. Capillary leak syndrome—movement of fluid from the vascular bed into tissues— end results are edema, weight gain, hypotension, and decreased urinary output; seen with interleukin-2 (IL-2) and GM-CSF.

    1. Administer supportive medical therapy such as albumin, diuretics, fluids, and vasopressors as ordered by physician.

    2. Instruct client to change positions from lying to sitting to standing slowly to avoid dizziness.

    3. Report significant changes to physician:

      a. Urinary output less than 30 ml/hour.

      b. Hypotension with systolic less than 80 mm Hg.

      c. Dyspnea.

      d. Weight gain greater than 10 pounds over 1 week.

IV. Interventions to enhance adaptation and rehabilitation.

  A. Teach strategies to manage chronic side effects of therapy—fatigue, anorexia, and mental status changes (see Chapter 7).

B. Teach client and family needed self-care skills for continuing biological response modifier therapy after discharge.

C. Provide with literature available for commercially available biological response modifiers.

D. Discuss changes in life-style resulting from side effects of therapy and continued need for follow-up care.

E. Use client logs to document the incidence and severity of side effects and type and effectiveness of self-care strategies used.

EVALUATION OF CLIENT AND FAMILY OUTCOMES

I. Describe type of and rationale for treatment with biological response modifiers.

II. List potential immediate and long-term complications of biotherapy—constitutional symptoms, bone pain, fatigue, anorexia, weight loss or gain, somnolence, confusion, psychosis, chest pain, hypotension, irregular heart beats, shortness of breath, decreased urinary output, and allergic reactions.

III. Describe self-care measures to decrease incidence and severity of complications of biological response modifier therapy.

IV. Demonstrate self-care skills required to administer biotherapy.

V. List changes in condition that should be reported to the health care team:
A. Fever uncontrolled with acetaminophen or unrelated to normal response to therapy.
B. Weight gain greater than 10 pounds in 1 week.
C. Marked changes in severity of shortness of breath.
D. Dizziness.
E. Marked changes in volume of urinary output.

VI. Identify potential community resources to meet unique demands of therapy and rehabilitation.

BIBLIOGRAPHY

Abernathy, E. (1987). Biotherapy: an introductory overview. *Oncol Nurs Forum 14*(suppl 6), 13-15.

Aistars, J. (1987). Fatigue in cancer patients: a conceptual approach to a clinical problem. *Oncol Nurs Forum 14*(6), 25-30.

Brogley, J.L. & Sharp, E.J. (1990). Nursing care of patients receiving activated lymphocytes. *Oncol Nurs Forum 17*(2), 187-193.

Clark, J. & Longo, D. (1986). Biological response modifiers. *Mediguide Oncol 6*(2), 1-10.

Collins, J.L. & Thaney, K.M. (eds) (1988). Biotherapy: a nursing challenge. *Semin Oncol Nurs 4*(2), 83-150.

Dillman, J.B. (1989). New antineoplastic therapies and inherent risks: monoclonal antibodies, biologic response modifiers, and interleukin-2. *J Intraven Nurs 12*(2), 103-113.

Dillman, R.O. (1989). Monoclonal antibodies for treating cancer. *Ann Intern Med 111*(7), 592-603.

Figlin, R.A. (1988). Biotherapy with interferon—1988. *Semin Oncol 15*(suppl 6), 3-9.

Foon, K.A. (1989). Biological response modifiers: the new immunotherapy. *Cancer Res 49*(7), 1621-1639.

Gabrilove, J.L. (1989). Introduction and overview of hematopoietic growth factors. *Semin Hematol 26*(suppl 2), 1-4.

Gallucci, B.B. (1987). The immune system and cancer. *Oncol Nurs Forum 14*(suppl 6), 3-12.

Glaspy, J.A. & Golde, D.W. (1989). Clinical applications of the myeloid growth factors. *Semin Hematol 26*(suppl 2), 14-17.

Gutterman, J.U. (1988). Overview of advances in the use of biological proteins in human cancer. *Semin Oncol 15*(suppl 5), 2-6.

Haeuber, D. & DiJulio, J.E. (1989). Hemopoietic colony-stimulating factors: an overview. *Oncol Nurs Forum 16*(2), 247-255.

Heberman, R.B. (1989). Interleukin-2 therapy of human cancer: potential benefits versus toxicity. *J Clin Oncol 7*(1), 1-4.

Hood, L.E. & Abernathy, E. (1991). Biologic response modifiers. In S.B. Baird, R. McCorkle, & M. Grant (eds). *Cancer Nursing: A Comprehensive Textbook*. Philadelphia: W.B. Saunders Co., pp. 321-343.

Irwin, M.M. (1991). The biotherapy of cancer—IV. *Oncol Nurs Forum 18*(suppl 1), 5-30.

Jassak, P.F. (ed) (1987). The biotherapy of cancer. *Oncol Nurs Forum 14*(suppl 6), 2-40.

Jassak, P.F. (1990). Biotherapy. In S.L. Groenwald, M.H. Frogge, M. Goodman, & C.H. Yarbro (eds). *Cancer Nursing: Principles and Practice*. Boston: Jones & Bartlett Publishers, pp. 284-306.

Jassak, P.F. & Ryan, M.P. (1989). Ethical issues in clinical research. *Semin Oncol Nurs 5*(2), 102-108.

Moldawer, N.P. (ed) (1989). The biotherapy of cancer. *Oncol Nurs Forum 15*(suppl 6), 2-40.

Oldham, R.K. (ed) (1987). *Principles of Cancer Biotherapy*. New York: Raven Press.

Oncology Nursing Society (1989). *Biological Response Modifiers: Guidelines and Recommendations for Nursing Practice*. Pittsburgh: Author.

Quesada, J.R., Talpaz, M., Rios, A., Kurzrock, R., & Gutterman, J.U. (1986). Clinical toxicity of interferons in cancer patients: a review. *J Clin Oncol 4*(2), 234-243.

Rieger, P.T. (1989). Infusing interleukin-2 and dopamine. *Oncol Nurs Forum 16*(2), 276.

Rieger, P.T. (1991). Biotherapy. In S. Otto (ed). *Oncology Nursing*. St. Louis: C.V. Mosby Co., pp. 318-348.

Rosenberg, S.A., Longo, D.L., & Lotze, M.T. (1989). Principles and applications of biologic therapy. In V.T. DeVita, Jr., S. Hellman, & S.A. Rosenberg (eds). *Cancer: Principles and Practice of Oncology* (3rd ed). Philadelphia: J.B. Lippincott Co., pp. 301-347.

Sherer, A. & Bohannon, P.A. (1989). Oncologic assessment tool. In C.E. Guzzetta, S.D. Bunton, L.A. Prinkey, A.P. Sherer, & P.C. Seifer (eds). *Clinical Assessment Tools for Use With Nursing Diagnoses*. St. Louis: C.V. Mosby Co., pp. 272-289.

Yasko, J.M. (ed) (1989). The biotherapy of cancer. *Oncol Nurs Forum 16*(suppl 6), 4-47.

Implications of Bone Marrow Transplantation for Nursing

Teresa Wilke, BA, BSN, RN, OCN

THEORY

I. Principles of bone marrow transplantation.
   A. Many malignancies exhibit a dose-related response to chemotherapy or radiation therapy; increasing the dose increases the number of cells that are destroyed.
      1. The dose of chemotherapy or radiation therapy that can be delivered is limited often by the degree of marrow toxicity.
      2. Bone marrow from either the client or compatible donor is infused and engrafts to "rescue" the marrow from the toxic effects of antineoplastic or radiation therapy.
      3. Therefore high doses of antineoplastic or radiation therapy may be administered and lethal marrow toxicity may be avoided.
   B. Process of bone marrow transplantation (Figure 24-1).
      1. Source of donor marrow is identified.
         a. Self—bone marrow biopsy done to determine if client is in remission or has metastatic cells in the marrow.
         b. Related or unrelated donor—histocompatibility testing done to determine if client and donor marrow are genetically compatible.
            (1) Human leukocyte antigen (HLA) testing—major histocompatibility complex encoded by genes (one from each parent) present on chromosome 6.
               (a) Major loci are HLA-A, HLA-B, HLA-C, HLA-D, and HLA-DR.
               (b) Results of allogeneic transplant are related to the degree of histocompatibility between the donor and the recipient.
               (c) Clients without an HLA-matched related donor have approximately a one in 30,000 chance of finding an HLA-matched unrelated volunteer donor from the National Bone Marrow Donor Registry.
            (2) Mixed lymphocyte culture testing–serum of recipient is mixed with lymphocytes of donor to measure the extent of reactivity against donor lymphocytes.
      2. Marrow recipient is prepared (Figures 24-2 and 24-3).
         a. Conditioning protocol established based on the primary disease and type of transplant.

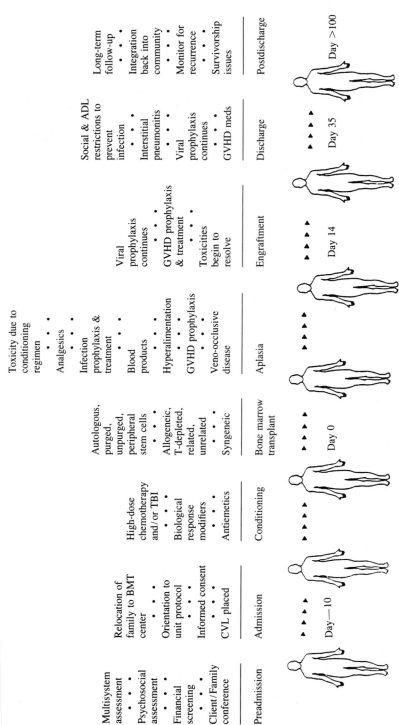

Figure 24-1 Usual Stages of the Transplant Process. *(Adapted from Ford, R., Eisenberg, S. Bone marrow transplant: Recent advances and nursing implications. Nursing Clinics of North America. 25[2]:406, 1990.)*

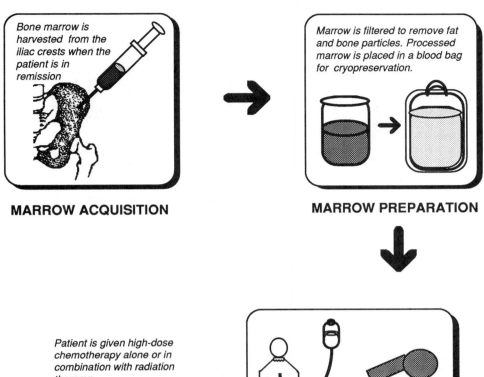

MARROW ACQUISITION

Bone marrow is harvested from the iliac crests when the patient is in remission

MARROW PREPARATION

Marrow is filtered to remove fat and bone particles. Processed marrow is placed in a blood bag for cryopreservation.

Patient is given high-dose chemotherapy alone or in combination with radiation therapy:

- *to kill remaining cancer cells,*
- *to suppress the immune system, and*
- *to open spaces within the marrow for donor marrow engraftment.*

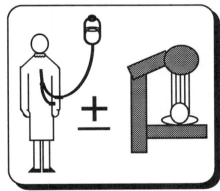

PREPARATION OF MARROW RECIPIENT

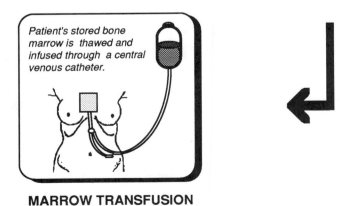

Patient's stored bone marrow is thawed and infused through a central venous catheter.

MARROW TRANSFUSION

Figure 24-2 Preparation of the recipient for an autologous bone marrow transplant.

Recipient is given high-dose chemotherapy alone or in combination with radiation therapy:

- *to kill remaining cancer cells,*
- *to suppress the immune system, and*
- *to open spaces within the marrow for donor marrow engraftment.*

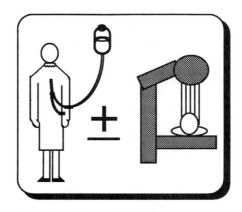

PREPARATION OF MARROW RECIPIENT

Bone marrow is harvested from the iliac crests of the donor.

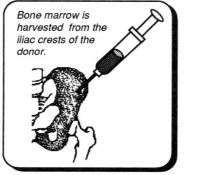
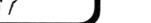

MARROW ACQUISITION

Bone marrow is filtered to remove fat and bone particles. Processed marrow is placed in a blood bag for transfusion.

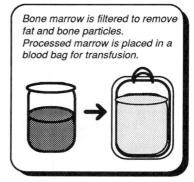

MARROW PREPARATION

Donor bone marrow is infused through a central venous catheter.

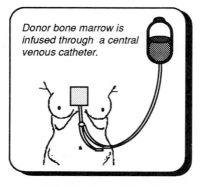
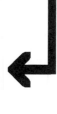

MARROW TRANSFUSION

Figure 24-3 Preparation of the recipient for an allogeneic bone marrow transplant.

      b. Goals of conditioning regimen are to:
        (1) Eradicate remaining malignancy in recipient.
        (2) Suppress the immune system of the recipient to allow for marrow engraftment.
        (3) Open spaces within the marrow compartment for donor marrow to engraft.
      c. Conditioning regimen may include high-dose chemotherapy alone or in combination with node-bearing or total body irradiation.
      d. Conditioning regimen is completed several days before marrow transplant.
   3. Marrow from donor is harvested and processed.
      a. Performed with client under general or regional anesthesia.
      b. Multiple incisions are made into the posterior iliac crests bilaterally.
        (1) Approximately 1 L of marrow is aspirated.
        (2) Marrow is filtered to remove bone particles and fat.
        (3) Processed marrow is placed in a blood administration bag for cryopreservation (autologous) or immediate infusion (allogeneic).
      c. If marrow harvesting is impossible, peripheral stem cells may be collected over a 5- to 10-day period by hemapheresis.
        (1) Cells are collected and cryopreserved.
        (2) When a sufficient number of cells are collected, the peripheral cells are thawed and infused into the recipient.
      d. If risk is high for recurrent disease from tumor cells in the transplanted marrow, the marrow may be purged.
        (1) Purging may be accomplished by antitumor monoclonal antibodies, chemotherapy, or other physical means.
        (2) Purging may increase the risk of prolonged time for engraftment.
   4. Marrow is infused through a central venous catheter.
      a. In autologous marrow transplant, marrow is brought to client's room, thawed, and infused over 4 to 6 hours.
      b. In allogeneic marrow transplant, freshly harvested marrow is brought to client's room and infused by intravenous push.
   5. Client is supported through period of pancytopenia (10 to 30 days), and preventive measures to decrease potential complications of bone marrow transplantation are instituted (Table 24-1).

II. Role of bone marrow transplantation in cancer care.
   A. Cure—each client is evaluated with curative intent.
   B. Palliation—some candidates will be treated to induce remission of disease.

III. Types of bone marrow transplants.
   A. Type of transplant is based on the source of donor marrow.
      1. Autologous—client receives own bone marrow that was harvested during remission or before treatment.
      2. Allogeneic—client receives bone marrow from another related or nonrelated donor.
      3. Syngeneic—client receives bone marrow from a genetically identical twin.
   B. Factors affecting source of donor marrow.
      1. Primary disease to be treated.
      2. Availability of a histocompatible donor.

DATA COLLECTION

I. Pertinent personal history.
   A. Diagnosis of leukemia, lymphoma, Hodgkin's disease, breast cancer, aplastic

Table 24-1
PREVENTIVE MEASURES FOR BONE MARROW TRANSPLANTATION–ASSOCIATED
COMPLICATIONS

Complication	Information
Graft-versus-host disease	Results from engraftment of immunocompetent donor T lymphocytes reacting against immunoincompetent recipient tissues (skin, gastrointestinal tract, and liver).
	Occurs in 30% to 60% of allogeneic bone marrow transplantation patients
	Can be either acute or chronic.
Pulmonary interstitial pneumonitis	Occurs more frequently in clients more than 30 yr old; with history of chest irradiation or bleomycin therapy; and cytomegalovirus (CMV) positive
	Causative agents
	CMV 50% *Pneumocystis carnii* 5%
	Idiopathic 30% Other 15%

anemia, neuroblastoma, multiple myeloma, thalassemia, or severe combined immunodeficiency disease.

B. High risk for recurrence of disease after standard therapy for a malignancy sensitive to either antineoplastic therapy or radiation therapy—breast cancer, small-cell carcinoma of the lung, Ewing's sarcoma, germ cell tumors of the testes, and glioblastoma multiforme.

C. Tumor refractory to standard doses of antineoplastic agents or radiation therapy.

D. Factors that may increase incidence of complications of marrow transplantation:
   1. Previous cancer therapy, length of time since last therapy, response to past therapy, and length of disease-free interval.
   2. Diagnosis of diseases of the kidney, lung, liver, or gastrointestinal tract.
   3. Patterns of bowel and bladder elimination.
   4. Previous infections and response to therapy.
   5. Age—older clients are more likely to develop transplant-related complications.

II. Physical examination.
   A. Pulmonary—respiratory rate, depth, and rhythm; lung expansion; adventitious breath sounds.
   B. Renal—color and odor of urine and urinary output.

Preventive Measures	Nursing Implications
T-cell depletion for non-identical human leukocyte antigen (HLA) donor marrow	Monitor for delayed marrow reconstitution.
Preventive immunosuppressive agents Cyclosporin A Methotrexate Monoclonal antibodies Immunotoxin	Monitor for prolonged lymphopenia and neutropenia. Evaluate cyclosporin levels and notify physician of significant abnormalities.
Therapeutic immunosuppressive agents Cyclosporin A High-dose steroids Antithymocyte globulin Azathioprine (Immuran) Thalidomide Monoclonal antibodies Immunotoxins Irradiate all blood products	Monitor for side effects of agents used for immunosuppression.
Use of CMV negative blood products in CMV negative patients with CMV negative donor marrow *Antimicrobial therapy* Gancyclovir Acyclovir Trimethoprim and sulfamethoxazole (Septra) Intravenous immunoglobulins	Monitor for side effects of antimicrobial therapy. Implement turn, cough, and deep breathe routine.

    C. Mobility—muscle strength and endurance; range of motion; gait; and activity level.

    D. Nutrition—weight, skin turgor; amount, content, and patterns of nutritional intake.

    E. Comfort level.

    F. Cardiovascular—heart rate and rhythm, blood pressure.

    G. Gastrointestinal—color, consistency, and caliber of stool.

    H. Integumentary—color and intactness of skin, condition of oral mucous membranes, dental evaluation, condition of perineum and rectum.

    I. Neurological—mental status, orientation, sensation, and reflexes.

III. Psychosocial examination.

    A. Psychological evaluation.

        1. Feelings on decision to have bone marrow transplantation.

        2. Understanding of aggressiveness of treatment, goals of therapy, and chances of survival.

        3. Number, type, and effectiveness of coping mechanisms used in past stressful situations by client and family members.

        4. Perceptions of client and family about isolation, prolonged hospitalization, living will, use of life-support technology, and potential death or survival.

B. Social evaluation.
  1. Previous roles and responsibilities within the family and community.
  2. Type, number, and history of use of support systems within the family and community.
  3. Financial status—employment, insurance coverage, and resources for daily living needs.
  4. Eligibility for community resources.

IV. Critical laboratory and diagnostic data unique to marrow transplantation.
  A. Hematological—complete blood count; differential; platelet count; coagulation studies; type and cross-match with marrow donor.
  B. Hepatic—lactic acid dehydrogenase (LDH) and bilirubin levels.
  C. Renal—electrolyte, blood urea nitrogen (BUN), and creatinine levels.
  D. Cardiovascular—electrocardiogram and cardiac ejection fraction.
  E. Pulmonary—chest x-ray examination, pulmonary function tests; arterial blood gas values.
  F. Immune—antibody titers for cytomegalovirus (CMV), herpes viruses, Epstein-Barr virus, toxoplasmosis, hepatitis B surface antigen, immunoglobulin levels, and anti-human T-cell lymphotropic virus III.

ASSOCIATED NURSING DIAGNOSES

I. Anxiety.

II. Potential for infection.

III. Alteration in comfort.

IV. Alteration in bowel elimination—diarrhea.

V. Diversional activity deficit.

VI. Alteration in growth and development.

NURSING PLANNING AND IMPLEMENTATION

I. Interventions to maximize safety for the client and family.
  A. Maintain aseptic techniques and level of protective isolation as identified by bone marrow transplantation program.
  B. Implement conditioning regimen as ordered by physician.
  C. Teach client and family strategies to decrease the risks of infection, bleeding, and injury during periods of pancytopenia following bone marrow transplantation.

II. Interventions to decrease the incidence and severity of complications unique to bone marrow transplantation.
  A. Anxiety.
    1. Assess changes in and perceived contributing factors to anxiety levels in client and family.
    2. Provide a thorough orientation to bone marrow transplantation unit and procedures in bone marrow transplantation.
    3. Implement strategies to encourage client and family to express concerns about bone marrow transplantation demands.
    4. Consult with occupational therapist to develop a plan for diversional activities during isolation.
    5. Teach new anxiety-relieving strategies as desired or needed by client and family.

B. Potential for infection (see Chapter 7).
   1. Notify physician of initial fever greater than 100.4° F or other symptoms of infection.
   2. Teach client and family strategies to decrease risk of endogenous infections:
      a. Meticulous hand washing (Table 24-2).

Table 24-2
CENTERS FOR DISEASE CONTROL RECOMMENDATIONS FOR HANDWASHING

Handwashing Indications

1. In the absence of a true emergency, personnel should *always* wash their hands
   a. **Before** performing invasive procedures
   b. **Before** taking care of particularly susceptible patients, such as those who are severely immunocompromised and newborns
   c. **Before** and **after** touching wounds, whether surgical, traumatic, or associated with an invasive device
   d. **After** situations during which microbial contamination of hands is likely to occur, especially those involving contact with mucous membranes, blood or body fluids, secretions, or excretions
   e. **After** touching inanimate sources that are likely to be contaminated with virulent or epidemiologically important microorganisms; these sources include urine-measuring devices or secretion-collection apparatuses
   f. **After** taking care of an infected patient or one who is likely to be colonized with microorganisms of special clinical or epidemiologic significance, for example, multiply-resistant bacteria
   g. **Between** contacts with different patients in high-risk units
2. Most routine, brief patient-care activities involving *direct* patient contact other than that discussed above (e.g., taking a blood pressure), do not require handwashing
3. Most routine hospital activities involving indirect patient contact (e.g., handing a patient medications, food, or other objects) do not require handwashing

Handwashing Technique

For routine handwashing, a vigorous rubbing together of all surfaces of lathered hands for at least 10 seconds, followed by thorough rinsing under a stream of water, is recommended

Handwashing with Plain Soap

1. Plain soap should be used for handwashing unless otherwise indicated
2. If bar soap is used, it should be kept on racks that allow drainage of water
3. If liquid soap is used, the dispenser should be replaced or cleaned and filled with fresh product when empty; liquids should not be added to a partially full dispenser

Handwashing with Antimicrobial-Containing Products (Health-Care Personnel Handwashes)

1. Antimicrobial handwashing products should be used for handwashing before personnel care for newborns and when otherwise indicated during their care, between patients in high-risk units, and before personnel take care of severely immunocompromised patients
2. Antimicrobial-containing products that do not require water for use, such as foams or rinses, can be used in areas where no sinks are available

Handwashing Facilities

1. Handwashing facilities should be conveniently located throughout the hospital
2. A sink should be located in or just outside every patient room; more than one sink per room may be necessary if a large room is used for several patients
3. Handwashing facilities should be located in or adjacent to rooms where diagnostic or invasive procedures that require handwashing are performed (e.g., cardiac, catheterization, bronchoscopy, sigmoidoscopy).

From the Centers for Disease Control (1985). *Guidelines: Nosocomial Infections in Handwashing and Hospital Environmental Control.* Washington, D.C.: Author.

      b. Routine oral and perineal care.

      c. Skin care.

   3. Teach client and family strategies to decrease risk of exogenous infections:

      a. Restrict visitors with suspected or known infections.

      b. Limit visitation of children.

      c. Place client on sterile or low bacteria diet.

      d. Avoid invasive procedures—peripheral intravenous catheters, catheterization, rectal examinations, or rectal temperatures.

   4. Administer prophylactic antibiotic therapy as ordered by physician.

      a. Nystatin for fungal infections.

      b. Trimethoprim-sulfamethoxazole (Septra) for prevention of *Pneumocystis carnii.*

      c. Acyclovir for prevention of herpes virus infection and CMV.

      d. Intravenous immunoglobulin for prevention of CMV.

      e. Oral nonabsorbable antibiotics for decontamination of the gastrointestinal tract.

   5. Perform routine surveillance cultures for bacteria, fungi, and viruses.

   6. Transfuse CMV-negative blood products for clients who are CMV negative and who have received CMV-negative marrow.

  C. Potential for injury (see Chapter 7).

   1. For clients receiving high-dose cyclophosphamide, hemorrhagic cystitis is a potential complication.

   2. Implement strategies to decrease risk of hemorrhagic cystitis:

      a. Administer continuous bladder irrigation as ordered by physician.

      b. If continuous irrigation is not ordered, push oral fluid intake and schedule voiding every 2 hours.

      c. Administer mesna, a uroprotective agent, as ordered by physician.

      d. Administer antispasmodics and analgesics as ordered by physician.

  D. Alteration in comfort related to keratitis (corneal irritation).

   1. Provide sunglasses and darken room to relieve discomfort from photophobia.

   2. Discourage client from rubbing eyes—use mittens.

   3. Administer artificial tears, steroid eye drops, and analgesics as ordered by physician.

   4. Encourage consultation with ophthalmologist.

  E. Altered oral mucous membrane (see Chapter 7).

III. Interventions to monitor for unique complications of bone marrow transplantation.

  A. Graft-versus-host disease (Table 24-3).

   1. Monitor condition of skin (erythema or rash) on palms of hands and soles of feet.

   2. Evaluate changes in liver function studies.

   3. Monitor amount, consistency, frequency, and color of stool.

  B. Hepatic veno-occlusive disease.

   1. Weigh client every day; notify physician of weight gain greater than 5 pounds.

   2. Monitor location of pain (right upper quadrant).

   3. Evaluate changes in mental status.

   4. Measure abdominal girth every day if other parameters indicate possible veno-occlusive disease.

  C. Pulmonary interstitial pneumonitis.

   1. Monitor temperature.

   2. Assess for presence of cough, chest pain, or adventitious breath sounds.

Table 24-3
STAGING OF GRAFT-VERSUS-HOST DISEASE

Stage	Skin	Liver	Gastrointestinal Tract
+	Maculopapular rash <25% of body surface	Bilirubin 2-3 mg/dl	>500-1000 ml diarrhea/day
+ +	Maculopapular rash 25% to 50% of body surface	Bilirubin >3-6 mg/dl	>1000-1500 ml diarrhea/day
+ + +	Generalized erythroderma	Bilirubin >6-15 mg/dl	>1500 ml diarrhea/day
+ + + + +	Generalized erythroderma with bullous formation and desquamation	Bilirubin >15 mg/dl	Severe abdominal pain with or without ileus

IV. Interventions to enhance adaptation and rehabilitation.
   A. Implement a program of range of motion and isometric exercises during isolation period.
   B. Initiate client/family teaching about care of central venous catheter early in course of hospitalization.
   C. Encourage client, donor, and significant others to express concerns related to transplant experience.
   D. Discuss potential changes in life-style and social interaction required immediately after discharge from the hospital.

EVALUATION OF CLIENT AND FAMILY OUTCOMES

   I. Describe the rationale for bone marrow transplantation.

   II. Participate in self-care strategies to decrease the risks and severity of predictable side effects of bone marrow transplantation.

   III. Describe recommended changes in self-care, life-style, and social interactions to minimize effects of bone marrow transplantation on health.

   IV. Discuss strategies to maintain valued roles and relationships during the transplant and post-transplant periods.

   V. List community resources available for assistance and support.

   VI. Discuss the rationale, schedule, and procedures required for continued follow-up after bone marrow transplantation.

BIBLIOGRAPHY

Berk, P.D., Popper, H., Krueger, G.R., Decter, J., Herzig, G., & Graw, R.G., Jr. (1979). Veno-occlusive disease of the liver after allogeneic bone marrow transplantation. Possible association with graft-versus-host disease. *Ann Intern Med 90*(2), 158-164.

Bortin, M.M., Horowitz, M.M., & Gale, R.P. (1988). Current status of bone marrow transplantation in humans: report from the International Bone Marrow Transplant Registry. *Nat Immun Cell Growth Regul 7*(5-6), 334-350.

Butturini, A. & Gale R.P. (1988). T-cell depletion in bone marrow transplantation for leukemia: current results and future directions. *Bone Marrow Transplant 3*(3), 185-192.

Butturini, A., Bortin, M.M., & Gale, R.P. (1987). Graft-versus-leukemia following bone marrow transplantation. *Bone Marrow Transplant 2*, 233-242.

Corcoran-Buchsel, P., & Parchem, C. (1988). Ambulatory care of the bone marrow transplant patient. *Semin Oncol Nurs 4*(1), 41-46.

Deeg, H.J. & Storb, R. (1986). Acute and chronic graft-versus-host disease: clinical manifestations, prophylaxis, and treatment. *J Nat Cancer Inst 76*, 1325-1328.

Durbin, M. (1988). Bone marrow transplantation: economic, ethical, and social issues. *Pediatrics 82*(5), 774-783.

Ford, R. & Ballard, B. (1988). Acute complications after bone marrow transplantation. *Semin Oncol Nurs, 4*(1), 15-24.

Ford, R. & Eisenberg, S. (1990). Bone marrow transplant: recent advances and nursing implications. *Nurs Clin North Am 25*(2), 405-422.

Ford, R.C. (1991). Bone marrow transplantation. In S.B. Baird, R. McCorkle, & M. Grant (eds). *Cancer Nursing: A Comprehensive Textbook*. Philadelphia: W.B. Saunders Co., pp. 385-406.

Freedman, S.E. (1988). An overview of bone marrow transplantation. *Semin Oncol Nurs 4*(1), 3-8.

Haberman, M.R. (1988). Psychosocial aspects of bone marrow transplantation. *Semin Oncol Nurs 4*(1), 55-59.

Hows, J., McKinnon, S., Brookes, P., Kaminski, E., Bidwell, J., Bradley, B., Batchelor, J., & Goldman, J. (1989). Matched unrelated donor transplantation. *Transplant Proc 21*(1), 2923-2925.

Hutchison, M.M. & Itoh, K. (1982). Nursing care of the patient undergoing bone marrow transplantation for acute leukemia. *Nurs Clin North Am 17*(4), 697-711.

Hutchison, M.M. & King, A.H. (1983). A nursing perspective on bone marrow transplantation. *Nurs Clin North Am 18*(3), 511-522.

Lindgren, P.S. (1983). The laminar air flow room: nursing practices and procedures. *Nurs Clin North Am 18*(3), 553-561.

McDonald, G.B., Sharma, P., Matthews, D.E., Shulman, H.M., & Thomas, E.D. (1984). Venoocclusive disease of the liver after bone marrow transplantation: diagnosis, incidence, and predisposing factors. *Hepatology 4*(1), 116-122.

Nims, J.W. & Strom, S. (1988). Late complications of bone marrow transplant recipients: nursing care issues. *Semin Oncol Nurs 4*(1), 47-54.

O'Quin, T. & Moravec, C. (1988). The critically ill bone marrow transplant patient. *Semin Oncol Nurs 4*(1), 25-30.

Patenaude A.F., Szymanski, L., & Rappeport, J. (1979). Psychological costs of bone marrow transplantation in children. *Am J Orthopsychiatry 49*(3), 409-422.

Paulin, T., Kingden, O., Wilsson, B., Lonnquist, B., & Gahrton, G. (1987). Variables predicting bacterial and fungal infections after allogeneic marrow engraftment. *Transplantation 43*(3), 393-398.

Ruggiero, M.R. (1988). The donor in bone marrow transplantation. *Semin Oncol Nurs 4*(1), 9-14.

Storb, R. (1987). Critical issues in bone marrow transplantation. *Transplant Proc 19*(1), 2774-2781.

Thomas, E.D. (1988). The future of marrow transplantation. *Semin Oncol Nurs 4*(1), 74-78.

Wikle, T. (1991). Cardiopulmonary complications of bone marrow transplantation. In M. Whedon (ed). *Bone Marrow Transplantation: Principles, Practice, and Nursing Insights*. Boston: Jones & Bartlett Publishers.

Wikle, T., Coyle, K., & Shapiro, D. (1990). Bone marrow transplant: today and tomorrow. *Am J Nurs 90*(5), 48-58.

Implications of Unproven Methods for Nursing

Nancy Kane, MS, RN, OCN

THEORY

I. Definition: methods that have not been shown active in tumor animal models or in acceptable clinical trials and yet are promoted as effective methods for the cure, palliation, and control of cancer.

II. Characteristics of unproven methods.
  A. Credentials of promoter.
    1. Lack of formal training in oncology.
    2. Alternative degrees such as chiropractor, naturalist, naprapathist.
    3. Meaningless letters after name.
  B. Lack of controlled studies.
    1. Report of experience in mass media, not scientific publications.
    2. Use of testimonials and anecdotal reports to market method.
    3. Disregard of nonresponders.
    4. Blame placed on client for treatment failures.
    5. Reproducible data not available.
  C. Classified information.
    1. "Cure" known only to promoter.
    2. Claims of conspiracy to keep cure from public.
    3. Poor record keeping.
  D. Marketed advantages of methods.
    1. Hope for a cure.
    2. Enhancement of personal control.
    3. Claims of treatment being harmless, painless, and nontoxic.
    4. Emphasis on providing a caring environment.

III. Classification of unproven methods.
  A. Nutritional approaches.
    1. Recommendations often contradictory to known nutritional needs of people with cancer.
    2. Emphasis on approaches of dietary manipulation and intestinal purification.
    3. Approach may include emphasis on vitamins, minerals, and enzymes.

4. Emphasis placed on a positive mental outlook and life-style changes.
5. Approach often discourages use of proven cancer therapies such as chemotherapy, radiation, or biotherapy.
6. Examples—Gerson's method and macrobiotic diet.
B. Psychological techniques.
1. Approach based on intense faith, promotion of hope, and increased personal control.
2. Examples—psychic surgery, Simonton method, and faith healing.
C. "Immune" therapy.
1. Purported to bolster the immune system.
2. Example—immune-augmentative treatment.
D. Drugs and chemicals.
1. Approach includes use of herbs, drugs, vaccines, and chemical preparations.
2. Based on unfounded concepts of carcinogenesis.
3. Examples—Kock and Hoxsey treatments, krebiozen, and Laetrile.
E. Machines and devices.
1. Devices used for both diagnosis and treatment.
2. Examples—oscillolast, and Hubbard E meter.

DATA COLLECTION

I. Pertinent personal history.
A. Education level—well educated more likely to seek unproven methods.
B. Socioeconomic status—middle to upper class more likely to seek unproven methods.
C. Phase of cancer trajectory—clients in whom cure or remission may be possible with standard therapies are more likely to seek unproven methods.

II. Psychosocial examination—perceptions of client/significant other about cancer and cancer treatment.
A. Fear of disease or poor prognosis.
B. Negative experiences with proven therapies and caregivers.
C. Misinformation.
D. Need for an increased level of emotional support, personal control, or caring from health professionals.
E. Feelings of helplessness or hopelessness.

ASSOCIATED NURSING DIAGNOSES

I. Knowledge deficit.

II. Hopelessness.

III. Fear.

NURSING PLANNING AND IMPLEMENTATION

I. Interventions to maximize client/family safety.
A. Encourage continuation of proven treatment plan.
B. Introduce enrollment in a legitimate clinical trial as an alternative to standard treatment.
C. Incorporate alternative support interventions such as relaxation, exercise, or nutrition.
D. Teach client/significant others critical side effects of the unproven method that should be reported to the health care team.

II. Interventions to include the client/significant other in care.
  A. Foster open communications with client/significant others.
    1. Clarify standard therapy options proposed.
    2. Use terminology that the client/significant other can understand.
    3. Maintain nonjudgmental, accepting attitude.
    4. Give client/significant other permission to ask questions about alternative therapies.
    5. Avoid guilt when a client or significant other inquires about unproven methods.
  B. Provide accurate information about unproven methods considered.
  C. Accept the right of the client/significant other to make personal decisions about care.

III. Interventions to educate the public about unproven methods.
  A. Support programs about advances in cancer treatment.
  B. Increase public awareness of dangers of unproven methods.
  C. Provide information to assist the public in identifying unproven methods.

EVALUATION OF CLIENT AND FAMILY OUTCOMES

  I. Describe criteria and methods used to evaluate the effectiveness of cancer therapies.

  II. List critical side effects of selected unproven methods to report to the health care team.

  III. Discuss alternatives to unproven methods.

BIBLIOGRAPHY

Cassileth, B. (1989). The social implications of questionable cancer therapies. *Cancer 63*(7), 1247-1250.

Cassileth, B. & Brown, H. (1988). Unorthodox cancer medicine. *CA 38*(3), 176-186.

Cassileth, B.R. & Kleinbart, J.M. (1991). Questionable cancer therapies. In S.B. Baird, R. McCorkle, & M. Grant (eds). *Cancer Nursing: A Comprehensive Textbook*. Philadelphia: W.B. Saunders Co., pp. 415-423.

Holland, J. (1981). Why patients seek unproven remedies: a psychological perspective. *Clin Bull 2*(11), 102-105.

Howard-Ruben, J. & Miller, N. (1984). Unproven methods of cancer management. II. Current trends and implications for patient care. *Oncol Nurs Forum 11*(1), 67-74.

Miller, N. & Howard-Ruben, J. (1984). Unproven methods of cancer management. I. Current trends and implications for patient care. *Oncol Nurs Forum 10*(4), 46-54.

Wojtalewicz-Friedberg, K., Flynn, B.A., Riley, M.B., Kelley, C.M., & Roth, E.L. (1991). Knowledge deficit related to unproven methods of cancer treatment. In J.C. McNally, E.T. Somerville, C. Miaskowski, & M. Rostad (eds). *Guidelines for Oncology Nursing Practice*. Philadelphia: W.B. Saunders Co., pp. 97-100.

Yarbro, C.H. (1990). Unproven methods of cancer treatment. In S.L. Groenwald, M.H. Frogge, M. Goodman, & C.H. Yarbro (eds). *Cancer Nursing: Principles and Practice*. Boston: Jones & Bartlett Publishers, pp. 1216-1227.

26

Nursing Implications of Supportive Therapies in Cancer Care

Lynn Erdman, MN, RN, OCN

Blood Component Therapy

THEORY

I. Use of blood component therapy in cancer care has increased with:
   A. Advancement of surgical oncology techniques.
   B. Use of more aggressive single and multimodality cancer therapy and resulting marrow suppression.
   C. Development of donor programs and hemapheresis technology.

II. Types of blood component therapy (Table 26-1).

III. Sources of blood components.
   A. Homologous blood—blood collected from donors for transfusion to another individual.
   B. Autologous blood—blood collected from the intended recipient:
      1. Self-donation usually made before elective surgery.
      2. Red blood cell salvage during surgery by use of automated "cell saver" device or manual suction equipment.
   C. Designated (directed) blood—blood collected from a donor designated by the intended recipient.

IV. Potential complications of blood component therapy.
   A. Allergic reactions.
   B. Febrile reactions.
   C. Hemolytic reactions.
   D. Bacterial contamination.
   E. Volume overload.
   F. Hypothermia.
   G. Air emboli.

DATA COLLECTION

I. All clients with a diagnosis of cancer may need some form of blood component therapy during the course of their illness.

374

Table 26-1
TYPES OF BLOOD COMPONENT THERAPY

Blood Component	Indications	Considerations
Whole blood	Replacement of blood volume Replacement of red blood cells	Contains plasma proteins to which client may develop sensitivity
Red blood cells (packed)	Replacement of red blood cells	
Platelet concentrates	Control or prevention of bleeding	Few red blood cells present; therefore ABO compatibility not required
Granulocytes	Treat infections unresponsive to conventional antibiotics	Long-term therapeutic benefit questionable
Fresh frozen plasma	Increase the level of clotting factors in client with a demonstrated deficiency	Plasma compatibility preferred If thawed, must be transfused within 24 hr
Cryoprecipitate	Increase levels of factors VIII and XIII, fibrinogen, and von Willebrand's factor	Plasma compatibility preferred If thawed, must be transfused within 6 hr If pooled, must be transfused within 4 hr
Coagulation factor concentrates	Increase levels of factors VIII and IX	Monitor factor assays at regular intervals
Colloid solutions	Expand blood volume	ABO compatibility not required
Immune serum globulins	Provide passive immune protection or treat hypogammaglobulinemia	Avoid transfusion for client with allergic reactions to plasma Intramuscular injections may be painful and irritating

II. Factors that increase the likelihood that blood component therapy will be needed:
   A. Cancer treatment—surgery, radiation therapy, and chemotherapy.
   B. Cancer that has invaded the bone marrow.
   C. Drugs that suppress bone marrow production such as chloramphenicol.
   D. Chronic infection.
   E. Aging.
   F. Malnutrition.
   G. Stress.

III. Physical assessment (see Chapter 7, discussion on thrombocytopenia, anemia, and neutropenia).

IV. Evaluation of laboratory data.
   A. ABO type.
   B. Hemoglobin—less than 9 g/dl.
   C. Platelet count:
      1. Less than 10,000/mm^3, with or without active bleeding.
      2. Less than 20,000/mm^3, with active bleeding.
      3. Less than 50,000/mm^3 and scheduled for surgical procedure.
   D. Neutrophils—less than 500/mm^3, with an infection unresponsive to antibiotic therapy.

ASSOCIATED NURSING DIAGNOSES

I. Fluid volume excess.

II. Hyperthermia.

NURSING PLANNING AND IMPLEMENTATION

I. Implement strategies to maximize client safety.
   A. Obtain blood component according to institutional protocol.
   B. Check blood component type with physician order.
   C. Check blood component type and identification numbers with another registered nurse.
   D. Compare blood component identification information with client identification information before administration.
   E. Examine blood product for clots, bubbles, and discoloration.
   F. Never add medications to blood products.

II. Implement interventions to decrease incidence and severity of side effects.
   A. Premedicate client with antipyretic and antihistamine as ordered by physician.
   B. Attach appropriate filter and/or blood component set to the blood product.
   C. Use 19-gauge or larger needle for infusion.
   D. Infuse component over time, according to institutional guidelines.
      1. Red blood cells—infuse slowly over initial 15 minutes then remainder over 1 to 2 hours per unit.
      2. Platelets—infuse 8 units of random donor platelets over 30 to 60 minutes.
      3. Granulocytes—infuse slowly over 2 to 4 hours.
   E. Observe for signs and symptoms of transfusion reactions.
      1. When a reaction occurs:
         a. Stop transfusion and keep intravenous line open with normal saline solution.
         b. Report reaction to the physician and the transfusion service or blood bank.
         c. Check identifying tags and numbers on the blood component at the bedside.
         d. Treat symptoms noted as ordered by the physician.
         e. Monitor vital signs.
         f. Send blood bag and attached administration set and labels to the transfusion service or blood bank.
         g. Collect blood and urine samples and send to laboratory.
      2. Document transfusion reaction:
         a. Date and time noted.
         b. Signs and symptoms observed.
         c. Actions taken.
         d. Response of client after transfusion discontinued.

III. Implement strategies to monitor for complications of blood component therapy.
   A. General—fever, chills, muscle aches and pain, back pain, chest pain, headache, and heat at site of infusion or along vessel.
   B. Respiratory—shortness of breath, tachypnea, apnea, cough, wheezing, and rales.
   C. Cardiovascular—bradycardia or tachycardia, hypotension or hypertension, facial flushing, cyanosis of extremities, cool, clammy skin, distended neck veins, and edema.
   D. Integumentary—rash, hives, swelling, itching, and diaphoresis.
   E. Gastrointestinal—nausea, vomiting, abdominal cramping and pain, and diarrhea.
   F. Renal—dark, concentrated, red- to brown-colored urine.

IV. Implement interventions to incorporate client and family into care.
   A. Teach client and family the purpose of the transfusion.
   B. Teach client and family the signs and symptoms of transfusion reaction to report to team.

 V. Implement measures to monitor for response to blood component therapy.
   A. Assess changes in laboratory values.
   B. Monitor changes in subjective responses of clients to blood component therapy.

EVALUATION OF CLIENT AND FAMILY OUTCOMES

 I. Describe personal risk factors for blood component therapy.

 II. Discuss the rationale for blood component therapy.

III. List signs and symptoms of reactions to blood component therapy that should be reported to the health care team.

IV. Describe community resources available to meet blood component therapy needs—American Red Cross, pheresis services, and blood banks.

Antimicrobial Therapy

THEORY

 I. Infections are a major complication of cancer and cancer therapy.
   A. Infections are the most common cause of death in persons with cancer.
   B. Sixty-five percent of clients with leukemia or lymphoma will die as a result of infectious complications.
   C. Forty percent of clients with solid tumors will die as a result of infectious complications.
   D. As a result of changes in immune functions, many of the usual signs and symptoms of infection are absent in the client diagnosed with cancer or receiving cancer treatment.

 II. Types of antimicrobial therapy (Table 26-2).

III. Principles of medical management.
   A. At the first sign of temperature greater than 100.4° F, a fever workup is initiated:
      1. Physical examination.
      2. Blood cultures.
      3. Central venous catheter or port cultures.
      4. Urine culture.
      5. Chest x-ray examination.
   B. Initiation of empiric antimicrobial therapy.
      1. Selection of antibiotics based on:
         a. Coverage for common infectious organisms among persons with cancer.
         b. Prevalence rates for microorganisms and the patterns of resistance within the institution.
      2. Most regimens include an antipseudomonal penicillin, an aminoglycoside, and a first- or third-generation cephalosporin.
      3. Intravenous doses and schedules are designed to provide bactericidal serum levels for as long as possible between each dose interval.
      4. Duration of treatment is sufficient for the resolution of the fever without exposure to unnecessary side effects of the agents.
         a. Negative cultures—if no organisms were isolated, treatment continues for a minimum of 7 days.

Text continued on p 384

Table 26-2
TYPES OF ANTIBIOTIC THERAPY

Antimicrobial Agent	Indications
Penicillins	
Penicillin G	*Streptococcus pneumoniae, S. pyogenes, S. viridens, S. bovis, Neisseria,* and most anaerobes
Methicillin sodium	*Staphylococcus aureus* and streptococci
Nafcillin sodium	
Oxacillin sodium	
Ampicillin	*Streptococcus fecalis, Listeria monocytogenes, Haemophilus, Escherichia coli, Salmonella,* and *Proteus*
Carbenicillin disodium	*Pseudomonas aeruginosa, Enterobacter, Proteus, Serratia* serraha, *Acinetobacter,* and *Providencia*
Ticarcillin	Anaerobes
Mezlocillin sodium	*Pseudomonas aeruginosa, Enterobacter, Proteus, Serratia* serraha, *Acinetobacter, Providencia, Klebsiella* spp.
Piperacillin sodium	Plus increased activity against *P. aeruginosa*
Azlocillin	Same as piperacillin
Cephalosporins	
First generation	
Cephalothin sodium	*E. coli, Klebsiella, Proteus, Haemophilus, S. aureus, Staphylococcus epidermidis,* streptococci
Cefazolin sodium	*Similar to cephalothin but more active against Klebsiella and E. coli*
Second generation	
Cephamandole	Most active against *Haemophilus, Klebsiella, E. coli, Enterobacter* spp., *Proteus,* and less active against gram-positive cocci
Cefoxitin sodium	Same as cephalotin plus *Proteus* spp. and anaerobes
Third generation	
Cefotaxime sodium	Same as cephalotin plus *Enterobacter* spp., *Proteus, H. influenzae, Citrobacter* spp., *Serratia* spp., and some *P. aeruginosa* and *Bacteroides* spp.
Moxalactam disodium	Same as cefotaxime but better anaerobe coverage

Potential Side Effects of Group	Nursing Interventions
Dizziness, neuromuscular hyperirritability, seizures, decreased sense of taste and smell, stomatitis, flatulence, diarrhea, pancytopenia, hypokalemia, and changes in liver and kidney function studies ↓ Nausea and vomiting Hypokalemia │ │ │ │ │ ↓ Prolonged bleeding	Monitor for neurological changes at regular intervals. Provide safety measures for client with dizziness. Evaluate the effect of changes in taste and smell, nausea, and stomatitis on nutritional intake. Implement strategies to control flatulence and diarrhea. Evaluate the effect of diarrhea on perineal skin and rectum. Evaluate laboratory studies as ordered by physician. Monitor volume, patterns, and character of urinary output. Monitor sites of invasive procedures for bleeding. Assess client for signs and symptoms of internal or external bleeding. Evaluate coagulation laboratory studies as ordered by physician.
Dizziness, vertigo, headache, nausea, vomiting, diarrhea, anorexia, abdominal cramping, pancytopenia, changes in SGOT, changes in SGPT, changes in alkaline phosphatase, changes in BUN and creatinine clearance, oliguria │ │ │ │ ↓ Hypersensitivity	Monitor for neurological changes at regular intervals. Provide safety measures for client experiencing dizziness and vertigo. Evaluate laboratory studies as ordered by physician. Monitor food and fluid intake and output. Evaluate effect of diarrhea on perineal skin and rectum. Monitor urinary output. Implement strategies to control pain, nausea, and diarrhea. See Chapter 7, discussion on thrombocytopenia, leukopenia, and anemia. Monitor for signs and symptoms of hypersensitivity reactions—respiratory status, itching, hives, fever, pain, changes in pulse rate, decrease in blood pressure, decrease in urinary output.
Transient leukopenia and thrombocytopenia Phlebitis Bleeding reactions	 Assess local reactions at site of infusion—pain, swelling, and redness. See Chapter 7, discussion on thrombocytopenia.

Table continued on following page

Table 26-2
TYPES OF ANTIBIOTIC THERAPY *Continued*

Antimicrobial Agent	Indications
Aminoglycosides	
Gentamicin sulfate	*P. aeruginosa*, Enterobacteriaceae, and enterococcus
Tobramycin sulfate	Similar to gentamicin except not as active against enterococcus
Amikacin sulfate	*Serratia, Proteus, Pseudomonas*, Enterobacteriaceae, and *Providencia*
Antifungals	
Amphotericin B	*Candida, Aspergillus*, Zygomycetes, *Torulopsis, Cryptococcus*, and *Histoplasma*
Flucytosine	*Cryptococcus, Candida, Torulopsis*, chromomycosis
Clotrimazole	*Candida* spp.
Miconazole nitrate	*Candida* spp., *Aspergillus* spp., Zygomycetes, *Torulopsis, Cryptococcus*, Petielldium, *Blastomyces, Histoplasma, Coccidioides*, Paracoccidiodes, *Sprorothrix*
Ketoconazole	Similar to miconazole

Potential Side Effects of Group	Nursing Interventions
Hearing loss, loss of balance, high-frequency deafness, peripheral neuritis, numbness, tingling of skin.	Evaluate neurological status before initiation of therapy. Assess hearing status before therapy.
Granulocytopenia, anema, thrombocytopenia purpura	See Chapter 7.
Proteinuria, changes in BUN, oliguria	Monitor urinary output. Evaluate laboratory studies as ordered by physician.
Changes in SGOT, SGPT, and LDH, pancytopenia, nausea, vomiting, headache, fever, lethargy	Implement measures to increase comfort. Monitor amount and type of fluid and food intake. Monitor amount and character of emesis output. Assist with activities of daily living as needed. Monitor for signs and symptoms of bleeding or infection.
Drowsiness, headache, unsteady gait, paresthesias, tremors	Provide assistance with activities of daily living and ambulation as needed. Teach client and family about use of assistive aids for ambulation.
Hypotension, tachycardia	Monitor blood pressure and pulse rate at regular intervals.
Oliguria, hematuria, thirst	Monitor amount and character of urinary output.
Ringing or buzzing in ears, high-frequency hearing loss	Assess levels of hearing before and periodically during treatment.
Bleeding reactions	Monitor for signs and symptoms of bleeding.
Fever, headache, sedation, weakness, paresthesia, flushing, arrhythmias, hypotension/hypertension, tinnitus, hearing loss, vertigo, nausea, vomiting, diarrhea, coagulation deficits, electrolyte imbalances (decreased potassium, magnesium, sodium), pancytopenia, and hepatic dysfunction	Monitor temperature, blood pressure, and pulse at regular intervals. Evaluate changes in sensory perception over time. Assess effect of vertigo, nausea, diarrhea, and neurological changes on ability to accomplish activities of daily living. Monitor changes in laboratory studies as ordered by physician. Assess client for signs and symptoms of electrolyte changes. See Chapter 7, discussion on thrombocytopenia, leukopenia, and anemia.
Erythema, stinging, blistering, peeling, edema, and pruritus with topical application	Evaluate condition of skin before initiation of treatment. Implement strategies to minimize symptoms of local skin reactions (see Chapter 7).
Gynecomastia and adrenal insufficiency	Monitor for signs of adrenal insufficiency—weakness, fever, abdominal pain, nausea, vomiting, diarrhea, decreased blood pressure, headache, and confusion. Assess changes in volume of breast tissue.

Table continued on following page

Table 26-2
TYPES OF ANTIBIOTIC THERAPY *Continued*

Antimicrobial Agent	Indications
Antivirals	
Vidarabine	Herpes simplex virus and varicella zoster virus
Acyclovir	Herpes simplex virus and varicella zoster virus
Interferons (alpha, beta, and gamma)	Herpes simplex virus and varicella zoster virus
Miscellaneous	
Chloramphenicol	*Haemophilus, Bacteroides fragilis, S. pneumonia, Neisseria, Salmonella, Klebsiella, Rickettsia,* and most anaerobes
Erythromycin	*Legionella* and *Mycoplasma*
Clindamycin	*B. fragilis,* clostridia, *S. pneumoniae, S. viridans, S. pyogenes,* and *S. aureus*
Vancomycin	*C. difficile, S. aureus, S. epidermidis, S. fecalis,* corynebacteria, and *S. bovis*
Trimethoprim-sulfamethoxazole	*P. carinii, S. aureus, S. pneumoniae, S. pyogenes, Salmonella, Listeria, E. coli, Proteus, Serratia, Haemophilus,* and *Neisseria*

SGOT, serum glumatic-oxaloacetic transaminase; SGPT, serum glutamate pyruvate transaminase; BUN, blood urea nitrogen; LDH, lactate dehydrogenase.
Modified from Pizzo, P.A. & Young, R.C. (1985). Infections in the cancer patient. In V.T. DeVita, Jr., S. Hellman, & S.A. Rosenberg (eds). *Cancer: Principles & Practice of Oncology,* vol 2 (2nd ed). Philadelphia: J.B. Lippincott Co., pp. 1969-1971.

Potential Side Effects of Group	Nursing Interventions
Anorexia, nausea, vomiting, diarrhea, myelosuppression, hallucinations, confusion, psychosis, dizziness, and metabolic encephalopathy	Assess nutritional intake. Monitor fluid intake and output. Evaluate effect of diarrhea on perineal skin and rectum. Provide safety measures for clients with neurological changes. Evaluate laboratory studies as ordered by physician.
Renal toxicity and neurotoxicity	Monitor flow rate for infusion and maintain hydration. Monitor blood pressure, pulse rate, and respiratory rate.
Local pain, fever, alopecia, fatigue, anorexia, and myelosuppression	Assess local reactions at site of infusion. Evaluate effect of fatigue on activities of daily living.
Headache, depression, confusion Nausea, vomiting, diarrhea, perianal irritation, stomatitis, xerostomia, abdominal distention, blotching skin, cyanosis, hypothermia, and bone marrow depression	Monitor for neurological changes at regular intervals. Provide safety measures if confusion is present. Encourage consultation with psychiatrist for evaluation of depression. Monitor food and fluid intake and output. Evaluate pulmonary status at least each shift—respiratory rate, effort. Assess rectal area for irritation. Teach perianal hygiene and protective measures. Monitor for signs and symptoms of bleeding or infection.
Abdominal cramping and distention, diarrhea, and phlebitis	Assess volume and character of stool. Encourage client to exercise in hallway, room, or bed.
Diarrhea, abdominal pain, bloating, nausea, vomiting, decreased taste, neutropenia, thrombophlebitis, jaundice, and abnormal liver function studies	Assess skin every day for changes in integrity, color, or texture. Evaluate liver function studies as ordered by physician.
Anaphylaxis, vertigo, dizziness, phlebitis, tinnitus, ototoxicity, increased BUN and creatinine, suprainfection	Provide for environmental safety with dizziness. Monitor client responses to changes in hearing. Evaluate renal function studies as ordered by physician.
Myelosuppression	Monitor signs and symptoms of infection or bleeding.

   b. Afebrile for 3 days.

   c. Neutrophil count greater than 500 cells/mm^3.

  5. If fever is unresponsive to initial antibiotic therapy, the risk of nonbacterial cause, infectious organism resistant to antimicrobial, inadequate serum and tissue levels of antimicrobial, or drug fever should be considered.

   a. Continue current antimicrobials if clinical condition is unchanged and evaluation reveals no new information.

   b. Change antimicrobial program if evidence of progressive disease is present.

   c. Add amphotericin B to the antimicrobial program.

    (1) One third of febrile neutropenic clients who do not respond to 1 week of antimicrobial therapy have a systemic fungal infection.

    (2) Most common organisms include *Candida* or *Aspergillus*.

 IV. Potential complications of antimicrobial therapy.

  A. Suprainfection.

  B. Renal toxicity—nephritis and electrolyte imbalances.

  C. Hematological—bleeding, neutropenia, and anemia.

  D. Hepatotoxicity.

  E. Cardiovascular—phlebitis, hypotension, and arrhythmias.

  F. Gastrointestinal—nausea, vomiting, anorexia, and colitis.

  G. Neurotoxicity.

DATA COLLECTION

 I. Identification of clients at risk.

  A. Disruption of primary barriers to organisms.

   1. Surgical disruption of skin.

   2. Extravasation of vesicant antineoplastic agents.

   3. Stomatitis.

   4. Rectal fissures.

   5. Burns.

  B. Alteration in phagocytic defenses.

   1. Neutropenia with granulocyte count less than 1000/mm^3.

   2. Length of time client has been neutropenic.

   3. Steroid use.

   4. Previous antibiotic therapy.

  C. Concurrent disease states.

   1. Diabetes.

   2. Renal disease.

   3. Liver disease.

   4. Stress.

  D. Tumor necrosis and invasion.

  E. Previous cancer therapy.

  F. History of drug allergies.

 II. Physical examination.

  A. Integumentary—rash, ulceration, redness, swelling, and warmth.

  B. Vital signs—temperature, blood pressure, pulse, and respirations.

  C. Pulmonary—respiratory rate, rhythm, effort, and presence of adventitious sounds.

  D. Renal—character of urine and urinary output.

  E. Neuromuscular—mental status.

III. Evaluation of laboratory data.
   A. Blood cultures.
   B. Chest x-ray examination.
   C. Complete blood count with differential.

NURSING PLANNING AND IMPLEMENTATION

   I. Implement strategies to maximize client safety (see Chapter 7).

   II. Implement interventions to decrease the incidence and severity of side effects of antimicrobial therapy (Table 26-2).

   III. Implement strategies to monitor for complications of antimicrobial therapy (Table 26-2).

   IV. Implement measures to monitor for response to antimicrobial therapy.
   A. Monitor temperature, pulse, respirations, and blood pressure.
   B. Evaluate subjective complaints of client.
   C. Assess changes in laboratory values.

EVALUATION OF PATIENT AND FAMILY OUTCOMES

   I. Describe personal risk factors for infection.

   II. Discuss the rationale for immediate evaluation of fever.

   III. List signs and symptoms of side effects of antimicrobial therapy to report to the health care team.

Nutritional Support Therapy

THEORY

   I. Nutritional complications are observed frequently in clients with a diagnosis of cancer.
   A. Effects of malignant tumors.
      1. Cancer cells compete with normal cells for nutrients needed for cellular division and growth. Although the exact demands of the tumor on the host are unknown, the following metabolic changes are proposed:
         a. Alteration in carbohydrate metabolism—glucose is mobilized for energy and results in glucose intolerance in selected clients.
         b. Alteration in protein metabolism—muscle tissue is mobilized to meet increased metabolic demands and results in muscle wasting.
         c. Alteration in fat metabolism—fat is mobilized as an energy source and results in depletion of fat stores.
      2. Cancer cells also produce biochemical substances that affect the desire for food.
      3. Malignant tumors may invade or compress structures and organs vital to the ingestion, digestion, and elimination of food and fluids.
         a. Fistular formation.
         b. Obstruction.
   B. Effects of cancer treatment.
      1. Structural changes in the gastrointestinal system may result from surgery and result in:
         a. Inability to feed oneself.
         b. Inability to masticate or swallow.
         c. Inability to move food through the stomach and bowel.

       d. Bowel diversion.

   2. Functional changes may occur as a result of surgery, radiation therapy, or chemotherapy and result in:

       a. Malabsorption of fat.

       b. Gastric hypersecretion.

       c. Water and electrolyte loss.

       d. Dumping syndrome.

       e. Xerostomia.

       f. Early satiety.

       g. Changes in taste and smell.

   3. Metabolic changes may occur as a result of treatment or side effects of treatment such as increased energy demands that result from fever, stress, diarrhea, vomiting, and cell division or destruction.

II. Principles of medical management.

   A. Controversy exists about the use of nutritional support for long-term management in clients with cancer.

     1. Nutritional support encourages tumor growth.

     2. Beneficial effects of nutritional support are temporary.

   B. Goals of nutritional therapy should be established.

     1. Increase weight.

     2. Maintain weight.

     3. Maintain fluid and electrolyte balance.

     4. Improve sense of well-being.

     5. Prolong life.

   C. Selection of type of nutritional therapy (enteral or parenteral) depends on:

     1. Function of gastrointestinal tract.

     2. Severity of nutritional problem.

     3. Ability of client to masticate and swallow.

     4. Length of proposed therapy and prognosis.

     5. Community resources for management at home.

     6. Cost.

   D. Type of nutritional support.

     1. Enteral therapy—provision of nutritional replacement through the gastrointestinal tract through an entry other than the mouth such as a gastrostomy or jejunostomy tube.

       a. Indicated if the need for nutritional support is anticipated for more than 1 month and attempts at oral intake have been unsuccessful.

       b. Requires surgical placement of feeding tube.

       c. Potential complications of enteral tube placement and feedings are included in Table 26-3.

     2. Parenteral therapy—provision of feeding through an intravenous route when the gastrointestinal tract cannot be used for nutritional replacement.

       a. Requires placement of a central venous line.

       b. Potential mechanical, metabolic, and infectious complications of parenteral therapy are presented in Table 26-4.

DATA COLLECTION

I. Nutritional assessment includes an evaluation of the desire and ability of the client to ingest and process nutritional products.

   A. Ingestion.

Table 26-3
POTENTIAL COMPLICATIONS OF ENTERAL TUBE PLACEMENT AND FEEDINGS

Complication	Nursing Interventions
Nasogastric	

Malpositioned tube	Verify proper placement via chest x-ray examination.
	Check placement each time before using by:
	    Aspirating gastric contents.
	    Observing for air bubbles by placing distal end of tube in water.
	Tape tube securely to nose.

Aspiration	Give bolus feeding rather than continuous feeding. Administer no more than 350-400 ml over 20 min every 3-4 hr while client is awake. Administer initial volume of 240 ml. Keep head of bed elevated 30 degrees during and 1 hr after infusion.
Contaminated equipment, clogged tube	Change feeding bag and tubing daily. Flush nasogastric tube with 30 ml of water or cranberry juice after each feeding. If tube is clogged, flush with 30 ml cranberry juice and ¼ teaspoon meat tenderizer.
Abdominal distention, vomiting, cramping, diarrhea	Regulate infusion accurately over 20 min. Give formula at room temperature; may need to decrease volume of formula given.
Nasoduodenal	
Aspiration	(Decreased risk of occurrence since tube is in the small bowel.) Give continuous rather than bolus feeding. Small bowel is sensitive to osmolarity; therefore administer at initial rate of 30-50 ml/hr for isotonic formula and increase by 25 ml/hr every 12 hr until desired volume is reached.
Contaminated equipment	Do not allow amount of formula in bag to exceed what can be administered in 8 hr. Change entire administration set every 24 hr.

Modified from Gordon A. (1987). Nutrition. In C. Ziegfeld (ed). *Core Curriculum for Oncology Nursing*. Philadelphia: W.B. Saunders Co., p. 253.

    1. Desire to eat.
    2. Patterns of dietary intake.
    3. Ability of client to prepare food and feed self.
    4. Food allergies and preferences.
    5. Dentation.
    6. Ability of client to moisten, chew, and swallow nutrients.
  B. Digestion.
  C. Metabolism.
    1. Presence of abnormal carbohydrate, fat, or protein metabolism.
    2. Presence of vitamin and mineral deficiencies.
    3. Presence of abnormal glucose metabolism.
  D. Excretion.

Table 26-4
POTENTIAL COMPLICATIONS OF PARENTERAL THERAPY

Complication	Nursing Interventions
Technical or Mechanical	
Pneumothorax	(May occur during insertion of subclavian catheter.) Observe client during insertion for chest pain, dyspnea, cyanosis. Obtain chest x-ray examination after insertion to verify placement. Verify blood return before connecting intravenous (IV) tubing to catheter. Administer D_5W solution at 30 ml/hr until chest x-ray examination confirms placement.
Arterial puncture	(May occur during insertion.) Observe for bright red blood pulsating from catheter. (Client may complain of pain at site.) Apply pressure to site for 15 minutes.
Malpositioned catheter	Monitor catheter for migration from the superior vena cava to another vein. Note client complaint of neck and shoulder pain, swelling in the surrounding area.
Clotted catheter	Note if unable to infuse solution through catheter and unable to obtain blood return. "Declot" catheter following institutional or agency procedure. Infuse $D_{10}W$ solution peripherally at the same rate as total parenteral nutrition (TPN) to prevent hypoglycemia.
Fluid overload	Regulate infusion on a volumetric pump for accuracy. Place a time tape on infusion, checking volume infused every hour. Obtain daily weights.
Air emboli	Secure all IV tubing connections with tape to prevent disconnection. If air emboli are suspected, clamp tubing immediately and place client on left side in Trendelenburg position.

    1. Bowel elimination patterns.
    2. Urinary elimination patterns.
    3. Characteristics of urine and stool.

II. Nutritional assessment includes evaluation of the effects of dietary intake on the person.
    A. Physical assessment.
        1. Skin turgor.
        2. Weight in comparison to ideal body weight.
        3. Muscle mass as measured by the mid-arm circumference.
        4. Fat stores as measured by triceps skin fold thickness.
    B. Evaluation of laboratory data.
        1. Serum albumin, total protein, and serum transferrin to assess protein stores.
        2. Nitrogen balance to assess energy balance.
        3. Creatinine height index to assess protein stores.
        4. Hemoglobin and hematocrit levels.
        5. Electrolyte levels.

Table 26-4
POTENTIAL COMPLICATIONS OF PARENTERAL THERAPY *Continued*

Complication	Nursing Interventions
Metabolic	
Hyperglycemia	Increase rate of infusion gradually. Check urine for sugar and acetone every 6 hr. Monitor serum glucose levels daily.
Hypoglycemia	Observe for signs and symptoms of hypoglycemia. Monitor serum glucose levels. If sudden cessation of TPN occurs, infuse $D_{10}W$ solution peripherally at same rate as TPN. Per physician's order, administer 50 ml of 50% dextrose intravenously.
Infections	
Contaminated solution	Do not leave solution unrefrigerated for longer than 4 hr. Check each bottle before and during infusion for color and clarity of solution.
Contaminated equipment	Change all IV tubing per institutional/agency procedure, using aseptic technique. Do not interrupt TPN for other infusions or blood collecting.
Local site infection	Change dressing, using aseptic technique, and following institutional procedure. Observe site for redness, tenderness, swelling, and exudate.
Fever	Monitor vital signs every 4 hr. Obtain both peripheral and central line blood cultures to identify source of infection.

Modified from Gordon, A. (1987). Nutrition. In C. Ziegfeld (ed). *Core Curriculum for Oncology Nursing.* Philadelphia: W.B. Saunders Co., p. 253.

ASSOCIATED NURSING DIAGNOSES

  I. Altered nutrition: less than body requirements.

 II. Fluid volume deficit.

III. Impaired swallowing.

IV. Self-care deficit: feeding.

 V. Anxiety.

NURSING PLANNING AND IMPLEMENTATION

  I. Implement strategies to maximize client safety.
   A. Administer nutritional therapy according to institutional protocol.
   B. Examine nutritional supplement for abnormalities in color or clarity.
   C. Check expiration date on nutritional supplement.
   D. Confirm placement of feeding tube or catheter before administering nutritional supplement.

 II. Implement interventions to decrease the incidence and severity of side effects of nutritional therapy (see Table 26-4).

III. Implement strategies to monitor for complications of nutritional therapy.
   A. Infection—fever and redness, swelling, pus, or pain along feeding tube, catheter tract, or exit site.

B. Respiratory complications—chest pain, dyspnea, cough, or cyanosis.
C. Fluid overload—weight gain, edema, shortness of breath, and distended neck veins.
D. Hyperglycemia—glucose monitoring every 6 hours and pattern of urinary elimination.
E. Gastrointestinal—character of stool, bloating, and pattern of bowel elimination.
F. Electrolyte abnormalities—changes in mental status, weakness, fatigue, and changes in neurological examination (restlessness and agitation).

IV. Implement interventions to incorporate client and family into care.
A. Teach client and family self-care procedures needed to manage the feeding tube or catheter.
B. Teach client and family signs and symptoms of complications of nutritional therapy.
C. Encourage participation of client and family in decision making about nutritional therapy.

EVALUATION OF CLIENT AND FAMILY OUTCOMES

I. Describe personal risk factors for malnutrition.

II. Participate in decision making about goals and methods of nutritional support.

III. List signs and symptoms of complications of nutritional support to report to the health care team—fever, diarrhea, changes in mental status, changes in urinary output, rapid weight gain, and signs of infection around feeding tube or catheter exit sites.

IV. Identify community resources available for management of nutritional support outside the acute care setting.

BIBLIOGRAPHY

Bodey, G.P. (1989). Evolution of antibiotic therapy for infection in neutropenic patients: studies at M.D. Anderson Hospital. *Rev Infect Dis 11*(suppl 7), S1582-S1590.
Burt, M.E., Gorschboth, C.M., & Brennan, M.F. (1982). A controlled prospective randomized trial evaluating the metabolic effects of enteral and parenteral nutrition in the cancer patient. *Cancer 49*(6), 1092-1105.
Deisseroth, A. & Wallerstein, R., Jr. (1989). Use of blood and blood products. In V.T. DeVita, Jr., S. Hellman, & S.A. Rosenberg (eds). *Cancer: Principles & Practice of Oncology* (3rd ed). Philadelphia: J.B. Lippincott Co., pp. 2045-2059.
Fry, S.T. (1986). Ethical aspects of decision-making in the feeding of cancer patients. *Semin Oncol Nurs 2*(1), 59-62.
Gordon, A. (1987). Nutrition. In C.R. Ziegfeld (ed). *Core Curriculum for Oncology Nursing*. Philadelphia: W.B. Saunders Co., pp. 245-258.
Grant, M. & Ropka, M.E. (1991). Alterations in nutrition. In S.B. Baird, R. McCorkle, & M. Grant (eds). *Cancer Nursing: A Comprehensive Approach*. Philadelphia: W.B. Saunders Co., pp. 717-741.
Haeuber, D. & Spross, J. (1991). Alterations in protective mechanisms: hematopoiesis and bone marrow depression. In S.B. Baird, R. McCorkle, & M. Grant (eds). *Cancer Nursing: A Comprehensive Textbook*. Philadelphia: W.B. Saunders Co., pp. 759-781.
Hathorn, J.W. (1989). Empiric antibiotics for febrile neutropenic cancer patients. *Eur J Cancer Clin Oncol 25*(suppl 2), S43-S51.
Ho, W.G. (1990). Transfusion and apheresis of blood cells. In C.M. Haskell (ed). *Cancer Treatment* (3rd ed). Philadelphia: W.B. Saunders Co., pp. 862-866.
Hughes, W.T. & Armstrong, D. (1990). Guidelines for the use of antimicrobial agents in neutropenic patients with unexplained fever. *J Infect Dis 161,* 381-396.
Jassak, P.F. & Godwin, J. (1991). Blood component therapy. In S.B. Baird, R. McCorkle, & M. Grant (eds). *Cancer Nursing: A Comprehensive Textbook*. Philadelphia: W.B. Saunders Co., pp. 370-384.
Klemm, P.R. & Hubbard, S.M. (1990). Infection. In S.L. Groenwald, M.H. Frogge, M. Goodman, & C.H. Yarbro (eds). *Cancer Nursing: Principles and Practice* (2nd ed). Boston: Jones & Bartlett Publishers, pp. 442-466.

Mayer, K.H. & DeTorres, O.H. (1985). Current guidelines on the use of antibacterial drugs in patients with malignancies. *Drugs 29,* 262-279.

Muscari-Lin, E. & Polomano, R.C. (1990). Inappropriate nutrition. In R.J. Daeffler & B.M. Petrosino (eds). *Manual of Oncology Nursing Practice: Nursing Diagnosis and Practice.* Rockville, Md.: Aspen Publishers, pp. 142-147.

Sandor, C. (1991). Nutrition, alteration in: less than body requirements related to disease process and treatment. In J.C. McNally, E.T. Somerville, C. Miaskowski, & M. Rostad (eds). *Guidelines for Oncology Nursing Practice.* Philadelphia: W.B. Saunders Co., pp. 165-172.

Szeluga, D.J., Groenwald, S.L., & Sullivan, D.K. (1990). Nutritional disturbances. In S.L. Groenwald, M.H. Frogge, M. Goodman & C.H. Yarbro (eds). *Cancer Nursing: Principles and Practice* (2nd ed). Boston: Jones & Bartlett Publishers, pp. 495-519.

Wade, J.C. (1989). Antibiotic therapy for the febrile granulocytopenic cancer patient: combination therapy vs. monotherapy. *Rev Infect Dis 11*(suppl 7), S1572-S1581.

Yarbro, C.H., McGuire, D.B., & Brain, H.G. (eds). (1990). Blood component therapy. *Semin Oncol Nurs 6*(2), 90-172.

Nursing Implications of Supportive Procedures in Cancer Care

Marcia Rostad, MS, RN, OCN, NS

Infusion Systems

THEORY

I. Infusion systems have become critical in the care of clients with cancer because of:
   A. Increased emphasis on timing of antineoplastic therapy.
   B. Increase in the number of intravenous therapies.
   C. Need to minimize entry into the system to minimize risk of infection.

II. Infusion systems are used for:
   A. Controlling the rate of infusions.
   B. Providing positive pressure for infusion.

III. Types of infusion systems.
   A. Large volume.
      1. Examples—controllers, volumetric pumps, and variable flow systems.
      2. Used to administer blood components, antibiotics, parenteral nutrition, and intravenous fluids.
   B. Small volume.
      1. Examples—intermittent syringe devices, continuous and intermittent peristaltic devices, and elastomeric and programmable portable infusion devices.
      2. Used to administer products similar to those in large volume systems except in smaller volumes.
   C. Patient controlled.
      1. Systems controlled by the client—deliver infusion at continuous, variable, intermittent, and basal rates.
      2. Used to administer antiemetics and analgesics.

IV. Potential complications associated with infusion systems.
   A. Occlusion.
   B. Severed or leaking infusion tubing.
   C. Mechanical errors—power failure, error in programming, insufficient fluid volume, or error in setting up the system.
   D. Infection.

DATA COLLECTION

I. Identification of potential candidates for infusion systems.
    A. Requires long-term or short-term, controlled-rate intravenous therapy.
    B. Has peripheral or central venous access established.

II. Physical examination.
    A. Site of venous access—color, temperature, contour, and drainage of entry site.
    B. Patency of venous access.

III. Psychosocial examination.
    A. Ability of client and family to care for infusion device if intended for home use.
    B. Concerns expressed about infusion device use.

ASSOCIATED NURSING DIAGNOSES

I. Potential for infection.

II. Potential for injury.

III. Anxiety.

NURSING PLANNING AND IMPLEMENTATION

I. Interventions to maximize safety for the client.
    A. Maintain aseptic technique when entering or manipulating the system.
    B. Teach client and family emergency procedures to use if system is disengaged.
    C. Maintain electrical safety—check all wiring, plugs, and accessory power packs; keep electrical equipment away from water hazards; and do not overload electrical outlets.

II. Interventions to minimize risks of complications of infusion system.
    A. Check patency of system with each system component change.
    B. Assess intactness of system, rate of infusion, remaining volume to be infused, and site of infusion at regular intervals.
    C. Use accessory components designed for the specific system.
    D. Operate infusion systems only for their intended use.
    E. Replace equipment and accessory components at intervals recommended by the manufacturer or institutional policy.

III. Interventions to monitor for complications of infusion system.
    A. Assess for redness, pain, swelling, and pus at infusion site.
    B. Assess client response to fluids being infused.
    C. Assess the system when any alarm sounds.

EVALUATION OF CLIENT AND FAMILY OUTCOMES

I. Participate in procedures to minimize risks of infection when manipulating the system.

II. Participate in strategies to limit electrical hazards from system use.

III. Participate in routine assessments to monitor for system malfunction.

IV. Report signs of potential complications to appropriate health personnel.

Venous, Arterial, and Peritoneal Access Devices

THEORY

I. Access devices have become critical in the care of the client with cancer.
    A. Increase in the use of intravenous therapy (antineoplastics and biological response modifiers) in the treatment of cancer.

  B. Increase in the use of supportive therapy (nutritional support, antibiotics, and blood component therapy) in cancer care.

  C. Increase in laboratory monitoring required with aggressive cancer treatment.

 II. Types of venous access devices.

  A. Short-term venous catheters.

   1. Description—single or multilumen catheters inserted peripherally.

   2. Inserted through the basilic or cephalic vein in the antecubital fossa or the subclavian or jugular veins.

   3. Made of soft, biocompatible silicone elastomer or silastic and polyurethane.

   4. Small size and peripheral insertion decrease risk for air embolism, sepsis, thrombosis, thrombophlebitis, and pneumothorax.

  B. Long-term venous catheters.

   1. Description—single or multilumen catheter tunneled subcutaneously and introduced into the cephalic, subclavian, or femoral vein.

   2. Tip of the catheter, which may be open or closed, is inserted near the right atrium.

   3. A Dacron cuff along the length of the catheter becomes embedded into the subcutaneous tissue:

    a. Stabilizes the catheter.

    b. Minimizes the risk of ascending infections.

  C. Implanted ports.

   1. Description—single or multiport units are inserted surgically.

   2. Port (reservoir and septum) is sutured into a subcutaneous pocket near the vessel in which the catheter is inserted.

   3. Size of the reservoir and gauge of the catheter vary.

   4. Entry to the port may be parallel or perpendicular to the skin.

   5. Port is accessed with a straight or angled, noncoring needle.

  D. Arterial catheters and implanted ports.

   1. Description—devices inserted surgically or percutaneously at a site proximal to the location of tumor (head and neck, liver, or extremity).

   2. Used for delivery of high concentrations of chemotherapy directly to the tumor and for limiting the systemic toxicity of the agent.

  E. Intraperitoneal catheters and implanted ports.

   1. Description—temporary, flexible silastic catheters inserted percutaneously or surgically into the peritoneal cavity.

   2. Tenckhoff catheters inserted into the peritoneal cavity for short-term intraperitoneal chemotherapy.

DATA COLLECTION

 I. Identification of potential candidates for venous, arterial, and peritoneal access devices (Table 27-1).

 II. Physical examination.

  A. Evaluate site of potential insertion.

  B. Evaluate condition of skin over potential insertion site.

 III. Psychosocial examination.

  A. Ability of client/family to care for the catheter or port.

  B. Knowledge of procedures for use of device for therapy.

  C. Concerns expressed about implications of insertion of device.

ASSOCIATED NURSING DIAGNOSES

 I. Potential for infection.

Table 27-1
IDENTIFICATION OF POTENTIAL CANDIDATES FOR VENOUS, ARTERIAL, AND
PERITONEAL DEVICES

Type of Device	Clinical Indications	Client Selection Criteria
Short-term venous catheters	Infusions of chemotherapy, antibiotics, nutritional support, blood components, and analgesics Infusions of vesicant or irritating agents that may damage peripheral veins Urgent need for establishing venous access	Limited venous access available Frequent venous access required Limited life expectancy
Long-term venous catheters	Infusions of chemotherapy, antibiotics, nutritional support, blood components, and analgesics Collection of blood samples	Limited venous access available Frequent venous access required Indefinite use of continuous or intermittent infusion therapy anticipated Long-term catheterization desired by client Ability of client/family to care for catheter determined
Implanted ports	Infusions of chemotherapy, antibiotics, nutritional support, blood components, and analgesics Collection of blood samples	Limited venous access available Frequent venous access required Indefinite use of continuous or intermittent infusion therapy anticipated Implanted port desired by client Client/family physically, mentally, or emotionally unable to care for external catheter
Arterial catheters and implanted ports	Delivery of high concentrations of chemotherapy directly to the tumor	Tumor with direct vascular access Tumor sensitive to antineoplastic agents
Intraperitoneal catheters and implanted ports	Delivery of high concentrations of chemotherapy to disease in peritoneal cavity	Metastatic cancer in the peritoneum Diagnosis of cancer of the ovary or colon, mesothelioma, or malignant ascites

II. Potential ineffective breathing pattern.

III. Alteration in comfort.

NURSING PLANNING AND IMPLEMENTATION
  I. Interventions to maximize safety for the client.
    A. Maintain aseptic technique when entering or manipulating the system.
    B. Teach client and family emergency procedures should catheter be severed.
    C. Await radiographic confirmation of catheter or port placement before using device.

  II. Interventions to minimize risks for complications of venous, arterial, or peritoneal devices (Table 27-2).

Table 27-2
COMPLICATIONS OF VENOUS, ARTERIAL, AND PERITONEAL DEVICES

Complication	Prevention	Restoration
Loss of blood return	Maintain flushing routines and techniques as outlined by institutional policy	Change position of client: roll to right or left side, sit up, lie flat Change intrathoracic pressures: have client inhale fully and hold breath, or exhale fully and hold breath Attempt "push-pull" maneuver using normal saline-filled syringe (avoid using force or high pressure) or a thrombolytic agent
Occlusion	Maintain flushing routines and techniques as outlined by institutional policy Flush system between administration of drugs Avoid mixing incompatible drugs	If occlusion is the result of clotted blood, urokinase may be instilled with a physician order
Infection	Wash hands thoroughly Follow strict aseptic techniques when using device	Administer antibiotics as ordered by the physician Remove device as ordered by the physician
Dislodgement	Avoid pulling on the catheters Tape catheters to the body Teach client to avoid manipulation of catheter or port Protect catheter or port from trauma	Refer to physician for resuturing if tip of the catheter remains in the vessel Remove device if cannot be used safely
Catheter migration	Protect device from trauma Avoid inserting device in an area with local disease	Refer to physician for repositioning catheter under fluoroscopy Remove device if cannot be used safely
Catheter pinholes, tracks, or cuts	Avoid use of scissors or sharp objects near the catheter Follow proper clamping procedures	Repair using the appropriate repair kit
Erosion of port through subcutaneous tissue	Maintain adequate nutrition status Avoid placing port at sites of actual or potential tissue damage (radiation fields) Avoid trauma or pressure over port	Refer to physician for removal of device
Port-catheter separation	Avoid trauma and high pressure infusions	Refer to physician for removal of device
Dislodgement of port access needle	Tape needle securely in place Avoid tension on the needle or tubing	Remove needle and reaccess the port using a sterile noncoring needle

III. Interventions to monitor for complications of venous or peritoneal devices.
   A. Occlusion—inability to infuse fluids with minimal pressure or inability to withdraw samples of blood or peritoneal fluid.
   B. Air embolism—presence of sudden onset of pallor or cyanosis, shortness of breath, cough, or tachycardia.
   C. Pneumothorax—presence of shortness of breath, chest pain, or tachycardia.
   D. Infection—presence of redness, pain, swelling, warmth, or drainage.
   E. Dislodgment—increase in the length of the external catheter, pain during infusion of fluids, or swelling along the catheter tract or insertion site.
   F. Migration—regional discomfort, pain, swelling, or difficulty in using device.

IV. Interventions to manage complications of venous, arterial, or peritoneal catheters or ports (Table 27-2).

EVALUATION OF CLIENT AND FAMILY OUTCOMES

I. Describe the rationale, benefits, and risks of venous, arterial, or peritoneal catheters or ports.

II. Participate in strategies to decrease the risks of complications of venous, arterial, or peritoneal catheters or ports.

III. List signs and symptoms of complications of venous, arterial, or peritoneal catheters or ports to report to a member of the health care team.

IV. Identify community resources for obtaining supplies for device care.

Infection Control

THEORY

I. Three factors are necessary for the development of infection—source of infectious organism, method of transmission, and susceptible host.
   A. Source of infectious organism.
      1. Endogenous organisms.
         a. People are colonized with a multitude of organisms in the nasopharynx, eyes, external ear, mouth, gastrointestinal tract, anterior third of the urethra, vagina, cervix, and skin.
         b. Normal flora help prevent colonization by pathogenic organisms.
      2. Exogenous organisms—pathogenic organisms present in the environment.
   B. Methods of transmission.
      1. Direct contact.
      2. Indirect contact.
      3. Airborne transmission.
   C. Susceptible host—determined by the presence or absence of mechanisms for preventing or fighting infection.
      1. Mechanical barriers—skin and mucous membranes.
      2. Chemical barriers—pH of tissues.
      3. Cellular elements of the inflammatory and immune responses such as white blood cells, monocytes, T lymphocytes, and B lymphocytes.
      4. Biochemical mediators of the inflammatory and immune responses such as antibody, complement, lymphokines, cytokines, and monokines.

II. Potential for a microorganism to cause infection depends on the:
   A. Degree of contamination of the object or person.
   B. Virulence of the organism.

Table 27-3
TYPES AND SITES OF INFECTIOUS ORGANISMS

Category	Organism
Gram positive	Staphylococci
	Clostridia
	Corynebacterium diphtheriae
	Listeria
Gram negative	*Klebsiella pneumoniae*
	Escherichia coli
	Salmonella
	Shigella
	Pseudomonas aeruginosa
	Neisseria
Fungi and yeasts	*Candida albicans*
	Nocardia
	Cryptococcus neoformans
	Aspergillus
	Coccidioides immitis
Parasites	*Giardia lamblia*
	Entamoeba histolytica
	Tapeworms
	Roundworms
	Flukes
Viruses	Influenza
	Adenovirus
	Enterovirus
	Poliovirus
	Cytomegalovirus
	Epstein-Barr virus
	Human immunodeficiency virus
	Hepatitis A, B, and non-A, non-B viruses

Common Sites of Infection

Oral cavity	*Sites of invasive procedures*
Respiratory tract	Intravenous sites
Rectum	Diagnostic biopsies
	Surgical wounds
Skin	Central venous catheters and ports

    C. Probability of transmission.
    D. Existence of a favorable environment for organism growth.
  III. Common sites of infection and infectious organisms in clients with cancer (Table 27-3).

DATA COLLECTION
  I. Identification of clients at risk.
    A. Myelosuppressive therapy.
      1. Antineoplastic agents.

2. Radiation therapy.
B. Disruption of natural barriers.
   1. Impaired skin integrity.
   2. Invasive procedures.
   3. Invasive equipment.
C. Diagnosis of cancer.
D. Recent exposure to infectious organism.

II. Physical examination.
A. Assess for signs and symptoms of infection—fever, redness, swelling, pain, and pus.
B. Assess skin integrity.
C. Assess oral mucosa integrity.
D. Assess perineal and rectal integrity.

III. Laboratory data—colonization of normal flora in another part of the body.

ASSOCIATED NURSING DIAGNOSES

I. Potential for infection.

II. Knowledge deficit related to infection control measures.

NURSING PLANNING AND IMPLEMENTATION

I. Implement an infection control program.
A. Surveillance of current immunization of employees.
   1. Tuberculosis vaccine required.
   2. Hepatitis B vaccine recommended.
B. Surveillance of infections present in the environment, employees, and clients.
C. Reporting of infections.

II. Implement procedures to protect clients and employees from infectious organisms.
A. Handwashing.
B. Isolation procedures.
   1. Universal precautions.
      a. Use of a barrier (gloves, gowns, face shields, goggles, masks, and protective bags) to prevent direct contact with body fluids.
      b. Type of barrier required depends on the activity being performed and the risk of accidental exposure.
   2. Respiratory isolation required for diseases transmitted by droplets such as pneumonia and *Haemophilus influenzae* meningitis.
C. Protective environments.
   1. Laminar air flow—sterilization of the room and contents; decontamination of the client with oral nonabsorbable antibiotics, skin antiseptics, and antibiotic sprays and ointments.
   2. HEPA filtration—forced air in a unidirectional pattern through a filter to remove particles such as bacteria, fungi, and large viruses.
D. Low bacterial diets—avoid fresh fruits, vegetables, and salads.

EVALUATION OF CLIENT AND FAMILY OUTCOMES

I. Participate in procedures to limit exposure to exogenous organisms in the environment.

II. Participate in strategies to minimize infection from endogenous organisms.

III. Report occurrences of infection to appropriate infection control personnel.

BIBLIOGRAPHY

Camp, L.D. (1988). Care of the Groshong catheter. *Oncol Nurs Forum 15*(6), 745-749.

Castle, M. & Ajemian, E. (1987). *Hospital Infection Control: Principles and Practice* (2nd ed). New York: John Wiley & Sons.

Jacobson, E. (1990). Hospital hazards. How to protect yourself. Part 2. *Am J Nurs 90*(4), 48-53.

Oncology Nursing Society (1989). *Access Device Guidelines: Modules I, II, III*. Pittsburgh: Author.

Tenenbaum, L. (1989). *Cancer Chemotherapy: A Reference Guide*. Philadelphia: W.B. Saunders Co.

Wenzel, R.P. (1987). *Prevention and Control of Nosocomial Infections*. Baltimore: Williams & Wilkins.

Nursing Principles Specific to the Major Cancers

28

Lung Cancer

Julena Lind, MN, RN

THEORY

I. Physiology and pathophysiology associated with lung cancer.
   A. Anatomy—see Figure 28-1 for schematic representation of the lungs, locations, and presenting symptoms of various types of tumors.
   B. Primary functions of the lungs are air exchange and filtering of microparticles from the air.
      1. Normal bronchial epithelial cells serve as a lining and have a protective function.
      2. Columnar epithelial cells line the tracheobronchial tree from the trachea to the terminal bronchioles.
      3. Columnar cells consist of ciliated cells that filter particles from the air and mucous-secreting cells that facilitate clearance of particles from the lungs.
   C. Changes associated with cancer.
      1. Long-term exposure to cigarette smoke or irritants such as coal dust damage the ciliated cells and mucus-producing cells and result in replacement by dysplastic cells.
      2. If the irritation continues, the atypia of the epithelial cells progresses to nuclear enlargement, nuclear variability, hyperchromatism, and abnormal mitotic activity.
   D. Histological types.
      1. Epidermoid (squamous)—incidence decreasing.
      2. Adenocarcinoma—incidence increasing; can occur without smoking history.
      3. Small cell (includes oat cell)—most rapidly growing.
      4. Large cell.
   E. Because treatment varies by histological types, lung tumors are classified as:
      1. Small cell tumors (SCLC).
      2. Non-small cell tumors (NSCLC):
         a. Epidermoid.
         b. Adenocarcinoma.
         c. Large cell.
   F. Presentation and metastatic patterns (see Figure 28-1).
      1. Squamous cell carcinoma typically arises in segmental bronchi and grows

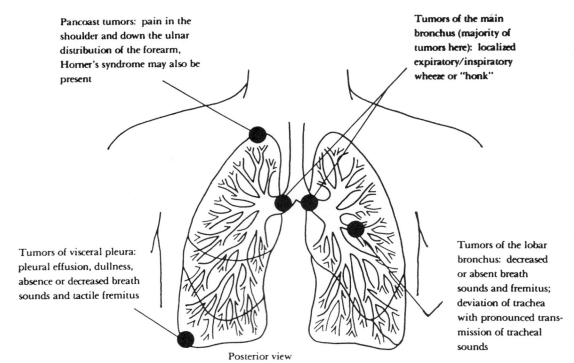

Pancoast tumors: pain in the shoulder and down the ulnar distribution of the forearm, Horner's syndrome may also be present

Tumors of the main bronchus (majority of tumors here): localized expiratory/inspiratory wheeze or "honk"

Tumors of visceral pleura: pleural effusion, dullness, absence or decreased breath sounds and tactile fremitus

Tumors of the lobar bronchus: decreased or absent breath sounds and fremitus; deviation of trachea with pronounced trans-mission of tracheal sounds

Posterior view

Figure 28-1 Anatomical relationships and tumor locations in the lung. *(From Frank-Stromborg, M. & Cohen, R. [1990]. Assessment and interventions for cancer prevention and detection. In S. Groenwald, M.H. Frogge, M. Goodman, & C.H. Yarbro [eds]. Cancer Nursing Principles and Practice. Boston: Jones & Bartlett Publishers, p. 128.)*

exophytically, causing bronchial obstruction or involvement of the adjacent lymph nodes.

2. Adenocarcinomas usually are located peripherally and spread more diffusely to brain, bones, other lung, and liver.

3. Small cell cancer usually occurs endobronchially in a segmental bronchus; however, because of its aggressiveness, hilar and mediastinal nodes are involved in 80% of cases at presentation.

4. Large cell lung cancer usually presents as bulky peripheral tumors and spreads as peripheral masses before metastasizing to brain, bones, adrenal glands, and liver.

5. In general, a 6:4 ratio of involvement of right versus left lung is reported.

G. Trends in epidemiology.

1. Lung cancer is the leading cause of cancer incidence and cancer death in the United States.

2. Age-adjusted lung cancer death rates in men in the United States increased from 11 per 100,000 population in 1940 to 73 per 100,000 in 1982.

3. Lung cancer rates started to decline in young white men ages 35 to 44 years in the 1970s and in white men 55 to 64 in the 1980s; incidence and mortality are increasing in all other groups.

4. Increase in lung cancer deaths in women is attributed to the increase in the number of women smoking.

   a. In 1950 the lung cancer ratio of women to men was 1:20.

   b. In 1974 the lung cancer ratio of women to men was 1:4.

   c. In 1980 the lung cancer ratio of women to men was 1:2.6.

5. Smoking-related disorders are estimated to cost the nation approximately $27 billion annually.

6. In addition to being a carcinogen, tobacco smoke promotes the carcinogenic effect of other carcinogens.

7. Smoking cessation is associated with a gradual decrease in the risk of lung cancer, but 5 or more years must elapse before an appreciable decrease in risk occurs.

8. Environmental and occupational factors.
   a. Asbestos exposure has been linked to the incidence of lung cancer (especially mesothelioma) in shipyard workers, miners, and pipe fitters.
   b. Uranium miners appear to have a particularly high incidence of small cell cancer of the lung (probably caused by radon, which is a radioactive gas that exists in the atmosphere).
   c. Indoor exposure to radon seems to present a risk for lung cancer, but current epidemiological studies are inconclusive in estimating risks of exposure to radon gas.

II. Principles of medical management.
   A. Screening tests.
      1. No reliable screening or early detection methods exist.
      2. Chest x-ray examinations, lung health questionnaires, and sputum cytology at regular intervals are ineffective in screening.
   B. Diagnostic tests.
      1. Tests to determine the size and location of the primary tumor:
         a. Chest x-ray examination.
         b. Thoracic computed tomographic (CT) scan (has revolutionized staging) (Table 28-1).
         c. Lung tomography.
         d. Bronchoscopy (with brush or needle biopsy) (Table 28-1).
      2. Tests that aid in determining the lymph node involvement:
         a. Mediastinoscopy (Table 28-1).
         b. Scalene node biopsy.
         c. Hilar tomography.
      3. Tests that aid in detecting distant metastases:
         a. Liver and spleen scans.
         b. Bone scan.
         c. CT scan of the brain.
         d. Thoracentesis (to detect tumor cells in pleural fluid).
   C. Staging methods and procedures.
      1. Stage I, II, III, IV (Appendix).
      2. TNM system (Appendix).
      3. Performance scales that measure physical status:
         a. Karnofsky scale (see Chapter 18, Table 18-3).
         b. Zubrod scale.
      4. Procedures as outlined above under "Diagnostic Tests."
   D. Standard therapies.
      1. Surgery—treatment of choice for non-small cell cancer of the lung.
         a. Lobectomy—removal of a lobe of the lung; associated with lower morbidity and mortality rates than pneumonectomy; generally the preferred treatment for small tumors.
         b. Pneumonectomy—removal of one lung; higher incidence of perfusion and ventilation problems, circulatory overload, and pulmonary hypertension.

Table 28-1
NURSING CARE RELATED TO PULMONARY TESTS

Procedure	Physical Alteration	Intervention
Bronchoscopy— to localize and/or perform a biopsy on a lesion		
Local anesthetic (duration 2-8 hr)	Gag reflex	Give client nothing by mouth. Maintain flat or semi-Fowler's position.
Hyperextended neck	Tension on neck muscles and vertebrae	Apply ice collar first 24 hrs, then heat. Provide lozenges and gargles when gag reflex returns. Administer analgesics if pain is severe.
Insertion of bronchoscope	Laryngeal edema Possible laryngospasms	Observe for and report respiratory distress. Administer oxygen.
Possible biopsy (brush or needle)	Possible bleeding and/or infection	Observe and report: Hemoptysis. Symptoms of upper respiratory infection.
	Possible pneumothorax	Report dyspnea, decreased breath sounds, cyanosis. Administer oxygen.
Mediastinoscopy— to evaluate lymph node involvement		
General anesthetic		Give client nothing by mouth before and after procedure.
Insertion of scope into intercostal space	Manipulation of trachea	Administer analgesics as needed.
	Possible air leaks into skin	Palpate for crepitus.
	Possible pneumothorax	Report dyspnea, decreased breath sounds, cyanosis. Administer oxygen.
	Possible bleeding	Check dressing.
	Possible mediastinitis	Report fever, cough.

(1) In the general population only approximately 50% of lung cancer clients are candidates for thoracotomy; only 25% are candidates for resection.
(2) Contraindications to thoracotomy:
  (a) Metastasis outside the lung.
  (b) Scalene node metastasis.
  (c) Metastasis to the other lung.
  (d) Inadequate pulmonary function.
(3) Palliative surgery may be used to control symptoms such as hemoptysis; laser surgery via bronchoscopy has been used to treat airway obstruction.
  2. Radiotherapy; external beam radiotherapy may be used:
  a. Alone with curative intent for Stage I or II non-small cell lung cancer if lung function is impaired or other conditions preclude surgery.

Table 28-1

NURSING CARE RELATED TO PULMONARY TESTS—*Continued*

Procedure	Physical Alteration	Intervention
Thoracic Computed Tomographic (CT) Scan— to localize lesion and/or detect node involvement		
Serial x-ray examinations of sectional planes of thorax and computer analysis to provide three-dimensional studies of the tissue	Noninvasive; client to lie still; rotation of large machine, making clicking noises, around client	Instruct client that procedure is painless. Tell client what to expect.
Possible use of contrast media containing iodides and/or radio-active materials	Intravenous administration Possible adverse reactions to contrast media	Warn client of immediate sensations of warmth, flushing, bitter or salty taste, nausea/vomiting, and itching and that pain at insertion site may occur.
	Possible hypersensitivity to contrast media (rare)	Perform cardiopulmonary resuscitation. Follow emergency procedures.
Sputum— to collect shedding endo-bronchial tissue for histological diagnosis		
Three containers with fixative given to client	None	Instruct client to collect daily specimens upon arising and before oral intake or brushing of teeth.
Collection of sputum and saliva for cytology		
Forwarding of specimen to laboratory for cytological studies		Inform client about time required to analyze tissue and complete report.

   b. As adjuvant to surgery, either preoperatively or postoperatively; the effect on survivorship is controversial.
   c. As prophylactic cranial irradiation to prevent or retard the incidence of brain metastases in small cell lung cancer (recent retrospective study that revealed the high incidence of central nervous system [CNS] toxicity associated with prophylactic cranial irradiation raises questions about the value of this treatment or therapy).
   d. As palliation for control of symptoms associated with lung cancer (severe cough, hemoptysis, pain, obstructive pneumonitis, superior vena cava syndrome) or to prolong the functional life of the client.
3. Chemotherapy.
   a. Treatment of choice for small cell lung cancer.
      (1) Improves survival rates (12- to 18-month median survival with chemotherapy versus 6 to 8 weeks without).
      (2) Has been combined with cranial irradiation to improve survival.
      (3) Combinations used include:
         (a) Etoposide-ifosfamide-cisplatin.
         (b) Cyclophosphamide-doxorubicin-vincristine.

(c) Cyclophosphamide-doxorubicin-etoposide.
(d) Cyclophosphamide-lomustine-methotrexate.
b. May be used as adjuvant therapy in non-small cell lung cancer.
(1) Not shown to improve survival.
(2) May improve disease-free survival.
(3) May be combined with surgery or radiotherapy.
(4) Combinations used include:
(a) Mitomycin-vindesine or vinblastine.
(b) Cyclophosphamide-doxorubicin-cisplatin (CAP).
c. Commonly used for advanced disease.
(1) Generally yields frequent but brief response rates (up to 40% in some studies).
(2) Combinations used:
(a) Cyclophosphamide-doxorubicin-methotrexate-procarbazine (CAMP).
(b) Vindesine-cisplatin.
(c) Etoposide-cisplatin (EC).
(d) Cyclophosphamide-doxorubicin-cisplatin (CAP).
d. Various types of chemotherapy commonly used alone or in combination in treating lung cancer—doxorubicin (Adriamycin), bleomycin (Blenoxane), lomustine (CCNU), cisplatin (CDDP, Platinol), hexamethylmelamine, M-AMSA (Amsacrine), methotrexate (Amethopterin), procarbazine (Matulane), vincristine (Oncovin), vindesine, etoposide (VP-16), ifosfamide (with mesna uroprotection), and carboplatin.
4. Immunotherapy—investigational; data inconclusive.
E. Trends in survival.
1. Overall survival rate at 5 years for all lung cancer is less than 10%.
2. Stage I 5-year survival rate is 40% to 60%.
3. Stage II 5-year survival rate is approximately 12%.
4. Survival depends on the size, location, and extent of metastases at the time of diagnosis.

DATA COLLECTION
I. Pertinent personal and environmental history (risk factors).
A. Tobacco use (number of packs per day multiplied by number of years smoked).
1. Smoking is responsible for approximately 80% of lung cancer cases.
2. At highest risk are people over 45 who have smoked two or more packs per day for 10 years or more (20 pack years); mortality rates are 15 to 25 times higher than for nonsmokers.
B. Occupational and environmental exposures (asbestos, uranium, radon).

II. Physical examination (may be asymptomatic).
A. Pulmonary manifestations:
1. Cough.
2. Hemoptysis.
3. Dyspnea.
4. Pneumonia.
B. Local manifestations (related to the growth of tumor and compression of adjacent structures):
1. Shoulder pain.
2. Arm pain.
3. Superior vena cava syndrome (distention of arm and neck veins; facial, neck and arm edema; suffusion of mucous membranes) (see Chapters 8 and 9).

III. Evaluation of laboratory data.
  A. Metabolic complications (small cell especially):
    1. Elevated antidiuretic hormone (ADH) level (because of ADH-mimic produced by the tumor).
    2. Elevated adrenocorticotropic hormone (ACTH) level (because of ACTH-mimic produced by the tumor).
  B. Blood gas values.
  C. Pulmonary function test results.

ASSOCIATED NURSING DIAGNOSES
  I. Knowledge deficit.

  II. Alteration in comfort; pain.

  III. Potential for impaired gas exchange.

  IV. Potential for impaired skin integrity.

  V. Potential alteration in fluid volume.

  VI. Grief; anticipatory.

NURSING PLANNING AND IMPLEMENTATION
  I. Interventions to maximize client safety by prevention and detection of hemorrhage, pneumothorax and/or mediastinal shift.
  A. Check the chest tube drainage system (if present; post-pneumonectomy clients may not have chest tubes or may have a clamped tube) for obstruction every 1 to 2 hours; observe and document:
    1. Absence of fluctuations in the waterseal chamber.
    2. Lack of drainage fluid in the drainage tubing or collection chamber.
  B. Reposition the chest tube drainage tubing as frequently as necessary.
    1. Secure chest tubes with a tight dressing.
    2. Minimize chest tube movement by securing tubes to body.
  C. Examine the drainage tubing and connections for clots and/or debris.
  D. Assess the drainage system for breaks in the system every 8 hours and as needed; document findings; immediately report:
    1. Continuous large amount of bubbling in the waterseal chamber.
    2. "Air leak" noises in the system.
  E. Assess for cause of air leak by checking:
    1. For occlusive seal at the insertion site.
    2. To determine if the chest tube has moved; if so, notify physician.
    3. For an improper fit at the connector site.
    4. For a defect in the equipment.
  F. Auscultate and document breath sounds every 2 to 4 hours.
  G. Monitor and document early signs of respiratory distress—increased respiratory rate, nasal flaring, use of accessory muscles.
  H. Instruct the client to report increase in shortness of breath.
  I. Document client teaching.
  J. Assess and document signs of pneumothorax every 2 to 4 hours—absent breath sounds unilaterally, tracheal deviation, increased shortness of breath.
  K. Obtain chest x-ray examination and blood gas values as ordered and monitor reports.
  L. Monitor position of trachea and report shift from midline.
  M. Avoid deep suctioning that may cause trauma to suture line.

II. Interventions to decrease severity of symptoms associated with the disease and/or treatment.
   A. Nursing interventions related to surgical treatment.
      1. Teach client and family preoperatively about equipment (may receive mechanical ventilation or supplemental oxygen immediately postoperatively), breathing exercises, and postoperative recovery.
      2. Apply elastic stockings and teach leg exercises to prevent postoperative emboli.
      3. Provide pain relief to promote comfort, early ambulation, and coughing and deep breathing.
      4. Position client to protect remaining lung tissue:
         a. After lobectomy—promote expansion to fill lung space by avoiding prolonged lying on operative side.
         b. After pneumonectomy—avoid positions that interfere with expansion of remaining lung (Trendelenburg, lying on surgery-free side).
      5. Promote optimal pulmonary function—coughing and deep breathing, hydrating, changing positions, ambulating.
      6. Teach breathing exercises and the need for cessation of smoking.
   B. Nursing interventions related to radiotherapy of pulmonary and/or cranial fields (see Chapter 20).
      1. Explain physiological effects of radiotherapy on selected field.
         a. Chest—hair loss, skin reactions (7 to 10 days after treatment is begun), dysphagia and esophagitis (approximately 3 weeks after initiation), tenacious bronchial secretions, pneumonitis (1 to 3 months later), pulmonary fibrosis, pericarditis, myelitis (long-term).
         b. Cranial—alopecia, desquamation of portion of ear, CNS syndrome (memory loss, tremor, sommolence, slurred speech, learning disability).
         c. General—bone marrow suppression, fatigue.
      2. Encourage rest periods and setting priorities to conserve energy.
      3. Provide foods that are easily swallowed (tepid, soft, not spicy).
      4. Provide or encourage frequent oral care and intake of at least 2 L of fluid daily.
      5. Monitor for decrease in platelet and granulocyte counts, which predisposes client to bleeding or infection.
      6. Promote mucus clearance—hydration, diaphragmatic breathing, postural drainage, percussion, and vibration.
      7. Teach client and/or family about half-life of radioisotopes (if getting implant treatment).
      8. Advise cutting hair and buying a wig (if getting cranial irradiation).
   C. Nursing intervention related to chemotherapy (see Chapter 21).

III. Interventions to monitor disease progression.
   A. Schedule follow-up care.
   B. Discuss purpose of brain, bone, and liver scans or other surveillance procedures for metastatic disease.
   C. Teach client and family signs and symptoms of metastatic disease.
      1. Changes in affect or personality.
      2. Bone pain.
      3. Changes in respiratory status.
      4. Jaundice.

IV. Interventions to enhance adaptation and rehabilitation.
   A. Pulmonary rehabilitation.
   B. Range of motion exercises on side of the thoracotomy.

V. Interventions to incorporate client/family in care.
  A. Help family to allow client to maintain roles and activities most important to him or her.
     1. Place emphasis on short-term goals in daily care and priority setting.
     2. Refer to local American Cancer Society or American Lung Association for respiratory program if available.
  B. Teach supportive care skills.
     1. Instruct client and family in the use of oxygen equipment, postural drainage, self-pacing program.
     2. Teach general strengthening exercises.
     3. Instruct in relaxation techniques.
     4. Assist to maintain realistic hope, yet prepare for changes in life-style if prognosis is poor.
     5. Assist to resume previous roles and responsibilities if prognostic factors are favorable (small, solitary, isolated lesion).

EVALUATION OF CLIENT AND FAMILY OUTCOMES

   I. Verbalize risks of smoking and the benefits of quitting.

  II. Name at least two smoking cessation resources in respective community (see Chapter 4).

 III. Discuss pain control strategies.

  IV. Demonstrate postural drainage techniques.

   V. Demonstrate the use of oxygen or other equipment.

  VI. Identify external and internal factors that increase risk of upper respiratory infection—exposure to crowds; inadequate rest, nutrition, or hydration.

 VII. List signs and symptoms of upper respiratory infection—fever, cough, expectoration (yellow or green in color).

VIII. Identify side effects of radiation therapy.

  IX. Verbalize methods to treat radiation skin reactions.

   X. Identify foods appropriate for dysphagia and/or esophagitis.

  XI. Verbalize indicators of hope (constitutional, psychological, and prognostic).

 XII. List signs and symptoms of metastatic disease.

XIII. List resources available for lung cancer clients.
  A. Local American Cancer Society (e.g., *Facts on Lung Cancer*).
  B. Local American Lung Association.
  C. Local hospice organizations.
  D. Visiting nurse agencies.

BIBLIOGRAPHY

Aisner, J. & Abrams, J. (1989). Cisplatin for small-cell lung cancer. *Semin Oncol 16*(4, suppl 6), 2-9.
Elpern, E.H. (1990). Lung cancer. In S.L. Groenwald, M.H. Frogge, M. Goodman, & C.H. Yarbro (eds). *Cancer Nursing: Principles and Practice* (2nd ed). Boston: Jones & Bartlett Publishers, pp 951-973.
Erickson, R.S. (1989). Mastering the ins and outs of chest drainage. Part 1. *Nursing 19*(5), 37-44.
Erickson, R.S. (1989). Mastering the ins and outs of chest drainage. Part 2. *Nursing 19*(6), 46-50.
Finley, R.S. (1989). Lung cancer: detection, prevention, and therapeutics. *Am Pharm NS 29*(11), 39-46.
Fleck, J.F., Einhorn, L.H., Lauer, R.C., Schultz, S.M., & Miller, M.E. (1990). Is prophylactic cranial irradiation indicated in small-cell lung cancer? *J Clin Oncol 8*(2), 209-214.

Garfinkel, L. & Silverberg, E. (1991). Lung cancer and smoking trends in the United States over the past 25 years. *CA 41*(3), 137-145.

Harley, N.H. & Harley J.H (1990). Potential lung cancer risk from indoor radon exposure. *CA 40*(5), 265-275.

Johnson, D.H. (1990). Overview of ifosfamide in small cell and non-small cell lung cancer. *Semin Oncol 17*(2, suppl 4), 24-30.

Lindsey, A.M. (1991). Lung cancer. In S.B. Baird, R. McCorkle, & M. Grant. *Cancer Nursing: a Comprehensive Textbook*. Philadelphia: W.B. Saunders Co., pp. 452-465.

Mackay, B., Lukeman, J.M., & Ordonez, N.G. (1991). *Tumors of the Lung*. Philadelphia: W.B. Saunders Co.

Sider, L. (1990). Radiographic manifestations of primary bronchogenic carcinoma. *Radiol Clin North Am 28*(3), 583-597.

Turris, A.T., III (1990). The nonsurgical management of lung cancer: a 1989 perspective for small cell and the non-small cell histologies. *Semin Roentgenol 25*(1), 117-122.

Wynder, E.L. (1972). Etiology of lung cancer: reflections on two decades of research. *Cancer 30*(5), 1332-1339.

Yesner, R. (1988). Histopathology of lung cancer. *Semin Ultrasound, CT MRT 9*(1), 4-26.

29

Breast Cancer

Nina Entrekin, MN, RN, OCN

THEORY

I. Physiology and pathophysiology associated with breast cancer.
  A. Anatomy of breast (Figure 29-1).
    1. Description.
      a. Adult female breast lies on anterior chest wall between sternum and mid-axillary line from second to sixth ribs.
      b. Twelve to 20 lobes occupy central and upper portion.
      c. Each lobe is connected by duct to nipple surface.
      d. Nipple is surrounded by circular, pigmented areola.
    2. Critical adjacent structures—pectoralis major and pectoralis minor muscles lie beneath the breast.
  B. Primary functions.
    1. Physiological function of the female breast, or mammary glands, is lactation.
    2. In Western culture the breast is associated more with sexuality and femininity than with infant feeding.
  C. Changes in function associated with cancer.
    1. If tumor is present during lactation, occlusion of lobule(s) and duct(s) could lead to hydrostasis, engorgement, mastitis.
    2. Extent of threat to sexuality and femininity is an individual response.
  D. Metastatic patterns.
    1. Regional spread.
      a. Axillary nodes receive 75% of lymph leaving the breast (Figure 29-2).
        (1) Nodes are positive at diagnosis in approximately 45% of clients.
        (2) Likelihood of axillary involvement increases with primary tumor size, regardless of location of primary tumor in breast.
      b. Internal mammary nodes receive 25% of lymph leaving breast.
        (1) Nodes are involved in 22% of clients at diagnosis.
        (2) Likelihood of involvement increases with inner quadrant or central primary tumors.
      c. Supraclavicular nodes receive most of lymph through axillary chain; involvement represents late stage of axillary spread.

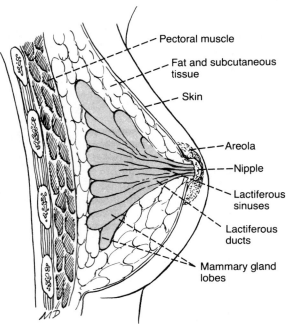

Figure 29-1 Female breast structure. *(From Luckman, J. & Sorenson, K.C. [1987]. Medical-Surgical Nursing: A Psychophysiologic Approach [3rd ed]. Philadelphia: W.B. Saunders Co., p. 1809.)*

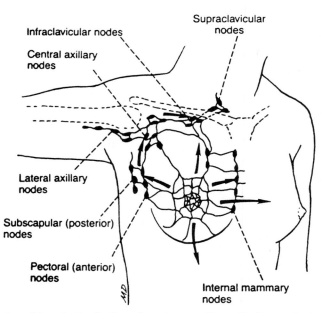

Figure 29-2 Routes of lymphatic drainage from breast. *(From Luckman, J. & Sorenson, K.C. [1987]. Medical-Surgical Nursing: A Psychophysiologic Approach [3rd ed]. Philadelphia: W.B. Saunders Co., p. 1809.)*

2. Distant spread.
    a. Metastasis can occur to any organ.
    b. Common sites:
        (1) Lymph nodes (76%).
        (2) Bone (71%).
        (3) Lung (69%).
        (4) Liver (65%).
        (5) Pleura (51%).
        (6) Adrenals (49%).
        (7) Skin (30%).
        (8) Central nervous system (CNS; 20%).
E. Trends in epidemiology.
    1. Information about changes in incidence over time:
        a. Incidence rates have increased approximately 3% per year since 1980.
        b. Increase is partially due to screening programs that detect more small tumors before clinical evidence of disease exists.
        c. Other reasons for increase are not fully understood.
    2. Characteristics of tumors.
        a. Most breast cancer arises in the epithelial tissues of the ducts (ductal carcinoma) or lobes (lobular carcinoma).
        b. More than 20 histological types exist (examples are in Table 29-1).

Table 29-1
SELECTED HISTOLOGICAL TYPES OF BREAST CANCER

Type	Incidence (%)	Characteristics	Prognosis
Infiltrating ductal carcinoma	70	Stony hard mass; gritty texture; may appear bilaterally	Poor; common involvement of axillary nodes
Medullary carcinoma	5-7	Soft mass; often reaches large size; may be circumscribed	Favorable
Mucinous, or colloid, carcinoma	3	Slow growing; can reach large size; may occur with other tumor type	Good if tumor is predominately mucinous
Invasive lobular carcinoma	5	Multicentricity common; may involve both breasts	Similar to ductal types
Paget's disease	3	Scaly, eczematoid nipple, with burning, itching, discharge; two thirds have palpable, underlying mass	Related to histological type of underlying tumor
Inflammatory breast cancer	<1	Skin red, warm, indurated, with obstructive lymphangitis (peau d'orange appearance)	Poor; often presents with palpable nodes and evidence of metastasis
Lobular carcinoma in situ	2.5	Usually found as incidental finding in benign breast specimens (high risk for development of invasive cancer in future)	Good

Table 29-2
BREAST BIOPSY TECHNIQUES

Time	Description	Indications	Potential Side Effects/Complications	Critical Symptoms to Report to Health Care Provider
Fine Needle Aspiration 15 min	Fine needle (21 gauge) inserted into localized mass and material aspirated by negative pressure Aspirate placed on slide, fixative applied, and slide sent to pathology department	Fluid aspirate indicative of benign, cystic mass Negative pathology of solid mass indicates need for open biopsy	Hematoma Infection Pneumothorax	Redness, warmth, swelling at site Dyspnea, sudden sharp chest pain
Needle Core Biopsy 15 min	Special needle with large lumen (Silverman or Tru-cut) used to remove core of tissue	Used when tumor is relatively large and located close to surface	Hematoma Infection Pneumothorax	Redness, warmth, swelling at site Dyspnea, sudden sharp chest pain
Open Biopsy 1 hr	Small tumor (excisional biopsy)—surgical removal of entire lump with margin of normal tissue Large tumor (incisional biopsy)—surgical removal of a small portion of tumor Frozen section done Remaining tissue of malignant samples sent for estrogen and progesterone receptor assay	Used for palpable masses within breast	Hematoma Infection Delayed wound healing	Redness, warmth, swelling at site Drainage, separation of incision, pain
Needle Localization* 2 hr	Radiologist locates suspicious area with needle, leaves in place a tiny wire with hook at end to guide surgeon to area of biopsy Removal of correct area is confirmed by x-ray test before tissue is sent to pathology	Used when suspicious area is seen on mammogram	Hematoma Infection Delayed wound healing	Redness, warmth, swelling at site Drainage, separation of incision, pain

*Needle localization biopsy technique is unique to the breast.

II. Principles of medical management.
   A. Screening and diagnostic procedures.
      1. General procedures.
         a. Breast self-examination (BSE)—critical self-care screening practice (see "Secondary Prevention," Chapter 5, Figure 5-1).
         b. Mammography—supplements, rather than replaces, physical examination by a skilled clinician and BSE by the individual.

    c. Ultrasonography—useful in distinguishing cystic from solid masses; ineffective in detecting small, nonpalpable cancers or in distinguishing benign from malignant solid lesions.

    d. Computerized axial tomography (CAT) scans—useful in supplementing mammography to evaluate dense breasts and to search for a primary lesion when mammogram is negative and axillary lymph node biopsy is positive.

    e. Biopsy—indicated for any discrete, palpable mass in the breast, regardless of mobility of mass, negative mammogram, age of the client, length of time the mass has been present, or benign nature of previous biopsies.

       (1) Breast biopsies are done with client under local anesthesia on outpatient basis; general anesthesia is used occasionally.

       (2) Four biopsy techniques are used (Table 29-2).

  2. Specific procedures unique to the site (Table 29-2).

B. Staging methods and procedures (see Chapter 18).

C. Treatment strategies.

  1. Standard therapies by stage.

    a. Stage 0—segmental mastectomy with or without irradiation.

    b. Stages I and II—segmental mastectomy with irradiation.

       (1) Adjuvant therapy dependent on menopausal status, axillary node involvement, and receptor status as determined by National Institutes of Health (NIH) Consensus Conference (Table 29-3).

       (2) If a woman with early stage disease is not a candidate for segmental mastectomy (e.g., diffuse microcalcifications or client preference), modified radical mastectomy may be done.

    c. Stages III and IV—modified radical mastectomy with or without breast reconstruction and adjuvant therapy as determined by NIH Consensus Conference; radical mastectomy may be done if mediastinal nodes or pectoral muscle is involved.

  2. Surgical options (Table 29-4).

    a. Surgical procedures, except segmental mastectomy for stage 0 disease, include axillary node dissection or sampling; nodal status essential to assess prognosis and need for adjuvant therapy.

    b. Estrogen receptor (ER) and progesterone receptor (PR) assays routinely are done on primary tumor specimens.

Table 29-3

RECOMMENDATIONS OF NATIONAL INSTITUTES OF HEALTH CONSENSUS CONFERENCE ON ADJUVANT CHEMOTHERAPY AND ENDOCRINE THERAPY FOR BREAST CANCER—1990

Nodal Status	Before Menopause	After Menopause
Negative	Adjuvant chemotherapy considered if client at high risk of recurrence	Adjuvant chemotherapy not recommended, regardless of hormone receptor status
Positive	Adjuvant chemotherapy recommended regardless of hormone receptor status	If hormone receptor is positive, antiestrogen is treatment of choice If hormone receptor is negative, adjuvant chemotherapy considered but is not standard practice

Table 29-4
BREAST CANCER SURGERIES

Procedure	Physical Alterations	Side Effects/Possible Complications
Segmental Mastectomy (lumpectomy, tylectomy, quadrant resection)		
Removal of tumor and clear tissue margin of 1 cm Axillary node dissection via second incision	Minimal breast disfigurement Disruption in skin integrity Disruption in lymphatic venous drainage	Psychological distress Infection Seroma Hematoma Nerve trauma (numbness, "pins and needles" sensation, itching) Arm edema Impaired arm mobility
Modified Radical Mastectomy		
Removal of entire breast Possible removal of pectoralis minor muscle Axillary node dissection via en bloc procedure	Loss of breast Disruption in skin integrity Disruption in lymphatic and venous drainage	Psychological distress Infection Seroma Hematoma Nerve trauma Phantom breast sensations Impaired arm and shoulder mobility Skin flap necrosis Chest wall tightness Altered body image
Radical Mastectomy		
Removal of entire breast Removal of pectoralis minor and pectoralis major muscles Axillary and possible mediastinal node dissection	Same as for modified radical mastectomy plus hollow chest wall defect, axillary defect, and shoulder abduction	Same as for modified radical mastectomy but with increased incidence

    c. National Surgical Adjuvant Breast Project (NSABP) Protocol B-06 was a landmark study, showing that 5-year survival of clients after segmental mastectomy plus irradiation was equivalent to survival of clients after modified radical mastectomy for stage I and stage II disease.

    d. Breast reconstruction.

        (1) Client options for cosmetic restoration of the breast include wearing of external prosthesis or having reconstructive surgery.

        (2) Reconstruction may be immediate (implant at time of modified mastectomy) or delayed (6 months to 1 year after surgery or until chemotherapy or irradiation is complete).

        (3) Procedures are covered by most insurance carriers (as are permanent external prostheses).

        (4) Reconstruction is contraindicated if disease is locally advanced or progressively metastatic or is an inflammatory breast cancer.

        (5) Common technique involves implanting silicone prosthesis under chest wall's musculofascial layer.

      (6) Procedures to transplant a flap of skin and muscle tissue to the chest are used if anterior chest wall is tight and concave.

      (7) To achieve symmetry, plastic surgery (mammoplasty) may be required on remaining breast:

         (a) Reduction mammoplasty if large.

         (b) Augmentation mammoplasty if underdeveloped.

         (c) Mastopexy if sagging.

      (8) Nipple-areolar complex can be reconstructed by sharing from the normal breast or grafting from the labia or upper inner thigh.

      (9) Complications include hematoma, infection, soft-tissue necrosis, seroma, capsular contracture, and extrusion of prosthesis.

3. Radiation therapy.

  a. Primary radiation.

      (1) Therapy begun 2 to 4 weeks after segmental mastectomy when incisions have healed and shoulder range of motion is adequate.

      (2) Total of 6000 cGy administered.

         (a) To entire breast over 4½ to 5 weeks by linear accelerator—4500 to 5000 cGy.

         (b) To the tumor site by either interstitial iodine-192 implants or electron beam "boost"—1000 to 1500 cGy.

      (3) Immediate side effects are fatigue, edema and tenderness of breast, skin reactions, and possibly sore throat.

      (4) Long-term effects are hyperpigmentation, rib fractures, breast fibrosis, pneumonitis.

      (5) May be administered concurrently with adjuvant chemotherapy.

  b. Palliative radiation.

      (1) Used for clients with inflammatory breast cancer.

      (2) Provides partial to complete relief of pain caused by bone metastasis.

4. Adjuvant chemotherapy.

  a. Combination drug regimens used to treat breast cancer generally are administered for 3 to 6 months:

      (1) Cyclophosphamide, methotrexate, 5-fluorouracil (CMF) is considered standard therapy.

      (2) Cyclophosphamide, doxorubicin (Adriamycin), 5-fluorouracil (CAF).

      (3) CMF with vincristine and prednisone (CMFVP).

      (4) Doxorubicin (Adriamycin) and cyclophosphamide (AC).

  b. Combinations of chemotherapy and hormones may result in an increased response rate but not necessarily an increased survival rate.

  c. Side effects and toxicities may be more pronounced in the client receiving concurrent irradiation to the breast.

5. Hormonal therapy.

  a. Goal of hormonal therapy is to increase survival time in women with metastatic breast disease.

  b. Estrogen receptor (ER) and progesterone receptor (PR) results predict those clients likely to respond to hormonal therapy.

      (1) Overall response rate of 65% in women with high positive ER results.

      (2) Only 10% response rate in those with negative ER results.

      (3) PR result is positive in approximately 75% of ER-positive tumors; may be more accurate predictor.

         (a) If both ER and PR results are positive, 77% response rate.

         (b) If both ER and PR results are negative, only 5% response rate.

  c. Additive hormonal therapies (increase level of circulating hormone):
   (1) Estrogen (35% response rate in women 5 or more years past menopause).
   (2) Androgens (infrequently used; have largely been replaced by antiestrogens).
   (3) Progestins (33% response rate to megesterol acetate).
  d. Ablative therapies (decrease level of circulating hormone).
   (1) Oophorectomy (32% response if ER result is positive); premenopausal or perimenopausal women with non–life-threatening recurrent disease are candidates.
    (a) Surgical castration (oophorectomy).
    (b) Ovarian radiation.
   (2) Adrenalectomy (32% response if ER result is positive); medical adrenalectomy with aminoglutethimide (Cytadren) is method used.
  e. Antiestrogens (53% response if ER result is positive).
   (1) First-line treatment in primary and metastatic disease in postmenopausal women.
   (2) Tamoxifen given along with chemotherapy increases survival rate in clients with metastatic disease.
   (3) A new research area is chemoprevention, involving the prophylactic use of tamoxifen in women at high risk for developing breast cancer.
 6. Use of autologous bone marrow transplantation and biological response modifiers in the treatment of breast cancer is investigational.
 D. Trends in survival.
  1. General survival rates for all cases by stage:
   a. Stage I—85%, 5-year survival; 75%, 10-year survival.
   b. Stage II—66%, 5-year survival; 52%, 10-year survival.
   c. Stage III—41%, 5-year survival; 28%, 10-year survival.
   d. Stage IV—10%, 5-year survival; 0%, 10-year survival.
  2. Determinants of survival.
   a. Strongest predictor of recurrence is number of positive axillary nodes at diagnosis:
    (1) 0 positive nodes—35% recurrence at 10 years.
    (2) 1-3 positive nodes—55% recurrence at 10 years.
    (3) 4-10 positive nodes—70% recurrence at 10 years.
    (4) 11-20 positive nodes—82% recurrence at 10 years.
    (5) More than 20 positive nodes—85% recurrence at 10 years.
   b. Hormone receptor status—women with ER- and PR-positive tumors have a lower risk of recurrence than women with ER- and PR-negative tumors.
   c. Cellular deoxyribonucleic acid (DNA) content and S-phase fraction (determined by flow cytometric analysis):
    (1) Abnormal amount of DNA content in tumor cells (aneuploid) indicates an aggressive cancer.
    (2) High percentage of S-phase cells indicates poor prognosis.

DATA COLLECTION

 I. Pertinent personal and family history (risk factors).
  A. Primary risk factors.
   1. Sex:
    a. Most common type of cancer in women; one out of every nine American women will have breast cancer at some point in her lifetime.

      b. Second leading cause of cancer deaths in women (44,500 deaths estimated in 1991).

      c. One percent of breast cancer occurs in men.

    2. Age—risk increases if more than 45 years of age.

    3. Personal history of breast cancer—15% develop breast cancer in the opposite breast.

    4. Family history of breast cancer:

      a. Risk is increased two to three times in daughters or sisters of women with breast cancer.

      b. Risk may be increased seven to eight times in daughters or sisters of women with premenopausal, bilateral breast cancer.

  B. Secondary risk factors.

    1. Parity:

      a. Risk is increased in women who have never had children.

      b. Woman who had first child after the age of 30 may be at even greater risk than the nulliparous woman.

    2. History of biopsy for fibrocystic changes in the breast that revealed atypical hyperplasia (ductal or lobular).

    3. Prolonged hormonal stimulation:

      a. Early menarche (before age 12 years).

      b. Late menopause (after age 50 years).

      c. Long-term use of exogenous estrogens in combination with progestin for menopausal symptoms (may be tumor-promoting factor).

    4. Exposure to excessive ionizing radiation such as multiple fluoroscopies for tuberculosis or radiation for mastitis or chest acne.

    5. History of endometrial, ovarian, or colon cancer.

    6. Obesity or high dietary fat intake, particularly after menopause.

  C. Women with high-risk profile account for only one third of all breast cancer.

  D. Pertinent history.

    1. Presence of risk factors identified in sections IA and IB.

    2. Health care practices—BSE and mammography.

II. Physical examination.

  A. Early signs and symptoms.

    1. Early—usually asymptomatic.

    2. Majority present with painless lump or thickening in the breast.

      a. Ninety percent discovered by the woman.

      b. Fifty percent occur in upper outer quadrant of the breast (more breast tissue in this quadrant).

      c. More often in left breast than in right.

      d. Only 25% of all breast lumps are malignant.

  B. Late signs and symptoms.

    1. Primary tumor changes:

      a. Dimpling of the skin.

      b. Nipple retraction or deviation.

      c. Asymmetry of breasts.

      d. Scaling of skin on nipple or areola.

      e. Peau d'orange skin—skin edema secondary to obstructed lymphatic drainage; thickened skin, prominent pores (similar to the peel of an orange).

      f. Bloody discharge from nipple.

      g. Ulceration of the breast.

2. Nodal involvement:
   a. Firm, enlarged axillary lymph nodes.
   b. Palpable supraclavicular nodes.
3. Distant metastasis:
   a. Pain in shoulder, hip, lower back, or pelvis.
   b. Persistent cough.
   c. Anorexia or unexplained weight loss.
   d. Digestive disturbances.
   e. Persistent dizziness or blurred vision.
   f. Headache.
   g. Difficulty walking.

III. Laboratory data specific to breast cancer.
   A. Biopsy report of breast lesion.
   B. Baseline biological tumor marker (see Chapter 5, Table 5-2) profile:
      1. Carcinoembryonic antigen (CEA).
      2. LASA-P.
      3. CA 15-3.
   C. Complete blood count.
   D. Liver chemistry results.

ASSOCIATED NURSING DIAGNOSES

I. Knowledge deficit related to breast cancer and breast cancer treatment options.

II. Potential altered peripheral tissue perfusion, related to removal of lymph nodes.

III. Potential impaired physical mobility, related to surgery.

IV. Potential for injury, related to infection.

V. Ineffective individual coping, related to diagnosis/treatment of breast cancer.

VI. Body-image disturbance, related to loss of part or all of the breast.

VII. Potential sexual dysfunction, related to disease process and treatment.

NURSING PLANNING AND IMPLEMENTATION

I. Interventions to maximize safety for client.
   A. Prevent fluid accumulation under chest wall incisions by maintaining patency of surgical drains.
      1. Drain(s) left in for 7 to 10 days or until output is less than 30 ml/24 hours.
      2. Client usually discharged with drain in place, so teach how to strip tubing, empty drain reservoir, measure and record output.
   B. Promote venous lymphatic drainage.
      1. Elevate affected arm with hand higher than elbow and elbow higher than shoulder to facilitate venous drainage.
      2. Place a sign on the bed advising that no blood pressure readings, injections, or blood testing should be done on the affected arm.
   C. Adduct arm first 24 hours to minimize tension on suture lines.
   D. Promote functional recovery of arm and shoulder.
      1. Perform limited exercise first 24 hours (squeezing ball; wrist and elbow flexion and extension).
      2. Begin active range of motion exercises, usually on second to third day or as ordered by physician (Figure 29-3).

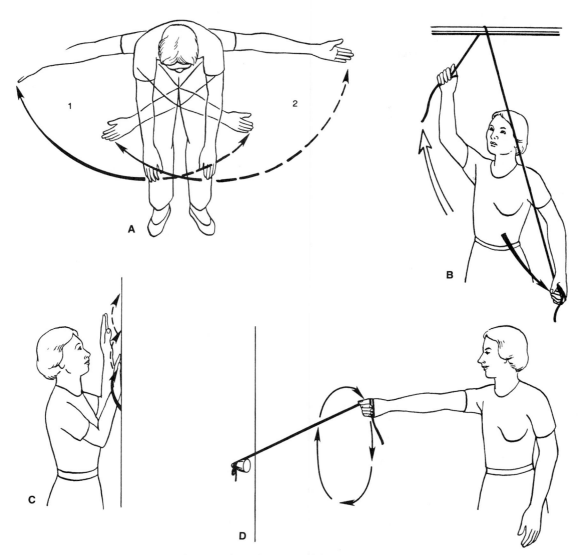

Figure 29-3 Post-axillary dissection exercises. **A,** Arm swings. Stand with feet 8 inches apart. Bend forward from waist, allowing arms to hang toward floor. Swing both arms up to sides to reach shoulder level. Swing back to center, then cross arms at center. Do not bend elbows. If possible, do this and other exercises in front of mirror to ensure even posture and correct motion. **B,** Pulley motion. Using affected arm, toss 6-foot rope over a shower curtain rod or over top of a door. Grasp one end of rope in each hand. Slowly raise affected arm as far as comfortable by pulling down on the rope on opposite side. Keep raised arm close to your head. Reverse to raise unaffected arm by lowering the affected arm. Repeat. **C,** Hand wall climbing. Stand facing wall with toes 6 to 12 inches from wall. Bend elbows and place palms against wall at shoulder level. Gradually move both hands up the wall parallel to each other until incisional pulling or pain occurs. (Mark that spot on wall to measure progress.) Work hands down to shoulder level. Move closer to wall as height of reach improves. **D,** Rope turning. Tie rope to door handle. Hold rope in hand of affected side. Back away from door until arm is extended away from body, parallel to floor. Swing rope in as wide a circle as possible. Increase size of the circle as mobility returns. *(From Luckman, J. & Sorenson, K.C. [1987]. Medical-Surgical Nursing: a Psycho-physiologic Approach [3rd ed]. Philadelphia: W.B. Saunders Co., p. 1823.)*

Table 29-5
PRECAUTIONS TO PREVENT LYMPHEDEMA

Avoid burns while cooking or smoking.

Avoid sunburns.

Have all injections, vaccinations, blood samples, and blood pressure tests done on the other arm whenever possible.

Use an electric razor with a narrow head for underarm shaving to reduce the risk of nicks or scratches.

Carry heavy packages or handbags on the other arm.

Wash cuts promptly, treat with antibacterial medication, and cover with a sterile dressing; check often for redness, soreness, or other signs of infection.

Never cut cuticles; use hand cream or lotion.

Wear watches or jewelry loosely, if at all, on the treated arm.

Wear protective gloves when gardening and when using strong detergents.

Use a thimble when sewing.

Avoid harsh chemicals and abrasive compounds.

Use insect repellent to avoid bites and stings.

Avoid elastic cuffs on blouses and nightgowns.

From (1987) *After Breast Cancer: a Guide to Followup Care.* NIH Pub. No. 87-2400.

    II. Interventions to decrease incidence and severity of symptoms specific to breast cancer; see Chapters 19, 20, and 21 for nursing interventions to manage problems associated with surgery, chemotherapy, and radiation.

    III. Interventions to monitor for unique side effects of treatment for breast cancer.
        A. Teach client to measure circumference of affected arm and to notify physician if the circumferential measurement is more than 5 cm larger than unaffected arm; see Chapter 7 for nursing interventions to manage lymphedema.
        B. Inform client about altered arm and breast sensations (numbness and tingling of arm, lack of sensation on chest wall, phantom breast sensation after mastectomy) that may persist for several years.

    IV. Interventions to enhance adaptation and rehabilitation.
        A. Promote communication between physician and client; alert physician to client's concerns about breast cancer and its treatment.
        B. Assess coping abilities, support systems, feelings about body image, sexual identity, role relationships; see Chapter 7, discussion on sexual dysfunction for interventions to manage problems with sexuality.
        C. Discuss breast prostheses, where permanent ones can be obtained, names of contact person(s) at the store(s), costs, insurance coverage; information has been compiled by Reach to Recovery (organization of American Cancer Society [ACS]) volunteers in local communities.
        D. Prepare client for long-term follow-up, with office visits every 3 months for first 2 to 3 years, every 6 months for next 2 to 3 years, and then at least annually.
        E. Teach mastectomy client the importance of practicing BSE of the remaining breast (see Chapter 5, Figure 5-1).
        F. Reevaluate client's BSE technique.

G. Teach client and family precautions to take with affected arm to prevent trauma and infection, which can lead to lymphedema (Table 29-5).

H. Use appropriate resources (see part VII of "Evaluation of Client and Family Outcomes").

V. Interventions to incorporate client/family in care.

A. Assess psychological status of spouse/significant other—level of distress, ability to serve as support system.

B. Include significant others in teaching (e.g., about surgical drain care, range of motion exercises).

C. Teach the daughters and sisters of client the importance of regular breast cancer screening.

EVALUATION OF CLIENT AND FAMILY OUTCOMES

I. Identify type of cancer and rationale for treatment.

A. Participate in ongoing decision making about breast cancer treatment options.

B. Describe breast cancer and rationale for treatment(s) received at a level consistent with educational and emotional status.

II. List signs and symptoms of immediate and long-term side effects of disease and treatment.

A. Immediate:
1. Infection
2. Seroma.
3. Hematoma.
4. Arm swelling.
5. Limited range of motion of arm.
6. Fatigue.

B. Long-term:
1. Nerve injury.
2. Lymphedema.

C. See Chapters 20 and 21 for immediate and long-term side effects of radiation and chemotherapy.

III. List self-care measures to decrease incidence and severity of symptoms associated with disease and treatment.

A. Communicate feelings about breast cancer and the selected therapy.

B. Identify potential alterations in perception of sexuality.

C. Identify plan for seeking health care assistance when alteration in health status occurs.

IV. Demonstrate skills in self-care demanded by structural or functional effects of disease and treatment.

A. Demonstrate appropriate care of incision(s) and surgical drain(s) at time of hospital discharge.

B. Demonstrate range of motion exercises of affected arm and shoulder.

C. Identify options for temporary and permanent cosmetic restoration of breast.

D. Demonstrate appropriate BSE techniques.

V. Describe schedule and procedures for routine follow-up.

A. Schedule:
1. Three-month intervals for first year.
2. Four-month intervals for second year.
3. Six-month intervals for third year.
4. Annually and as needed after third year.

B. Procedures:
   1. Physical examination and interview.
   2. Chest x-ray examination.
   3. Complete blood count, blood chemistry results.
   4. CEA, LASA-P, CA 15-3 testing.
   5. Bone scan if tumor markers or chemistry results indicate need.
   6. Mammography at 6 months, 1 year, and then annually.

VI. List signs and symptoms of recurrent disease.
   A. Changes in breast or in incision scar (lumps, thickening, inflammation).
   B. Pain in breast, shoulder, hip, lower back, or pelvis.
   C. Persistent cough or hoarseness.
   D. Persistent digestive disturbances (nausea, vomiting, diarrhea, heartburn).
   E. Loss of appetite or unexplained weight change.
   F. Persistent dizziness, blurred vision, headache, or gait disturbances.

VII. Identify potential community resources to meet unique demands of breast cancer, treatment, and survivorship.
   A. Self-help organizations:
      1. Reach to Recovery, sponsored by ACS.
         a. Volunteer visitors who are successful breast cancer survivors make hospital visits and provide a kit of practical information and a temporary breast form.
         b. Contact local ACS unit for free service.
      2. Encore, program offered by Young Women's Christian Association (YWCA).
         a. Includes support groups and pool and floor exercise program for women after breast surgery.
         b. Contact local YWCA for availability and cost.
      3. Y-ME, largest breast cancer support program in United States.
         a. Program includes telephone hotline, counseling, group meetings, workshops, speakers bureau, resource library, newsletter.
         b. Call (800) 221-2141 weekdays.
      4. *Look Good—Feel Better,* developed by Cosmetic, Toiletry, and Fragrance Association Foundation in partnership with ACS and National Cosmetology Association.
         a. Helps women deal with side effects on appearance resulting from chemotherapy and radiation therapy.
         b. Call (800) 395-LOOK for referral to local programs.
   B. Booklets and pamphlets.
      1. Selected National Cancer Institute (NCI) publications (call (800) 4-CANCER):
         a. *Breast Biopsy: What you Should Know* (publication number 7-657).
         b. *Breast Cancer: Understanding Treatment Options* (publication number 87-2675).
         c. *Breast Reconstruction: A Matter of Choice* (publication number 88-2151).
         d. *Mastectomy: A Treatment for Breast Cancer* (publication number 87-658).
         e. *Radiation Therapy: A Treatment for Early Stage Breast Cancer* (publication number 87-659).
         f. *After Breast Cancer: A Guide to Follow-up Care* (publication number 87-2400).
         g. *Breast Exams: What you Should Know* (publication number 84-2000).
      2. Resource available from Women's Breast Cancer Advisory Center, Inc.,

P.O. Box 224, Kensington, MD 20895—*If You've Thought About Breast Cancer. . .*, by Rose Kushner.
3. Selected ACS publications (contact local unit):
   a. *How to Do Breast Self Exam* (publication number 2088) (available in English and Spanish).
   b. *Special Touch* (publication number 2095) (available in English and Spanish).
   c. *Cancer Facts for Women* (publication number 2077).
   d. *What is Reach to Recovery?* (publication number F312).

BIBLIOGRAPHY

American Cancer Society (1991). *Cancer Facts and Figures*. (Pub. No. 5009.91-LE). Atlanta: Author.

American Joint Committee on Cancer (1988). *Manual for Staging of Cancer* (3rd ed). Philadelphia: J.B. Lippincott Co.

Brown-Daniels, C.J. & Blasdell, A. (1990). Early-stage breast cancer: adjuvant drug therapy. *Am J Nurs 90*(11), 32-33.

Collins-Hattery, A.M. & Blumberg, B.D. (1991). S phase index and ploidy prognostic markers in node negative breast cancer: information for nurses. *Oncol Nurs Forum 18*(1), 59-62.

Dianon Systems (1986). *Dianon Systems Oncology Tests* (No. 140MP). Stratford, Conn: Author.

(1990) Early stage breast cancer. *NIH Consensus Development Conference Consensus Statement. 8*(6), 1-19.

Fisher, B. (1991). A biological perspective of breast cancer: contributions of the National Surgical Adjuvant Breast and Bowel Project clinical trials. *CA 41*(2), 97-111.

Frank-Stromborg, M. & Savela, B. (1990). Yellow pages for the cancer nurse. In S.L. Groenwald, M.H. Frogge, M. Goodman, & C.H. Yarbro (eds). *Cancer Nursing: Principles and Practice* (2nd ed). Boston: Jones & Bartlett Publishers, pp 1281-1308.

Goodman, M. (1988). Concepts of hormonal manipulation in the treatment of cancer. *Oncol Nurs Forum 15*(5), 639-647.

Goodman, M. & Harte, N. (1990). Breast cancer. In S.L. Groenwald, M.H. Frogge, M. Goodman, & C.H. Yarbro (eds). *Cancer Nursing: Principles and Practice* (2nd ed). Boston: Jones & Bartlett Publishers, pp 722-750.

Harris, J.R., Hellman, S., Canellos, G.P., & Fisher, B. (1985). Cancer of the breast. In V.T. DeVita, Jr., S. Hellman, & S.A. Rosenberg (eds). *Cancer: Principles & Practice of Oncology,* vol 2 (2nd ed). Philadelphia: J.B. Lippincott Co., pp 1119-1177.

Hassey, K.M. (1988). Pregnancy and parenthood after treatment for breast cancer. *Oncol Nurs Forum 15*(4), 439-444.

Kinne, D.W. (1991). The surgical management of primary breast cancer. *CA 41*(2), 71-84.

Knobf, M.T. (1991). Breast cancer. In S.B. Baird, R. McCorkle, & M. Grant (eds). *Cancer Nursing: A Comprehensive Textbook*. Philadelphia: W.B. Saunders, pp 425-451.

Knobf, M.T. (1990). Early-stage breast cancer: the options. *Am J Nurs 90*(11), 28-30.

Pierce, S.M. & Harris, J.R. (1991). The role of radiation therapy in the management of primary breast cancer. *CA 41*(2), 85-96.

Schwarz-Appelbaum, J., Dedrick, J., Jusenius, K., & Kirchner, C.W. (1984). Nursing care plans: sexuality and treatment of breast cancer. *Oncol Nurs Forum 11*(6), 16-24.

30

Genitourinary Cancers

Julena Lind, MN, RN

Kidney Cancer

THEORY

I. Physiology and pathophysiology of cancer of the kidney.
   A. Anatomical placement of a kidney (Figures 30-1 and 30-2).
   B. Primary function.
      1. Pair of organs approximately 4½ inches long lying behind the peritoneum in a mass of fatty tissue.
      2. Consists chiefly of nephrons (parenchyma) in which urine is secreted, collected, and discharged into a main cavity (pelvis) and then conveyed by the ureters to the bladder.
   C. Changes associated with cancer—excessive cell production results in growth into adjacent organs and gradual loss of function in the affected kidney.
   D. Pathophysiology.
      1. Two major types of kidney cancer.
         a. Renal cell:
            (1) Most common—75% to 85% of all kidney tumors.
            (2) Occurs in parenchyma.
            (3) Often associated paraneoplastic syndromes (e.g., inappropriate antidiuretic hormone [ADH], parathyroid; see Chapter 16) occur.
         b. Cancer of the renal pelvis:
            (1) Comprises 5% to 9% of all kidney tumors.
            (2) Generally arises from epithelial tissue anywhere in renal pelvis; may be multifocal.
            (3) Because of the relative infrequent occurrence, cancer of the renal pelvis will not be discussed in this text.
      2. Renal cell cancers tend to grow toward the medullary portion of the kidney and spread in direct extrusion to the renal vein and sometimes into the vena cava.
      3. Between 30% and 50% of kidney cancers have metastasized by the time of diagnosis; mean survival time with metastasis is approximately 4 months.
   E. Trends in epidemiology.
      1. Kidney cancer is relatively rare in the United States, accounting for only 3% of all cancers.

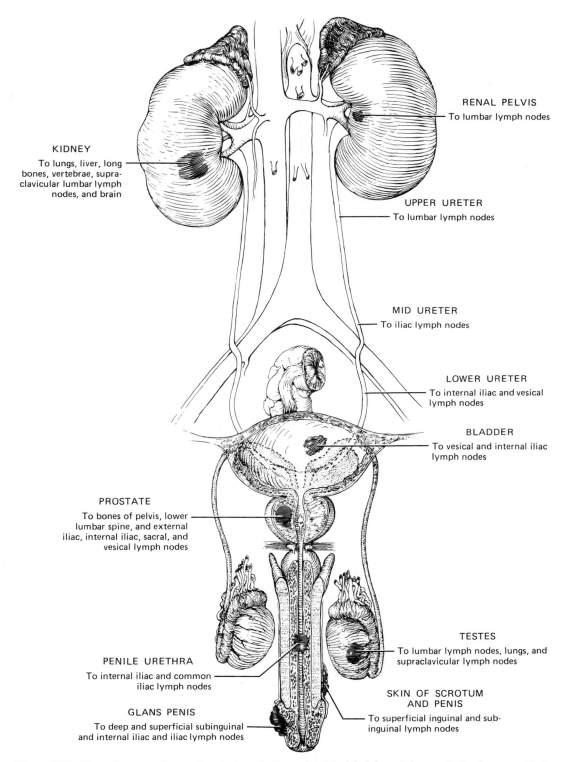

RENAL PELVIS
To lumbar lymph nodes

KIDNEY
To lungs, liver, long
bones, vertebrae, supra-
clavicular lumbar lymph
nodes, and brain

UPPER URETER
To lumbar lymph nodes

MID URETER
To iliac lymph nodes

LOWER URETER
To internal iliac and vesical
lymph nodes

BLADDER
To vesical and internal iliac
lymph nodes

PROSTATE
To bones of pelvis, lower
lumbar spine, and external
iliac, internal iliac, sacral, and
vesical lymph nodes

TESTES
To lumbar lymph nodes, lungs, and
supraclavicular lymph nodes

PENILE URETHRA
To internal iliac and common
iliac lymph nodes

**SKIN OF SCROTUM
AND PENIS**
To superficial inguinal and sub-
inguinal lymph nodes

GLANS PENIS
To deep and superficial subinguinal
and internal iliac and iliac lymph nodes

Figure 30-1 Sites of tumor origin and metastases in the male. *(Modified from Johnson, D.E., Swanson, D.A., & von Eschenbach, A.C. [1987]. Tumors of the genitourinary tract. In E.A. Tanagho & J.W. McAninch [eds]. Smith's General Urology [12th ed]. San Mateo, Calif.: Appleton & Lange, p. 332.)*

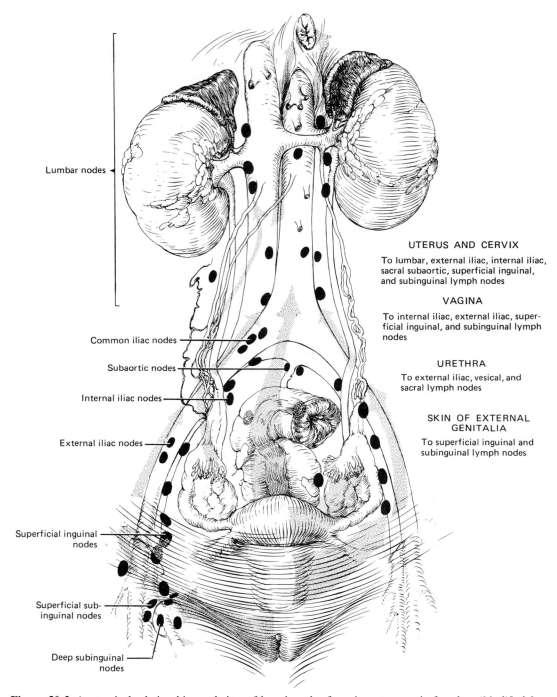

Lumbar nodes

UTERUS AND CERVIX

To lumbar, external iliac, internal iliac, sacral subaortic, superficial inguinal, and subinguinal lymph nodes

VAGINA

To internal iliac, external iliac, superficial inguinal, and subinguinal lymph nodes

URETHRA

To external iliac, vesical, and sacral lymph nodes

SKIN OF EXTERNAL GENITALIA

To superficial inguinal and subinguinal lymph nodes

Common iliac nodes

Subaortic nodes

Internal iliac nodes

External iliac nodes

Superficial inguinal nodes

Superficial sub-inguinal nodes

Deep subinguinal nodes

Figure 30-2 Anatomical relationships and sites of lymph nodes for urinary tumors in females. *(Modified from Johnson, D.E., Swanson, D.A. & von Eschenbach, A.C. [1987]. Tumors of the genitourinary tract. In E.A. Tanagho, J.W. McAninch [eds]. Smith's General Urology [12th ed]. San Mateo, Calif.: Appleton & Lange, p. 333.)*

2. A slight steady increase in kidney cancer among males has been reported.

II. Principles of medical management.
   A. Screening and diagnostic tests—no screening tests are available for kidney cancer; diagnostic tests include:
      1. Kidney, ureter, and bladder (KUB) radiography (Table 30-1).
      2. Nephrotomography.
      3. Excretory urography (test of choice) (Table 30-1).
      4. Retrograde urography (Table 30-1).
      5. Renal ultrasound.
      6. Renal computerized tomography (CT).
      7. Renal angiography.
      8. Magnetic resonance imaging (MRI).
   B. Staging methods and procedures.
      1. Based on factors that influence survival—regional lymph node involvement, invasion through the renal capsule, extension to contiguous organs, and distant metastases.

Table 30-1

UROLOGICAL DIAGNOSTIC TESTS AND NURSING INTERVENTIONS

Test	Physical Alteration	Nursing Interventions
X-ray examination of kidneys, ureter, bladder (KUB)	None—plain film of abdomen	Explain client will lie flat on x-ray examination table. Do not schedule after barium studies (will obscure kidneys).
Excretory urography	Dye is excreted unchanged by kidneys; therefore hydration is important, followed by nothing by mouth 6 to 8 hr before test Dye is injected intravenously; anaphylactic or allergic reaction to dye may occur; may premedicate with antihistamines	Assess history of allergy to iodine dyes or contrast media before test; pretesting may be indicated. Use of iodine dyes may be contraindicated in clients with severe renal or hepatic disease or clinical hypersensitivity (severe allergies, asthma). Have emergency equipment and personnel available before injection (anaphylaxis and cardiovascular reactions may occur) and 30-60 min after test (delayed reactions). Observe for adverse reactions to dye—angina, chest pain, arrhythmias, hypotension, dizziness, blurred vision, headache, fever, convulsions, dyspnea, rhinitis, laryngitis, nausea.
Retrograde urography	General anesthesia or narcotic analgesia may be used; cystoscope is inserted; iodinated dye is injected via urethral catheter Laxatives at bedtime before test may be used to cleanse bowel	Observe for reaction to anesthetic or analgesic. Monitor for bleeding, symptoms of urinary tract infections, dysuria, or difficulty voiding after test.

2. Size of the primary tumor is not correlated strongly with survival and may not be a significant factor in staging.
3. Systems most often used for classifying renal cell carcinoma—modification of the system of Flocks and Kadesky and the TNM system (see Appendix).

C. Treatment strategies.
1. Renal cell cancer is usually treated by surgical removal via a radical nephrectomy, including removal of the lymph nodes in the renal hilar area.
2. Regional lymphadenectomy remains controversial.
   a. Improved survival rate has not been demonstrated conclusively.
   b. Lymphadenectomy provides a more meaningful staging of the disease and probably offers the best chance of survival to those for whom radical nephrectomy is potentially curative.
3. Radiotherapy and chemotherapy.
   a. Renal cell cancers are usually radioresistant.
   b. Metastatic bone pain can be treated by radiotherapy.
   c. Adjuvant chemotherapy has not improved survival.
4. Treatment of advanced disease.
   a. Approximately 30% of clients present with metastases at diagnosis.
   b. Adjunctive or palliative nephrectomy has been used.
   c. Hormonal therapy, using progesterone such as medroxyprogesterone acetate (Depo-Provera) or megesterol acetate (Megace), testosterone, or antiestrogens such as tamoxifen, has been used.
   d. Immunotherapy using high doses of interleukin-2 (IL-2) and large number of lymphokine activated killer cells (LAK) has shown promise in treating metastatic renal cancer.

D. Five-year survival rate:
1. Stages I and II—50% to 70%.
2. Stage III—approximately 50%.
3. Stage IV—less than 10%.

DATA COLLECTION

I. Identification of clients at high risk.
   A. Kidney cancer accounts for approximately 3% of all cancers.
   B. A 2:1 male predominance exists.
   C. Geographical differences have been reported:
      1. Scandinavian countries have a relatively high incidence (approximately 11% of all cancers).
      2. Japan has a low incidence.
      3. United States and Western European countries have an intermediate risk.
   D. Average age at diagnosis is 55 to 60 years.

II. Pertinent history.
   A. Carcinogens linked to kidney cancer:
      1. Cigarette smoking, nicotine, and coal tars.
      2. Exposure to cadmium, lead pigment in colored printing ink, and asbestos.
      3. Heavy use of analgesics, specifically phenacetin-containing products, increases the risk of cancer of the renal pelvis.
   B. Association between renal cell cancer and obesity in women was first identified in 1974.

III. Physical examination.
   A. In 40% of people with renal cell cancer the initial, but not early, symptom is gross hematuria.

B. Pain (dull, aching) and a palpable abdominal mass are late signs.

C. More generalized late signs—fever, weight loss, elevated erythrocyte sedimentation rate (ESR), and/or anemia.

IV. Evaluation of diagnostic data.

A. Gross hematuria found on urinalysis.

B. Elevated ESR.

C. Obstruction or blockage related to tumor presence as demonstrated in excretory urogram.

D. Differential diagnosis of renal cysts versus neoplasms demonstrated by nephrotomogram and/or renal ultrasound.

ASSOCIATED NURSING DIAGNOSES

I. Airway clearance, ineffective.

II. Potential fluid volume deficit.

III. Alteration in comfort: pain.

IV. Alteration in bowel elimination.

V. Knowledge deficit.

VI. Anxiety.

NURSING PLANNING AND IMPLEMENTATION

I. Interventions to maximize safety.

A. Prevention of atelectasis and pneumonia.

1. Because of the close proximity of the nephrectomy incision to the diaphragm, deep breathing and coughing can be extremely uncomfortable.

2. Clients should be taught proper splinting and instructed to take at least 10 deep breaths every hour while awake.

3. Incentive spirometer and intermittent positive pressure breathing may be beneficial.

B. Observation for signs of hemorrhage.

1. Bleeding is a danger (but not a frequently observed complication) after nephrectomy because the kidney is highly vascular.

2. Acute massive hemorrhage is manifested by profuse drainage and distention at the suture line or by internal bleeding.

3. The nephrectomy dressing and underlying sheet should be examined frequently for blood.

C. Observation for toxicity to immunotherapy.

1. Toxicities—flulike symptoms (fever and rigors <2 to 4 hours after administration); myalgias, headaches; acute or chronic nausea, vomiting, diarrhea; pruritis; mental status changes; hypotension, dyspnea, anemia, and thrombocytopenia.

2. Client may be treated in intensive care unit if toxicity rate is high.

D. Maintenance of water seal drainage for chest tubes if thoracoabdominal incision is used (see Chapter 28).

II. Interventions to decrease severity of symptoms associated with treatment.

A. Pain relief measures.

1. Pain can be severe after nephrectomy because of incisional pain and muscular aches and pains (related to lithotomy position on operative table).

    2. Pain medication should be given on a regular basis and titrated to the needs of the client (see Chapter 7).

  B. Prevention and observation for paralytic ileus.

    1. Paralytic ileus occurs fairly commonly after nephrectomy (kidneys are retroperitoneal; thus the intestines are manipulated in surgery).

    2. Ambulation and encouragement to turn from side to side may help expel flatus and promote comfort.

    3. Observe for abdominal distention and auscultate bowel sounds frequently.

  C. Prevention of loss of function of remaining kidney.

    1. Teach client and family the importance of continuing liberal oral intake (up to 2500 ml/day).

    2. Teach client and family to avoid high-fat diets (see Chapter 4), which may result in protein catabolism.

III. Interventions to monitor for unique side effects of treatment.

  A. Follow-up monitoring:

    1. Frequent blood pressure and renal function tests to monitor function of remaining kidney.

    2. Excretory urography to detect contralateral tumors.

    3. Lung x-ray examination to rule out lung metastases.

    4. Bone scans to detect bony metastasis.

  B. Teach client and family to report signs of respiratory distress, hemoptysis, pain, or pathological fracture of an extremity (related to bony metastasis).

IV. Interventions to monitor for response to medical management.

  A. Monitoring renal function immediately postoperatively for volume (at least 30 ml/hour).

  B. Monitoring urinary output for excessive external bleeding and vital signs for internal hemorrhage.

EVALUATION OF CLIENT AND FAMILY OUTCOMES

  I. Identify the disease and rationale for treatment.

 II. List signs and symptoms of immediate and long-term side effects of disease and treatment.

  A. Verbalize methods to control pain.

  B. Demonstrate aseptic wound care techniques.

III. Describe self-care measures.

  A. List signs of abdominal distention.

  B. Describe the importance of liberal oral fluid intake (up to 2500 ml/day).

  C. Discuss diet.

  D. List phenacetin-containing drugs.

  E. Identify smoking cessation techniques if applicable.

  F. Cite strategies to deal with fatigue or other responses to biological response modifiers (BRM), if applicable.

  G. List resources—local American Cancer Society (ACS), CanSurmount.

IV. Participate in follow-up care.

  A. Verbalize the schedule for follow-up appointments and the rationale for blood pressure checks, excretory urograms, chest x-ray examinations, and other diagnostic tests.

  B. Report signs and symptoms of recurrence—abdominal or flank pain, hematuria, bone pain, respiratory changes.

C. Report signs and symptoms of renal dysfunction—decreased urinary output, fluid retention, hypertension.

Bladder Cancer

THEORY

I. Physiology and pathophysiology associated with bladder cancer.
  A. Anatomy of the bladder.
    1. Consists of a membranous sac that serves as temporary retainer for urine, which is then discharged through the urethra.
    2. In men, in addition to the local lymph nodes, critical adjacent structures include the prostate, seminal vesicles, urethra, and nerves at the base of the penis (Figure 30-1).
    3. In women the critical adjacent structures include the uterus, ovaries, fallopian tubes, urethra, and local lymph nodes (Figure 30-2).
  B. Changes associated with cancer.
    1. Proliferation of abnormal tissue in one or more places inside the bladder.
    2. Clinical changes—bleeding if the tumor has produced a bladder wall lesion and, occasionally, urethral obstruction.
  C. Histology.
    1. In North America 90% to 95% of bladder tumors are transitional cell carcinomas.
      a. Transitional cell tumors arise in the epithelial layer of the bladder, which rests on the basement membrane.
      b. If the basement membrane remains intact, metastasis to the vascular or lymphatic system is unlikely.
      c. Within the transitional cell classification, the tumors are further subdivided—carcinoma in situ (confined to urothelial lining), papillary infiltrating, papillary noninfiltrating, and solid tumors.
        (1) Papillary tumors have a propensity for recurrence.
        (2) Transitional cell tumors are usually multifocal.
        (3) High recurrence and multicentricity necessitate aggressive follow-up.
    2. Squamous cell carcinoma account for 6% to 8% of bladder cancers.
    3. Adenocarcinomas are rare (2%).
  D. Metastatic patterns.
    1. Many of these tumors arise on floor of bladder and can involve one or both ureteral orifices.
    2. Most important prognostic feature—depth of penetration into the bladder wall; the deeper the penetration, the greater is the risk of metastases.
    3. Some tumors spread rapidly to the pelvic lymph nodes; others grow slowly and spread into the pelvic tissues.
    4. Metastasis takes place via direct extension from the muscle of the bladder into the perivesical fat (or serosa).
      a. Tumor can obstruct ureters or bladder neck.
      b. Can spread by direct extension to involve other adjacent structures such as the sigmoid colon, rectum, prostate, uterus, or vagina.
    5. The grade (or degree of tumor cell differentiation) is a key predictor of the aggressive nature of the cancer.
  E. Trends in epidemiology.
    1. The incidence of bladder cancer has been gradually increasing over the past 30 years.

2. The rate of diagnosis in the localized stage has increased over the past 20 years.
3. The higher male-to-female ratio is diminishing, probably as a result of increased smoking rates among females.

II. Principles of medical management.
  A. Screening and diagnostic tests.
    1. No good early screening test for bladder cancer exists.
    2. Urinary cytology—for best results specimens are obtained from late morning or early afternoon urine.
    3. Bladder washings provide even more reliable results.
    4. Flow cytometry—technique used to examine the deoxyribonucleic acid content of urinary cells; useful in identifying high-grade, high-stage tumors.
    5. Excretory urography (intravenous pyelography)—done before cystoscopy to help evaluate the upper tracts (Table 30-1).
    6. Cystoscopy—for tumor visualization, for possible biopsy, and to allow bimanual examination of the bladder (to determine fixation and extent of tumor).
    7. Imaging:
       a. Computerized tomography (CT)—aids in defining the extent of local tumor and in identifying pelvic lymph node metastasis.
       b. Transurethral ultrasound—used to define local extension and the degree of involvement of the bladder wall.
       c. Magnetic resonance imaging (MRI)—to distinguish the tumor from the normal bladder wall and to identify the presence of pelvic lymph node involvement.
  B. Staging methods and procedures.
    1. Most common systems used in the United States—Jewett-Strong system (modified by Marshall) and the TNM system developed by the American Joint Committee on Cancer (Appendix).
    2. Another factor often considered in treatment but not actually included in the staging systems—grade of the tumor (grades 1, 2, 3, 4); refers to the degree of tumor cell differentiation and helps to determine the aggressiveness of therapy.
  C. Standard therapies.
    1. Carcinoma in situ is usually treated by fulguration and administration of intravesical thiotepa or radical cystectomy.
    2. Superficial low-grade tumors are treated by transurethral surgery with resection and fulguration (if multiple small lesions are found).
       a. Because the chance of recurrence is so great, intravesical chemotherapy, using thiotepa or mitomycin C, has been used; controversy persists regarding the efficacy of this treatment.
       b. Small superficial bladder tumors also have been treated with laser therapy.
    3. High-stage, high-grade tumors need more aggressive treatment because of the invasion to the bladder muscle.
       a. Definitive radiotherapy—according to some experts, can cure no more than 16% to 30% of clients with invasive bladder cancer, a rate not comparable to that for surgery.
       b. Preoperative radiation—used to decrease both pelvic lymph node recurrence and dissemination during surgical excision.
       c. Radical cystectomy.
          (1) In men includes excision of the bladder with the perivesical fat, the attached peritoneum, and the entire prostate and seminal vesicles.

(2) Aggressive surgery in women includes removal of the bladder and entire urethra, the uterus, ovaries, fallopian tubes, and anterior wall of the vagina (not all surgeons remove the reproductive organs); pelvic lymph node dissection also may be performed.

d. Urinary diversion.

(1) Ileal conduit (Figure 30-3)—popular urinary diversion performed with cystectomy.

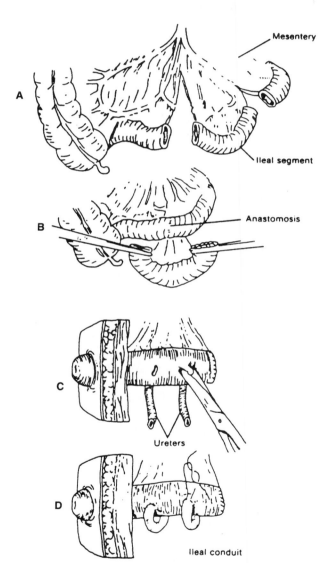

Figure 30-3 Ileal conduit. **A,** Segment of ileum is isolated from the gastrointestinal tract with its mesenteric blood flow. **B,** Gastrointestinal tract is reanastomosed. One end is sutured closed, and the other end will be used to form an abdominal stoma. **C,** Ureters, which are located retroperitoneally, are brought into the abdominal cavity. Incisions are made in the conduit for ureteral implantation. **D,** Abdominal stoma is matured, and ureters are anastomosed to the ileal segment in an end-to-side fashion. *(From Broadwell, D.C. & Jackson, B.S. [eds] [1982]. St. Louis: C.V. Mosby Co.)*

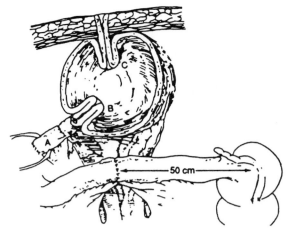

Figure 30-4 Continent ileal reservoir. **A,** Original ileal conduit with implanted ureters. **B,** Reflux-preventing nipple valve. **C,** Continence-maintaining nipple valve. *(From Gerber, A. [1983]. The Kock continent ileal reservoir for supravesical urinary diversion. Am J Surg 146, 16.)*

          (a) Portion of the terminal end of the ileum is isolated, the proximal end is closed, the distal end is brought out through a hole in the abdominal wall and is sutured to the skin, creating a stoma.

          (b) Ureters are implanted into the ileal segment, urine flows into the conduit, and peristalsis propels urine out through the stoma.

       (2) Continent ileal reservoir (Figure 30-4)—technique that provides an intra-abdominal pouch for storage of urine.

          (a) Typically has nipple valves created to maintain and prevent ureteral reflux.

          (b) No external collecting device is needed.

    e. Radical cystectomy can damage the nerves responsible for erectile ability; therefore in many centers a penile prosthesis is implanted at the time of surgery or soon thereafter.

  4. Advanced bladder cancer is often treated with single agents or combination chemotherapy:

    a. Single agents—doxorubicin (Adriamycin), bleomycin, etoposide, methotrexate, cisplatin, and vinblastine.

    b. Combination chemotherapy—doxorubicin and cyclophosphamide; doxorubicin and cisplatin; doxorubicin and 5-fluorouracil; methotrexate and cyclophosphamide plus cisplatin.

D. Trends in survival show an increase in survival rates, with overall rates higher for whites than blacks (Table 30-2).

Table 30-2
FIVE-YEAR SURVIVAL RATE WITH BLADDER CANCER

Stage	Whites (%)	Blacks (%)
Localized	88	80
Disseminated	41	25
All stages	77	56

Data from Silverberg, E. & Lubera, J.A. (1989). Cancer statistics, 1988. *CA* 39:3-32.

DATA COLLECTION

I. Pertinent personal and family history to identify risk factors.
   A. Bladder cancer accounts for 2% to 5% of all cancer in the United States.
   B. Four major variables are related to bladder cancer incidence:
      1. Race—age-adjusted bladder cancer rate in white men in the United States is twice the rate of black men.
      2. Gender—in whites the male-female ratio is 4:1.
      3. Age—most tumors occur in men over 50 years old.
      4. Geographical location—areas with a high incidence of bladder cancer include Africa and Egypt (attributed to the parasite *Schistosoma haematobium*; higher rate of squamous cell type); more prevalent in highly industrialized urban areas than rural areas.
   C. Assess occupational risks—exposure to dyes, rubber, leather, paint, and organic chemicals (latency period may be 20 years).
   D. Determine smoking history—rate is twice as high in smokers versus nonsmokers.
   E. Artificial sweeteners act as both initiators and promoters in rats, but risk in humans is inconclusive.

II. Physical examination.
   A. Early signs and symptoms.
      1. Gross painless hematuria—most common presenting symptom but not usually considered an early sign.
      2. Irritability of the bladder (dysuria, urinary frequency, urgency, and burning on urination)—common.
   B. Later signs and symptoms.
      1. If the tumor is large, compression of the internal urethral orifice may occur and cause decrease in force and caliber of the stream.
      2. Obstruction of the ureters can cause flank pain and result in hydronephrosis.

III. Laboratory data.
   A. DNA flow cytometry of urine specimen (higher DNA content indicates more aggressive tumor).
   B. Serum carcinoembryonic antigen (CEA) levels are moderately elevated in 50% of late stage bladder cancer cases.

ASSOCIATED NURSING DIAGNOSES

I. Knowledge deficit.

II. Potential for infection (pyelonephritis).

III. Alteration in comfort: pain.

IV. Impairment of skin integrity.

V. Body image disturbance.

NURSING PLANNING AND IMPLEMENTATION

I. Interventions to maximize safety for the client.
   A. Teach client and family the importance of a low-residue diet 2 days before surgery, followed by clear liquid diet on day before surgery.
   B. Teach client and family the importance of using the prescribed antibiotics and cathartics before surgery (incomplete adherence to the preoperative regimen increases the risk of infection); unlike a fecal diversion that is subject to an adynamic ileus, the urinary diversion should produce urine from the time of surgery.

1. Maintain current input and output records; the urinary flow should be rather continuous.
2. Monitor for significant imbalances in weight and electrolyte values.
3. Monitor for bleeding.

C. Participate with or initiate referral to enterostomal therapist to assist in marking preoperative stomal site to avoid skin folds, scars, bony prominences, and belt lines that interfere with adherence of appliance.
   1. Consider vocational and recreational activities and visibility to the client when lying, sitting, standing.
   2. Preferable site is 3 inches in diameter, without folds or prominences, and slightly convex.

D. Monitor signs of urinary tract infection—elevated temperature, flank pain, malodorous urine, and/or hematuria.

C. Attach straight drainage bag to pouch when client is in bed or at bedtime to prevent infections and damage to stomal tissue.

II. Interventions to decrease severity of symptoms (pain) associated with the disease and/or treatment.
   A. After evaluation of pain status, medicate client routinely for pain.
   B. Splint abdomen with pillow when coughing.
   C. Position with pillows when turning.

III. Interventions to monitor for unique side effects of treatment.
   A. Monitor and document color of stoma through a clear pouch.
      1. Color of the intestinal stomal tissue can be compared to the mucosal lining of the mouth.
      2. Stoma may bleed when rubbed because of the capillaries in the area.
      3. Ideally, stoma should protrude ½ to ¾ inch above the skin to allow the urine to drain into the aperture of the appliance.
      4. Normal color of the stoma is a deep pink to dark red; a dusky appearance ranging from purple to black may develop if circulation is seriously impaired.
   B. Assess client for signs of peritonitis related to anastomotic leak:
      1. Abdominal distention or tenderness.
      2. Elevated temperature.
      3. Sudden decrease in urinary output or presence of abdominal wound drainage.
   C. Monitor urinary output—at least 30 ml per hour.
      1. Stomal edema is normal in the early postoperative period.
      2. Edema should not interfere with stomal functioning, but a larger opening in appliances is needed initially to prevent pressure or constriction of the stoma.
      3. Edema should resolve during the first 1 or 2 weeks after surgery.

IV. Interventions to enhance adaptation and rehabilitation.
   A. Assess client and family for signs of readiness to learn self-care of stoma (Table 30-3).
      1. Write all instructions.
      2. Encourage the client to observe pouch change and gradually to participate in self-care.
      3. Encourage client and family to empty the pouch when one third full.
      4. Follow-up with phone calls after discharge.
      5. Refer to home health nursing agency if indicated.
   B. Teach client and family care of stoma and schedule return demonstrations until proper technique is achieved.
   C. Teach client and family preventive elements of care.

Table 30-3
MANAGEMENT OF COMMON COLOSTOMY, ILEOSTOMY, OR UROSTOMY PROBLEMS

Problem	Cause or Sign	Treatment	Manufacturer
Odor			
Fecal	Food	Topical, in appliance	United Surgical
	Oral medicines	Banish, 10 drops in pouch as needed	
	Active disease	Odour-guard	Marlen
		Oral medication	
		Bismuth subgallate 250 mg four times daily	Parthenon
		Bismuth subcarbonate 0.6 g four times daily	Lilly
		Derifil, one three times daily	Rystan
Urinary	Poor hygiene		
	Infection	Avoid rubber pouch	
		Soak appliance in vinegar/water 1:4	
Crystals	Encrustation of stoma, skin, or appliance	Acidification of urine	
		8 to 16 ounces cranberry juice daily	
		Ascorbic acid, 1 g four times daily	
	Bleeding stoma	Acetic acid in pouch, solution 1:8	
Skin irritation	Appliance leaks or fits badly or im-properly	Large karaya gum ring of Colly-seel	Mason Labs
		Stomahesive	Squibb
		Temporary appliance	United Surgical
		New, proper permanent appliance	Marlen, Torbot
	Allergy to adhesive or material	Patch test to find cause of allergy	
	Flush stoma	Deep convex appliance	Permatype
		Consider revision or stoma at a new site	
Fistula	Deep infection	Revision or stoma at a new site	
Ulcer of peri-stomal skin	Rigid appli-ance disk	Colly-seel and temporary appliance	Hollister
		Flexible mounting ring of appliance	
Cut stoma	Sliding or small appli-ance	Colly-seel and temporary appliance, then proper appliance	
		Nonallergic tape to help hold appliance	
Hyperkeratosis	Peristomal skin overex-posed to urine	Apply pressure to area with a firm mounting ring measured to exact stoma size	

Modified from Rowbotham, J.L. (1982). *Managing Colostomies* (Pub No. 3422-PE). Atlanta: American Cancer Society.

1. Ways to avoid malodorous urine:
   a. Avoid ingestion of large quantities of alkaline liquids such as carbonated beverages.
   b. Drink fluids with vitamin C content.
   c. Clean reusable pouch regularly with soap and water, rinsing with vinegar if desired.
   d. Avoid foods (e.g., fish, asparagus) that cause urinary odors.

2. Ways to prevent urinary tract infection:
   a. Drink at least 2 L of fluid per day.
   b. Use straight drainage bag at bedtime and clean the system each morning.
3. Ways to prevent ammonia salt encrustation—ingest food and fluid (cranberry juice) that keep the urine acid.
4. Ways to prevent peristomal skin breakdown:
   a. Use a skin barrier if irritation is present.
   b. Use appropriate stoma opening in the barrier and the pouch.
   c. Remove pouch if burning or itching occurs.
   d. Change pouch on a regular basis (e.g., every 3 to 7 days).
   e. Do not use preparations that are greasy or that contain benzoin or alcohol on irritated skin.
D. Arrange preoperative and/or postoperative visit by rehabilitated client with similar diversion.

EVALUATION OF CLIENT AND FAMILY OUTCOMES

I. Describe a low-residue and clear liquid diet.

II. Describe antibiotic regimen and sources for obtaining medications.

III. Verbalize pain control strategies.

IV. Describe a viable stoma (i.e., pink and moist).

V. Describe desired urinary output (>30 ml/hour).

VI. List the signs and symptoms of urinary tract infection and measures to prevent it.

VII. Describe strategies to prevent ammonia salt encrustation.

VIII. Demonstrate pouch change.

IX. Describe the use of skin barriers.

X. Demonstrate the steps of peristomal skin care.

XI. Describe schedule and rationale for aggressive follow-up care (as frequent as every 2 to 4 months for first 3 years).

XII. Identify selected resources—enterostomal therapy, home care, and support services (CanSurmount, ACS Transportation Services, ACS Look Good–Feel Better Program).

Prostate Cancer

THEORY

I. Physiology and pathophysiology associated with prostatic cancer.
   A. Anatomy and physiology—the prostate is:
      1. A small, firm organ shaped like an inverted and flattened pyramid.
      2. Made of glands and musculature enclosed in a fibrous capsule.
      3. Approximately the size of a walnut (4 to 6 cm long).
      4. Located posterior to the symphysis pubis, inferior to the bladder, and in front of the rectum (Figure 30-1).
      5. Inverted so that the base is at the neck of the bladder.
      6. Penetrated by a portion of the urethra (prostatic urethra).
      7. Controlled by sex hormones (growth and function).
      8. A secondary sex organ that secretes a component of seminal fluid.

B. Pathophysiology and metastatic patterns.
   1. Primary type is adenocarcinoma.
   2. More common in the posterior lobe, although some researchers believe that the tumors are multifocal.
   3. Grows and spreads locally to the seminal vesicles, bladder, and peritoneum (Figure 30-1).
   4. Varies in histology and differentiation; most prostatic tumors are extremely slow growing and indolent, but an unusually wide range of biological malignancy exists.
   5. May be detected accidentally and may never grow and spread (a minority of tumors).
   6. Spreads via the blood vessels and lymphatic system:
      a. Spreads into the perineural lymphatics, involving the seminal vesicles and the sacral, external iliac, and lumbar lymph nodes.
      b. One third of men with early cancer have evidence of metastases to the pelvic lymph nodes.
      c. From the pelvis the lymphatic fluids travel to the thoracic duct and into the venous system at the junction of the left internal jugular and the left subclavian veins; the supraclavicular nodes lie adjacent to the veins that communicate with the thoracic duct; therefore clients with widespread cancer often have scalene or supraclavicular node involvement.
      d. Hematogenous spread of prostatic cancer typically involves the lung, liver, kidneys, and bones.
C. Trends in epidemiology:
   1. Accounts for approximately 18% of all cancer in men in the United States; second to skin cancer in incidence among males.
   2. Accounts for 11% of all cancer deaths in men.
   3. A significant relative rise in the incidence of prostatic cancer in American men has been reported.
   4. A significant increase has been noted in the 5-year survival rate.

II. Principles of medical management.
   A. Screening tests.
      1. Early detection is not common; rectal examination may reveal small asymptomatic nodule (50% of prostatic nodules are malignant).
      2. ACS recommends annual digital examination for men over 40 years old.
      3. Transrectal ultrasonography for high-risk groups—initially believed a useful screening modality, but re-evaluation of this technique is being weighed in light of expense of equipment and training required.
   B. Diagnostic tests.
      1. Rectal examination by which the prostate may be palpated for firm, hard lesions.
      2. Biopsy.
         a. Needle—perineal or transrectal; transrectal preferred.
         b. Open—in selected cases (i.e., if size of prostate demands removal).
      3. Histological diagnosis—may be found in asymptomatic specimens removed for benign prostatic hypertrophy.
      4. Cytological examination of urine and expressed prostatic fluid (which is positive in as many as 85% of men with prostate cancer).
      5. CT scans to diagnose pelvic lymph node involvement.
      6. MRI to determine involvement of the seminal vesicles and changes in the contour of the prostate.

7. Laboratory studies:
   a. Acid phosphatase—elevated serum levels; trauma to prostate causes release into bloodstream.
      (1) Wait 48 hours after rectal examination or catheterization to draw serum for acid phosphatase study.
      (2) Elevated acid phosphatase level in a client suspected of having prostatic cancer may indicate metastatic disease.
   b. Prostatic acid phosphatase level can be measured by radioimmunoassay; 80% of men with stage D have increased levels.
   c. Alkaline phosphatase—elevated serum level.
      (1) Elevated in presence of bone metastasis.
      (2) Many clients with cancer of prostate have bone metastasis on presentation.
   d. Prostatic specific antigen—increased levels may be significant as an adjunct in differential diagnosis or as a marker for disease progression.
C. Staging methods and procedures.
   1. Staging workup may include:
      a. Chest x-ray examination to assess hilar node, lung, and rib involvement.
      b. Excretory urography (see Table 30-1) to detect obstruction caused by pelvic lymph node metastasis or direct invasion by tumor.
      c. Liver scan and brain scan to detect distant metastases.
      d. Lymphangiography to detect presence of pelvic lymph nodes.
   2. Staging systems (see Appendix A).
      a. Stage A—incidental microscopic focus (not clinically palpable); 5% of all cases.
      b. Stage B—localized, palpable macroscopic nodule confined to prostate gland; 5% of all cases.
      c. Stage C—local extension to adjacent structures; 45% of all prostatic cancers at diagnosis.
      d. Stage D—extrapelvic or distant metastases; 40% of all prostatic cancers at diagnosis.
D. Standard therapies.
   1. Stage A.
      a. If low grade (well differentiated), may leave untreated.
         (1) Fifteen-year survival rate is equal to that in the general population.
         (2) Age of client and morbidity of treatment must be considered.
         (3) Common treatment for well-differentiated stage A tumors is radical perineal or retropubic prostatectomy.
         (4) Radiation, with curative intent, also is used.
      b. High-grade anaplastic tumors may respond to megavoltage radiation.
   2. Stage B.
      a. Surgery—radical prostatectomy for cure.
         (1) Perineal approach is generally treatment of choice.
         (2) Retropubic approach may be associated with lower incidence of urethral stricture formation.
         (3) Suprapubic approach may be used.
         (4) Walsh technique for radical retropubic prostatectomy minimizes damage to pelvic nerves needed to achieve erection and to preserve potency.
      b. Lymph node dissection may be performed with prostatectomy.
         (1) May not increase survival, but benefits have been reported.
         (2) Involves considerable morbidity.
      c. Complications associated with surgical treatment:

(1) Impotence (some centers implant penile prosthesis at time of prostatectomy; others allow 6 to 12 months before considering an implant).

(2) Incontinence.

(3) Stricture formation in urethra.

d. Radiation therapy is becoming more widely used.

(1) Reported lower incidence of impotence than with surgery.

(2) Types of radiation used:

(a) Interstitial implants (temporary or permanent)—lower incidence of
impotence reported than with external beam.

(b) External beam therapy of 6000 to 7000 rads to extended field—
25% to 30% have gradual loss of erectile function within 6 to 12
months.

e. Large (>1.5 to 2 cm) stage B and stage C lesions may be treated by
multimodality approach:

(1) Transurethral resection of the prostate (TURP).

(2) Megavoltage radiation therapy:

(a) Administration of 6500 to 7000 rads over 6 to 7 weeks.

(b) Delayed for 6 weeks after TURP to allow urothelial healing.

3. Palliative treatment for stage C and D disease.

a. Radiation therapy—for local extension and distant metastases.

(1) May be primary treatment for stage D lesions if hormonal manipulation
is ineffective or contraindicated.

(2) Used for palliation of pain from bone metastasis.

(3) Emergency treatment for spinal cord compression.

b. Hormonal manipulation—to counter effects of male hormones (androgens);
prompt initiation for palliation may prevent or alleviate symptoms.

(1) Estrogen therapy—generally diethylstilbestrol, 1 mg/day by mouth (or
intravenously for central nervous system symptoms or emergencies),
will result in decreased pain, weight gain, decreased tumor size, and
decreased urinary symptoms; primary disadvantages are breast enlargement (gynecomastia), cardiovascular complications, and relapse (usually within 2 to 3 years) to hormone-resistant form.

(2) Antiandrogens (cyproterone acetate, megestrol acetate, flutamide)—
interfere with intracellular androgen activity; effects may be delayed
1 to 2 months.

(3) Gonadotropin releasing hormone (Gn-RH analogues)—decreases production of testosterone; may produce fewer side effects than estrogens.

(4) Orchiectomy—surgical removal of testicles; used for prompt response,
for clients unreliable in taking medications, or for clients in whom side
effects of estrogens contraindicate continued use.

(5) Adrenalectomy—surgical or "chemical" (aminoglutethimide); removes
secondary source of androgens; effect occurs in 3 to 5 days with drug
use.

E. Trends in survival.

1. Stage A—5-year survival rate, 84%.

a. Low-grade tumor—15-year survival rate closely approximates actual life
expectancy.

b. High-grade tumor—prognosis may be as poor as with metastatic disease.

2. Stage B—10-year survival rate, as high as 72%.

3. Stage C.

a. Average life expectancy, 2 to 3 years.

b. Survival rate at 5 years, 45%; 10 years, 26%.

4. Stage D—usual prognosis, 1 to 2 years.

DATA COLLECTION

I. Pertinent personal and family history.
   A. Age.
      1. More than 14% of men age 50 have cancer of prostate.
         a. Incidence increases with each decade.
         b. Occurs in 50% of men over 75 years old.
      2. Some theorize that prostate cancer is normal part of the aging process since 95% of men who die over the age of 90 years have some foci of disease in the prostate at autopsy.
   B. Ethnicity.
      1. Native Orientals are at low risk; however, incidence increases markedly in those who adopt Western habits, particularly dietary ones.
      2. Highest rate of prostatic cancer in the world is among black Americans; much lower in African blacks.
   C. Pertinent history.
      1. Exposure to cadmium may lead to its accumulation in the prostate and, in turn, to interruption of cell growth.
      2. Transmission of viruslike particles has been investigated but not substantiated as an environmental factor.
      3. Endocrine factors may play a role; testosterone given to rats can produce prostatic cancers.

II. Physical examination.
   A. Localized disease is generally asymptomatic—digital rectal examination reveals nodule; with tumor growth, client will report:
      1. Dysuria.
      2. Urinary hesitancy.
      3. Straining to start stream; narrowing of urinary stream.
      4. Urgency, frequency.
   B. Later signs:
      1. Hematuria.
      2. Chronic urinary retention, with dribbling.
   C. Clients with widespread disease on presentation appear generally debilitated and older than chronological age and may present with:
      1. Bone and neuritic pain secondary to osseous involvement or nerve compression.
      2. Weight loss, lethargy, and secondary disease (e.g., bronchopneumonia).

III. Evaluation of laboratory data—serum alkaline phosphatase, serum acid phosphatase, prostatic acid phosphatase, and prostatic specific antigen.

ASSOCIATED NURSING DIAGNOSES

I. Related to radical prostatectomy.
   A. Potential for fecal incontinence.
   B. Potential for sexual dysfunction.

II. Related to external beam radiation.
   A. Alteration in urinary elimination.
   B. Alteration in bowel elimination.

III. Related to hormonal therapy.
   A. Alteration in tissue perfusion, cardiovascular.
   B. Sexual dysfunction.

NURSING PLANNING AND IMPLEMENTATION

I. Interventions to maximize safety for client.

A. Maintain closed urinary catheter drainage system and aseptic technique during irrigation to prevent infection.

B. Apply antiembolic hose; teach client proper application technique.

C. Maintain positioning and patency of urethral catheter (serves as splint for urethral anastomosis and for bladder drainage after radical prostatectomy).

D. Facilitate healing of perineal wound (with perineal prostatectomy):

1. Irrigate wound.

2. Provide sitz baths.

3. Apply heat lamp to perineum.

4. Minimize pressure on perineal wound:

a. Administer low-residue diet and stool softeners to avoid straining at stool.

b. Avoid and teach client to avoid use of rectal tubes, rectal thermometers, or enemas until healing is complete.

c. Bed rest may be extended to lessen pressure on suture line.

E. Protect skin integrity (e.g., use of T-binder versus tape to hold dressing in place after perineal proctectomy).

F. Assess for symptoms of hypercalcemia (polyuria, polydipsia, confusion, weakness) with initiation of hormonal therapy (see Chapter 9).

II. Interventions to promote comfort.

A. Maintain patency of urinary and/or bladder irrigation systems.

1. Maintain continuous or intermittent bladder irrigation to remove blood clot and/or mucous plugs.

2. Avoid kinked tubing by positioning of client and securing of tubes.

B. Administer antispasmodics and/or analgesics for bladder spasms; initiate use of stool softeners with antispasmodics to avoid constipation.

C. Consult with enterostomal therapist as indicated for perineal wound care, radiation reactions, or management of incontinence.

D. Administer antidiarrheal medications as ordered for proctitis and teach client to avoid a high-residue diet.

III. Interventions to monitor and decrease incidence or severity of symptoms of prostatic cancer or recurrence.

A. Teach client to report symptoms of urinary obstruction promptly—diminished stream, abdominal pain and distention, dysuria, retention with dribbling, bladder spasms.

B. Teach client to report early symptoms of urinary tract infection—fever, dysuria, urgency, hematuria.

C. Teach client to report symptoms of recurrence—hematuria, urinary obstruction, bone pain, abdominal pain, neuritic pain, weight loss, debilitation, back pain.

D. Describe follow-up schedule as determined by physician.

IV. Interventions to monitor effects of treatment of prostatic cancer.

A. Facilitate physician-nurse-client discussion of potential impact of treatment on sexual functioning and interventions to minimize effects.

1. Give permission before and after treatment to discuss functional and anatomical changes with treatment and resultant sexual concerns (having testicles removed as an adult does not affect masculinity).

2. Provide information on potential effects of treatment (e.g., impotence after radical prostatectomy; feminization after hormonal therapy).

3. Provide specific suggestions related to treatment used and alternatives (e.g.,

penile implants after radical prostatectomy; testicular implants after orchiectomy; or to ask physician if alternative hormonal therapy may be used if estrogens cause severe decrease in libido).
    4. Initiate referral for sexual counseling if indicated.
  B. Record amount and frequency of voiding after removal of urethral catheter.
  C. Inform clients to report lymphedema of legs, scrotum, or penis after lymph node dissection.
  D. Teach clients symptoms of proctitis, which may occur with radiotherapy—diarrhea, cramps, rectal pain.
  E. Teach side effects of hormonal therapy (edema, mood changes) as indicated; possible therapies (fluid restriction, diuretics); and need for continued medical follow-up for laboratory tests (serum sodium and calcium levels) and blood pressure monitoring.

  V. Interventions to enhance adaptation and rehabilitation.
  A. Teach care of Foley catheter, three-way irrigation equipment, or other equipment.
  B. Instruct to drink at least 2 L of fluid per day to alleviate cystitis associated with radiotherapy.
  C. Initiate appropriate referrals for home care (e.g., visiting nurse, enterostomal therapist).
  D. Teach perineal exercises to manage dribbling, urgency, or urinary incontinence (in most cases, problem gradually diminishes).

  VI. Interventions to incorporate client/family in care.
  A. Assess resources and coping strategies of client/family.
  B. Incorporate personal and cultural values of client/family in discussing sexual concerns.
    1. Respect reticence in discussing sexual concerns (most clients are elderly and socialized not to discuss sexuality).
    2. Use terminology appropriate to social and cultural level.
    3. Provide written information and anatomical drawings as indicated for clarity and to reinforce teaching.
  C. Identify resources, as needed, for home care, follow-up, reconstructive treatment, or palliation.

EVALUATION OF CLIENT AND FAMILY OUTCOMES

  I. List signs and symptoms of immediate and long-term side effects of treatment—wound infection, fecal incontinence, sexual dysfunction (impotence, decreased libido), urinary bleeding, urinary tract infection, side effects of hormonal therapy.

  II. List self-care measures to decrease incidence and severity of symptoms associated with disease and treatment:
  A. Description of exercises to strengthen perineal muscles and decrease urinary dribbling or incontinence.
  B. Importance of drinking 2 L of fluid daily.
  C. Need for sexual counseling if problem is present.

  III. Identify a follow-up schedule of every 6 months to every year (or as prescribed).

  IV. List signs and symptoms of recurrent disease.
  A. Bone pain.
  B. Further changes in urinary habits.
  C. Abdominal pain.

V. Identify resources to deal with disease and treatment—American Cancer Society (*Cancer of the Prostate, Cancer Facts for Men, Sexuality and Cancer for the Man Who Has Cancer and His Partner*, loan closets, transportation services); National Cancer Institute (*Radiation Therapy and You*); local home health care and/or hospice agencies.

BIBLIOGRAPHY

deKernion, J.B. (1983). Treatment of advanced renal cell carcinoma: traditional methods and innovative approaches. *J Urol 130*(1), 2-7.

Dudjak, L.A. & Yasko, J.M. (1990). Biological response modifier therapy. In J.M. Yasko & L. Dudjak (eds). *Biological Response Modifier Therapy: Symptom Management*. Pittsburgh: Park Row Publishers, pp 3-24.

Flocks, R.H. & Kadesky, M.C. (1958). Malignant neoplasms of the kidney; an analysis of 353 patients followed five years or more. *J Urol 79*(2):196-198.

Fowler, J.E., Jr. (1988). Adoptive immunotherapy using lymphokine-activated killer cells. *J Urol 139*(1), 148-149.

Lind, J. (1991). Urinary tract cancers. In S.B. Baird, M.G. Donehower, V.L. Stalsbroten, & T.B. Ades (eds). *A Cancer Source Book for Nurses* (6th ed). Atlanta: American Cancer Society, pp 208-215.

Lind, J. & Irwin, R.J., Jr. (1991). Genitourinary cancers. In S.B. Baird, R. McCorkle, & M. Grant (eds). *Cancer Nursing: A Comprehensive Textbook*. Philadephia: W.B. Saunders Co., pp 466-484.

Lind, J.M. & Nakao, S.L. (1990). Urologic and male genital cancers. In S.L. Groenwald, M.H. Frogge, M. Goodman, & C.H. Yarbro (eds). *Cancer Nursing: Principles and Practice* (2nd ed). Boston: Jones & Bartlett Publishers, pp. 1026-1073.

Paganini-Hill, A., Ross, R.K., & Henderson, B.E. (1988). Epidemiology of renal cancer. In D.G. Skinner & G. Lieskovsky (eds). *Diagnosis and Management of Genitourinary Cancer*. Philadelphia: W.B. Saunders Co., pp. 32-39.

Pritchett, T.R., Lieskovsky, G., & Skinner, D.G. (1988). Clinical manifestations and treatment of renal parenchymal tumors. In D.G. Skinner & G. Lieskovsky (eds). *Diagnosis and Management of Genitourinary Cancer*. Philadelphia: W.B. Saunders Co., pp. 337-361.

Rosenberg, S.A., Lotze, M.T., Muul, L.M., Chang, A.E., Avis, F.P., Leitman, S., Linehan, W.M., Robertson, C.N., Lee, R.E., Rubin, J.T., Seipp, C.A., Simpson, C.G., & White, D.E. (1987). A progress report on the treatment of 157 patients with advanced cancer using lymphokine-activated killer cells and interleukin-2 or high-dose interleukin-2 alone. *N Engl J Med 316*(15), 889-897.

Wynder, E.L., Mabuchi, K., & Whitmore, W.F., Jr. (1974). Epidemiology of adenocarcinoma of the kidney. *J Natl Cancer Inst 53*(6), 1619-1634.

Bladder Cancer

Catalona, W.J., Dresner, S.M., & Haaff, E.O. (1988). Management of superficial bladder cancer. In D.G. Skinner & G. Lieskovsky (eds). *Diagnosis and Management of Genitourinary Cancer*. Philadelphia: W.B. Saunders Co., pp 281-294.

Lieskovsky, G., Ahlering, J., & Skinner, D.G. (1988). Diagnosis and staging of bladder cancer. In D.G. Skinner & G. Lieskovsky (eds). *Diagnosis and Management of Genitourinary Cancer*. Philadelphia: W.B. Saunders Co., pp 264-280.

Marini, F., Signori, G.B., & Valente, R. (1988). The relationship between transurethral ultrasound and pathological findings in 16 cases of tumor of the bladder. *Prog Clin Biol Res 260*, 271-274.

Paulson, D.F. (1988). Role of endocrine therapy in the management of prostatic cancer. In D.G. Skinner & G. Lieskovsky (eds). *Diagnosis and Management of Genitourinary Cancer*. Philadelphia: W.B. Saunders Co., pp 464-472.

Ross, R.K., Paganini-Hill, A., & Henderson, B.E. (1988). Epidemiology of prostatic cancer. In D.G. Skinner & G. Lieskovsky (eds). *Diagnosis and Management of Genitourinary Cancer*. Philadelphia: W.B. Saunders Co., pp 40-45.

Silverberg, E. & Lubera, J.A. (1989). Cancer statistics, 1989. *CA 39*(1), 3-20.

Skinner, D.G., Boyd, S.D., & Lieskovsky, G. (1988). Creation of the continent Kock ileal reservoir as an alternative to cutaneous urinary diversion. In D.G. Skinner & G. Lieskovsky (eds). *Diagnosis and Management of Genitourinary Cancer*. Philadelphia: W.B. Saunders Co., pp 653-674.

Skinner, D.G. & Lieskovsky, G. (1988). Management of invasive and high-grade bladder cancer. In D.G. Skinner & G. Lieskovsky (eds). *Diagnosis and Management of Genitourinary Cancer*. Philadelphia: W.B. Saunders Co., pp 295-312.

Williams, R.D. (1987). Magnetic resonance in the diagnosis and staging of urologic cancer. In Williams, R.D. (ed). *Advances in Urologic Oncology*, vol 1. New York: Macmillan, pp 69-88.

Prostate Cancer

Gittes, R.F. (1991). Carcinoma of the prostate. *N Engl J Med 324*(4), 236-245.

Lee, F., Littrup, P.J., Torp-Pedersen, S.T., Mettlin, C., McHugh, T.A., Gray, J.M., Kumasaka, G.H., & McLeary, R.D. (1988). Prostate cancer: comparison of transrectal US and digital rectal examination for screening: *Radiology 168*(2), 389-394.

Lieskovsky, G. (1988). Technique of radical retropubic prostatectomy (Campbell's procedure) with limited pelvic lymph node dissection. In D.G. Skinner & G. Lieskovsky (eds). *Diagnosis and Management of Genitourinary Cancer*. Philadelphia: W.B. Saunders Co., pp 735-752.

McClennan, B.L. (1988). Transrectal US of the prostate: is the technology leading the science? *Radiology 168*(2), 571-575.

McCullough, D.L. (1988). Diagnosis and staging of prostatic cancer. In D.G. Skinner & G. Lieskovsky (eds). *Diagnosis and Management of Genitourinary Cancer*. Philadelphia: W.B. Saunders Co., pp 405-416.

Redmond, M. (1991). Cancers of the male genital organs. In Baird, S.B., Donehower, M.G., Stalsbroten, V.L., & Ades, T.B. (eds). *A Cancer Source Book for Nurses* (6th ed). Atlanta: American Cancer Society, pp 242-251.

Ross, R.K., Paganini-Hill, A., & Henderson, B.E. (1988). Epidemiology of prostatic cancer. In D.G. Skinner & G. Lieskovsky (eds). *Diagnosis and Management of Genitourinary Cancer*. Philadelphia: W.B. Saunders Co., pp 40-45.

Sogani, P.C. & Fair, W.R. (1987). Treatment of advanced prostatic cancer. *Urol Clin North Am 14*(2), 353-371.

Walsh, P.C. & Donker, P.J. (1982). Impotence following radical prostatectomy: insight into etiology and prevention. *J Urol 128*(3), 492-497.

Reproductive Cancers

Marie Flannery, MS, RN

Cervical Cancer

THEORY

I. Physiology and pathophysiology associated with cervical cancer.
  A. Anatomy of the cervix (Figure 31-1).
    1. Consists of the lower portion of the uterus and is contiguous with the upper portion of the vagina.
    2. Composed of the exocervix and the endocervix.
    3. Surrounded by paracervical tissues rich in lymph nodes.
  B. Changes associated with cancer of the cervix.
    1. Cellular changes exist on a continuum from premalignant changes (mild to moderate to severe cervical intraepithelial neoplasia [CIN]) to carcinoma in situ (CIS) to invasive disease.
    2. The majority of invasive cervical cancers (ICC) arises in the transformation zone at the squamocolumnar junction (Figure 31-1).
      a. Exophytic, fungating, or cauliflower-like lesions protrude from the cervix.
      b. Excavating or ulcerative, necrotic lesions replace the cervix or upper vagina.
      c. Endophytic lesions extend within the cervical canal.
    3. The two main histological types of cervical cancer are squamous and adenocarcinoma.
      a. Squamous carcinoma is most common (80% to 95%) and occurs in older women.
      b. Adenocarcinoma occurs in younger women and carries a poorer prognosis.
        (1) Presents as bulky endocervical tumor.
        (2) Is aggressive in nature.
        (3) Is less responsive to treatment.
  C. Metastatic patterns.
    1. Direct extension to other pelvic structures.
    2. Lymph node metastases.
    3. Metastasis to lung, liver, and bone through hematological route.
  D. Trends in epidemiology.

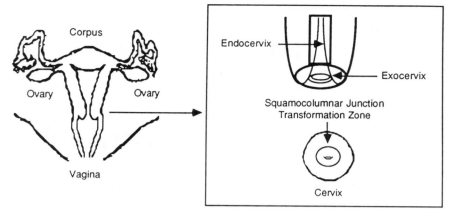

Figure 31-1 Female reproductive organs.

1. Invasive cervical cancer is the sixth most common cancer among women in the United States and the most commonly occurring cancer among women worldwide.
2. Incidence of invasive cervical cancer has decreased 50% since 1945, with a corresponding increase in the diagnosis of preinvasive disease.

II. Principles of medical management.
    A. Screening and diagnostic procedures.
        1. Screening procedures.
           a. Papanicolaou (Pap) smear with bimanual pelvic examination is recommended as the screening test for premalignant and malignant cervical disease.
              (1) Initial Pap smear at age 18 years or initiation of sexual intercourse.
              (2) After three consecutive annual normal Pap smears, every 3 years at discretion of physician.
           b. Cervicography (photographing the cervix after application of acetic acid) is used in some settings as an adjunct to the Pap smear and pelvic examination in screening.
        2. Diagnostic procedures.
           a. Colposcopy (examination of the cervix under magnification after application of acetic acid) is recommended as a component of evaluation of the cervix after obtaining an abnormal result from a Pap smear.
           b. Cervical biopsy is recommended when abnormalities are identified on the cervix by colposcopy.
           c. Endocervical curettage is recommended when:
              (1) The upper limits of cervical abnormalities are not visualized.
              (2) The transformation zone within the endocervical canal is not visualized completely.
           d. Cone biopsy may be recommended to obtain a larger wedge of tissue to rule out invasive cancer (Figure 31-2).
    B. Staging methods and procedures.
        1. Examination with the client under anesthesia may be done to evaluate the extent of the disease with abdominal relaxation.
        2. Evaluation of extension of disease to the bladder or rectum is determined by a cystoscopy, intravenous pyelogram (IVP), sigmoidoscopy, proctoscopy, or barium enema examination.

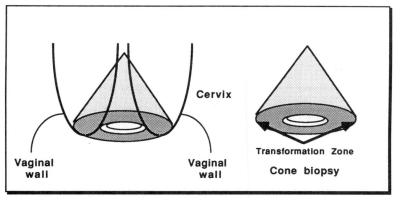

Figure 31-2 Cone biopsy of the cervix.

3. Abdominal or pelvic computed tomographic (CT) scan, ultrasound, or magnetic resonance imaging (MRI) may be done to evaluate the extent of the local lesion and metastasis to regional lymph nodes.
4. Chest x-ray examination is used to rule out lung metastasis.
5. Clinical staging is not altered by subsequent surgical findings (see Appendix).

C. Treatment strategies.
  1. Preinvasive disease—biopsy, cautery, cryotherapy, laser therapy, conization, or hysterectomy; treatment depends on:
    a. Size and location of CIN visualized (Figure 31-3).
    b. Client desire for preservation of childbearing capacity.
    c. Physician skills and preference.

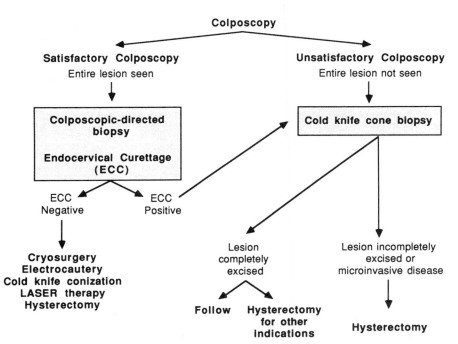

Figure 31-3 Treatment options for cervical intraepithelial neoplasia.

2. Invasive disease—surgery or radiation.
   a. Treatment choice depends on client age, physical condition, percent of ideal body weight, tumor volume, and desire to maintain ovarian function.
   b. Primary surgical treatment—early stage disease:
      (1) Radical hysterectomy with pelvic lymphadenectomy and para-aortic lymph node dissection.
      (2) Bilateral salpingo-oophorectomy included in postmenopausal women over age 40 years.
   c. Primary radiation therapy treatment—early or advanced stage disease.
      (1) Combination of external and intracavitary brachytherapy implants.
      (2) Intracavitary implants may be given before or after external radiation therapy.
   d. Combination of surgery and radiation therapy for advanced stage disease or early stage disease with positive lymph nodes or surgical margins at surgery.
3. Recurrent disease presents a treatment challenge.
   a. Recurrent local disease—anterior, posterior, or total pelvic exenteration.
      (1) Extensive preoperative workup done to rule out extrapelvic disease.
      (2) Initial lymph node frozen sections to rule out metastatic disease.
      (3) Anterior pelvic exenteration—radical hysterectomy, pelvic lymph node dissection, removal of bladder, and creation of ileal conduit.
      (4) Posterior pelvic exenteration—radical hysterectomy, pelvic lymph node dissection, removal of rectosigmoid colon, and creation of a colostomy.
   b. Recurrent disseminated disease—chemotherapy.
      (1) Chemotherapy is primarily palliative.
      (2) Cisplatin most commonly used agent.
D. Trends in survival (Table 31-1).
   1. No overall change in survival rate has occurred for clients with invasive cervical cancer, although mortality rate has decreased because of decreased incidence.
   2. Prognosis is related to stage of disease.
   3. Thirty-five percent of women will have recurrent disease within 3 years of initial therapy.
   4. Cause of death associated most often with uremia, infection, or hemorrhage.

Table 31-1
FIVE-YEAR SURVIVAL RATES FOR CLIENTS WITH CERVICAL CANCER

Stage	5-Year Survival Rate (%)
0	95-100
IA	85-90
IB	80
IIA	70-75
IIB	60
III	30
IV	>10

DATA COLLECTION

I. Pertinent personal and family history.
  A. Bimodal peak of occurrence at 35 to 39 years and 60 to 64 years.
  B. Initiation of sexual intercourse during teenage years.
  C. Multiple sexual partners and sexual partners who have had multiple sexual partners.
  D. History of cervical intraepithelial neoplasia.
  E. Cigarette smoking.
  F. Presence of selected viruses—human papilloma viruses 16 and 18 and herpes simplex type 2.

II. Physical examination.
  A. Early signs and symptoms—most women are asymptomatic until disease is advanced.
    1. Thin, watery vaginal discharge.
    2. Painless, intermittent, postcoital, intramenstrual, or postmenopausal vaginal bleeding.
    3. Increase in the length and amount of menstrual flow.
  B. Late signs and symptoms:
    1. Dyspareunia.
    2. Urinary symptoms—dysuria, urinary retention, urinary frequency, or hematuria.
    3. Bowel symptoms—rectal bleeding, constipation, or bowel obstruction.
    4. Abdominal or pelvic pain referred to flank or leg.
    5. Lower extremity edema.

III. Evaluation of laboratory data.
  A. Elevated blood urea nitrogen (BUN) or creatinine levels.
  B. Decreased hemoglobin or hematocrit levels.
  C. Increased white blood cell count.

ASSOCIATED NURSING DIAGNOSES

I. Body image disturbance.

II. Sexual dysfunction.

III. Altered bowel elimination.

IV. Altered urinary elimination.

NURSING PLANNING AND IMPLEMENTATION

I. Interventions to maximize safety for the client.
  A. Teach changes in life-style that can modify risks of cervical cancer.
    1. Use of barrier-type contraceptive—diaphragm or condom.
    2. Discontinuation of cigarette smoking.
    3. Screening with a Pap smear as recommended to detect premalignant changes.
  B. See Chapters 19 and 20 for safety concerns with surgery and radiation therapy.

II. Interventions to decrease the severity of symptoms associated with disease and treatment.
  A. Teach client about possible symptoms associated with treatment modality options (see Chapters 19, 20, 21, and 23).
  B. Primary symptoms related to surgery.

1. Inability to void—innervation to the bladder can be disrupted during radical hysterectomy and can result in an inability to sense the need to void and an inability to empty the bladder completely; a suprapubic catheter usually will be in place postoperatively.
   a. Initiate bladder training by clamping the catheter for 2 to 3 hours.
   b. Encourage client to drink fluids unless contraindicated by physiological status.
   c. Have client try to void after 3 hours.
   d. After client has voided, unclamp catheter and measure residual urine in bladder.
   e. When residual urine is less than 50 ml consistently, obtain an order from the physician to remove the catheter.
2. Constipation—bowel is manipulated during radical surgery; peristalsis does not return for several days (see Chapter 7, constipation).
3. Shortened vagina—small portion of vagina is excised with hysterectomy; remaining margins are sutured to form vaginal cuff (see Chapter 7, sexual dysfunction).
4. Urinary and stool diversions with pelvic exenteration (see Chapters 30 and 32).
C. Primary symptoms related to radiation therapy (see Chapter 20, Table 20-4, for nursing implications of radiation therapy to the ovary, urinary bladder, uterus, gastrointestinal tract, hair, and skin).

III. Interventions to monitor for sequelae of disease or treatment.
   A. Surgery:
      1. Assess changes in bowel pattern—constipation, bowel obstruction, and rare fistula formation.
      2. Evaluate changes in bladder pattern—recurrent urinary tract infection and fistula formation.
   B. Radiation therapy:
      1. Assess changes in bowel pattern—diarrhea, bowel obstruction, rectal ulcers, and rectovaginal fistulas.
      2. Assess changes in bladder pattern—urinary retention, cystitis, and vesico-vaginal fistulas.
      3. Evaluate changes in vaginal tissues—atrophy, stenosis, and dryness.
   C. Recurrent disease:
      1. Assess for history of vaginal bleeding.
      2. Evaluate occurrence of new pain, particularly in hips or lower back.
      3. Evaluate lower extremities for edema.
      4. Assess for changes in appetite with weight loss.

IV. Interventions to incorporate client and family in care.
   A. Encourage open communication about impact of disease and treatment on the client and significant others.
   B. Teach client and significant other new self-care skills required during or after treatment.
   C. Identify concerns client and sexual partner may have about resuming intercourse after treatment.

EVALUATION OF CLIENT AND FAMILY OUTCOMES

I. Describe personal risk factors for cervical cancer.

II. Discuss rationale, schedule, and personal demands of treatment and follow-up care.

III. List potential side effects of disease and treatment.

IV. Describe self-care measures to decrease the incidence, severity, and complications of treatment.

 V. List signs and symptoms of recurrent disease to report to the health care team—pain in hips or lower back, vaginal bleeding, swelling of lower extremities, or unexplained weight loss.

VI. Describe potential community resources to meet demands of treatment and survivorship—American Cancer Society and National Coalition for Cancer Survivorship.

Endometrial Cancer

THEORY

 I. Physiology and pathophysiology associated with endometrial cancer.
   A. Anatomy of the endometrium (see Figure 31-1).
      1. Inner layer of three layers of the uterus (endometrium, myometrium, and parietal peritoneum).
      2. Highly vascular mucous membrane lining.
   B. Primary function of the endometrium.
      1. Provides vascular and nutrient supply for developing fetus.
      2. Responds to variations in estrogen and progesterone levels in a cyclic fashion.
   C. Changes associated with cancer of the endometrium.
      1. Underlying cause of endometrial cancer is believed to be abnormal production and metabolism of endogenous estrogen.
      2. Premalignant phases of endometrial cancer include atypia and adenomatous hyperplasia.
   D. Metastatic patterns.
      1. Invades inner one third of the endometrium and progresses to the full thickness of the endometrium.
      2. Metastasis occurs through local extension to adjacent structures such as cervix and vagina.
      3. Metastasis occurs in femoral, iliac, and hypogastric lymph nodes.
      4. Hematological metastasis is uncommon except in rare sarcoma.
   E. Trends in epidemiology.
      1. Most common gynecological malignancy among women in the United States.
      2. Fourth most common cancer in women in the United States.
      3. Incidence has increased over the past several decades and has been associated with an increase in estrogen replacement therapy.

II. Principles of medical management.
   A. Screening procedures.
      1. Endometrial aspiration or biopsy.
      2. Bimanual pelvic examination to palpate the size and shape of the uterus.
   B. Diagnostic procedures.
      1. Endocervical curettage to rule out cervical cancer.
      2. Fractional dilation and curettage (D and C) if previous endometrial biopsies have been negative and abnormal bleeding persists.
   C. Staging methods and procedures.
      1. Procedures.
         a. Bladder involvement—cystoscopy or IVP.
         b. Bowel involvement—barium enema examination, proctoscopy, or sigmoidoscopy.

      c. Chest x-ray examination to rule out metastasis.

      d. Hysterography, hysteroscopy, lymphangiography, ultrasound, CT scan, or MRI to evaluate size of tumor and extension to lymph nodes.

    2. Surgical staging based on findings from exploratory laparotomy, total abdominal hysterectomy–bilateral salpingo-oophorectomy (TAH-BSO), and peritoneal washings.

    3. Results of staging reported as anatomical stage, histopathological grade, depth of myometrial invasion, and evaluation of peritoneal cytology (see Appendix).

  D. Treatment strategies.

    1. Treatment decisions based on stage of disease, grade, depth of myometrial invasion, and client characteristics.

    2. Preinvasive disease—administration of progesterone or simple hysterectomy.

    3. Invasive disease—surgery and/or radiation therapy.

      a. Surgery:

        (1) Surgical staging procedure (TAH-BSO) serves as primary surgical treatment for early stage disease.

        (2) Pelvic and para-aortic lymphadenectomy included for grade 2 and 3 lesions.

      b. Radiation therapy:

        (1) Primary treatment for high-risk surgical candidates.

        (2) Adjuvant radiation therapy.

          (a) Preoperative therapy for clients with extensive lesions involving the cervix or high-grade lesions.

          (b) Postoperative therapy for clients with risk factors for recurrent disease—high-grade, deep myometrial invasion or cervical involvement.

          (c) Intraperitoneal radioactive phosphorus 32 for clients with positive pelvic cytology.

      c. Hormonal therapy for disseminated disease:

        (1) Synthetic progestational agents—megestrol acetate or medroxyprogesterone acetate.

        (2) Tamoxifen citrate used as a second-line treatment.

    4. Recurrent disease—surgery or radiation therapy to previously untreated areas.

  E. Trends in survival (Table 31-2).

    1. Most curable gynecological malignancy.

    2. Prognostic factors include stage, grade, and depth of myometrial invasion.

    3. Twenty-five to 35% of clients will have recurrent disease.

DATA COLLECTION

  I. Pertinent personal and family history.

    A. Age—peak incidence, 50 to 59 years.

    B. Menopausal status—80% of clients are postmenopausal.

Table 31-2
FIVE-YEAR SURVIVAL RATES FOR CLIENTS WITH ENDOMETRIAL CANCER

Stage	5-Year Survival Rate (%)	Grade	5-Year Survival Rate (%)
I	76	1	92
II	50	2	74
III	30	3	48
IV	9	—	—

C. Socioeconomic status—higher status places at increased risk.
D. History of changes in hormone levels—obesity, nulliparity, late menopause, infertility, irregular menstrual history, Stein-Leventhal syndrome, and estrogen replacement therapy without progestational agents.
E. Personal history of endometrial hyperplasia or breast, ovarian, or colorectal cancers.
F. Family history of multiple endocrine-related cancers.
G. Triad of obesity, diabetes, and hypertension.

II. Physical examination.
   A. Early signs and symptoms:
      1. Bleeding in postmenopausal women.
      2. Irregular or heavy menstrual flow in premenopausal women.
      3. Vaginal discharge.
      4. Lumbosacral pain.
   B. Late signs and symptoms:
      1. Hemorrhage.
      2. Ascites.
      3. Jaundice.
      4. Bowel obstruction.
      5. Respiratory distress.

III. Evaluation of laboratory data.
   A. Decreased hemoglobin or hematocrit level.
   B. Abnormal liver enzyme levels.
   C. Abnormal chemistry profile results.

ASSOCIATED NURSING DIAGNOSES
I. Body image disturbance.
II. Sexual dysfunction.
III. Potential for ineffective individual coping.
IV. Fear.

NURSING PLANNING AND IMPLEMENTATION
I. Interventions to maximize safety for the client.
   A. Teach changes in life-style that can modify risks of endometrial cancer.
      1. Encourage client to maintain ideal body weight.
      2. Suggest combination of estrogen and progesterone hormone replacement post-menopausally if uterus is present.
   B. See Chapters 19 and 20 for safety concerns about surgery and radiation therapy.

II. Interventions to decrease the severity of symptoms associated with disease and treatment (see Chapters 19, 20, and 21).
   A. Venous stasis.
      1. Encourage turning in bed and ambulation as soon as possible.
      2. Teach isometric leg exercises to do while in bed.
      3. Apply antiembolic stockings.
      4. Monitor for discomfort in legs and thighs.
      5. Avoid use of knee gatch in bed.
   B. Urinary retention.
      1. Monitor urinary output.

2. Assess for bladder distention above the symphysis pubis.
3. Assess for lower abdominal discomfort.

III. Interventions to monitor for sequelae of disease and treatment.
  A. See Chapters 19, 20, and 21 for sequelae of treatment.
  B. See Chapter 7, diarrhea, sexual dysfunction, body image, fear, and anemia.
  C. Assess for signs of recurrent disease:
    1. Vaginal bleeding.
    2. Change in bowel habits—constipation.
    3. Pelvic pain.

EVALUATION OF CLIENT AND FAMILY OUTCOMES

  I. Describe personal risk factors for endometrial cancer.

 II. Discuss rationale, schedule, and personal demands of treatment and follow-up care.

III. List potential side effects of disease and treatment.

IV. Describe self-care measures to decrease the incidence, severity, and complications of treatment.

 V. List signs and symptoms of recurrent disease to report to the health care team—vaginal bleeding, constipation, and pelvic pain.

VI. Describe potential community resources to meet demands of treatment and survivorship.

Ovarian Cancer

THEORY

  I. Physiology and pathophysiology of ovarian cancer.
  A. Anatomy of the ovary (see Figure 31-1).
    1. Ovaries are located on each side of the uterus behind the fallopian tubes.
    2. Ovarian lymphatics drain into the iliac and periaortic lymph nodes.
  B. Primary functions of the ovary.
    1. Production and release of ova.
    2. Production of hormones to meet needs of female for development, growth, and function—estrogen, progesterone, and testosterone.
  C. Metastatic patterns.
    1. Local extension to adjacent organs.
    2. Exfoliation over the ovarian capsule.
    3. Serosal seeding by tumor nests throughout the peritoneal cavity.
    4. Hematological spread to the lungs and liver.
  D. Trends in epidemiology.
    1. Steady increase in the incidence of ovarian cancer.
    2. Increase in disease-free intervals but no significant increase in survival data.

 II. Principles of medical management.
  A. Screening procedures.
    1. Bimanual pelvic examination.
      a. Increase in size or irregularity of the ovary.
      b. Palpable ovary in a postmenopausal woman.
    2. Serial CA_{125} determinations in high-risk women.
  B. Diagnostic procedures.
    1. Laparoscopy or exploratory laparotomy to obtain tissue for diagnosis.

2. Paracentesis of ascitic fluid.
C. Staging procedures and methods.
  1. Bowel involvement—barium enema examination, proctosigmoidoscopy, and upper gastrointestinal series.
  2. Bladder involvement—cystoscopy and IVP.
  3. Pulmonary involvement—chest x-ray examination.
  4. Liver involvement—liver enzyme values.
  5. Surgical staging laparotomy is mandatory to evaluate pelvic and abdominal contents—TAH-BSO; peritoneal cytology; omentectomy; lymph node biopsies or removal; multiple biopsies of bladder, bowel, liver, and diaphragm surfaces; appendectomy; and debulking cytoreduction of all visible tumor (see Appendix).
  6. Majority of clients with ovarian cancer are diagnosed with late-stage disease.
D. Treatment strategies.
  1. Primary surgical treatment:
    a. Cytoreduction, with removal of all tumor or tumors less than 2 cm in size so that minimal residual disease remains.
    b. Surgery may be used alone to treat early stage disease or borderline tumors with "low malignant potential."
    c. Surgery may be used to evaluate the response to chemotherapy treatment ("second-look" procedures).
      (1) Goals are to detect residual tumor; debulk remaining tumor; and determine further treatment.
      (2) Second-look procedures are done only in the presence of a complete response clinically.
      (3) One fourth to one third of clients with a complete response clinically will have evidence of disease on second look.
  2. Adjuvant radiation therapy:
    a. Pelvic or whole abdominal extended fields may be used for treatment of metastic disease to the pelvis or abdomen.
    b. Acute and chronic gastrointestinal complications are common.
    c. Radioactive isotopes such as P^{32} may also be given intraperitoneally to treat abdominal metastases.
  3. Adjuvant chemotherapy:
    a. Treatment of clients with late-stage disease.
    b. Cisplatin, cyclophosphamide, carboplatin, and melphalan (alkeran) have been used effectively to increase disease-free intervals, but increases in survival have not been demonstrated.
    c. Chemotherapy may be administered intravenously and intraperitoneally; advantages of intraperitoneal method include:
      (1) Higher concentrations of drug to surface of tumor.
      (2) Decreased systemic side effects.
      (3) Systemic tolerance of higher doses of drug.
    d. Hormonal therapy may be used for salvage therapy—megestrol acetate and tamoxifen citrate.
  4. Biological response modifers are used as single agents and in combination with chemotherapy as adjuvant therapy.
    a. Biological response modifiers can be administered intravenously or intraperitoneally.
    b. Interferon, interleukin-2, and monoclonal antibodies are under investigation.
E. Trends in survival (Table 31-3).

Table 31-3
FIVE-YEAR SURVIVAL RATES FOR CLIENTS WITH OVARIAN CANCER

Stage	5-Year Survival Rate (%)
I	80
II	60
IIIa	60
IIIb	30
IIIc	5-10
IV	5

1. Overall 5-year survival rate ranges from 30% to 35%.
2. Stage and grade are important prognostic factors.
3. Abdominal carcinomatosis commonly occurs and results in intestinal obstruction, malabsorption, and fluid and electrolyte imbalances.

DATA COLLECTION
I. Pertinent personal and family history.
  A. Age.
    1. Occurs commonly in premenopausal women ages 40 to 65 years old.
    2. Peak incidence at age 55 to 59 years.
    3. Germ cell tumors are more common in children and adolescents.
  B. Infertility.
  C. Nulliparity.
  D. Personal history of breast, endometrial, or colon cancers.
  E. Family history of breast, endometrial, or colon cancers.

II. Physical examination.
  A. Early signs and symptoms:
    1. Gastrointestinal distress.
    2. Dyspepsia.
    3. Abdominal discomfort.
    4. Flatulence.
    5. Eructation.
    6. Increased pelvic pressure.
  B. Late signs and symptoms:
    1. Palpable abdominal or pelvic mass.
    2. Increased abdominal girth.
    3. Ascites.
    4. Pleural effusions.
    5. Intestinal obstruction.
    6. Weight loss.

III. Evaluation of laboratory data.
  A. CA_{125} may be used to monitor treatment response or disease recurrence.
  B. Beta-human chorionic gonadotropin (hCG) levels may be used to detect and monitor germ cell tumors.

ASSOCIATED NURSING DIAGNOSES
I. Body image disturbance.

II. Altered bowel elimination—constipation.

III. Altered nutritional status.

IV. Ineffective individual coping.

V. Ineffective family coping.

NURSING PLANNING AND IMPLEMENTATION

See Chapters 7, 19, 20, 21, and 22.

EVALUATION OF CLIENT AND FAMILY OUTCOMES

I. Describe personal risk factors for ovarian cancer.

II. Discuss rationale, schedule, and personal demands of treatment and follow-up care.

III. List potential side effects of disease and treatment.

IV. Describe self-care measures to decrease the incidence, severity, and complications of treatment.

V. List signs and symptoms of recurrent disease to report to the health care team.

VI. Describe potential community resources to meet demands of treatment and survivorship.

Testicular Cancer

THEORY

I. Physiology and pathophysiology associated with testicular cancer.
   A. Anatomy of the testes.
      1. Testes are ovoid glands located in the scrotal sac.
      2. Testes descend from the abdomen through the inguinal canal during the seventh month of fetal life.
   B. Primary functions of the testes.
      1. Spermatogenesis.
      2. Production of hormone (testosterone) to meet the needs of male development, growth, and function.
   C. Changes associated with cancer of the testes.
      1. Testicular cancers arise from germinal epithelium.
      2. Proposed cause is abnormal exposure to estrogen in utero.
      3. Behavior of testicular cancer varies with histological subtype.
         a. Seminomas.
            (1) Occur in approximately 40% of cases.
            (2) Spread slowly, primarily through the lymphatics.
            (3) Are responsive to radiation therapy.
         b. Nonseminomatous malignancies—embryonal, teratoma, interstitial cell, and gonadal stromal.
            (1) Embryonal tumors (25% of cases) invade spermatic cord and metastasize to lung.
            (2) Embryonal tumors are not responsive to radiation therapy.
   D. Metastatic patterns.
      1. Direct extension to adjacent structures.
      2. Metastasis to lymphatics—pelvis and para-aortic and supraclavicular areas.
      3. Hematological metastasis to the brain, lung, bone, and liver.
   E. Trends in epidemiology.
      1. Most commonly occurring cancer among men ages 20 to 40 years.
      2. Incidence increasing among white males.

II. Principles of medical management.
  A. Screening and diagnostic procedures.
    1. Screening procedures:
        a. Monthly testicular self-examination.
        b. Annual bimanual palpation and examination of the testes by health care provider.
    2. Diagnostic procedures—tissue biopsy by high inguinal orchiectomy.
  B. Staging methods and procedures.
    1. IVP to evaluate displacement of ureter or kidney.
    2. Chest x-ray examination, CT scan, and/or tomography to evaluate lung metastasis.
    3. Abdominal CT scan and ultrasound to evaluate lymph node involvement.
    4. Multiple staging systems are used currently (see Appendix).
  C. Treatment strategies.
    1. Surgery:
        a. Transinguinal orchiectomy is primary treatment for seminomas and non-seminomas.
        b. Retroperitoneal lymph node dissection on the affected side may be done.
        c. Surgery may be used to resect isolated metastatic lesions of lung, liver, and retroperitoneum.
    2. Radiation therapy:
        a. Adjuvant treatment for seminomas.
        b. Fields may include iliac, retroperitoneal, and para-aortic lymph nodes or whole abdomen.
        c. Use of radiation therapy to lung fields limits use of bleomycin for recurrent disease because risk of pulmonary fibrosis increases.
    3. Chemotherapy:
        a. Treatment for clients with elevated tumor markers, advanced stage disease, or recurrent disease.
        b. Agents commonly used include cisplatin, vinblastine, bleomycin, etoposide, ifosfamide, and doxorubicin.
        c. Response rates are excellent—complete response (70%) and partial response (30%).
  D. Trends in survival (Table 31-4).
    1. Survival from testicular cancer has increased dramatically over the past 10 years.
    2. Testicular cancer is considered curable, and the prognosis for clients is excellent.
    3. Prognosis depends on bulk of disease at diagnosis.

Table 31-4
FIVE-YEAR SURVIVAL RATES FOR CLIENTS WITH TESTICULAR CANCER

Seminomas		Non-seminomas	
Stage	5-Year Survival Rate (%)	Stage	5-Year Survival Rate (%)
A	98	A	90-100
B1-B2	75-94	B	90
B3-C	71	C	80-85

4. Recurrences usually occur within 2 years; however, recurrent disease is also responsive to treatment.

DATA COLLECTION

I. Pertinent personal and family history.
  A. Age.
    1. Most commonly occurs in men age 20 to 40 years.
    2. Incidence decreases for men age 40 to 60 years and increases again after age 60 years.
  B. Cryptorchidism (undescended testicle) increases risk twentyfold to fortyfold; if orchipexy is done after 6 years of age, protection is lost.
  C. Polythelia (multiple nipples) increases risk.

II. Physical examination.
  A. Early signs and symptoms are absent usually.
    1. Asymptomatic mass.
    2. Gynecomastia.
    3. Infertility.
    4. Testicular fullness, heaviness, swelling, or pain.
  B. Late signs and symptoms:
    1. Back pain.
    2. Bony pain.
    3. Respiratory distress.

III. Evaluation of laboratory data; serum tumor markers—α-fetoprotein and beta-hCG to establish a differential diagnosis, assess response to treatment, and monitor long-term responses.

ASSOCIATED NURSING DIAGNOSES

I. Body image disturbances.

II. Altered sexuality.

III. Ineffective individual coping.

IV. Ineffective family coping.

V. Knowledge deficit related to risk or diagnosis of testicular cancer.

NURSING PLANNING AND IMPLEMENTATION

I. See Chapters 7, 19, and 20.

II. Interventions decrease the severity of symptoms associated with disease and treatment.
  A. Edema.
    1. Apply ice bags to scrotal area for first 12 hours after surgery.
    2. Apply compression dressing to surgical site.
    3. Teach client to avoid standing for long periods of time.
    4. Advise client to take 20-minute tub baths three times a day for 1 week after discharge.
    5. Instruct client to avoid heavy lifting for 4 to 6 weeks after surgery.
  B. Comfort.
    1. Encourage bed rest for 24 to 48 hours after surgery.
    2. Encourage use of athletic supporter when ambulating.

C. Body image.
  1. Discuss use of prosthetic devices before surgery.
  2. Encourage open discussion about changes in body image between the client and sexual partner.

EVALUATION OF CLIENT AND FAMILY OUTCOMES

 I. Describe personal risk factors for testicular cancer.

 II. Discuss rationale, schedule, and personal demands of treatment and follow-up care.

III. List potential side effects of disease and treatment.

IV. Describe self-care measures to decrease the incidence, severity, and complications of treatment.

 V. List signs and symptoms of recurrent disease to report to the health care team.

VI. Describe potential community resources to meet demands of treatment and survivorship.

Penile Cancer

THEORY

 I. Physiology and pathophysiology associated with penile cancer.
   A. Anatomy of the penis (Figure 31-4).
     1. Composed of the shaft and the glans.
     2. Shaft has three cylindrical layers—bilateral corpus spongiosum, corpora cavernosa, and erectile tissues.
   B. Primary functions of the penis.
     1. Urination.
     2. Copulation.
   C. Changes associated with cancer of the penis.
     1. Smegma has been associated with carcinogenesis in animal models.
     2. Penile cancer rarely occurs in males who have been circumcised as neonates.
   D. Metastatic patterns.
     1. Direct extension to adjacent tissues.
     2. Metastasis to regional lymphatics—inguinal and iliac nodes.

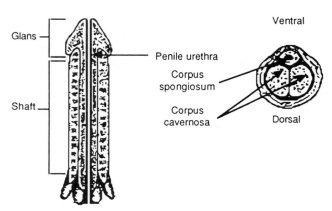

Figure 31-4 Anatomy of the penis. *(Adapted from Broadwell, D.C. & Jackson, B.S. [eds]. [1982]. Principles of Ostomy Care. St. Louis: C.V. Mosby Co., p. 52.)*

II. Principles of medical management.
   A. Diagnostic procedures—biopsy of penile lesion.
   B. Staging methods and procedures (see Appendix).
      1. Abdominal CT scan and x-ray examination to evaluate regional lymph nodes.
      2. Intravenous urography.
      3. Lymphangiography.
      4. Chest x-ray examination.
      5. Liver and bone scans.
      6. Staging is done clinically.
   C. Treatment strategies.
      1. Premalignant lesions—local excision, topical fluorouracil or laser therapy.
      2. Invasive cancer:
         a. Surgery:
            (1) Partial or total penectomy.
            (2) Total penectomy requires creation of perineal urostomy for urination.
            (3) Radical lymphadenectomy or lymph node sampling may be done, depending on stage of disease.
         b. Radiation therapy:
            (1) Interstitial, surface mold, or external beam therapy may be used for small penile lesions.
            (2) Radiation therapy also may be used for palliative treatment.
         c. Chemotherapy:
            (1) May be used as palliative treatment for clients with stage III and IV disease.
            (2) Cisplatin, methotrexate, and bleomycin are used commonly.
   D. Trends in survival—since the number of cases diagnosed annually is small (500), accurate trends in survival are not available (Table 31-5).

DATA COLLECTION

I. Pertinent personal and family history.
   A. Age—60 years or older.
   B. Penile hygiene practices—poor hygiene increases risk.
   C. Circumcision status—no circumcision increases risk.

II. Physical examination.
   A. Early signs and symptoms:
      1. Mass, nodule, or ulceration of the penis.
      2. Foul-smelling penile discharge.
      3. Inguinal lymphadenopathy.
      4. Bleeding on the surface of the penis.

Table 31-5
FIVE-YEAR SURVIVAL RATES FOR CLIENTS WITH PENILE CANCER

Stage	5-Year Survival Rate (%)
I	80
II	60
III	25
IV	0

    B. Late signs and symptoms:
      1. Fungating lesion of the penis.
      2. Bone pain.
      3. Respiratory distress.
III. Evaluation of laboratory data—none specific to penile cancer.

ASSOCIATED NURSING DIAGNOSES

  I. Body image disturbance.

 II. Sexual dysfunction.

III. Ineffective individual coping.

IV. Ineffective family coping.

NURSING PLANNING AND IMPLEMENTATION

  I. Interventions to maximize safety for the client.
    A. Discuss option of circumcision before puberty for protective effect.
    B. Instruct high-risk clients in penile self-examination.
    C. Teach penile hygiene practices:
      1. Retraction of foreskin for cleansing.
      2. Washing penis with mild soap and water.

 II. Interventions to decrease severity of symptoms associated with disease and treatment (see Chapter 7, sexual dysfunction; Chapters 19, 20, and 21 for sequelae of treatment).

III. Interventions to enhance adaptation and rehabilitation.
    A. Encourage open discussion of sexual concerns.
      1. Reinforce information that clients with partial penectomy maintain sexual desire and the ability to penetrate, reach orgasm, and ejaculate.
      2. Discuss prosthetic options with clients who have had a total penectomy.
    B. Discuss alternate forms of sexual expression with client and sexual partner.

EVALUATION OF CLIENT AND FAMILY OUTCOMES

   I. Describe personal risk factors for penile cancer.

  II. Discuss rationale, schedule, and personal demands of treatment and follow-up care.

 III. List potential side effects of disease and treatment.

 IV. Describe self-care measures to decrease the incidence, severity, and complications of treatment.

  V. List signs and symptoms of recurrent disease to report to the health care team.

 VI. Describe potential community resources to meet demands of treatment and survivorship.

BIBLIOGRAPHY

Berek, J.S. & Hacker, N.F. (1989). *Practical Gynecologic Oncology*. Baltimore: Williams & Wilkins.
Blackmore, C. (1988). The impact of orchiectomy upon the sexuality of the man with testicular cancer. *Cancer Nurs 11*(1), 33-40.
Casciato, D.A. & Lowitz, B.B. (1988). *Manual of Clinical Oncology* (2nd ed). Boston: Little, Brown & Co.
DeVita, V.T., Jr., Hellman, S., & Rosenberg, S.A. (1985). *Cancer Principles & Practice of Oncology* (2nd ed). Philadelphia: J.B. Lippincott Co.
DiSaia, P.J. & Creasman, W.T. (1989). *Clinical Gynecologic Oncology* (3rd ed). St. Louis: C.V. Mosby Co.

Groenwald, S.L., Frogge, M.H., Goodman, M., & Yarbro C.H. (eds). (1990). *Cancer Nursing Principles and Practice* (2nd ed). Boston: Jones & Bartlett Publishers.

Hampton, B.G. (1986). Nursing management of a patient following pelvic exenteration. *Semin Oncol Nurs 2*(4), 281-286.

Higgs, D.J. (1990). The patient with testicular cancer: nursing management of chemotherapy. *Oncol Nurs Forum 17*(2), 243-249.

Jenkins, B. (1988). Patients' reports of sexual changes after treatment for gynecological cancer. *Oncol Nurs Forum 15*(3), 349-354.

Morrow, C.P. & Townsend, D.E. (1987). *Synopsis of Gynecologic Oncology* (3rd ed). New York: John Wiley & Sons.

Pocinki, K.M. (1989). *Cancer of the Ovary*. Bethesda, Md.: National Institutes of Health.

Rieker, P.P., Fitzgerald, E.M., & Kalish, L.A. (1990). Adaptive behavioral responses to potential infertility among survivors of testis cancer. *J Clin Oncol 8*(2), 347-355.

Rosenthal, S.N., Carignan, J.R., & Smith, B.D. (1987). *Medical Care of the Cancer Patient*. Philadelphia: W.B. Saunders Co.

Silverberg, E., Bering, C.C., & Squires, T.S. (1990). Cancer statistics, 1990. *CA 40*(1), 9-26.

Walczak, J.R. (ed). (1990). Gynecologic cancers. *Semin Oncol Nurs 6*(3), 179-243.

Yoder, L.H. (1990). The epidemiology of ovarian cancer: a review. *Oncol Nurs Forum 17*(3), 411-415.

32

Colorectal Cancers

Roberta Anne Strohl, MN, RN

THEORY

I. Anatomy of organs.
   A. Colon (Figure 32-1).
      1. Extends from the terminal ileum to anal canal.
      2. Consists of four parts—ascending or right colon, transverse or middle colon, descending or left colon, and sigmoid colon.
   B. Rectum (Figure 32-1).
      1. Is continuous with sigmoid colon and terminates at distal anal canal.
      2. Contains transitional zone between keratinized and nonkeratinized stratified squamous epithelium at anal verge.
      3. Is covered with peritoneum.
   C. Anus—landmarks of anorectal ring, pectinate line, and anal verge represent transitions in epithelium.
   D. Critical adjacent structures.
      1. Venous drainage from colon and upper to middle third of rectum enters portal system to liver.
      2. Lower third of rectum drains to portal and inferior vena cava.
      3. Colon, rectum, and anus lie in proximity to the vagina in females and to the bladder, seminal vesicles, prostate, and urethra in males.

II. Physiology and pathophysiology associated with colorectal cancers.
   A. Primary functions include:
      1. Processing of ileal contents.
         a. Colon receives 800 to 1000 ml of ileal contents per day.
         b. Absorption of water and electrolytes occurs primarily in the proximal or right colon.
         c. Feces in right colon is more fluid than in the sigmoid colon.
      2. Movement of ileal contents through bowel.
         a. Innervation of gut responds to both parasympathetic and sympathetic signals.
         b. Secretion, blood flow, and sensory perception are controlled by submucosal structures.
         c. Ileal contents are moved through the colon by a mixture of circular constrictions and longitudinal contractions.

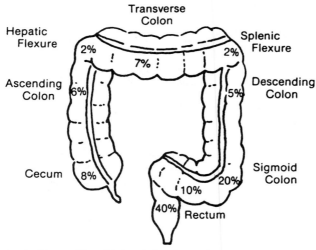

Figure 32-1 Cancer incidence. Two thirds of all colorectal cancers occur in the rectosigmoid and the rectum. Many of these cancers are within reach of the examining finger, and 50% are within the reach of a sigmoidoscope. *(From Otte, D.M. [1988]. Nursing management of the patient with colon and rectal cancer.* Semin Oncol Nurs 4*[4], 286.)*

       d. Fecal material is exposed to bowel wall for absorption of nutritional elements.

       e. Feces are pushed into the rectum.

   3. Storage of feces—in the left colon until defecation.

   4. Defecation:

       a. Rectal wall is distended by feces.

       b. Peristalsis is initiated; anal sphincter relaxes; and defecation occurs.

       c. External anal sphincter is controlled by conscious mind and can inhibit defecation.

       d. If impulse for defecation is ignored, reflex fades.

  B. Changes in function associated with colorectal cancers.

   1. Increase or decrease in consistency of stool.

   2. Changes in color of stool.

   3. Inability to move stool through bowel (obstruction).

  C. Metastatic patterns.

   1. Colorectal cancers.

       a. Local extension through penetration of layers of bowel.

       b. Deeper penetration increases chance of spread.

       c. Tumors that have invaded beyond submucosal layer have direct access to vascular and lymphatic systems.

       d. Distant metastases most frequently occur in the liver and lungs and less frequently in the brain, bone, and adrenal glands.

   2. Anal cancers.

       a. Local extension to sphincter ani muscles, prostate, urethra, and bladder in males and vagina in females.

       b. Distant metastases occur in lung and liver.

III. Trends in epidemiology.

  A. Colorectal cancer is a common tumor, second only to lung cancer in the number of new cases.

Table 32-1
DIAGNOSTIC TESTS FOR COLORECTAL CANCERS

Description/ Purpose	Time Required for Test	Sensations Experienced	Potential Side Effects/ Complications	Self-Care Measures	Critical Symptoms to Report to Health Care Team
Barium Enema Identify extent of lesion in colon Identify obstruction	30-45 min	Fullness, abdominal pain, discomfort, urge to defecate	Perforation Bowel obstruction	Preparation includes liquid diet day before, and low residue diet 1-3 days before test Bowel preparation—laxatives or enema before and after examination Client must hold anal sphincter against tube and breathe slowly to minimize discomfort	Failure to pass barium Signs of gastrointestinal obstruction
Computed Axial Tomographic (CAT) Scan Identify lymph node involvement, liver metastases	45-60 min	May be claustrophobic when in scanner Sound of machine going on and off Warm feeling with injection of dye	Allergic reaction to dye Nausea from dye Blood samples for determining blood urea nitrogen (BUN) and creatinine levels are drawn first to assess renal function	May receive nothing by mouth or be instructed to eat lightly before examination because of potential nausea from dye	With contrast, immediately report any discomfort, breathing difficulty, itching
Stool for Occult Blood	Preparation—48-72 hr		False-positive results: Results from meat in diet, hemorrhoids, fissures, peroxidases in skin of vegetables and fruits (cherries, tomatoes), gastritis from aspirin False-negative results: Failure to use high-residue, high-fiber diet 72 hr before test Vitamin C in diet Delay between collection and examination Failure to prepare slides properly Lesion not bleeding at time of examination	No red meat, poultry, fish, turnips, horseradish for 72 hr before and during test Withhold iron and aspirin Collect three specimens Client urinates first into toilet, uses bedpan to collect stool Send specimen to laboratory or return as instructed	
Colonoscopy, Sigmoidoscopy, Proctoscopy Visualize gastrointestinal tract	15-30 min	Pressure discomfort Intravenous infusion with sedation Lying on left side Scope feels cool Sensation of need to defecate	If tissue removed, bleeding Adverse effects from sedatives	Clear liquid diet for 24 hr, laxative evening before, cleansing enema 3-4 hr before test Deep breathing during examination Expect a large amount of flatus after examination	Pain Bleeding

B. Age-adjusted death rates per 100,000 population compared between 1955 to 1957 and 1985 to 1987 indicate:
  1. Decrease in the death rate related to colon cancer among women.
  2. No change in the death rate related to colon cancer among men.
  3. Decrease in the death rate related to rectal cancer among both men and women.
C. Over 30-year period the population-adjusted incidence is unchanged—47 cases per 100,000 persons.

IV. Principles of medical management.
  A. Screening and diagnostic procedures (Table 32-1).
    1. Digital examination detects 10% of anorectal lesions.
    2. Stool for occult blood is controversial with respect to cost effectiveness as a screening test.
    3. Flexible fiberoptic sigmoidoscopy allows examination of up to 60 cm of colon.
  B. Laboratory tests.
    1. Hemoglobin and hematocrit levels to evaluate anemia commonly found with lesions on right side.
    2. Carcinoembryonic antigen (CEA)—although not valuable as a diagnostic or screening test, CEA has been used to monitor the response to therapy and follow-up care.
  C. Staging methods and procedures.
    1. Colon (see Appendix A).
      a. Staging may be based on clinical data or on surgical data.
      b. Depth of penetration into the wall of the colon or rectum is basis for staging.
    2. Anus (see Appendix A)—staging based on involvement of sphincter ani muscles, pelvic tissue, and lymph nodes.
  D. Treatment strategies.
    1. Surgery.
      a. Surgical resection is primary treatment for 75% of clients with colorectal cancers.
      b. Surgical procedures for colorectal and anal cancers are presented in Table 32-2.
    2. Radiation therapy.
      a. Preoperative radiation therapy used to:
        (1) Decrease tumor size and render tumor resectable.
        (2) Eradicate microscopic disease.
        (3) Decrease the incidence of local recurrence.
      b. Postoperative radiation therapy used to eradicate remaining disease if:
        (1) Surgical margins are positive.
        (2) Residual tumor is present.
        (3) Duke's B or C lesion is present.
      c. Combined preoperative and postoperative radiation therapy may be used.
      d. Early rectal cancers in the low and midrectal regions and anal cancer have been treated with endocavitary radiation (three treatments to a total dose of 8000 to 15,000 rads):
        (1) High complication rate secondary to superficial effect of high doses of radiation, although delivered with low energy sources.
        (2) Complications—radionecrosis, anal canal ulcers, strictures, bleeding.
    3. Chemotherapy.
      a. Used in combination with surgery and radiation therapy.

Table 32-2
SURGICAL MANAGEMENT OF COLORECTAL CANCERS

Site	Procedure	Technique	Physical Alterations	Possible Complications
Rectum	Low anterior resection— for lesions more than 10 cm from anal verge	Resect tumor and 2- to 5-cm margins; staple or suture bowel, conserving sphincter	Sphincter preserved	Anastomatic leak Abscess infection irregular bowel function
	Abdominal incision—remove tumor and adjacent involved or potentially involved structures	Performed through abdomen and perineum; perineal wound closed with drain or open to heal by granulation	Colostomy Perineal wound Foley catheter postoperatively Nasogastric tube postoperatively until peristalsis returns	Urinary dysfunction Wound infection Stomal complications Impotency in males Sexual dysfunction related to scarring in females
Anus	Removal of perianal skin, anal canal	Wide excision; anterior-posterior resection may include total pelvic exenteration if lesions involve bladder or urethra	Colostomy Urinary diversion if total pelvic exenteration	As above
Colorectum	Hemicolectomy	Small tumors may be resected with enough margin so that permanent colostomy not needed; may have temporary colostomy	Temporary colostomy possible	Anastomatic leak
	Single-barreled colostomy	Proximal colon brought out and sutured to abdominal wall Defunctionalized colon removed or placed into abdomen (Hartmann's pouch).	Permanent colostomy Type of stool depends on location of stoma—*ascending,* fluid, semifluid; *transverse,* mush, semimush; *descending,* solid; *rectum,* solid; *anus,* hard solid	Stomal complications Herniation Prolapse Hemorrhage
	Double-barreled colostomy	Two stomas Defunctionalized colon not removed Proximal portion sutured to abdominal wall end Stoma Distal mucous fistula		
All sites	Relief of obstruction May be done for palliation of symptoms	Debulking	May have temporary colostomy, nasogastric tube	

    b. Agents used for colorectal cancer—5-fluorouracil (5-FU), levamisole, methotrexate, 5-fluorouracil deoxyribonucleoside (FUDR), and cisplatin.

    c. Agents used for anal cancer—mitomycin C and 5-FU.

V. Trends in survival.

  A. Survival is determined by the stage of disease, grade of tumor, histological type of tumor, and the general health status of the client.

  B. Colon cancer—general 5-year survival rate by stage:

    1. Duke's A, 90%.

    2. Duke's B, 60% to 80%.

    3. Duke's C, 20% to 50%.

    4. Duke's D, 5%.

  C. Anal cancer—overall 5-year survival rate for all clients, 48% to 66%.

DATA COLLECTION

I. Pertinent client and family history.
   A. Age—incidence increases slightly at 40 years; increases sharply at 50 years; doubles each decade thereafter.
   B. Genetic factors.
      1. Familial polyposis.
      2. Gardner's syndrome.
      3. Turcot syndrome.
      4. Peutz-Jeghers syndrome.
      5. Juvenile polyposis.
      6. Family cancer syndrome.
   C. Preexisting bowel disease.
      1. Villous adenoma.
         a. Polyps most likely to become malignant.
         b. Excision of polyps recommended, with annual colonoscopy follow-up.
      2. Ulcerative colitis.
         a. Increased duration of colitis increases risk for malignant change.
         b. The longer the length of involved bowel, the greater is the risk for malignancy.
      3. Crohn's disease—risk of malignancy is related to duration and extent of disease.
   D. Other cancers such as breast and gynecological cancers.
   E. Diet.
      1. High-fat intake is proposed as increased risk for colorectal cancer.
      2. Low-fiber diet increases transit time in colon; therefore, fecal bile acids and carcinogens in stool have a longer time to interact with mucosa.
   F. Irritation of anal canal related to condylomata, fistula, fissures, abscesses, and hemorrhoids.

II. Physical examination.
   A. Early signs and symptoms:
      1. Malaise and fatigue.
      2. Signs and symptoms depend on location of cancer (Table 32-3).
      3. Palpation of mass in transverse or right colon.
   B. Late signs and symptoms:
      1. Pain.
      2. Weight loss.
      3. Presence of symptoms of metastatic disease:
         a. Pulmonary—cough, chest pain, dyspnea, hemoptysis, wheezing, or dysphagia.
         b. Hepatic—ascites, abdominal distention, nausea, anorexia, increasing abdominal girth, changes in color of urine and stool, or pruritus.

III. Laboratory data.
   A. Decreased hemoglobin and hematocrit levels.
   B. Elevated results of liver function tests—lactate dehydrogenase (LDH), serum glutamate pyruvate transaminase (SGPT), or serum glutamic-oxaloacetic transaminase (SGOT).
   C. Elevated CEA.

ASSOCIATED NURSING DIAGNOSES

I. Anxiety.

II. Altered nutrition: less than body requirements.

Table 32-3
CHARACTERISTICS OF COLORECTAL CANCERS

Site	Pathology	Characteristics	Presentation
Colon	Adenocarcinoma (95%)	Most are relatively slow growing, poorly differentiated, more aggressive; lymph node involvement common with progression	
Ascending			Anemia, nausea, weight loss, pain (vague and dull); palpable mass uncommon Late symptoms—diarrhea, constipation, anorexia
Transverse			Palpable mass, blood in stool, change in bowel habits, obstruction
Descending			Obstruction, pain (cramps), change in bowel habits
Sigmoid			Blood in stool, constipation, pencil-like stool, obstruction
Rectum	Adenocarcinoma	Same as above	Mucous discharge, bright red rectal bleeding (most common), tenesmus, sense of incomplete evacuation, mucous diarrhea, pain Late symptoms—feeling of rectal fullness, constant ache
Anus	Adenocarcinoma	Higher incidence in fifth through seventh decades; tend to be highly malignant; increasing incidence in male homosexuals	Rectal bleeding, pruritus, mucous discharge, tenesmus, pain or pressure in rectal region
	Squamous cell	May be multifocal; generally well differentiated and slow growing	
	Basal cell	Local spread only but may be highly malignant; does not behave like basal cell in skin—may metastasize	Sensation of lump, bleeding, pruritus, mucous discharge
	Kaposi's sarcoma (see Chapter 37)		

III. Potential sexual dysfunction.

IV. Potential impaired skin integrity.

V. Body image disturbance.

NURSING PLANNING AND IMPLEMENTATION

I. Interventions to decrease the incidence and severity of complications of treatment unique to colorectal cancer.
   A. Stomal placement to decrease the incidence of skin reactions.
      1. Mark site at least 2 inches below the waist and away from leg creases.
         a. Avoid stoma placement near scars, bony prominences, skin folds, fistulas, pendulous breasts, or belt line.
         b. Allow for 2 inches of smooth skin around stoma for appliance adherence.
      2. Mark site while client is lying flat, sitting, standing, and bending.
      3. Mark site within borders of rectus muscles to minimize risk of herniation and prolapse.
   B. Appliance selection based on character of stool, contour of skin surrounding stoma, manual dexterity, and cost.
   C. Stoma care.
      1. Change appliance every week.
      2. Use skin barriers cut to fit stoma exactly.
      3. Avoid use of skin products and appliances that contain materials that cause allergic reactions.
      4. Assess stoma and skin around stoma for complications with each appliance change—erythema, edema, erosion, bleeding, and stomal protrusion, retraction, herniation, or narrowing.
   D. Management of common problems associated with an ostomy (see Table 30-3).
      1. Avoid odor-producing foods—legumes, cabbage, onions, carbonated beverages, beer, alcohol, and fatty foods.
      2. Discuss use of odor-absorbing pouches or products such as charcoal.

II. Interventions to monitor for side effects of treatment.
   A. Monitor for postoperative complications related to bowel surgery.
      1. Obstruction or paralytic ileus—pain, constipation, diarrhea, nausea, vomiting, or abdominal distention.
      2. Bleeding—pulse rate, respiratory rate, blood pressure, amount and color of drainage from wound and/or stoma.
      3. Infection—fever, pain, redness at incision site, edema, or changes in amount or color of wound drainage.
      4. Stomal complications—retraction, changes in color of stoma, protrusion of stoma onto abdomen, narrowing of stomal opening, herniation, or drainage from fistulous tracts around stoma.
      5. Changes in sexual function.
         a. Males—may have erectile and ejaculatory problems with severing of nerves (S2 to S4 and L2 to L4).
         b. Females—enervation not a problem but may have a decrease in length of vagina, lack of lubrication, or discomfort with intercourse.
   B. Monitor for return of bowel function.
      1. Presence of bowel sounds, passage of flatus, and passage of stool.
      2. Tolerance of progressive oral diet.
   C. Monitor for complications of radiation therapy to the gastrointestinal tract.
      1. Inflammation of the bowel or bladder.

2. Blood in stool or urine.
3. Ulceration of gastrointestinal mucosa—pain.
4. Necrosis.
5. Changes in sexual activity related to inflammation of perineal skin.
D. Monitor for complications of chemotherapy for colorectal cancers—5-FU, leucovorin, cisplatin, methotrexate, and semustine (MeCCNU).
   1. Mucositis.
   2. Diarrhea.
   3. Nausea and vomiting.
   4. Pancytopenia.
   5. Decreased libido.

III. Interventions to incorporate client and family in care.
   A. Prevention and early detection.
      1. Instruct family members about familial risks for colorectal cancers.
      2. Discuss recommended screening guidelines for high-risk individuals.
      3. Suggest dietary modifications to reduce risks of colorectal cancers (see Chapter 4).
      4. Teach family to recognize early signs and symptoms of colorectal cancers.
   B. Treatment and follow-up demands.
      1. Educate client and family about self-care measures to reduce complications of disease and treatment.
      2. Inform about written and service resources available for client and family facing a diagnosis of colorectal cancer.
         a. National Cancer Institute publications.
         b. American Cancer Society (ACS).
            (1) Address—Clifton Road, NE, Atlanta, GA 30329; check telephone book for state divisions or local units.
            (2) Services—education and support groups (I Can Cope, CanSurmount, ostomy clubs), Service and Rehabilitation (ACS) direct aid program for ostomy supplies, and publications, including *Sexuality and Cancer*.
         c. United Ostomy Association.
            (1) Address—36 Executive Park, Suite 120, Irvine, CA 92714, (714) 660-8624.
            (2) Services—local chapters; *Ostomy Quarterly*; other publications, including *Sex, Courtship, and the Single Ostomate*; *Sex and the Female Ostomate*; and *Sex and the Male Ostomate*.
         d. International Ostomy Association, c/o Maria Siegel, 73 Widdicombe Hill Boulevard, Suite PH2, Western Ontario, Canada M9R 4B3.
      3. Teach client and family signs and symptoms to report immediately to health care team.

EVALUATION OF CLIENT AND FAMILY OUTCOMES

I. Describe personal risk factors for colorectal cancers.

II. Discuss rationale, schedule, and personal demands of treatment and follow-up plan.

III. List potential side effects of disease and treatment.

IV. Describe self-care measures to decrease the incidence, severity, and complications of treatment.

V. Demonstrate competence in self-care measures demanded by structural or functional effects of disease or treatment.

VI. Specify symptoms to report immediately to the health care team:
   A. Changes in structure or function of ostomy.
   B. Symptoms of obstruction.
   C. Blood in stool.
   D. Symptoms of metastatic disease to lung or liver.

BIBLIOGRAPHY

Adjuvant therapy for patients with colon and rectum cancer (1990). *Natl Inst Health Consensus Dev Conf Consensus Statement 8*(4), 1-75.

Alterescu, K.B. (1987). Colostomy. *Nurs Clin North Am 22*(2), 281-289.

American Cancer Society (1991). *Cancer Facts and Figures.* Atlanta: Author.

Baird, S.B., McCorkle, R. & Grant, M., (eds). (1991). *Cancer Nursing: A Comprehensive Textbook.* Philadelphia: W.B. Saunders Co.

Boarini, J. (1990). Gastrointestinal cancer: colon, rectum, and anus. In S.L. Groenwald, M.H. Frogge, M. Goodman, & C.H. Yarbro (eds). *Cancer Nursing: Principles and Practice* (2nd ed). Boston: Jones & Bartlett Publishers, pp. 792-805.

Broadwell, D.C. (1987). Peristomal skin integrity. *Nurs Clin North Am 22*(2), 321-332.

Cohen, A.M., Shank, B., & Friedman, M.A. (1989). Colorectal cancer. In V.T. DeVita, Jr., S. Hellman, & S.A. Rosenberg (eds). *Cancer: Principles & Practice of Oncology,* vol 1 (3rd ed). Philadelphia: J.B. Lippincott Co., pp. 895-964.

Gloeckner, M. (1991). Perceptions of sexuality after ostomy surgery. *J Enterostom Ther 18*(1), 36-38.

Harms, B.A. & Starling, J.R. (1990). Current status of sphincter preservation in rectal cancer. *Oncology 4*(8), 53-60.

Holyoke, E.D. (1988). The role of the carcinoembryonic antigen in the management of colorectal cancer. In V.T. DeVita, Jr., S. Hellman, & S.A. Rosenberg (eds). *Cancer: Principles Pract Oncol Update 2*(3), 1-11.

American Joint Committee on Cancer (1988). *Manual for Staging of Cancer* (3rd ed). Philadelphia: J.B. Lippincott Co., pp. 75-85.

Messner, R.L., Gardner, S.S., & Webb, D.D. (1986). Early detection—the priority in colorectal cancer. *Cancer Nurs 9*(1), 8-14.

Rheaume, A. & Gooding, B.A. (1991). Social support, coping strategies, and long-term adaptation to ostomy among self-help group members. *J Enterostom Ther 18*(1), 11-15.

Shank, B., Cohen, A.M., & Kelsen, D. (1989). Cancer of the anal region. In V.T. DeVita, Jr., S. Hellman, & S.A. Rosenberg (eds). *Cancer: Principles & Practice of Oncology,* vol 1 (3rd ed). Philadelphia: J.B. Lippincott Co., pp. 965-978.

Shipes, E. (1987). Sexual function following ostomy surgery. *Nurs Clin North Am 22*(2), 303-310.

Stevens, K.R., Jr. (1989). The colon and rectum. In W.T. Moss & J.D. Cox (eds). *Radiation Oncology: Rationale, Technique, Results* (6th ed). Baltimore: C.V. Mosby Co., pp. 388-408.

33

Leukemias

Maryellen Maguire-Eisen, MSN, RN
Katharine Sibley Edmonds, BSN, RN, OCN

THEORY

I. Physiology and pathophysiology associated with leukemia.

   A. Hematopoietic system is composed of undifferentiated, pluripotential stem cells.

      1. As biochemical messages are received by the marrow, the stem cells divide and begin the process of differentiation.

      2. The cell goes through several stages of differentiation and ultimately forms a mature hematopoietic cell (red blood cell, granulocyte, monocyte, lymphocyte, or platelet).

   B. The primary functions of specific hematopoietic cells are described in Table 33-1.

   C. Leukemia is a malignant disorder of the blood and blood-forming organs (bone marrow, lymph nodes, and spleen).

      1. Malignant stem cells result in cells that have lost cell division regulation and the ability to differentiate to mature, functional cells.

      2. Immature cellular elements accumulate in the marrow spaces, peripheral vasculature, and selected organs and tissues (spleen, gums, and lymph nodes).

      3. As immature cellular elements accumulate, the production of normal hematopoietic cells is limited by lack of space in the marrow and by lack of nutrients.

         a. Symptoms of leukemia reflect a decrease in the number of mature, functional white blood cells, platelets, and red blood cells (Table 33-2).

         b. Symptoms may also be attributed to the effects of immature cellular accumulation in other organs and tissues.

      4. Classification of leukemia (Table 33-3) is based on predominant cell line affected (lymphocytic or granulocytic) and the level of differentiation reached (acute or chronic).

II. Trends in epidemiology.

   A. Leukemia accounts for 8% of all cancers diagnosed in the United States.

   B. Most common form of cancer affecting children; represents 30% of all childhood malignancies.

Table 33-1
PRIMARY FUNCTIONS OF SELECTED HEMATOPOIETIC CELLS

Type of Cell	Function
Red blood cell	Transportation of oxygen and excretion of carbon dioxide
Platelet	Formation of hemostatic plug Provision of phospholipid surface necessary for the interaction of clotting factors of the intrinsic pathyway Production of platelet factor IV to neutralize the action of heparin
Granulocyte	Removal of foreign substances from the blood and tissues (bacteria) Release of substances (histamine, heparin, bradykinin, serotonin) in hypersensitivity reactions
Lymphocyte	Recognition of antigen Regulation of humoral (B lymphocyte) and cellular (T lymphocyte) immune responses
Monocyte	Removal of foreign substances from the blood and tissues (mycobacteria, fungi, and large molecules) Synthesis and secretion of complement components, transferrin, interferon, colony-stimulating factors Recognition of antigen, activation of cellular immune response, and humoral antibody production

III. Principles of medical management.
  A. Diagnostic procedures.
    1. Complete blood count with differential.
    2. Bone marrow aspirate and biopsy.
  B. Treatment strategies.
    1. Phases of therapy.
      a. Remission induction—initial treatment phase when multiple antineoplastic agents are given at high doses to "empty" the bone marrow of abnormal hematological elements and to allow normal constituents to repopulate the marrow.
        (1) Goal of treatment—to achieve a complete remission.
        (2) Complete remission requires:
          (a) Absence of all clinical signs and symptoms of leukemia.
          (b) Normal peripheral blood differential without blasts (immature cells).
          (c) Restoration of a normal bone marrow with less than 5% blasts, adequate numbers of maturing myeloid cells, megakaryocytes, and adequate numbers of erythroid and lymphoid precursors.
      b. Postremission therapy.
        (1) Successful induction regimens reduce the leukemic cell population to an undectable level.
        (2) Goals of treatment—to reduce further or eliminate the remaining population of undetectable cells.
      c. Intensification or consolidation therapy.
        (1) Intensive therapy given during remission to reduce the remaining leukemic cell population.

Table 33-2
CLINICAL SIGNS AND SYMPTOMS OF THE LEUKEMIAS

Clinical Symptoms	Clinical Signs	Laboratory Findings	Cause
Malaise, fatigue, weakness	Pallor	Anemia	Marrow failure
Weight loss	Decreased weight	Hypoalbuminemia	Anorexia, increased metabolism
Easy bruising, gum bleeding, visual difficulties, tarry stools	Petechiae, ecchymosis, microscopic hematuria, hypertrophy or bleeding of gums, retinal hemorrhage, guaiac-positive stools	Thrombocytopenia Abnormal clotting	Marrow failure
Prolonged or recurrent viral or bacterial infection	Sinusitis, pneumonitis, urinary tract infection, decreased wound healing	Granulocytopenia	Marrow failure
Headache, nausea, vomiting	Meningismus Papilledema	Increased cerebrospinal fluid (CSF) protein, decreased CSF sugar, leukemic cells in CSF	Meningeal or central nervous system leukemic involvement
Bone pain	Bone tenderness	Abnormal roentgenogram	Leukemic infiltration
Swollen glands	Lymphadenopathy	Abnormal biopsy or scans	Leukemic infiltration
Abdominal fullness or pain	Splenomegaly or hepatomegaly	Abnormal liver function tests	Leukemic infiltration
Testicular swelling	Testicular mass	Abnormal biopsy	Leukemic infiltration

Modified from Williams, W.J. et al. (1977). *Hematology.* Reproduced with permission of McGraw-Hill, Inc., New York.

    (2) Sequencing of treatment is designed for optimal effect and tolerable toxicity.

    (3) Bone marrow transplantation (see Chapter 24) is a form of consolidation therapy (Table 33-4).

  d. Maintenance.

    (1) Administration of long-term therapy in moderate doses to "maintain" a disease-free state.

    (2) Maintenance therapy has not been shown as beneficial in treatment of acute myelogenous leukemia (AML).

2. Relapse is the reappearance of clinical and hematological evidence of leukemia.

  a. Marrow relapse.

  b. Extramedullary site relapse—central nervous system (CNS), testes, or skin.

    (1) Most clients that relapse have a poor prognosis.

Table 33-3
CLASSIFICATION OF LEUKEMIA

Cell Line	Level of Differentiation	High-Risk Clients	Induction Therapies	Effects of Treatment
Myelogenous	Acute	Adults	Daunorubicin and cytarabine Mitoxantrone and cytarabine	Long-term, disease-free interval in 10% to 40% of adults Prognosis related to duration of remission
Myelocytic				
Promyelocytic				
Myelomono-cytic	Chronic	Adults Chromosome abnormality (Philadelphia chromosome)	Busulfan or hydroxyurea Interferon Blast crisis: Vincristine and predni-sone Spleenectomy Radiation therapy	Three phases of disease—chronic, accelerated, and blastic Differentiated by total leukocyte count, presence of symptoms, and complications
Monocytic				
Erythrocytic				
Megakaryocytic				
Lymphocytic	Acute	Children	Vincristine, prednisone, an anthracycline, 6-mercapto-purine, cyclophosphamide, daunorubiein, doxorubicin, L-asparaginase, teniposide, and mitroxanthrone CNS prophylaxis: Intrathecal medication Whole brain irradiation	Long-term remissions in 80% of clients Late effects associated with cen-tral nervous system (CNS) pro-phylaxis, type of treatment, and intensity of treatment
	Chronic	Adults Fifth decade of life	Chlorambucil, prednisone, cyclophosphamide, vincris-tine, interferon, and doxo-rubicin Radiation therapy to spleen and lymph nodes	Median survival, 71 mo Treatment initiated secondary to granulocyte count greater than 200,000; hemolytic anemia; in-fection; increased splenomegaly

Table 33-4
BONE MARROW TRANSPLANTATION: LONG-TERM SURVIVAL RATES*

Type of Leukemia	Remission Status at Time of Transplant	Type of Transplant (%)	
		Allogeneic	**Autologous**
Acute lymphocytic	Remission	25-50	43
	Relapse	10-20	15
Acute myelogenous	Remission	20-70†	40-48
	Relapse	20-34	30
Chronic myelogenous	Chronic phase	45-70	5-15
	Accelerated	15-28	
	Blast	5-15	

*Defined as alive 3 years without evidence of disease.
†First and subsequent remission rates combined
Modified from Ford, R. & Eisenberg, S. (1990). Bone marrow transplantation. *Nurs Clin North Am 25*(2), 408.

    (2) Predictors of outcomes of future therapy—site of relapse, timing of
      the relapse, and duration of remission.

 C. Trends in survival.

  1. Improved survival rates in clients with acute leukemia over past three decades.

  2. Factors influencing increased survival rate include:

   a. Introduction of combined and multimodality treatment regimens.

   b. Improvement in support services such as blood banking, nutritional support, and antimicrobial therapy.

   c. Coordinated and cooperative research efforts (Figure 33-1).

  3. Increased survival rate has resulted in identification of late effects of therapy.

   a. Neuropsychiatric—deficits in attention span, concentration, and short-term memory and decrease in level of intellectual functioning as compared to siblings and peers.

   b. Cardiac—cardiomyopathy accompanied by congestive heart failure and pericarditis.

   c. Delayed growth and development among children.

   d. Secondary malignancies.

   e. Psychosocial—anxiety, depression, decreased self-concept, poor school performance, and fear of intimacy because of concerns about infertility.

DATA COLLECTION

 I. Pertinent client and family history.

  A. Exposure to radiation.

   1. Treatment of neoplastic or benign disease with radiation therapy.

   2. Accidental radiation exposure.

  B. Exposure to chemicals.

   1. Cytotoxic drugs—alkylating agents.

   2. Benzene.

   3. Chloramphenicol.

   4. Phenylbutazone.

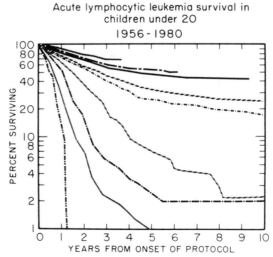

Acute lymphocytic leukemia survival in
children under 20
1956-1980

Figure 33-1 Results of successive clinical trials. Each line designates a different clinical trial. Successive controlled clinical trials in 3072 children demonstrate the incremental steps to the cure of acute lymphocytic leukemia. *(From Holland, J. [1983]. Breaking the cure barrier. J Clin Oncol 1:75.)*

C. Genetic abnormalities—Down syndrome, Turner's syndrome, Bloom syndrome, Klinefelter's syndrome, and Fanconi's anemia.

D. Exposure to viruses—human immunodeficiency virus associated with T-cell lymphocytic leukemia.

II. Physical examination.
  A. Oral cavity—swollen, friable, pale gums.
  B. Abdomen—enlarged liver or spleen.
  C. Supraclavicular, cervical, axillary, mediastinal, or groin lymphadenopathy.
  D. Neurological—headache, papilledema, meningismus, or abnormal cranial nerve responses.
  E. Musculoskeletal—joint pain and inflammation.
  F. Genitourinary—hematuria, signs and symptoms of urinary tract infection, or testicular mass.
  G. Integumentary—bruising, ecchymoses, and petechiae.

III. Evaluation of laboratory data.
  A. Decreased hemoglobin and hematocrit levels.
  B. Increased white blood cell count with abnormal differential.
  C. Decreased platelet count.
  D. Increased cerebrospinal fluid (CSF) protein; decreased CSF glucose; leukemic infiltrates of CSF.
  E. Elevated liver function test values.

ASSOCIATED NURSING DIAGNOSES

I. Potential for injury.

II. Impaired social interaction.

III. Altered oral mucosa.

IV. Potential for infection.

V. Fatigue.

VI. Body image disturbance.

NURSING PLANNING AND IMPLEMENTATION

I. Interventions to maximize client safety.
  A. See Chapter 7 (leukopenia, thrombocytopenia, anemia, fever, and stomatitis, esophagitis, and mucositis).
  B. See Chapter 9 (tumor lysis syndrome, disseminated intravascular coagulation, and septic shock).

II. Interventions to decrease the incidence and severity of symptoms unique to leukemia.
  A. See Chapter 7 (leukopenia, thrombocytopenia, anemia, fever, and stomatitis, esophagitis, and mucositis).
  B. See Chapter 9 (tumor lysis syndrome, disseminated intravascular coagulation, and septic shock).

III. Interventions to monitor for unique side effects of disease or treatment.
  A. Leukostasis—absolute leukocyte count greater than $100,000/mm^3$.
    1. Physiological effects—capillary plugging, vessel rupture, bleeding, and organ damage.
    2. Clients at risk—diagnosis of acute leukemia or chronic leukemia in blast crisis.

3. Signs and symptoms—increased intracranial pressure and respiratory distress.
4. Medical management:
   a. Treat disease with chemotherapy.
   b. Administer intravenous fluids.
   c. Administer prophylactic radiation to CNS.
   d. Initiate leukopheresis.
5. Nursing interventions:
   a. Assess neurological status every 4 hours when white blood count is greater than $100,000/mm^3$.
   b. Institute additional environmental and personal safety measures as client becomes confused.
   c. Assess for signs of bleeding every 4 hours.
   d. Assess respiratory rate, depth, effort, and effectiveness every 4 hours.
B. Infection.
   1. Clients at risk—absolute granulocyte count less than $500/mm^3$.
   2. Signs and symptoms:
      a. Fever may be the first and only sign of infection.
      b. Redness, swelling, pain, and pus may also be present.
   3. Medical management (Table 33-5).
   4. Nursing interventions:
      a. Institute measures to minimize exposure from exogenous organisms.
         (1) Admit client to a private room.
         (2) Limit visitors.
         (3) Avoid invasive procedures.
         (4) Avoid contact with persons with viral and bacterial infections.
      b. Institute measures to minimize exposure from endogenous organisms.
         (1) Teach client prophylactic oral hygiene measures.
         (2) Institute perineal hygiene measures.

Table 33-5
EVALUATION OF FEBRILE, NEUTROPENIC CLIENT

Temperature of 101° F (38.5° C) lasting more than 2 hr, unassociated with administration of pyrogenic substances, indicates presence of infection until proven otherwise

Thorough history and physical examination
   Particular attention paid to oropharynx, axillae, groins, perianal area, sinuses, indwelling catheters, any suspected area of infection
   Characteristic signs and symptoms of infection may be absent

Blood cultures
   Two sets (at least 10-15 ml each) before antibiotics begun
   Culture of both central line and peripheral intravenous site
   Repeat cultures daily while febrile

Cultures of nose, throat, urine, sputum, stool, rectum, axilla, obvious lesions as a baseline; repeat as indicated

Urinalysis (looking for bacteriuria, not pyuria)

Chest radiograph (may initially be negative; repeat)

Reexamine client on a regular basis until site of infection is documented or is resolved

---

Modified from Oniboni, A. (1990). Infection in the neutropenic patient. *Semin Oncol 6(1)*, 54.

(3) Teach handwashing guidelines.

(4) Encourage client to bathe each day with attention to skin-fold areas.

EVALUATION OF CLIENT AND FAMILY OUTCOMES

I. Describe the type of leukemia and rationale for treatment.

II. List signs and symptoms of immediate and long-term side effects of leukemia and treatment—infection, bleeding, stomatitis, fatigue, and sterility.

III. List self-care measures to decrease the incidence and severity of symptoms associated with disease and treatment.

IV. Demonstrate skills in self-care demanded by structural or functional effects of disease and treatment.

V. Describe schedule and procedures for routine follow-up care—peripheral blood counts, bone marrow biopsy, and evaluation of spinal fluid.

VI. List signs and symptoms of recurrent disease—bruising; bleeding from nose, gums, bladder, or bowel; fatigue; recurrent or persistent infection.

VII. Describe potential community resources to meet the unique demands of leukemia, treatment and survivorship.

    A. Leukemia Society of America.

    B. American Cancer Society.

    C. American Red Cross.

    D. National Coalition for Cancer Survivorship.

BIBLIOGRAPHY

Baird, S.B., McCorkle, R., & Grant, M. (eds). (1991). *Cancer Nursing: A Comprehensive Textbook:* Philadelphia: W.B. Saunders Co.

Bavier, A.R. (1985). Alterations in hemostasis. In B.L. Johnson & S. Gross, (eds). *Handbook of Oncology Nursing.* New York: John Wiley & Sons, pp. 511-516.

Bodey, G.P. (1985). Infectious complications of leukemia—seven principles of treatment. *Prim Care Cancer* 5(3), 41-50.

Campbell, J.B., Preston, R., & Smith, K.Y. (1983). The leukemias: definition, treatment, and nursing care. *Nurs Clin North Am* 18(3), 523-541.

Collins, P.M. (1990). Diagnosis and treatment of chronic leukemia. *Semin Oncol Nurs* 6(1), 31-43, 1990.

Coping With Survival Support for People Living with Adult Leukemia and Lymphoma (1988). Leukemia Society of America.

Dow, K.H. (1990). The enduring seasons in survival. *Oncol Nurs Forum* 17(4), 511-516.

Ellerhorst-Ryan, J.M. (1985). Complications of the myeloproliferative system: infection and sepsis. *Semin Oncol Nurs* 1(6), 244-250.

Erickson, J.M. (1990). Blood support for the myelosuppressed patient. *Semin Oncol Nurs* 6(1), 61-66.

Fuller, A.K. (1990). Platelet transfusion therapy for thrombocytopenia. *Semin Oncol Nurs* 6(2), 123-128.

Goodman, M. (1989). Managing the side effects of chemotherapy. *Semin Oncol Nurs* 5(2), 29-52.

Karp, J.E., Merz, W.G., Dick, J.D., Saral, R., & Burke, P.J. (1990). Management of infectious complications of acute leukemia and antileukemia therapy. *Oncology* 4(7), 45-53.

Levenson, J.A. & Lesko, L.M. (1990). Psychiatric aspects of adult leukemia. *Semin Oncol Nurs* 6(1),76-83.

Maguire-Eisen, M. (1990). Diagnosis and treatment of adult acute leukemia. *Semin Oncol Nurs* 6(1), 17-24.

Martocchio, B.C. (1985). Family coping: helping families help themselves. *Semin Oncol Nurs* 1(4), 292-297.

Oniboni, A.C. (1990). Infection in the neutropenic patient. *Sem Oncol Nurs* 6(1), 50-60.

Wujcik, D. (1990). Options for postremission therapy in acute leukemia. *Semin Oncol Nurs* 6(1), 25-30.

34

Skin Cancer

Alice Longman, EdD, RN, FAAN

THEORY

I. Physiology and pathophysiology associated with skin cancers.
  A. Anatomy of the skin.
    1. Epidermis is the uppermost layer—its inner layer contains basal keratinocytes (skin cells) and melanocytes (pigment cells).
    2. Dermis, or corneum, is the underlying layer—contains collagen-producing fibroblasts, giving skin strength.
    3. Melanin, a brownish-black pigment, protects the epidermis and is nature's sunscreen.
  B. Primary organ functions.
    1. Protects body from mechanical, chemical, and thermal injuries and from infection-causing microorganisms.
    2. Helps maintain homeostasis and temperature regulatory function.
  C. Changes in function associated with cancer.
    1. Ultraviolet portion of the solar spectrum affects incidence of skin cancer.
    2. Aging skin.
      a. Epidermis flattens and thins with age.
      b. Decrease in melanin production, with changes in skin and hair color.
  D. Metastatic patterns.
    1. Basal cell carcinoma.
      a. Rarely metastasizes but has the possibility of creating extensive damage.
      b. Metastases develop under or next to previous treatment sites.
      c. Recurrence rates vary, depending on size of tumor and length of follow-up.
    2. Squamous cell carcinoma.
      a. Metastasizes almost exclusively via lymphatics.
      b. Degree of metastasis varies according to causative factors, morphological characteristics, and size and depth of penetration.
      c. Recurrence rates vary, but most develop within 2 years of diagnosis.
    3. Malignant melanoma.
      a. Metastasizes to regional lymph nodes and then to other distant sites.

    b. Most important prognostic features are the size and depth of the lesion at the time of removal.

    c. Difficult and unpredictable problem of hematogenous dissemination has not been solved.

E. Trends in epidemiology.

  1. Changes in incidence.

    a. Nonmelanoma skin cancer.

      (1) Most common malignant neoplasm in U.S. Caucasian population.

      (2) Incidence has been increasing for several decades.

      (3) Estimated 600,000 cases in 1990 in United States.

    b. Cutaneous malignant melanoma.

      (1) Accounts for 3% of all skin cancers.

      (2) Estimated 27,600 cases in 1990 in United States.

      (3) Accounts for an estimated 6000 deaths annually.

      (4) Highest rates are found in southern Arizona.

  2. Characteristics of tumors.

    a. Nonmelanoma skin cancers (basal cell carcinoma and squamous cell carcinoma) (Table 34-1).

      (1) Nodular basal cell carcinoma.

        (a) Bulky growth caused by lack of keratinization in the epidermis.

        (b) Masses of tumor cells.

        (c) Elevated lesion moderately firm to the touch.

        (d) Ulcerated center with elevated margins.

      (2) Superficial basal cell carcinoma.

        (a) Irregular proliferating tumor tissue.

        (b) Center usually crusted, scaly, and erythematous.

        (c) Superficial, sharply marginated plaque.

        (d) Raised, pearly, threadlike border.

      (3) Pigmented basal cell carcinoma.

        (a) Melanin in the epidermis and dermis and in the tumor itself.

        (b) Blue, black, or brown appearance.

        (c) Contains telangiectases and has a raised, pearly border.

      (4) Morphea-like basal cell carcinoma.

        (a) Fingerlike projections of fibroepitheliomatous strands of tumor.

        (b) Flat or depressed scarlike plaque that is pale yellow or white.

        (c) Nodularity, ulceration, and bleeding may occur.

Table 34-1
COMMON SITES OF NONMELANOMA SKIN CANCERS

Type of Skin Cancer	Common Sites
Nodular basal cell carcinoma	Face, head, neck
Superficial basal cell carcinoma	Trunk, extremities
Pigmented basal cell carcinoma	Face, head, neck
Morphea-like basal cell carcinoma	Head, neck
Squamous cell carcinoma	Head, nose, border of lips, hands

      (5) Squamous cell carcinoma.

         (a) Arises from the keratinizing cells of the epidermis.

         (b) Varies from an ulcerated, infiltrating mass to an elevated, erythematous nodular mass.

         (c) Usually an opaque plaque.

   b. Malignant melanoma (Table 34-2).

      (1) Major features.

         (a) Arises from melanocytes, which are cells specializing in the biosynthesis and transport of melanin.

         (b) Characterized by radial and/or vertical growth phases.

         (c) Precursor lesions:

            i. Dysplastic nevi that may be familial (B-K moles) or nonfamilial (sporadic dysplastic nevi).

            ii. Pigmented congenital nevi covering large areas of the body.

      (2) Classification of malignant melanoma.

         (a) Lentigo maligna melanoma (LMN):

            i. Most often occurs on a premalignant lesion.

            ii. Large, frecklelike lesion, tan in color, with shades of brown and dark areas.

            iii. Raised nodule with notched border.

         (b) Superficial spreading melanoma (SSM):

            i. Usually arises in preexisting nevus.

            ii. Variety of colors, ranging from tan, brown, or black to a characteristic red, white, and blue.

            iii. Flat lesion with a fine crust or scaly, surface-notched border.

         (c) Nodular melanoma (NM):

            i. Raised, dome-shaped, blue-black or red nodule.

            ii. Elevated lesion with well-demarcated borders.

            iii. Aggressive and metastasizes early.

         (d) Acral-lentiginous melanoma (ALM):

            i. Irregular in shape and size.

            ii. Variegated colors in shades of blue and black.

            iii. Smooth or ulcerated lesion, which may be raised or flat.

      (3) Features of early malignant melanoma (Table 34-3).

         (a) Asymmetry.

         (b) Border irregularity.

         (c) Color variegation.

         (d) Diameter generally greater than 6 mm.

Table 34-2

COMMON SITES OF MALIGNANT MELANOMA

Type of Melanoma	Common Sites
Lentigo maligna melanoma	Face, neck, trunk, dorsum of hands
Superficial spreading melanoma	Backs of men; legs of women
Nodular melanoma	Head, neck, trunk
Acral-lentiginous melanoma	Palms of hands, soles of feet, nail beds, mucous membranes

Table 34-3

DANGER SIGNS OF MALIGNANT MELANOMA ON THE SKIN SURFACE

Changes in color	Changes in surface
Changes in size	Changes in surrounding skin
Changes in shape	Changes in sensation
Changes in elevation	Changes in consistency

II. Principles of medical management.
  A. Screening and diagnostic procedures.
    1. General procedures.
      a. Nonmelanoma skin cancers.
        (1) Excisional biopsy and histology with 0.5- to 1-cm margins are recommended if a lesion is small.
        (2) Incisional biopsy, including 1-cm margin, is justified for larger lesion.
      b. Malignant melanoma.
        (1) Most important characteristic in the staging of melanoma is the vertical depth of melanotic penetration through the skin.
        (2) Refinement of classification relates the prognosis of melanoma to the actual measured depth or thickness of invasion.
    2. Specific procedures.
      a. Accurate histological diagnosis.
        (1) Excisional biopsy, yielding a specimen with a few millimeters of normal tissue.
        (2) Step sections of biopsy specimen at 3 mm or closer.
      b. Microstaging describes the level of invasion of malignant melanoma and maximal tumor thickness.
  B. Staging methods and procedures—parameters assessing the depth of invasion of malignant melanoma (Table 34-4).
    1. Anatomical level of invasion or Clark's level (five histological levels).
    2. Maximal vertical tumor thickness or Breslow's measurement (five measures in millimeters).
  C. Treatment strategies.
    1. Nonmelanoma skin cancers—definitive treatment depends on location and

Table 34-4

PARAMETERS OF MICROSTAGING TO EVALUATE MALIGNANT MELANOMA

Skin Layer	Clark's Level	Breslow's Measurement
Epidermis	I and II	0.10-0.75
Basal cell level	III (thin)	0.76-1.40
Papillary dermis	III (thick)	1.20-2.5
Reticular dermis	IV	2.6-4.00
Subcutaneous tissue	V	>4.00

size of the lesion, exact histological type, possible extension into nearby structures, metastases, previous treatment, anticipated cosmetic results, age, and general condition of the client.

   a. Surgery.

     (1) Excision of lesion, may be simple or complex.

     (2) Curettage and electrodesiccation for small, superficial, or recurrent lesions.

     (3) Mohs' micrographic controlled surgery or chemosurgery (surgically removes tissue in multiple, progressively thin layers).

   b. Radiotherapy.

     (1) Recommended for lesions that are inoperable and greater than 1 cm but less than 10 cm.

     (2) Administered in fractional doses.

   c. Cryotherapy.

     (1) Tumor destruction by use of liquid nitrogen to freeze and thaw tumor tissue.

     (2) Lesions with well-defined margins benefit from treatment.

   d. Chemotherapy.

     (1) Topical 5-fluorouracil (5-FU) for premalignant keratosis.

     (2) For recurrent skin cancers, particularly squamous cell carcinoma, no longer manageable by surgery or irradiation, cisplatin and doxorubicin have been used.

2. Malignant melanoma.

   a. Surgery.

     (1) Wide, local excision, leaving a 3- to 5-cm margin if anatomically possible.

     (2) Split-thickness skin grafting may be required for cosmetic reasons.

     (3) Regional lymph node dissection may be indicated but is controversial.

     (4) Used for palliative management in relief of symptoms or solitary metastasis.

   b. Radiotherapy.

     (1) Most effective when tumor volume is low.

     (2) Used for palliative management when subcutaneous, cutaneous, and nodal metastases are inaccessible for surgical removal.

   c. Chemotherapy—agents with consistent activity include dacarbazine (DTIC) and the nitrosureas (carmustine [BCNU], lomustine [CCNU], semustine [Me-CCNU], and chlorozotocin).

   d. Hormonal therapy/biotherapy.

     (1) Trials with hormonal therapy such as tamoxifen and diethylstilbestrol remain inconclusive.

     (2) Agents such as interferon, interleukins, tumor necrosis factors, monoclonal antibodies, and retinoids are being studied.

3. Special considerations.

   a. Primary melanoma of the eye.

     (1) Melanoma primarily in the iris responds well to local resection.

     (2) Ciliary body and choroidal melanoma require enucleation.

     (3) Success of treatment for metastatic disease from eye melanoma is uniformly poor.

   b. Local advanced disease.

     (1) Development of massive, local disease, frequently in the neck and in axillary or inguinal nodal areas.

     (2) Combination of radiotherapy and hyperthermia offers palliation.

D. Trends in survival.
  1. General survival.
    a. Nonmelanoma skin cancers.
      (1) Basal cell carcinoma.
        (a) Equally high cure rates with either surgery or radiation.
        (b) Possibility of creating extensive local destruction if left untreated.
      (2) Squamous cell carcinoma.
        (a) Equally high cure rates with either surgery or radiation.
        (b) Recurrence of lesion is major complication.
    b. Malignant melanoma.
      (1) Most important prognostic features are the size and the depth of the lesion at the time of removal.
      (2) Evaluation at 3 to 6 months for 2 years; every 6 months for up to 5 years; yearly thereafter.
      (3) Survival rates have been increasing because of earlier stage at diagnosis.
  2. Determinants of survival.
    a. High-risk clients are advised to do monthly skin self-examination.
    b. Survival rates are based on recurrence rates for melanomas of different thickness.

DATA COLLECTION

I. Pertinent personal and family history.
  A. Risk factors (basal cell carcinoma and squamous cell carcinoma) (Table 34-5).
    1. Exogenous factors.
      a. Ultraviolet radiation from sunlight over a long period of time.
      b. Exposure to ionizing radiation, arsenic, or petroleum.
      c. Scars following injury.
    2. Endogenous factors.
      a. Fair or freckled complexion.
      b. Red, blonde, or light brown hair.
      c. Light-colored eyes.
      d. Xeroderma pigmentosum or albinism.
      e. Immunological deficiency or suppression.

Table 34-5
MAJOR RISK FACTORS FOR SKIN CANCERS

Risk Factor	Skin Cancer Risk
Personal factors	Excessive exposure to sunlight Easily burned Increasing age Premalignant states
Life-style	Outdoor work Outdoor recreational activities Chronic exposure to chemical agents, uranium, arsenic
Drugs	Treatment for psoriasis (psoralen ultraviolet A [PUVA])
Immunological factor	Organ transplant recipients

     3. Premalignant states or lesions.
       a. Actinic, or senile, keratosis.
       b. Seborrheic keratosis.
       c. Bowen's disease.
  B. Risk factors (malignant melanoma) (see Table 34-5).
     1. Exogenous factors.
       a. Ultraviolet radiation from sunlight.
       b. Poor tolerance of sunlight.
       c. Intense, intermittent exposure to sunlight.
     2. Endogenous factors.
       a. Dysplastic nevi.
       b. Congenital nevi.
  C. Pertinent history.
     1. Skin exposure to sunlight.
       a. Time of day during exposure.
       b. Geographical area of residence(s) or recreation.
       c. Altitude or overcast weather conditions.
       d. Time of year exposed to the sun.
       e. Length of exposure(s).
     2. Skin type (Table 34-6).
       a. Pigmentation or erythema type.
       b. Genetic history.
II. Physical examination.
  A. Skin assessment (Table 34-7).
     1. Inspection and palpation of all accessible skin surfaces.
     2. Assessment of preexisting lesions such as nevi on the skin.
     3. Inspection of the scalp and entire hairline.
     4. Inspection of the face, lips, and neck.
     5. Inspection and palpation of all surfaces of upper extremities.
     6. Inspection and palpation of the skin of the back, buttocks, and back of the legs.
  B. Signs and symptoms—changes in existing moles.
     1. Size.
     2. Shape.
     3. Color.

Table 34-6
SKIN TYPES AND SKIN REACTIONS

Skin Type	Skin Reactions
1	Burns easily and severely; tans little or not at all
2	Burns easily and severely; tans minimally or lightly
3	Burns moderately; tans approximately average
4	Burns minimally; tans easily
5	Burns rarely; tans easily and substantially
6	Never burns; tans profusely

Table 34-7
COMPARISON OF NORMAL MOLES AND DYSPLASTIC NEVI

Feature	Normal Moles	Dysplastic Nevi
Color	Usually one shade of tan or brown	Variation in color; speckles of tan, brown, or black
Shape	Round or oval	Irregular or hazy
Diameter	Usually less than ¼ inch	Usually more than ¼ inch
Border	Sharp and well-defined	Irregular or hazy
Location	Sun-exposed skin	Most common on sun-exposed skin; occur anywhere on body

    4. History of itching in existing moles.
    5. History of burning in existing moles.

ASSOCIATED NURSING DIAGNOSES

 I. Knowledge deficit related to prevention and early detection of skin cancer.

 II. Knowledge deficit related to warning signs of early malignant melanoma.

 III. Knowledge deficit related to skin self-assessment.

 IV. Ineffective individual coping related to being newly diagnosed with malignant melanoma.

 V. Ineffective individual coping related to changes in recreational activities or work because of skin cancer.

 VI. Ineffective family coping: compromised, related to changes in life-style as a result of the diagnosis of malignant melanoma.

NURSING PLANNING AND IMPLEMENTATION

 I. Nonmelanoma skin cancers (basal cell carcinoma and squamous cell carcinoma).
   A. Preventive measures (Table 34-8).
     1. Minimize skin exposure to sunlight between the hours of 10 AM and 3 PM.
     2. Use protective clothing such as a hat, long-sleeved shirt, and long pants during prolonged exposure to the sun.
     3. Use sunglasses during prolonged exposure to the sun.
     4. Use sunscreens (absorbers) and sunblocks (reflectors).
       a. Commercial sunscreens with a sun protection factor (SPF) of 15 or more.
       b. Reapply sunscreen every 2 to 3 hours during prolonged exposure to the sun; reapply sunscreen after swimming.
     5. Use sunscreen with benzophenones because of photosensitivity if taking thiazides, sulfonamides, and antineoplastic agents.
     6. Avoid tanning parlors.
     7. Keep infants out of the sun.
   B. Screening and early detection measures.
     1. Obtain history of any recent changes in lesion(s).

Table 34-8
SUN-INTENSITY PREDICTION: MINUTES IN SUN TO REDDEN SKIN*

Time	Minutes
9 AM	60
10 AM	39
11 AM	26
Noon	21
1 PM	19
2 PM	23
3 PM	31
4 PM	60

Data from Arizona SunAwareness Project, University of Arizona Cancer Center (602-626-6044).
*Predictions are for untanned Caucasians, assuming no clouds.

    2. Teach systematic assessment of skin for suspicious lesions.
    3. Do a family pedigree to determine family history of skin cancers.
    4. Use educational resources:
        a. American Academy of Dermatology—*The Sun and Your Skin*.
        b. American Cancer Society—*Cancer of the Skin*.
        c. Skin Cancer Foundation—*Sun and Skin Needs*.
  C. Rehabilitative measures.
    1. Assess impact of treatment for skin cancer.
    2. Stress importance of evaluation at regular intervals for potential recurrence.

II. Malignant melanoma.
  A. Preventive measures (see Table 34-8).
    1. Teach importance of assessing for early signs of changes of nevi.
    2. Stress importance of monthly, systematic assessment of the skin to detect suspicious lesions.
  B. Screening and early detection.
    1. Do a family pedigree to determine family history of malignant melanoma.
    2. Use educational resources:
        a. American Academy of Dermatology—*Melanoma Skin Cancer*.
        b. National Cancer Institute—*What You Need to Know About Melanoma*.
        c. Skin Cancer Foundation—*The Melanoma Letter*.
    3. Arrange an ophthalmic examination for those at risk for uveal melanoma.
  C. Therapeutic measures.
    1. Prepare client and family for extensive surgical intervention and treatment.
    2. Use open, optimistic approach in discussing feelings and attitudes about the diagnosis.
    3. Attend to implications of life-threatening cutaneous melanoma.
  D. Rehabilitative measures.
    1. Stress importance of evaluation at regular intervals for potential recurrence.
    2. Teach importance of change in life-style in relation to sun exposure for high-risk individuals and families to reduce chances of further development of malignant melanoma.

EVALUATION OF CLIENT AND FAMILY OUTCOMES

I. Identify type of cancer and rationale for treatment.
   A. Describe the effects of treatment for basal cell carcinoma and squamous cell carcinoma.
   B. Describe the type of malignant melanoma and the treatment modalities.

II. List signs and symptoms of immediate and long-term effects of disease and treatment.
   A. State early signs of basal cell carcinoma and squamous cell carcinoma.
   B. State potential risks and problems associated with the treatment of malignant melanoma.

III. List self-care measures to decrease incidence and severity of symptoms associated with disease and treatment.
   A. Demonstrate psychomotor skills in doing a careful assessment of the sites affected by basal cell carcinoma and squamous cell carcinoma.
   B. Demonstrate psychomotor skills inherent in skin self-examination (see Chapter 5, Figure 5-2).

IV. Demonstrate skills in self-care demanded by structural or functional effects of disease and treatment.
   A. Describe use of sunscreen and/or sunblock for recreational activities or work.
   B. State protective measures necessary for continued care of the skin cancer site.

V. Describe schedule and procedures for routine follow-up.
   A. State time sequence for checkups.
   B. State modification of behaviors to enhance health promotion.

VI. List signs and symptoms of recurrent disease.
   A. Describe warning signs such as change in skin around site of original skin cancer.
   B. State feelings of well-being related to skin cancer.

VII. Identify potential community resources to meet unique demands of site-specific disease, treatment, and survivorship.
   A. State resources available in the community.
   B. State activities available for cancer clients and families in the community.

BIBLIOGRAPHY

American Cancer Society (1990). *Cancer Facts and Figures—1990*. Atlanta: Author.

Arizona Sun Awareness Project (1985). *Sun Awareness*. Tucson, Ariz.: Arizona Cancer Center.

Balch, C.M. (1987). Cutaneous melanoma: a review of clinical management. *Tex Med 83*(3), 70-78.

Berkman, S. (1985). The skin remembers. *Cancer News 39*(2), 2-4.

Berliner, H. (1986). Aging skin. *Am J Nurs 86*(10), 1138-1141.

Berliner, H. (1986). Aging skin: part two. *Am J Nurs 86*(11), 1259-1261.

Berwick, M., Bolognia, J.L., Heer, C., & Fine, J.A. (1991). The role of the nurse in skin cancer prevention, screening, and early detection. *Semin Oncol Nurs 7*(1), 64-71.

Frank-Stromborg, M. (1986). The role of the nurse in cancer detection and screening. *Semin Oncol Nurs 2*(3), 191-199.

Fraser, M.C., Hartge, P., & Tucker, M.A. (1991). Melanoma and nonmelanoma skin cancer: epidemiology and risk factors. *Semin Oncol Nurs 7*(1), 2-12.

Fraser, M.C. & McGuire, D.B. (1984). Skin cancer's early warning system. *Am J Nurs 84*(10), 1232-1236.

Friedman, R.J., Rigel, D.S., & Kopf, A.W. (1985). Early detection of malignant melanoma: the role of physician examination and self-examination of the skin. *CA 35*(3), 130-151.

Johnson, B.L. (1987). Malignant melanoma. In S.L. Groenwald, M.H. Frogge, M. Goodman, & C.H. Yarbro (eds). *Cancer Nursing: Principles and Practice*. Boston: Jones & Bartlett Publishers, pp. 684-692.

Lawler, P.E. (1991). Cutaneous malignant melanoma. *Semin Oncol Nurs 7*(1), 26-35.

Lawler, P.E. & Schreiber, S. (1989). Cutaneous malignant melanoma: nursing's role in prevention and early detection. *Oncol Nurs Forum 16*(3), 345-352.

Loescher, L.J. & Booth, A. (1990). Skin cancer. In S.L. Groenwald, M.H. Frogge, M. Goodman, & C.H. Yarbro (eds). *Cancer Nursing: Principles and Practice* (2nd ed). Boston: Jones & Bartlett Publishers, pp. 999-1014.

Longman, A. (1987). Skin cancer. In C.R. Ziegfeld (ed). *Core Curriculum for Oncology Nursing*. Philadelphia: W.B. Saunders Co., pp. 117-127.

Longman, A.J. (1991). Skin cancers. In S.B. Baird, R. McCorkle, & M. Grant (eds). *Cancer Nursing: A Comprehensive Textbook*. Philadelphia: W.B. Saunders Co., pp. 637-646.

McGuire, D.B. (1985). Preventive health practices and educational needs in families with hereditary melanoma. *Cancer Nurs 8*(1), 29-36.

Stewart, D.S. (1987). Indoor tanning: the nurse's role in preventing skin damage. *Cancer Nurs 10*(2), 93-99.

Vargo, N.L. (1991). Basal and squamous cell carcinoma: an overview. *Semin Oncol Nurs 7*(1), 13-25.

Head and Neck Cancers

Leonita H. Cutright, MSN, RN

THEORY

I. Anatomy of head and neck.
- A. The head and neck area is composed of a variety of different anatomical structures.
  1. Incidence, staging, and treatment of cancer in this area are dependent on the specific location of the tumor.
  2. Although the incidence of cancer occurring in this area is relatively small in number (5% of all cancers), the devastation of this disease in terms of dysfunction and body image changes calls for intensive nursing interventions to promote adaptation.
- B. Description of head and neck anatomy (Figure 35-1).
  1. Oral cavity—extends from the lips to the hard palate above and the circumvallate papillae below; structures include lips, buccal mucosa, floor of mouth, upper and lower alveoli, retromolar trigone, hard palate, and anterior two thirds of the tongue.
  2. Oropharynx—extends from the circumvallate papillae below and hard palate above to the level of the hyoid bone; structures include the base of tongue (posterior one third), soft palate, tonsils, and posterior pharyngeal wall.
  3. Nasal cavity and paranasal sinuses—include nasal vestibule; paired maxillary, ethmoid, and frontal sinuses; and a single sphenoid sinus.
  4. Nasopharynx—located below the base of skull and behind the nasal cavity; continuous with the posterior pharyngeal wall.
  5. Larynx—extends from the epiglottis to the cricoid cartilage; protected by the thyroid cartilage, which encases it; subdivided into three anatomical areas:
     - a. Supraglottis—located below the base of tongue, extending to but not including the true vocal cord; structures include epiglottis, aryepiglottic folds, arytenoid cartilages, and false vocal cords.
     - b. Glottis—area of the true vocal cord.
     - c. Subglottis—area below the true vocal cord, extending to the cricoid cartilage.
  6. Hypopharynx—extends from the hyoid bone to the lower border of the cricoid cartilage; structures include pyriform sinuses, postcricoid region, and the lower posterior pharyngeal wall.

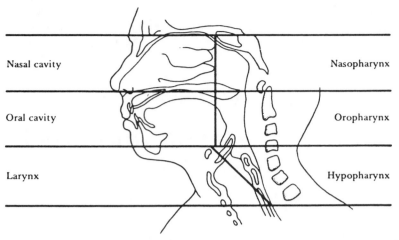

Figure 35-1 Major anatomical subdivisions of the upper aerodigestive tract. *(From Goodman, M. [1990]. Head and neck cancer. In S.L. Groenwald, M.H. Frogge, M. Goodman & C.H. Yarbo [eds]. Cancer Nursing: Principles and Practice [2nd ed]. Boston: Jones & Bartlett Publishers, p. 891.)*

C. Critical adjacent structures.
    1. Regional lymph nodes of the neck drain the anatomical structures of the head and neck; area includes submental submaxillary, upper and lower jugular, posterior triangle (spinal accessory), and preauricular nodes (Figure 35-2).
    2. Head and neck structures are contiguous with the lower aerodigestive tract— trachea, lungs, and esophagus.

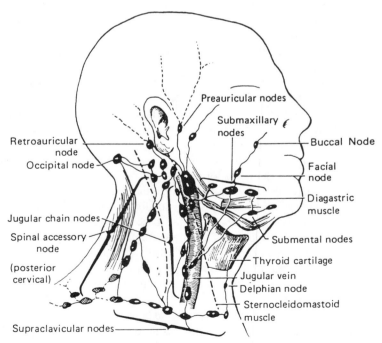

Figure 35-2 Areas of drainage to cervical lymph nodes. *(From Schleper, J.R. [1989]. Prevention, detection, and diagnosis of head and neck cancers. Semin Oncol Nurs 5[3], 146. Drawing by Greg Patterson.)*

3. The nasopharynx and paranasal sinuses are in close approximation to the brain.

II. Primary functions of the head and neck—structures of the head and neck are responsible for the mechanics of respiration, speech, and swallowing.
   A. Respiration—the upper respiratory tract serves as the passageway for transporting air into the lungs by the following process:
      1. The diaphragm descends, increasing the intrathoracic pressure.
      2. Negative pressure results in air entering the mouth and nose where it is warmed, filtered, and humidified.
      3. Air enters the upper air passageways of the pharynx, larynx, and trachea, then enters the lung.
   B. Speech—speech is formed from sound waves created as air is expelled from the lungs, passes through the vocal cords and is mechanically perfected through the processes of:
      1. Phonation—achieved by the larynx.
      2. Articulation—achieved by the lips, tongue, and soft palate.
      3. Resonation—resonators (pharynx, mouth, nose, and nasal sinuses) create the tone and quality of speech.
   C. Swallowing—complex process wherein 26 muscles and six cranial nerves orchestrate the transport of food from the mouth to the stomach in four phases of swallowing:
      1. Oral preparatory—bolus of food is prepared for initiating the swallow by mastication of the food into smaller particles and secretion of saliva into the oral cavity to lubricate the bolus.
      2. Oral—bolus is propelled into the pharynx by the front-to-back movement of the tongue.
      3. Pharyngeal—bolus moves through the pharynx and is propelled toward the esophagus; the vocal cords close, and the larynx moves upward and forward, preventing aspiration.
      4. Esophageal—bolus moves through the esophagus and enters the stomach.

III. Changes in function associated with head and neck cancer.
   A. Respiration:
      1. Head and neck cancer affects primarily the structures of the upper airway, which serve to transport warmed, filtered, and humidified air into the lungs.
      2. Disease and treatment in this area may result in bypassing the natural air-conditioning function of the upper air passageways, causing a cooling, drying effect on the trachea and lungs that can lead to infection.
   B. Speech:
      1. Removing part or all of the *larynx* results in loss of the vibrating component for speech; thus sound waves cannot be produced (total laryngectomy) or are diminished (partial).
      2. Surgery to the *mouth, tongue,* or *palate* causes changes in the individual's ability to articulate clear, understandable speech.
      3. Cancer or treatment of the *nose* or *sinuses* influences the tone and quality of the speech.
   C. Swallowing:
      1. *Supraglottic laryngectomy* affects the pharyngeal phase of swallowing, resulting in decreased protection of the glottis; aspiration is a danger until swallowing techniques are learned.
      2. Extensive resections of structures in the *oral cavity* and *oropharynx* requiring flap reconstruction affect the oral preparatory and oral phase of swallowing

and may result in drooling of saliva, decreased mastication, aspiration, pooling of food and fluids; radiation to this area will cause decreased salivary production (xerostomia), with loss of the lubricating effect on the bolus.

IV. Metastatic patterns.
   A. Head and neck cancer is a locally aggressive disease that spreads regionally to the lymphatics of the neck (Figure 35-2).
   B. Most clients present with stage III and IV disease, which indicates tumor spread to the lymphatics and/or a very large invasive primary tumor.
   C. The incidence of local regional failure is as high as 60%, with clinically detected distant metastasis occurring at a rate of 20%.
   D. Autopsy studies indicate the incidence of distant metastasis is 50%; however, 90% of these clients die with uncontrolled primary tumors or neck disease (i.e., regional disease).
   E. Most common sites of distant metastasis—lung, liver, and bone (in approximately 50% of clients with distant metastasis).

V. Trends in epidemiology.
   A. Changes in incidence and treatment.
      1. Usually occurs in the 50- to 70-years age group.
      2. No appreciable increase in 5-year survival rates has been achieved over the last 30 years, but advances made since the early 1970s include more conservative surgical techniques and reconstruction, increasing the quality of life, and decreasing the airway, communication, and swallowing dysfunctions.
      3. Use of prosthetic devices and surgical flaps (myocutaneous and free) has resulted in improved cosmetic effects and reduced deformities.
      4. Chemotherapy for head and neck tumors has not proved effective, but future research in this area holds the best hope for increased survival.
   B. Histology and incidence.
      1. Histology of head and neck tumors—90%, squamous cell; 10%, adenocarcinoma (salivary glands), melanoma, sarcoma, or lymphoma.
      2. Majority of head and neck tumors occur in the oral cavity (48%), larynx (25%), and oropharynx (10%).

VI. Principles of medical management.
   A. Screening and diagnostic procedures.
      1. General procedures—clients with head and neck cancer are at an increased risk for synchronous primary tumors as a result of prolonged exposure of the mucosal surface to carcinogens; therefore the initial workup includes evaluation to rule out multiple primary tumors.
         a. No definitive screening examination or test is recommended for early detection; however, a thorough oral examination should be included in a cancer-related checkup conducted every 3 years for those 20 to 40 years of age and every year for those 40 and over.
         b. Radiological studies:
            (1) Computed tomographic (CT) scan—to assist in determining the extent of the primary tumor and in identifying metastasis to the cervical lymph nodes.
            (2) Chest x-ray examination—to identify disease in the lung, a second primary tumor, or distant metastasis.
            (3) Panorex—panoramic views to evaluate mandibular invasion from oral cavity and oropharyngeal lesions.

(4) Magnetic resonance imaging (MRI) scan—superior to the CT scan in staging nasopharyngeal primaries, but value in comparison to the CT scan for detecting cancer in other sites is still under investigation.

(5) Cine-esophagography / barium swallow—to identify the extent of lesions in the oropharynx that may extend into the hypopharynx.

(6) Bone and liver scans—to evaluate distant metastasis among high-risk clients (elevated liver enzymes or bone pain).

c. Evaluation of suspected head and neck tumors includes a thorough history and examination of all structures of the upper aerodigestive tract:

(1) History of risk factors (Table 35-1).

(2) Physical examination:

(a) Visualization.

(b) Mirror examination of the pharynx and larynx.

(c) Palpation via a bimanual examination to assess the oral cavity and upper neck.

(3) Signs and symptoms of disease (Table 35-2).

d. Histological diagnosis—mandatory before definitive treatment and obtained by:

(1) Fine-needle aspiration—performed on suspicious neck nodes and accessible lesions in the oral cavity.

(2) Excisional biopsy of the entire lesion—for diagnostic or curative purposes.

(a) Performed on small oral cavity, lip, or skin lesions.

(b) As a rule, an open or excisional biopsy of suspicious neck nodes is contraindicated (to avoid seeding of the tumor) except when all other examinations fail to identify a primary site or when lymphoma is suspected.

(3) Incisional biopsy—taking a small sample of tumor along with adjoining normal tissue.

e. Panendoscopy (passing an endoscope along the entire mucosa of the upper aerodigestive tract)—to examine and perform a biopsy on suspicious areas, determine the full extent of disease, and identify synchronous primary tumors.

f. Specific procedures unique to head and neck evaluation (Table 35-3).

Table 35-1
RISK FACTORS FOR HEAD AND NECK CANCER

Personal / Environmental	Tobacco use—All Forms
	Cigarettes, cigars, pipe, smokeless tobacco
	Alcohol
	Poor oral hygiene
	Long-term sun exposure
Occupational	Asbestos, coke, nickel, textile, wood, or leather workers; machinists
Ethnicity	Southern Chinese population
Viruses	Epstein-Barr
	Possibly herpes simplex and human papilloma

Table 35-2
SIGNS AND SYMPTOMS OF HEAD AND NECK CANCER

Early	Late
Oral Cavity and Oropharynx	
Leukoplakia	Dysphagia
Erythroplakia	Aspiration (oropharyngeal)
Pain or ulcer that fails to heal	Speech difficulties
Painless, persistent mass	Trismus (lockjaw)
Difficulty with dentures	Referred otalgia (ear pain)
	Weight loss
	Cervical adenopathy
Larynx and Hypopharynx	
Persistent hoarseness	Pain
Throat pain	Dysphagia
	Dyspnea and stridor
	Hemoptysis
	Referred otalgia (supraglottic)
	Aspiration (supraglottic)
	Cervical adenopathy
Nose and Paranasal Sinuses	
Nasal stuffiness	Bloody nasal discharge
Headache	Pain in teeth
	Asymmetry, pain, and/or numbness over involved sinus
	Trismus
	Proptosis (eyes protrude)
	Diplopia (cranial nerves III, IV, VI)
Nasopharynx	
No early symptoms	Bloody nasal discharge
	Unilateral nasal obstruction
	Unilateral serous otitis media
	Unilateral hearing loss
	Poorly localized headaches
	Cranial nerve compression
	Presence of an enlarged posterior, high-cervical lymph node (most common presenting symptom)

B. Staging methods and procedures—TNM classification system, defined by the American Joint Committee on Cancer (AJCC) in 1988, is used for staging head and neck tumors (see Appendix).
  a. T designation of head and neck malignancies varies, depending on anatomical site.
  b. As a general guide, the T classification applies to most sites except larynx and maxillary sinus.
C. Treatment strategies—surgery and radiation are the primary treatment modalities for managing malignant head and neck tumors.
  1. As a rule, treatment based on the T and N classification is as follows:
    a. T1 and T2 lesions of the oral cavity, larynx, nose, and paranasal sinuses

Table 35-3
SPECIFIC DIAGNOSTIC PROCEDURES IN EVALUATION OF HEAD AND NECK TUMORS

Description	Time Required	Sensations Experienced	Potential Side Effects/ Complications	Self-Care Measures	Symptoms to Report to Health Care Team
Panoramic X-ray (Panorex)					
Examination of an entire dental arch viewed on one film To evaluate mandibular invasion	10 min	None	None	None	N/A
Cine-esophagography					
Video x-ray examination of oral and pharyngeal stages of swallowing To identify extension of lesions into hypopharynx	30 min	Vary, depending on degreee of dysphagia	Aspiration	None	Temperature elevation Productive cough
Barium Swallow and X-ray Examination of Upper Gastrointestinal Tract					
To evaluate tumor invasion of hypopharynx and cervical esophagus	15 min	Chalky taste	Constipation secondary to use of barium	Assess bowel function Take laxative as needed Force fluids	No bowel movement within 3 days Abdominal distention
Panendoscopy					
Surgical procedure in which a lighted scope is passed along the upper aerodigestive tract to inspect and obtain biopsy specimens from areas of the entire mucosa (includes bronchoscopy, esophagoscopy, nasopharyngoscopy, and laryngoscopy) To detect metastasis or second primary tumor	1 hr	Related to general anesthesia	Reactions to general anesthesia Airway obstruction Tracheoesophageal fistula Sore throat Aspiration Hemorrhage from biopsy site Pneumothorax	Deep breathe, turn, ambulate	Difficulty breathing Excessive bleeding Inability to swallow (nurse should check for return of gag reflex) Increased temperature, cough, or sputum production

are treated with primary surgery or radiation, whereas T3 and T4 tumors are treated with combination therapy.

b. Surgery and radiation (usually external beam is used 6 weeks after surgery, but preoperative radiation or permanently placed iodine-125 seeds may be used to debulk large or unresectable lesions).

(1) Advantage of postoperative radiation—fewer wound complications than with untreated preoperative lesions.

(2) Preoperative dental evaluations, removal of diseased teeth, and prophylactic fluoride are indicated.

(3) Postoperative radiation is initiated after the wounds heal (3 to 6 weeks) and is administered over a 6-week period.

2. Table 35-4 identifies the common surgical procedures used in treating head and neck malignancies, the physical alterations expected, and nursing implications.

   a. Classification and location of the primary tumor influence treatment strategies. Table 35-5 summarizes treatment by site for T0; T1 and T2; and T3 and T4.

      (1) Clinically negative neck disease and a large primary lesion (T2, N0) of the oral cavity, oropharynx, hypopharynx, or larynx generally are treated with either lymphadenectomy or radiation because of the propensity to spread.

      (2) Treatment of N1, N2, and N3 disease is outlined in Table 35-6.

   b. Extensive disease.

      (1) Palliation—use of surgery, radiation, and/or chemotherapy for unresectable lesions, recurrent tumors, or clients who are a high surgical risk.

      (2) Short courses of radiation (3000 cGy over 3 to 4 weeks) may be used to relieve pain, bleeding, or obstruction.

3. Special considerations:

   a. Cancers of the nasopharynx are treated primarily with radiation.

      (1) Close proximity to vital structures of the brain precludes surgery.

      (2) Carefully selected clients who fail after radiation therapy may be treated with skull base resection.

   b. Large doses of radiation (6000 to 7000 rads) are used when radiation is the primary treatment modality.

      (1) Radiation as primary treatment is selected to control the primary tumor and adjacent lymph nodes yet maintain structure and function.

      (2) Adjuvant treatment dose for stage III and IV disease and tumors that have a tendency to spread toward the midline (oropharyngeal lesions) is 5000 rads.

   c. Brachytherapy (implanted iodine 192 or cesiun 137) may be used to treat lesions of the anterior and posterior tongue, floor of mouth, and nasal vestibule to maximize dose to the tumor bed and minimize exposure to surrounding tissue.

   d. Single agent or combination (cisplatin, bleomycin, 5-fluorouracil [5-FU], and methotrexate) chemotherapy regimens may be given as adjuvant and neoadjuvant therapy; may be used as palliative therapy for recurrent or unresectable lesions.

   e. Potentiating effect of chemotherapy on radiation treatment is investigational.

      (1) Trends in survival have not increased in the last 30 years.

      (2) Chemotherapy in combination with surgery and/or radiation serves as the best hope for increasing survival rates.

D. Trends in survival rates.

1. Five-year relative survival rate for all head and neck tumors approximates 50%.

   a. For early stage I and II cancers—40% to 95%.

Table 35-4
SURGICAL PROCEDURES FOR HEAD AND NECK CANCER

Procedure	Physical Alteration	Nursing Implications
Laser	Little to none	Minimal bleeding
Composite resection	Resection of oral cavity/oropharyngeal lesion in continuity with neck dissection Portion of mandible is resected Reconstruction with myocutaneous flaps is usually required, with resections of large amounts of tissue	May experience problems with speech (decreased articulation with tongue involvement), swallowing (impaired mastication, salivary drooling, aspiration), altered facial contour
Supraglottic laryngectomy	Resection of structures above the false vocal cords, including the epiglottis (preserves the true vocal cords)	Aspiration until swallowing techniques are learned Maintains a relatively normal voice
Hemilaryngectomy	Vertical excision of one true and one false cord and underlying cartilage	Hoarse voice Minimal or no swallowing problems
Total laryngectomy	Excision of entire larynx from the hyoid bone to the second tracheal ring	Permanent tracheostomy Aphonia Decreased sense of smell Unable to perform Valsalva maneuver
Maxillectomy	Partial or total en bloc resection of the cavity May include the ethmoid sinus, lateral nasal wall, palate, and floor of orbit	Preoperatively, orthodontist makes dental obturator to fill the large surgical defect and to facilitate swallowing Requires daily care to cavity and placement of obturator
Orbital exenteration	Resection of orbit secondary to extension of maxillary sinus tumor or recurrent disease	Facial defect Unilateral vision loss Requires daily care and cleansing of cavity
Craniofacial/skull base dissection	Surgical approach to inaccessible midfacial and extensive paranasal sinus and nasopharyngeal lesions	May have facial defect and cranial nerve (III, IV, V) deficits
Radical neck dissection	Resection of sternocleidomastoid muscle, jugular vein, spinal accessory nerve, and cervical lymph nodes	Shoulder droop Concave contour of neck
Modified neck dissection	Radical neck dissection with preservation of either the sternocleidomastoid muscle, jugular vein, or spinal accessory nerve	Shoulder droop if spinal accessory nerve resected Concave contour of neck
Lymphadenectomy	Resection of lymph nodes in neck	Surgical scars

   b. For stage III and IV lesions—0% to 50%.
2. Five-year survival (all stages) varies by site: oral cavity (40% to 70%), oropharynx (35% to 50%), larynx (50% to 80%), nasopharynx (26%), and nose and sinuses (15% to 40%).
3. Eliminating aggravating life-style factors (smoking and alcohol) decreases the chance of developing recurrent disease.

Table 35-5

TREATMENT STRATEGIES FOR HEAD AND NECK CANCER BY TUMOR CLASSIFICATION AND SITE

	T0	T1 and T2	T3 and T4
Oral cavity and oropharynx	Laser excision	Radiation (4500-5500 cGy), with 500-2500 cGy boost to primary site *or* Simple excision with primary closure	Composite resection, with primary closure *or* Myocutaneous flap closure *and* Adjuvant radiation (5000 cGy)
Larynx	Laser excision	Glottic lesions—radiation (5500-6500 cGy) Supraglottic lesions—supraglottic laryngectomy Lesions confined to one side of glottis, with posterior extension—hemilaryngectomy	Total laryngectomy *and* Adjuvant radiation (5000 cGy)
Nose and paranasal sinuses	—	Maxillectomy Excision of nasal vault and lesion *or* Radiation	Maxillectomy (may include orbital exenteration) Excision of nasal vault lesions *and* Radiation
Nasopharynx	—	Excision Radiation	Radiation to nasopharynx, retropharyngeal nodes, lymph nodes in both sides of neck Skull base surgery in selected cases that fail with radiation therapy

Table 35-6

TREATMENT STRATEGIES FOR NODAL INVOLVEMENT IN HEAD AND NECK CANCER

N0	N1	N2 and N3
No treatment *or* Lymphadenectomy *or* Modified neck dissection *or* Radiation	Modified neck dissection if tumor has not compromised cranial nerve XI *with* Radiation *or* Radiation (if node <2 cm) *or* Radical neck dissection *without* Radiation	Radical neck dissection *with* Radiation

DATA COLLECTION

I. Pertinent personal and family history (risk factors).
   A. Assess risk factors (Table 35-1), that are thought to account for approximately 90% of head and neck cancers.
   B. Assess client for signs and symptoms of the disease (Table 35-2).
   C. Assess health history and previous history of carcinoma and/or treatment of the head and neck.

II. Physical examination.
   A. Direct visualization of the oral cavity, oropharynx, and nasal vault for signs and symptoms (Table 35-2).
   B. Indirect visualization of the larynx and base of tongue via mirror examination to assess for ulcerative and exophytic lesions and to determine vocal cord mobility.
   C. Endoscopic evaluation to assess laryngeal, nasal, paranasal sinus, and nasopharyngeal tumors.
   D. Bimanual palpation of lesions in the floor of mouth, base of tongue, and lymph nodes to assess the extent of disease.
   E. Assessment of lymph nodes (size, number, mobility, and degree of tenderness); malignant nodes generally are not tender, are greater than 1 cm, have decreased mobility or are fixed, and are spherical or matted in shape.

III. Laboratory data.
   A. Complete blood count, electrolyte values, liver and renal function tests.
   B. Liver scan is indicated if liver functions are abnormal.

ASSOCIATED NURSING DIAGNOSES

I. Ineffective airway clearance related to tracheostomy.

II. Impaired communication related to tracheostomy (temporary) or laryngectomy (permanent).

III. Alteration in nutrition: less than body requirements related to swallowing dysfunction and disease process.

IV. Alteration in mobility related to resection of spinal accessory nerve XI.

V. Body image-disturbance related to surgical procedure or radiation response.

VI. Potential impaired skin integrity related to fistula formation.

NURSING PLANNING AND IMPLEMENTATION

I. Interventions to maximize safety for the client.
   A. Close proximity to the nurses' station to monitor clients with altered airway.
   B. An extra tracheostomy tube of the same size (inner and outer cannula and obturator), scissors, and a tracheal dilator at the bedside of all tracheostomy clients.
   C. Call bell within reach at all times.
   D. Label intercommunication system if client has a tracheostomy in place.
   E. Observe for signs and symptoms of delirium tremens in clients with recent history of alcohol abuse.
   F. Observe for signs and symptoms of aspiration in clients who have had a supraglottic laryngectomy, resection of structures in the oropharynx, or cranial nerve (IX, X, XII) deficits.
   G. Implement carotid precautions for clients at risk for carotid rupture.

II. Interventions to decrease the severity of symptoms associated with cancers of the head and neck.

A. Preoperative teaching.
   1. Initiate at the time of diagnosis and incorporate the treatment team (nursing, speech and language pathologist, social worker, physicians).
   2. Discuss information about the disease, treatment, side effects, and anticipated dysfunction with the client and family.
   3. Give instructions and demonstrate the use of various types of equipment (tracheostomy tube, drains, nasogastric tube).
   4. Counsel and support client and family as needed.
   5. Discuss economic and rehabilitation resources.
   6. Arrange a preoperative and a postoperative visit with a Lost Chord or Laryngectomy Club member if indicated (call American Cancer Society [ACS] or local agencies).
B. Communication.
   1. Determine client's reading ability preoperatively and choose communication mechanisms to use postoperatively:
      a. Paper and pencil.
      b. Magic slate.
      c. Picture board.
      d. Nonverbal cues.
      e. Electronic communication board or device.
C. Airway management related to tracheostomy.
   1. Permanent tracheostomy (total laryngectomy) (Figure 35-3).
      a. Airway.
         (1) Use a cuffed tracheostomy tube while the client requires mechanical

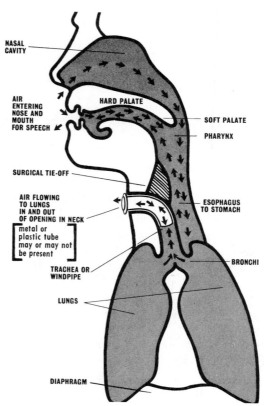

Figure 35-3 Physiology of the head and neck after total laryngectomy. *(From* First Aid for [Neck-breathers] Laryngectomees. *Atlanta: American Cancer Society, p. 3, phone 404-320-3333.)*

ventilation; may be removed by day 2 or 3, with the stoma remaining open.

    (2) Laryngectomy tube may be used if the stoma begins to narrow.

  b. Humidity.

    (1) Provide humidified air or oxygen via a tracheostomy collar to prevent drying of the mucosa and crusting of secretions.

    (2) Apply moistened 4 × 4 gauze pads to cover the stoma to provide humidity yet allow greater client mobility.

    (3) Advise that stoma bib worn over the stoma may lessen drying.

    (4) Teach symptoms of inadequate humidity—thick, tenacious secretions that are difficult to expectorate.

  c. Stoma care.

    (1) Cleanse stoma with peroxide and normal saline solution, freeing all crustings, twice each day and as needed.

    (2) Remove visible plugs with a Kelly clamp.

    (3) Apply a thin layer of bacitracin around the stoma twice each day.

2. Temporary tracheostomy (Figure 35-4).

  a. A cuffed tube (generally placed in the operating room and kept in place for 5 days)—should be kept inflated if mechanical ventilation is needed or if client is at risk for aspiration.

  b. Initial tracheostomy is changed by the physician to a non-cuffed tube (unless the client is aspirating); thereafter it may be changed by trained

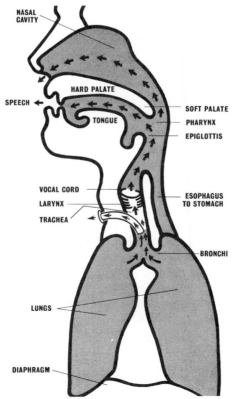

Figure 35-4 Physiology of the head and neck after a temporary tracheostomy. *(From* First Aid for [Neck-breathers] Laryngectomees. *Atlanta: American Cancer Society, p. 4.)*

nursing personnel as ordered by the physician or by hospital protocol.
  c. As edema decreases, the client may be able to breathe without the tracheostomy.
    (1) Tube is downsized to a number 4 or 5 or fenestrated tube is placed.
    (2) Tube is plugged for 24 hours.
    (3) If the client is able to breathe with the tube corked for prolonged time periods and to expectorate secretions through the mouth, the cannula may be removed.
    (4) Dressing over stoma is changed every day and as needed.
    (5) Client is instructed to place finger over stoma dressing when coughing or speaking until tract has sealed.
  d. Suctioning (all tracheostomies) is based on the need for airway clearance.
    (1) Routine suctioning, if unnecessary, causes irritation to the tracheal mucosa.
    (2) Hyperoxygenate and/or hyperinflate the lungs before and after suctioning to prevent hypoxemia and arrhythmia:
      (a) The optimal amount of oxygen and the best method remain in question.
      (b) If respiratory expansion is impaired, hyperinflation with a resuscitation bag may be necessary.
      (c) Postoperative clients without respiratory problems can breathe deeply with the oxygen collar next to the tracheostomy.
      (d) Clients with a healed tracheostomy can hyperoxygenate by deep breathing before and after suctioning.
    (3) Limit each pass to 10 seconds or less with 120 mm HG suctioning pressure.
    (4) Instill 2 to 5 ml of normal saline solution to lavage and stimulate the trachea and bronchi if needed to precipitate coughing and to mobilize secretions.
    (5) Use an incentive spirometer attached via a female adapter to a plastic tracheostomy tube and/or chest physical therapy, as indicated, to mobilize secretions and prevent atelectasis.
    (6) Chart the color, amount, and odor of sputum produced and how frequently suctioning is required.
  D. Tracheostomy care.
    1. Remove the inner cannula and cleanse of all mucus and crusts with peroxide and normal saline solution (half and half) every 4 to 8 hours initially, then twice daily and as needed.
    2. Replace soiled tracheostomy ties as needed; allow one finger breadth underneath when determining tightness.
    3. Cuffed tube with the disposable inner cannula is cleansed by removing the soiled tube and inserting a new one.
  E. Wound care.
    1. Assess the surgical wounds, noting color (pink versus cyanotic), temperature, and capillary refill (immediately after blanching) of skin and muscle flaps.
    2. Avoid excessive pressure that interferes with flap perfusion (tight tracheostomy ties, oxygen collars, hyperextension of the neck, and clients' lying on the flap), to assure flap viability.
    3. Assess integrity of suture lines, both external and intraoral (if applicable); breakdown may be the first sign of wound infection or fistula formation.
    4. Clean external suture lines with peroxide and normal saline solution; then apply bacitracin every 4 to 8 hours.

5. If myocutaneous flaps are sutured intraorally to close the surgical defect resulting from large tumor resections, inspect flaps and suture lines every 3 to 4 hours for assessment of:
   a. Flap viability.
   b. Wound dehiscence.
   c. Crust formation.
   d. State of hygiene.
   e. Pooling of secretions.
6. If client has nasal surgery, a maxillectomy, and/or an orbital exenteration, gently cleanse the cavities to remove accumulated crusts as ordered by the physician; a solution of normal saline and sodium bicarbonate (half and half) or normal saline solution alone can be used.
7. Assess wound drains for color, amount, and odor of drainage; clotting and air leaks can lead to wound infections if not prevented or treated early.

F. Oral care.
1. Use or instruct the client, if able, to use a tonsil suction catheter to rid the oral cavity of excess secretions.
2. Perform oral care with peroxide and normal saline solution (half and half) at least every 4 hours once ordered by the physician.
3. A gravity gavage or a jet-spray dental system may be used for gentle cleansing of the cavity.
4. A Kelly clamp or toothette may be used to remove crusts that develop on immobile suture lines and flaps.
5. Avoid the use of lemon glycerin swabs and commercially prepared mouthwashes that contain alcohol to minimize drying of the mucosa.

G. Nutrition.
1. Assess nutritional status preoperatively (60% of head and neck clients present with a fair or poor nutritional status; subsequent treatment with surgery, radiation, or chemotherapy further increases risks for nutritional problems).
2. Communicate with dietary personnel in the outpatient, inpatient, and radiation therapy areas to identify clients with nutritional deficiencies that necessitate oral, enteral, or parental nutritional supplements:
   a. Greater than 10% body weight loss during any treatment phase.
   b. More than 20% below ideal body weight.
3. Confer with physician if enteral support is required for more than 6 weeks to determine feasibility of placement of gastrostomy tube (percutaneous if possible).
4. Assess surgically treated head and neck clients for dysfunction in the swallowing mechanism (see Chapter 7).
5. Assess clients treated with radiation for mucositis, pain, dysphagia, and taste changes that may interfere with adequate oral intake (see Chapters 7 and 20).
6. Assess clients receiving chemotherapy for nausea and vomiting, malabsorption, diarrhea, and pain in the mouth and tongue (see Chapters 7 and 20).

H. Mobility.
1. If a neck dissection is performed (stages III and IV), often the spinal accessory nerve and the sternocleidomastoid muscles are resected, resulting in shoulder droop, atrophy of the trapezius muscle, forward curvature of the spine, and limited range of motion (approximately 90 degrees) of the shoulder.
2. Passive and active range of motion exercises are initiated after the wound drains are removed and clients are progressed to resistive exercises, with the ultimate goal of a range of 150 degrees, which is considered a functional range.

I. Body image and sexuality changes.
   1. Arrange preoperative and postoperative visits by support group members (Lost Chord Club, Laryngectomee Association).
   2. Avoid personal reactions to the disfigurement that convey negative verbal and nonverbal expressions.
   3. Provide and teach wound, oral, and tracheostomy care techniques to promote control of secretion and odors.
   4. Encourage self-care activities (tracheostomy care, tube feeding, suctioning) and activities of daily living (grooming, hair combing, shaving, applying makeup).
   5. Encourage resocialization through progressive ambulation, interaction with others, and support group participation (Voice Masters, Lost Chord Club, I Can Cope, CanSurmount).
   6. Involve social worker to assist with counseling and financial, vocational, and adjustment issues.
   7. Assist with purchase of tracheostomy covers, scarves, makeup, or other cosmetic assistance; consult ACS Look Good, Feel Better program for further suggestions (hair care, scarves).
   8. Support clients and family through the normal grieving process.
J. Observe and advise about other possible alterations in functioning:
   1. Loss of sense of smell and/or taste.
   2. Loss of ability to blow nose (may need suctioning with nasal congestion or a cold).
   3. Loss of ability to perform Valsalva maneuver may predispose to constipation, often requiring use of stool softeners.
   4. Loss of normal airway.
      a. Advise to wear Medic Alert bracelet identifying client as a neck breather and to carry cards and/or windshield stickers for emergency use (Figure 35-5).
      b. Establish emergency plans with local emergency system (tape recorder at phone with prerecorded call for help).
      c. Teach client, family, public, and professionals first aid for individuals with a laryngectomy (Figure 35-6).
   5. Loss of ability to blow air from their mouth (cannot extinguish candles on a birthday cake).

III. Interventions to monitor for unique side effects of treatment for head and neck cancers.
   A. Fistula formation.
      1. Fistula formation is more common if client has received preoperative radiation.
      2. Breakdown of suture lines (pharyngeal, tracheoesophageal) allows secretions to leak into the wounds or under skin flaps.
      3. Usually occurs 3 to 5 days postoperatively.
      4. Signs and symptoms—erythema, drainage, tenderness of the suture line, low-grade temperature of 100° to 101° F, fluctuance below the neck skin, local edema.
      5. Treatment to allow natural healing—nothing by mouth with enteral nutrition; dressing changes and wound packing every 4 to 8 hours or as needed to promote granulation and wound healing.
   B. Carotid artery rupture (see Chapter 8, "Oncological Emergencies").
      1. Rupture of the carotid artery occurs in 3.5% of head and neck clients treated with radical surgery.
      2. Radiation therapy effects or fistula formation increases risks of carotid artery rupture.

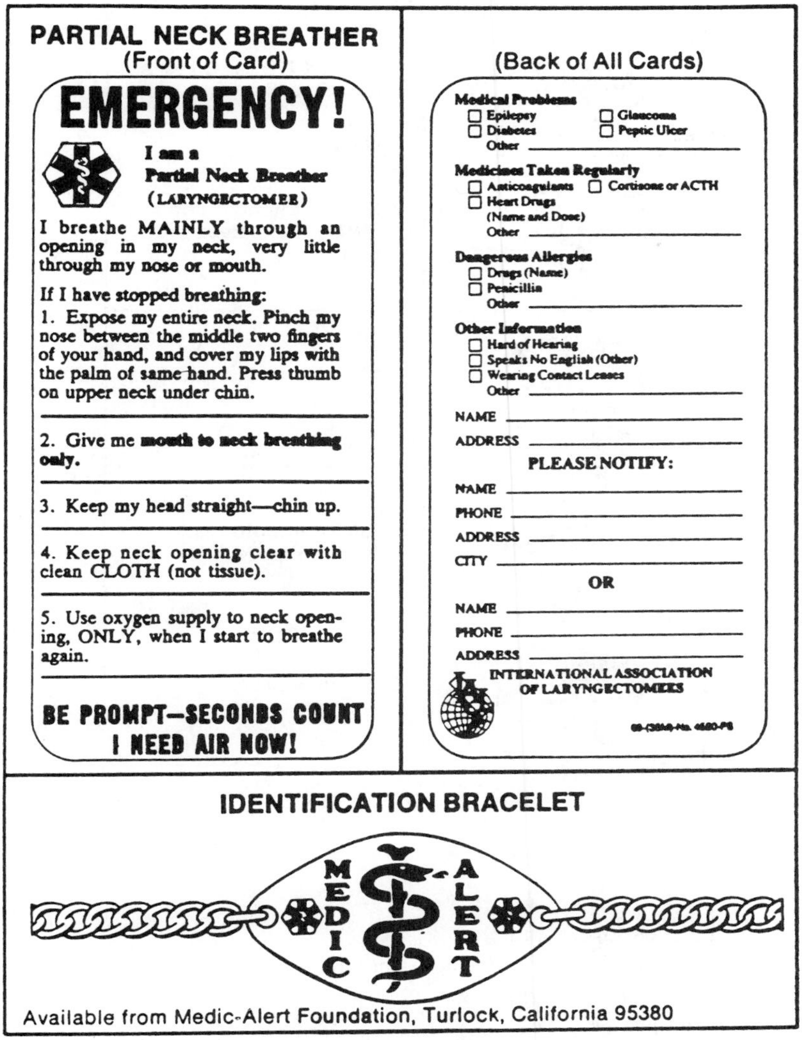

Figure 35-5 Medic Alert information. *(From* First Aid for [Neck-breathers] Laryngectomees. *Atlanta: American Cancer Society, p. 4.)*

3. Clients with an exposed carotid artery are placed on "Carotid Precautions"; supplies placed at the bedside include:

Three bath towels

Six packs of 4 × 4 sponges

Six 5 × 9 combine dressing pads

One cuffed tracheostomy tube

Ten-milliliter syringe

Alcohol swabs

Four packs of 4-inch rolled gauze (e.g., Kling)

Intravenous solutions (normal saline, lactated Ringer's)

Type and crossmatch–stamped requisitions for 2 units of blood

Suction apparatus and setup

Arterial blood gases kit

Blood drawing equipment

Latex gloves, disposable gowns, goggles

4. An intact heparin lock is kept in place.
5. Clients are placed on stool softeners to avoid straining.
6. Wet-to-wet dressing changes are used to avoid débriding the artery.

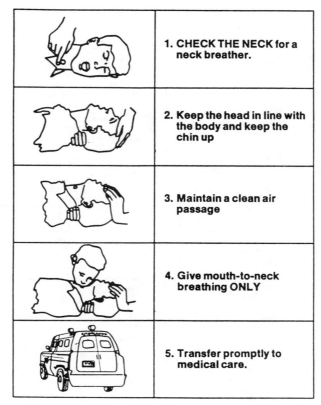

	1. CHECK THE NECK for a neck breather.
	2. Keep the head in line with the body and keep the chin up
	3. Maintain a clean air passage
	4. Give mouth-to-neck breathing ONLY
	5. Transfer promptly to medical care.

Figure 35-6 First aid for laryngectomee. *(From* First Aid for [Neck-breathers] Laryngectomees. *Atlanta: American Cancer Society, p. 13.)*

       7. In the event of a rupture:
         a. Apply pressure if bleeding externally or pack gauze in mouth if bleeding internally and *call for assistance.*
         b. Establish an airway.
         c. Inflate cuff on the tracheostomy tube to prevent aspiration and to apply internal pressure on the artery.
         d. Suction oral and tracheal secretions.
         e. Infuse intravenous fluids through the heparin lock.
         f. Obtain blood from the blood bank and determine arterial blood gas values.
         g. Call operating room personnel to alert about emergency.
         h. Prepare client and transfer to the operating room.
         i. Initiate universal precautions (as quickly as possible).
         j. Client is alert; therefore provide supportive and explanatory information throughout the situation.
  IV. Interventions to enhance adaptation and rehabilitation—speech and swallowing are the major foci of rehabilitation, are usually performed by the speech and language pathologist, and are reinforced by hospital and home care nurses.
    A. Communication.
      1. Cancers in the oral cavity affect the function of *articulation;* therapy includes:
        a. Exercises to increase strength, range of motion, coordination, and accuracy of tongue movement.

      b. Use of oral prostheses to compensate for tissue loss and to allow for greater contact of the tongue with the palate, creating more intelligible speech.

   2. Cancers in the larynx affect *phonation;* therapy includes:

      a. After a partial laryngectomy, exercises to improve voice quality, pitch, and loudness.

      b. After a total laryngectomy:

         (1) Use of artificial larynx that transmits sound into the vocal tract (family and friends must learn how to listen actively to this mechanized speech).

         (2) Use of esophageal speech—technique wherein air is taken in and trapped in the esophagus, then released, allowing air to vibrate against the walls of the esophagus.

         (3) Use of tracheoesophageal puncture, with placement of a prosthesis in a surgically created tracheoesophageal fistula; sound is formed by air from the lungs, creating a better quality of esophageal speech.

B. Swallowing.

   1. Surgeries in the head and neck region can affect swallowing in the oral preparatory, oral, and pharyngeal stages.

   2. A thorough clinical evaluation of the oral preparatory and pharyngeal stages of swallowing is conducted.

   3. A barium swallow and x-ray examination or cine-esophagography is performed to assess the oral and pharyngeal stages of the swallow.

   4. An individual swallowing plan is developed and instructions placed at the bedside; the plan includes:

      a. Compensatory strategies—postural changes that facilitate passage of food into the oral cavity and pharynx (head elevated); changes in food consistency (i.e., thin versus thick fluids, semisolids versus pureed foods).

      b. Indirect swallowing therapy—jaw and tongue range of motion exercises; adduction of tongue exercises to improve laryngeal closure.

      c. Direct swallowing therapy using supraglottic swallow:

         (1) Prepare the bolus of food in the oral preparatory phase.

         (2) Before initiating the swallow, hold breath to close vocal cords.

         (3) Swallow while still holding breath.

         (4) Cough while exhaling after the swallow to expectorate remaining food or fluids on top of vocal cords.

         (5) Repeat 3 and 4 (swallow/cough).

C. Other nursing roles in rehabilitation and adaptation:

   1. Support the client and family during practice sessions while relearning speech and swallowing skill.

   2. Partially or totally inflate the cuff on the tracheostomy tube during meals and 30 minutes afterward to avoid aspiration.

   3. For some clients removal of the tracheostomy tube improves swallowing by allowing the larynx to elevate.

   4. Until the client can take adequate amounts by mouth, use enteral feeding to maintain nutritional requirements.

V. Interventions to incorporate client/family in care.

A. Complete preoperative teaching with all available family present.

B. Teach postoperative and home care skills to both client and an individual readily available to the client; return demonstrations are evaluated.

C. Begin discharge teaching immediately after surgery and include care of the tracheostomy tube; stoma care; suctioning techniques; enteral/supplemental feeding;

alternative methods of providing humidity (bedside humidifier at bed time and as needed); swallowing techniques; speech, occupational, and physical therapy.

D. Teach self-examination of lips, mouth, and oral cavity and palpation of adjacent nodes (Figure 35-2) to monitor disease progression or recurrence.

E. Include discharge teaching about alleviation of risk factors to minimize risk of recurrence (use of smoking cessation programs, Alcoholics Anonymous).

F. Initiate inpatient head and neck support group to discuss fears and help clients and families cope with the disease and treatment.

G. Provide literature to reinforce or augment teaching (ACS booklets—*Cancer of the Larynx, Don't Bite Off More Than You Can Chew, First Aid for Laryngec-tomees, How To Quit Cigarettes;* National Cancer Institute [NCI] booklets—*Quit for Good, Progress Against Cancer of the Larynx;* International Association of Laryngectomees' Laryngectomy Kit).

EVALUATION OF CLIENT AND FAMILY OUTCOMES

I. Identify type of cancer, rationale for treatment, alterations in anatomy and physiology that will result from treatment, and the specific side effects of treatment.

II. List signs and symptoms and treatment of immediate and long-term side effects of disease and treatment (see Chapter 7).
A. Altered airway.
B. Altered swallowing mechanism.
C. Aphonia.
D. Inability to project voice.
E. Xerostomia.
F. Stomatitis.
G. Taste changes.
H. Anorexia; nutritional deficits.

III. Discuss self-care measures to decrease incidence and severity of symptoms associated with disease and treatment.
A. Refrain from further tobacco use and drinking of alcoholic beverages.
B. Maintain prophylactic oral care during and after radiation treatment (removal of diseased teeth, daily fluoride treatments).
C. Maintain high-residue diet and high fluid intake to prevent constipation that may result from absence of Valsalva maneuver (after total laryngectomy).

IV. Discuss coping strategies.
A. Independence in activities of daily living and new skills (tracheostomy care, esophageal speech).
B. Socialization with family and friends.
C. Return to previous work or activities or occupational training for alternative work and leisure activities.
D. Participation in support groups and informational systems to aid in problem solving, life-style changes, and adjustment (Lost Chord Club, I Quit Clinics, I Can Cope educational programs).

V. Demonstrate skill in self-care demanded by structural or functional effects of disease and treatment by return demonstration of the following:
A. Wound care—clean suture line (maxillary, nasal, or oral cavity); apply antibiotic ointment; perform dressing care.
B. Airway management:

1. Tracheostomy care:
   a. Clean inner and outer cannula twice daily and as needed.
   b. Replace tracheostomy tube every week and as needed.
2. Stoma care:
   a. Inspect stoma for erythema, drainage.
   b. Clean stoma with peroxide and normal saline solution or soap and water as needed to keep clean and free of crustings.
   c. Use protective covering to prevent water and soap from entering stoma when showering.
3. Suctioning:
   a. Suction tracheostomy as needed.
   b. Instill 1.5 ml saline solution as needed to loosen and mobilize secretions.
4. Humidity:
   a. List symptoms indicative of inadequate humidity.
   b. Apply stoma bib or protective covering over open stoma to warm and filter air.
   c. Maintain bedside humidifier at night and as needed to moisten air.
C. Nutrition—list supplements ordered (for use orally, enterally, or parentally) and resources for follow-up or home care.
D. Disease progression or recurrence:
   1. Demonstrate self-examination of head and neck area.
   2. List symptoms to report—red areas (erythroplakia), white areas (leukoplakia), ulcers that do not heal in 2 weeks, lymph node enlargement or changes.

VI. Describe plan for follow-up care.
   A. To detect recurrence or a second primary tumor:
      1. Cite schedule for clinical evaluation (e.g., every month for the first year; every 2 months the second year; every 3 months the third year; every 4 months the fourth year; every 5 months the fifth year; and every year thereafter).
      2. List signs and symptoms of recurrence—pain, dysphagia, neck nodes, ulceration, bleeding, hemoptysis, airway obstruction, bone pain.
   B. To promote physical and psychosocial adjustment—use of physical therapist, occupational therapist, speech therapist, CanSurmount or Laryngectomy Club.
   C. To change life-styles—stop smoking and/or alcohol cessation programs.

VII. Discuss community resources to meet unique demands of head and neck disease, treatments, and survivorship.
   A. Lost Chord Club, I Can Cope, CanSurmount (contact the local ACS office).
   B. International Association of Laryngectomees (Contact local American Cancer Society or national American Cancer Society office.)
   C. American Cancer Society
      1599 Clifton Road, N.E.
      Atlanta, GA 30329
      404-320-3333
   D. (Booklet) *Self-Help for the Laryngectomee*
      Edmund Lauder, author
      11115 Whisper Hollow
      San Antonio, TX 78230
      512-492-1984

    E. Bruce Medical Supply (information about stoma bibs and shower shields)
       411 Waverly Oaks Road
       P.O. Box 9166
       Waltham, MA 02254
       1-800-225-8446

    F. Medic-Alert Foundation International
       2323 Colorado Ave.
       Turlock, CA 95381-1009
       1-800-ID-ALERT
       (1-800-432-5378)

    G. (Rehabilitation booklet) Keith, R.L. (1991). *Looking Forward . . . a Guidebook for the Laryngectomee* (2nd ed). New York: Thiene Medical Publishers.

       Available from publisher:
       Thiene Medical Publishers
       381 Park Ave., S.
       New York, NY 10061

       or from the author:
       Dr. Robert L. Keith
       Mayo Comprehensive Cancer Center
       Speech Pathology, E-8A
       Rochester, MN 55905
       507-284-3112

    H. National Coalition for Cancer Survivorship
       1010 Wayne Ave.
       Silver Spring, MD 20910
       301-230-0831

BIBLIOGRAPHY

Adams, G.L., Boies, L.R., & Hilger, P.A. (1989). *Boies Fundamentals of Otolaryngology* (6th ed). Philadelphia: W.B. Saunders Co.

Corbett, J.V. (1983). *Diagnostic Procedures in Nursing Practice.* Norwalk, Conn.: Appleton-Century-Crofts.

Dropkin, M.J. (1989). Coping with disfigurement and dysfunction after head and neck cancer surgery: a conceptual framework. *Semin Oncol Nurs 5*(3), 213-219.

Fee, W.E., Jr., Goepfert, H., & Johns, M.E., et al (eds). (1990). *Head and Neck Cancer: Proceedings of the Second International Conference* (vol 2). Philadelphia: Brian C. Decker.

Goodman, M. (1990). Head and neck cancer. In S.L. Groenwald, M.H. Frogge, M. Goodman, C.H. Yarbro (eds). *Cancer Nursing: Principles and Practice* (2nd ed). Boston: Jones & Bartlett Publishers, pp. 889-929.

Grant, M., Rhiner, M., & Padilla, G.V. (1989). Nutritional management in the head and neck cancer patient. *Semin Oncol Nurs 5*(3), 195-204.

Guyton, A.C. (1987). *Human Physiology and Mechanisms of Disease* (4th ed). Philadelphia: W.B. Saunders Co.

Hannon, L.M. (1989). Cancer of the oral cavity. *Semin Oncol Nurs 5*(3), 150-159.

Harris, L.L. & Smith, S. (1989). Chemotherapy in head and neck cancer. *Semin Oncol Nurs 5*(3), 174-181.

(1988). Lip and oral cavity, pharynx (including base of tongue, soft palate, and uvula), larynx. In American Joint Committee on Cancer. *Manual for Staging of Cancer* (3rd ed). Philadelphia: J.B. Lippincott Co., pp. 27-44.

Logemann, J.A. (1989). Swallowing and communication rehabilitation. *Semin Oncol Nurs 5*(3), 205-212.

Mahon, S.M. (1987). Nursing interventions for the patient with a myocutaneous flap. *Cancer Nurs 10*(1), 21-31.

Martin, L.K. (1989). Management of the altered airway in the head and neck cancer patient. *Semin Oncol Nurs 5*(3), 182-190.

McQuarrie, D.G., Adams, G.L., Shons, A.R., & Browne, G.A. (eds). (1986). *Head and Neck Cancer: Clinical Decisions and Management Principles.* Chicago: Year Book Medical Publishers.

Norris, C.M. & Blake, C. (1991). Head, Neck, and Thyroid Cancer. In A.I. Holleb, D.J. Fink, & G.P. Murphy (eds). *American Cancer Society Textbook of Clinical Oncology*. Atlanta: American Cancer Society, pp. 306-328.

Reese, J.L. (1991). Head and neck cancers. In S.B. Baird, R. McCorkle, & M. Grant (eds). *Cancer Nursing: A Comprehensive Textbook*. Philadelphia: W.B. Saunders Co., pp. 567-583.

Rice, D.H. & Spiro, R.H. (1989). *Current Concepts in Head and Neck Cancer*. Atlanta: American Cancer Society.

Schleper, J.R. (1989). Prevention, detection, and diagnosis of head and neck cancers. *Semin Oncol Nurs 5*(3), 139-149.

Schwartz, S.S. & Yuska, C.M. (1989). Common patient care issues following surgery for head and neck cancer. *Semin Oncol Nurs 5*(3), 191-194.

Sievers, A.E.F. & Donald, P.J. (1989). Staging system for head and neck cancer. *J Soc Otorhinolaryngol Head-Neck Nurses 7*(3), 5-9.

Sigler, B.A. (1989). Nursing care of patients with laryngeal carcinoma. *Semin Oncol Nurs 5*(3), 160-165.

Silver, C.E. & Moisa, I.I. (1990). The role of surgery in the treatment of laryngeal cancer. *CA 40*(3), 134-149.

Strohl, R.A. (1989). Radiation therapy for head and neck cancers. *Semin Oncol Nurs 5*(3), 166-173.

Yuska, C.M. (1987). Head and neck cancer. In C.R. Ziegfeld (ed). *Core Curriculum for Oncology Nursing*. Philadelphia: W.B. Saunders Co., pp. 153-161.

Zagars, G. & Norante, J.D. (1983). Head and neck tumors. In P. Rubin (ed). *Clinical Oncology for Medical Students and Physicians: a Multidisciplinary Approach* (6th ed). New York: American Cancer Society, pp. 230-261.

36

Neurological Cancers

Betty Owens, MS, RN

Brain Tumors

THEORY

I. Physiology and pathophysiology associated with brain tumors.
   A. Anatomy of the brain.
   1. Description of structures (Figure 36-1).
       a. Cerebrum—two hemispheres consisting of pairs of lobes: frontal, temporal, parietal, occipital; thalamus and hypothalamus located at the base of the cerebrum.
       b. Cerebellum—located in posterior fossa at the back of the head below the cerebrum.
       c. Brainstem—located at the top of the spinal cord; consists of midbrain, pons, and medulla.
   2. Identification of critical adjacent structures (Figure 36-2).
       a. Meninges—membranes that cover brain and spinal cord; outermost layer is the dura, a thick, whitish, inelastic covering.
       b. Cerebral spinal fluid (CSF)—clear, colorless, odorless fluid that bathes the brain and spinal cord within the dural covering.
       c. Ventricles—four connected cavities in the brain through which CSF flows.
       d. Cerebral blood vessels.
          (1) Two vertebral arteries and two internal carotid arteries supply blood to the brain.
          (2) Circle of Willis supplies alternate flow if vessels are blocked.
          (3) Venous drainage is accomplished via dural sinuses, vascular channels created by two dural layers.
       e. Blood-brain barrier.
          (1) Tighter junctions in the brain capillaries that selectively allow substances to cross neuronal membranes.
          (2) Movement across the barrier is dependent on particle size, lipid solubility, chemical dissociation, and protein-binding potential of the substance.
       f. Skull.
          (1) Bony framework encasing the brain to protect from injury.

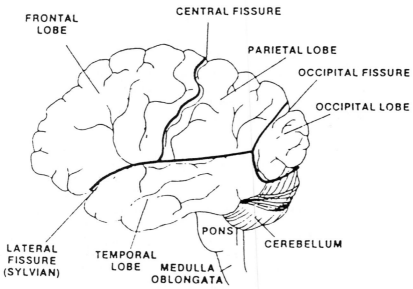

Figure 36-1 Lobes of the cerebral hemispheres. *(From [1988]. A Primer of Brain Tumors [4th ed]. Chicago: Association for Brain Tumor Research, p. 18.)*

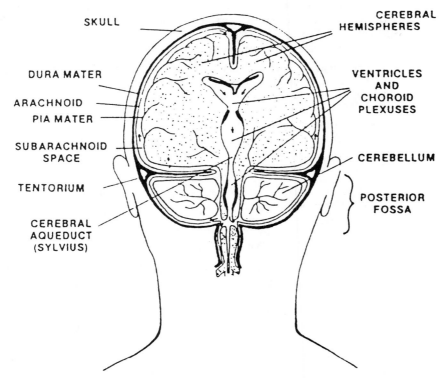

Figure 36-2 Ventricles and cerebrospinal fluid flow (arrows show direction). *(From [1988]. A Primer of Brain Tumors [4th ed]. Chicago: Association for Brain Tumor Research, p. 14.)*

Table 36-1
EXAMINATION OF CRANIAL NERVES

Cranial Nerve	Method of Testing	Desired Response
I Olfactory	Inhalation of commonly recognized aromatic substance such as cloves; avoid the use of ammonia or alcohol because they stimulate the trigeminal nerve and evoke a pain response	Identification of the substance with each nostril
II Optic	Direct ophthalmoscopy; use finger movement and eye charts to test visual acuity and fields	Note the appearance of the optic disk, macula, vessels, and retina; correct eye movement and chart identification with each eye separately
III Oculomotor IV Trochlear VI Abducens	Individual follows the examiner's finger with the eyes to test eye movement; check pupil response to light; observe for ptosis of the eyelid, which indicates destruction of cranial nerve III	Movement of eyes should be equal in all six cardinal directions of gaze; pupils react to direct and consensual response to light: eyes are symmetrical at rest and move conjugatively
V Trigeminal	Individual clamps the jaw, opens the mouth against resistance, and masticates to check motor division of the nerve; touch both sides of the person's face, checking for pain, touch, and temperature response; gently touch the person's cornea with a cotton wisp to check the corneal reflex	Correct identification of sensations; rapid blinking
VII Facial	Observe for facial symmetry and the person's ability to contract muscles to check motor division; individual tastes sweet, sour, salty, and acidic flavors	Person smiles and frowns with symmetry; correct identification of tastes
VIII Acoustic	Test hearing ability with the use of whispered voice and tuning fork at various distances from the ear to check the cochlear nerve; check the vestibular nerve by having the person stand on one foot with eyes closed	Recognition of sound; maintains balance
IX Glossopharyngeal	Check the gag reflex by touching the pharynx with a tongue depressor	Gag response
X Vagus	Check the individual's swallowing ability; ask the person to cough and speak; glossopharyngeal and vagus nerves are easily examined together because of overlapping innervation of the pharynx	Speaks without hoarseness or weakness
XI Spinal accessory	Ask the individual to elevate the shoulders, turn the head, and resist the examiner's attempts to pull the chin back to midline; check the symmetry of the trapezius and sternocleidomastoid muscles	Equal bilateral muscle strength; atrophy may indicate nerve dysfunction
XII Hypoglossal	Ask the individual to protrude the tongue	Absence of deviations, atrophy, or tremors

From Groenwald, S.L., Frogge, M., Goodman, M., & Yarbro, C.H. (eds) (1990). *Cancer Nursing: Principles and Practice* (2nd ed). Boston: Jones & Bartlett Publishers, p. 647.

(2) Brain and CSF are in a closed space, making tumors, whether benign or malignant, lethal.

   g. Cranial nerves.

     (1) Twelve pairs.

     (2) Part of the peripheral nervous system; the majority is attached to the brainstem.

     (3) Evaluation of brainstem determined by cranial function (Table 36-1).

B. Brain functions.

  1. Cerebrum.

    a. Right hemisphere controls left side of body; left hemisphere controls right side of body.

    b. Cerebral dominance.

     (1) One hemisphere (usually the left in right-handed individuals) controls performance of speech and understanding of language.

     (2) Speech and handedness often, but not always, are related.

     (3) Dominant hemisphere is responsible for verbal and analytical skills.

     (4) Nondominant hemisphere is responsible for creative arts and spatial relations.

    c. Lobes (Table 36-2 and Figure 36-3).

Table 36-2
CLINICAL MANIFESTATIONS OF INTRACRANIAL TUMORS

Location	Function	Abnormality
Frontal lobes	Intellect	Intellectual deterioration
	Personality	Personality changes
	Judgment	Impaired judgment
	Abstract thinking	Bowel and bladder incontinence
	Mood and affect	Emotional lability
	Memory	Memory loss
	Motor activity (contralateral)	Muscle weakness or paralysis
		Babinski's sign
		Decreased deep tendon reflexes
	Expressive speech (left hemisphere)	Expressive aphasia
Parietal lobes	Sensory input (contralateral)	Decreased or lost sensation (pain, temperature, pinprick, light touch, proprioception, vibration, two-point discrimination, double simultaneous stimulation, stereognosis, graphesthesia)
Occipital lobes	Sight	Visual field defects, hallucinations, inability to identify objects or symbols
	Visual identification of objects	
Temporal lobes	Hearing	Hearing changes, hallucinations
	Memory	Memory loss
	Receptive speech	Receptive aphasia
Cerebellum	Coordination	Ataxia, action tremor
		Nystagmus
	Balance (ipsilateral)	Loss of balance, wide-base gait
		Decreased deep, tendon reflexes

From Groenwald, S.L., Frogge, M., Goodman, M., & Yarbro, C.H. (eds) (1990). *Cancer Nursing: Principles and Practice* (2nd ed). Boston: Jones & Bartlett Publishers, p. 762.

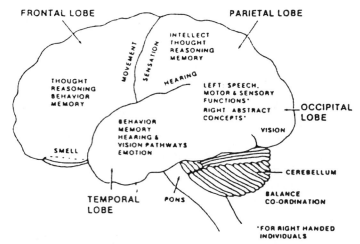

Figure 36-3 Lobes of the brain. *(From [1987].* Coping with a Brain Tumor. *Chicago: Association for Brain Tumor Research, p. 5.)*

       d. Thalamus.
          (1) Monitors sensory input.
          (2) Acts as a relay station for sensory information.
       e. Hypothalamus.
          (1) Controls water balance, sleep, temperature, appetite, and blood pressure.
          (2) Coordinates overall patterns of activity.
    2. Cerebellum.
       a. Coordinates movement.
       b. Controls balance.
    3. Brainstem—controls basic functions of involuntary activities such as blood pressure, heartbeat, and respiration.
  C. Changes in function associated with brain tumors.
    1. Cerebral edema caused by compression of surrounding brain tissue.
    2. Obstruction of flow of CSF (hydrocephalus).
    3. Increased intracranial pressure (ICP) related to increased intracranial volume (tumor plus edema) in a closed space.
    4. Seizure activity.
       a. Brain injured by tumor causes abnormal firing of neurons.
       b. Develops in 30% of clients.
       c. Seizures may be focal or generalized.
    5. Focal neurological deficits.
       a. Damage to specialized tissue in the brain from compression, infiltration, invasion, or edema.
       b. Sensorimotor deficits, visual deficits, speech and language problems, and memory and cognitive problems.
    6. Displacement of brain structures (herniation).
       a. Emergency situation likely resulting in death unless immediately relieved (Figure 36-4).
       b. Signs and symptoms of impending herniation:
          (1) Decreased level of consciousness.
          (2) Pupillary abnormalities.
          (3) Motor dysfunction (hemiplegia, decortication, or decerebration).

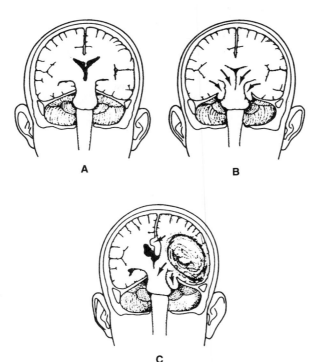

Figure 36-4 Intracranial shifts caused by supratentorial lesions. **A,** Normal. **B,** Central transtentorial herniation. **C,** Uncal herniation. *(From Groenwald, S.L., Frogge, M.H., Goodman, M., & Yarbro, C.H. [eds] [1990].* Cancer Nursing: Principles and Practice *[2nd ed]. Boston: Jones & Bartlett Publishers, p. 760.)*

        (4) Impaired brainstem reflexes (corneal, gag, swallowing).

        (5) Alterations in vital signs, including respiratory irregularities.

  D. Metastatic patterns.

    1. Primary central nervous system (CNS) tumors rarely metastasize outside CNS.

    2. Some CNS tumors (e.g., medulloblastoma) seed to distant parts of CNS (down the spinal cord).

  E. Trends in epidemiology.

    1. Incidence of primary brain tumors is believed increasing, but this increase may be due to improved diagnostic methods.

    2. Characteristics of tumors.

      a. Adult primary brain tumors.

        (1) Histology—common types.

          (a) Gliomas—general classification of tumors (with many subtypes) arising from glial cells, the supporting tissue of the brain.

            i. Astrocytoma—arises in cerebral hemispheres, may be cystic, is infiltrative, and lacks encapsulation.

            ii. Oligodendroglioma—arises in frontal lobes, is circumscribed, and often is slow growing (often not a "pure" oligodendroglioma but a mixture of astrocytoma and oligodendroglioma).

          (b) Medulloblastoma—arises in cerebellum.

            i. Most often occurs in children.

            ii. Frequently metastasizes around brain and down spinal cord.

        (2) May be benign by histology but malignant by location.

        (3) Most common presenting symptom—headache or seizure.

    b. Pediatric primary brain tumors.
      (1) Astrocytomas and medulloblastomas—most common.
      (2) Second most common neoplasm and most common solid tumor in children.
    c. Metastatic tumors.
      (1) Approximately one fourth of persons who die from cancer have brain metastases.
      (2) Metastases occur at three sites—skull and dura, brain, and subarachnoid space.
      (3) Occur by hematogenous spread.
      (4) One third originate in lung.
      (5) Other frequent originating sites—breast, colon, and kidney.
      (6) Cortex most common site; supplied by three main cerebral arteries.

II. Principles of medical management.
  A. Screening and diagnostic procedures.
    1. General procedures.
      a. Computed tomography (CT).
      b. Magnetic resonance imaging (MRI).
      c. Skull x-ray examinations.
      d. Lumbar puncture.
      e. CT myelography (only if spine metastasis suspected).
      f. Spine x-ray examinations (only if spine metastasis suspected).
    2. Specific procedures unique to neurological malignancies (Tables 36-3 and 36-4).
      a. Cerebral angiography—method to visualize cerebral blood flow.
      b. Stereotactic biopsy—method to obtain biopsy specimen from lesion without performing open craniotomy (Figure 36-5).
  B. Staging methods and procedures (see Appendix).
    1. Performing biopsy is imperative—histopathology is most critical information.
    2. Pathological staging is based on histopathology, grade, and microscopic evidence of completeness of removal of resected tumor.
    3. Pathological findings are classified in ascending grades of malignancy.
    4. Clinical staging is based on neurological signs.
    5. Spine is assessed for metastases from some tumors, especially pediatric ones.
  C. Treatment strategies.
    1. Surgery.
      a. Indications for surgery.
        (1) Tumor size and location (e.g., can be removed with little risk of neurological injury).
        (2) General medical condition acceptable for surgery.
        (3) Deteriorating neurological status.
      b. Unfavorable factors for surgery.
        (1) Tumor location presents too great a risk (e.g., brainstem, motor strip, speech area).
        (2) Poor medical condition.
        (3) Multiple intracranial tumors.
        (4) Major neurological deficits not responsive to steroid therapy.
        (5) Rapidly growing and spreading tumor.
      c. Types of surgery.
        (1) Stereotactic biopsy (see Table 36-4 and Figure 36-5).
        (2) Open craniotomy for biopsy and tumor debulking.
        (3) Open craniotomy for complete tumor removal.

Text continued on page 533.

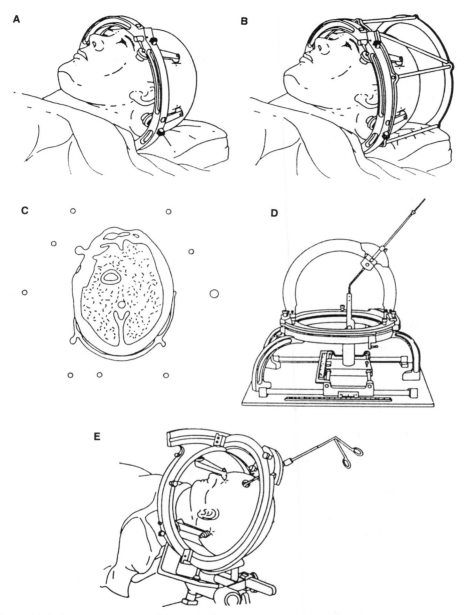

Figure 36-5 Stereotactic surgery. Diagrams show sequence of steps using the Brown-Roberts-Wells (BRW) stereo-tactic guidance system. **A,** Head ring is fixed to the skull. **B,** Localizing rod system is attached to the head ring for scanning. **C,** Sample localizing scan from which x-y coordinates of nine localizing rod and intracranial target images are determined for computation by the calculator. **D,** Computed arc settings are verified for correct trajectory and depth to target on the simulator. **E,** Arc guidance system is attached to the head ring, and intracranial procedure is performed. *(From Heilbrun, P., Roberts, T., Apuzzo, M., Wells, T., & Sabshin, J. [1983]. Preliminary experience with Brown-Roberts-Wells [BRW] computerized tomography stereotaxic guidance system. J Neurosurg 59, 218.)*

Table 36-3
NEUROLOGICAL DIAGNOSTIC TESTS

Description/Purpose	Time Required for Test	Sensations Experienced
Cerebral Angiography Contrast agent injected into cerebral blood vessels; approach usually through femoral artery; computed tomographic scan of head performed at certain time intervals after injection to visualize cerebral flow Purpose—to determine abnormal blood flow	1 hr	Needle stick is felt when local anesthetic is administered before catheter insertion Nausea and headache during injection of contrast agent are possible After injection of contrast agent, burning sensation for 4-6 sec may be felt behind eyes or in jaws, teeth, tongue, lips
Stereotactic Biopsy Frame secured to client's head with screw pins; computed tomography (CT) or magnetic resonance imaging (MRI) is performed with frame in place; using CT or MR film and known points of frame and location of the lesion on film, coordinates of lesion are calculated; with frame in place, client is taken to operating room and mildly sedated; arc portion is attached to frame; burr hole is made, and needle is passed through calculated coordinates of lesion to obtain biopsy Purpose—surgical method to target and obtain biopsy specimen from lesion in brain without an open craniotomy and subsequent risks	3 to 4 hr for whole procedure	Discomfort with frame application Needle stick when local anesthetic administered Feeling of pressure when biopsy specimen taken Drowsiness from premedication
Electromyography (EMG) Recording of electrical activity of the muscle and peripheral nerve; insertion of needle electrodes; records electrical activity of muscle at rest and during contraction Purpose—to detect neuromuscular disorders	1-2 hr	Uncomfortable sensation when needle electrode inserted Client asked to contract and relax particular muscles during test If needle must be repositioned, may experience a slight dull ache when adjusted
Computed Tomographic (CT) Myelogram CT images of spinal cord and vertebral column taken after injection of a contrast medium into subarachnoid space; subarachnoid puncture (usually lumbar) performed; 2-3 ml cerebrospinal fluid (CSF) removed for analysis; water-soluble contrast agent injected (usually 5-18 ml), and CT performed Purpose—any partial or complete obstruction can be visualized	1 hr	Mild to severe pain or feeling of pressure After procedure—headache, nausea and vomiting

Potential Side Effects/Complications	Self-Care Measures	Critical Symptoms to Report to Health Care Team
Allergic reaction to contrast agent (flushing, hives, dyspnea) Vasospasm Thrombosis Embolism Hematoma, hemorrhage Renal toxicity from contrast agent	Follow instructions about correct positioning	Difficulty breathing Weakness or dizziness Neurological changes Hemorrhage from puncture site
Intraoperative and/or postoperative bleeding requiring open craniotomy to remove clot Neurological damage resulting from bleed Missed target	None	Sleepiness Change in mental status Drainage from burr hole site
None	None	None
Allergic reaction to contrast agent (flushing, hives, dyspnea) Meningeal irritation Seizure Infection Headache Herniation if increased intracranial pressure Cord compression, leading to neurological deficit Nausea and vomiting	Follow instructions regarding correct positioning after procedure	Change in sensation or strength Headache Stiff neck Fever Pain during hip flexion Seizure

Table 36-4

NURSING IMPLICATIONS OF NEUROLOGICAL DIAGNOSTIC TESTS

Procedure	Actual or Potential Physical Alteration	Nursing Goals	Nursing Interventions
Cerebral Angiography	Potential for allergic reaction to contrast medium Potential for stroke (embolic or hemorrhagic) Potential for hemorrhage from puncture site Potential for seizure Potential for neurological deficit	Early detection of problems Prevention of hemorrhage at puncture site	Report preprocedure serum creatinine level; if elevated, notify physician Before procedure, advise client to lie still and try not to cough during procedure Provide adequate hydration before and after angiogram Administer premedication if ordered Provide nothing by mouth (or clear liquids) for 8 hr before procedure Perform baseline vital sign and neurological check After procedure, check extremities of puncture site for color, temperature, presence of pulse Check vital and neurological signs frequently Notify physician of any change or problem Apply sandbag or ice bag to puncture site should bleeding occur Immobilize extremity for 16 hr to minimize risk of bleeding
Stereotactic Biopsy	Potential for infection Potential for alteration in neurological status caused by intracranial hemorrhage Alteration in comfort related to frame	Early assessment and intervention for hemorrhage Prevention of infection Minimization of discomfort	Before procedure, instruct client about expectations during procedure Assess neurological status frequently for 24 hr after procedure Notify physician of any change Assess biopsy site for drainage from frame pin sites or biopsy site Instruct client to keep area clean and dry for 3 or 4 days until well healed Instruct client to call if fever, redness, drainage, or tenderness develops or change in mental status occurs

Table 36-4
NURSING IMPLICATIONS OF NEUROLOGICAL DIAGNOSTIC TESTS *Continued*

Procedure	Actual or Potential Physical Alteration	Nursing Goals	Nursing Interventions
Electromyography	Alteration in comfort	Minimization of discomfort and anxiety	Before the test, advise client to expect some discomfort when needle electrodes inserted Inform client he or she will be asked to contract and relax particular muscle groups Advise about importance of test in diagnosing neurological problem
CT Myelogram	Alteration in comfort Potential for meningeal irritation Potential for infection Potential for allergic reaction Potential for neurological deficits	Maintenance of comfort Early recognition of any problem or allergic reaction or infection	Keep client supine, with head slightly elevated 15 to 30 degrees for 6-8 hr after procedure Advise client to rest for 24 hr after procedure Perform frequent assessment of vital signs and neurological status Observe for back pain, spasms, nuchal rigidity, nausea and vomiting, seizure activity, or headache Encourage fluid intake Administer mild analgesics Observe puncture site for CSF drainage Keep puncture site clean Assess for motor and sensory changes

    (4) Ventriculoperitoneal shunt placement to relieve hydrocephalus—shunts CSF from blocked ventricles to peritoneal cavity. (Figure 36-6).
  d. Objectives of surgery.
    (1) Remove tumor as primary treatment.
    (2) Facilitate radiation and chemotherapy treatment by reducing tumor burden.
    (3) Improve or maintain quality of life by removing pressure causing neurological deficits.
  e. Surgical complications.
    (1) Intracranial bleeding.
    (2) Cerebral edema.
    (3) Infection.

            (4) Venous thrombosis.
            (5) Hydrocephalus.
            (6) Neurological injury.
    f. Signs and symptoms of postoperative complications.
            (1) Decreased level of consciousness (LOC).
            (2) Increased ICP.
            (3) Progressive neurological deficit.
            (4) Seizures.
    g. Acute postoperative management.
            (1) Monitoring in surgical intensive care unit until stable, usually 24 to 48 hours.
            (2) ICP maintained at less than 20 mm Hg via medication, ventriculostomy draining, hyperventilation, and activity limitation.
            (3) Systolic blood pressure maintained with medication, if necessary, to reduce risk of intracranial bleeding.
            (4) Therapeutic blood levels of anti-convulsants maintained to prevent seizures (Table 36-5).
            (5) Fluid balance maintained (use of steroids and mannitol as needed to prevent cerebral edema; use of colloids as needed to prevent hypovolemia); electrolyte values monitored closely.
            (6) Narcotics avoided because of respiratory and sensorium depression.
            (7) Frequent monitoring of neurological status.
    h. Postoperative discharge concerns.
            (1) Incision clean and dry until sutures and/or staples removed.
            (2) Activity—no heavy lifting.
            (3) No driving if seizures not controlled.
            (4) Discharge teaching about seizures, wound care, shunt function, and medication.
2. Radiotherapy.
    a. Radiosensitivity depends on histology.
            (1) Medulloblastoma—highly radiosensitive.
            (2) High-grade astrocytoma—minimally responsive but more so in younger age group.
            (3) Breast and lung metastatic tumors—responsive.
            (4) Melanoma and sarcoma metastatic tumors—minimally responsive.
    b. Recommended dose and schedule.
            (1) Usually focal to tumor plus 2-cm margin, but whole brain radiation also used.
            (2) Usual dose—5000 to 6000 rads in divided doses over 5 to 6 weeks.
            (3) Radiation damage resulting in cognitive deficits is a major concern.
            (4) Pediatric considerations.
                (a) Not recommended for children less than 2 years old because of potential cognitive and developmental problems.
                (b) Reduced dosage for children less than 5 years of age.
                (c) Baseline neuropsychological testing before beginning radiation.
                (d) Evaluation of pituitary hormonal function, especially growth hormone, after radiation therapy.
3. Chemotherapy.
    a. Usually palliative.
    b. Response rate low (usually 20% to 40%).
    c. Nitrosoureas—most commonly used drugs because of lipid solubility and ability to pass through blood-brain barrier.

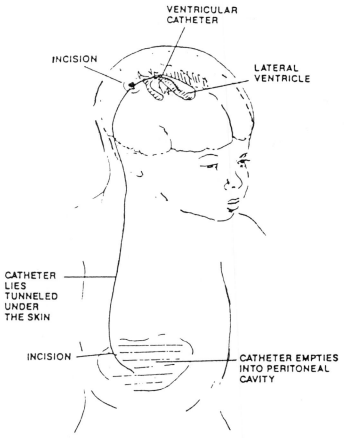

Figure 36-6 Ventriculoperitoneal shunt. *(From [1989]. Shunts. Chicago: Association for Brain Tumor Research.)*

      d. Used only in high-grade tumors; not effective in low-grade tumors because of slow rate of cell division.

      e. Agents commonly used.

        (1) Alkylating agents—cisplatin, nitrosoureas, cyclophosphamide, nitrogen mustard.

        (2) Antibiotics—bleomycin.

        (3) Plant alkaloids—vincristine, etoposide.

        (4) Procarbazine.

   4. Investigative treatment modalities for brain tumors.

      a. Immunotherapy.

      b. Interstitial brachytherapy.

      c. Hyperthermia.

      d. Photodynamic therapy.

      e. Regional infusion of chemotherapy.

      f. Bone marrow transplant.

      g. Radiosensitizers.

D. Trends in survival.

   1. General survival times for clients with primary brain tumors (Table 36-6).

Table 36-5
COMMON ANTICONVULSANT MEDICATIONS

Medication	Dose	Therapeutic Blood Level (μg/ml)	Side Effects/Toxicities
Barbituates			
Phenobarbital	60-400 mg/day	10-30	Drowsiness, mental dullness, nightmares, dizziness, fever, depression, irritability, rash, loss of libido, ataxia, anemia, nystagmus
Mephobarbital (Mebaral)	400-600 mg/day	25-50	Same as phenobarbital plus facial edema and possible hypersensitivity reactions
Primidone (Mysoline)	250-1500 mg/day	5-15	Same as phenobarbital plus diplopia, alopecia, impotence, lupus-like syndrome
Hydantoin			
Phenytoin (Dilantin)	300-600 mg/ml	10-20	Gastrointestinal upset, ataxia, diplopia, nystagmus, gingival hyperplasia, dermatitis, hirsutism, hypocalcemia, osteomalacia, agranulocytosis, leukopenia, megaloblastic anemia, insulin suppression, increased cholesterol, lupus-like syndrome, low bound thyroxin level
Others			
Carbamazepine (Tegretol)	600-1200 mg/day	2-8	Drowsiness, psychotic behavior, ataxia, dizziness, diplopia, nystagmus, dry mouth, skin eruptions, jaundice, edema, leukopenia, aplastic anemia, pancytopenia
Valproic acid (Depakene)	15-60 mg/kg/day	50-100	Drowsiness, ataxia, altered bleeding times, liver toxicity, transient hair loss, leukopenia, nausea and vomiting, depression, hallucinations, bone marrow depression
Clonazepam (Klonopin)	3-12 mg/day		Drowsiness, ataxia, dizziness, thick speech, hypotonia, hyperactivity, anorexia, rash, thrombocytopenia, palpitations, bradycardia, hirsutism, hysteria

Modified from Rudy, E. (1984). *Advanced Neurological and Neurosurgical Nursing.* St. Louis: C.V. Mosby Co.

Table 36-6
SURVIVAL TIMES FOR CLIENTS WITH PRIMARY BRAIN TUMORS BY HISTOLOGY
AND GRADE

Histology	Grade	Survival with Conventional Treatment
Astrocytoma		
Pilocytic astrocytoma	I	Close to normal life expectancy
Astrocytoma	II	Years
Anaplastic astrocytoma	III	18-24 mo
Glioblastoma multiforme	IV	9-12 mo
Medulloblastoma		
		2-5 yr (some cures)
Oligodendroglioma		
Oligodendroglioma	II	Years
Anaplastic oligodendroglioma	III/IV	Similar to high-grade astrocytoma

2. Determinants of survival.
   a. Younger clients survive longer.
   b. Neurologically intact clients survive longer.
   c. Survival decreases as grade of tumor increases.
   d. Amount of residual tumor influences survival.
   e. Pediatric client prognosis varies with age at diagnosis, location of tumor, and histology.
      (1) Medulloblastoma—the more advanced the stage at diagnosis, the worse the prognosis.
      (2) Children older than 10 years of age survive longer than those under 10.
      (3) Brainstem tumors—very poor prognosis.

DATA COLLECTION

I. Pertinent personal and family history (risk factors).
   A. Risk factors for primary brain tumors.
      1. Incidence highest in young children and middle-aged adults in fifties and sixties.
      2. Incidence slightly higher in males than females.
      3. Chemical exposure implicated but not confirmed:
         a. Vinyl chloride or radiation.
         b. Exposure of petrochemical and rubber workers to acrylonitrile.
         c. Chemicals used in experimental induction of brain tumors in animals.
         d. Exposure to ink and solvents by artists.
         e. Exposure to lubricating oils and solvents by machinists.
      4. Heredofamilial disorders.
         a. Neurofibromatosis.
         b. Tuberous sclerosis.
         c. Von Hippel-Lindau disease.

      5. Familial medulloblastoma in children with nevoid basal cell carcinoma syndrome.
      6. Coexistence of astrocytoma and colonic carcinoma in clients with Turcot syndrome.
      7. Cancer family syndrome in which breast carcinoma, soft-tissue sarcoma and leukemia are most frequently associated malignancies.
      8. Prophylactic radiation therapy in children (e.g., with leukemia).
      9. Immunosuppressed clients at increased risk.

B. Pertinent history.
  1. Adult.
    a. Familial disorders.
    b. Exposure to chemicals.
    c. History of headaches.
    d. Personality change.
    e. Report of seizures, visual changes, nausea and vomiting.
    f. Memory problems.
    g. Cognitive changes.
    h. Sensorimotor changes.
  2. Pediatric population.
    a. Prenatal or perinatal history.
    b. Neonatal and postnatal problems.
    c. Developmental history.
    d. Family history.

II. Physical examination.
  A. Early signs and symptoms.
    1. Adult.
      a. Common symptoms of tumor.
        (1) Headache.
        (2) Seizure.
        (3) Mental changes—personality change, short-term memory loss, confusion or dementia.
        (4) Visual changes—diplopia, blurred vision, ptosis, visual field defect.
        (5) Speech or language disorders.
        (6) Sensorimotor deficits.
      b. Focal symptoms (Table 36-2).
        (1) Cerebral tumors of motor and sensory strip cause contralateral (other side) deficits.
        (2) Cerebellar tumors cause ipsilateral (same side) deficits.
        (3) Dominant hemisphere tumor affects:
          (a) Reading, arithmetic, writing.
          (b) Initiation of speech and comprehension of speech.
        (4) Nondominant hemisphere tumor results in:
          (a) Loss of right-left discrimination.
          (b) Neglect of one side of body.
          (c) Astereognosis (inability to recognize objects by touch).
          (d) Inability to process sensory information.
      c. Early increased ICP (Table 36-7).
    2. Pediatric population.
      a. Early increased ICP (Table 36-7).
      b. Focal deficits related to location of tumor (e.g., abnormal gait with cerebellar tumors) (Table 36-2).

Table 36-7
SYMPTOMS OF INCREASED INTRACRANIAL PRESSURE

Early Signs	Late Signs
Adult	
Drowsiness	Headache
Decreased attention span	Vomiting
Mood changes	Papilledema
Poor judgment	Decreased level of consciousness
Impaired cognitive skills	Changes in vital signs
	Pulse pressure widens
Pediatric	Bradycardia
Irritability	Slowed, irregular pulse
Lethargy	
Vomiting	
Anorexia	
Headache	
Papilledema	
Behavioral changes	
Bulging fontanelles in infant	

    B. Late signs and symptoms (adult and pediatric populations).
        1. Increased ICP.
        2. Displacement of brain structures (herniation) (Figure 36-4).
  III. Laboratory data—brain tumors.
    A. CSF—for cytology only when checking for CSF spread of cells—glial, medulloblastoma, or systemic cancer.
    B. CSF—for elevated protein level.

ASSOCIATED NURSING DIAGNOSES

  I. Knowledge deficit related to brain tumors and treatment.

 II. Potential for injury related to neurological deficits from effects of tumor and/or subsequent treatment.

III. Knowledge deficit related to postcraniotomy discharge instructions about wound care, medication, response to seizures, and activity limitations.

IV. Potential for injury related to postoperative complications from craniotomy.

 V. Cognitive dysfunction related to brain injury from tumor or effects of treatment.

VI. Ineffective individual and family coping related to client's change in cognitive functioning and subsequent family role changes.

NURSING PLANNING AND IMPLEMENTATION

  I. Interventions to maximize safety for client and family.
    A. Observe for seizures.
        1. Document and communicate to other health personnel—date, time of onset, duration, client activity at time of onset, aura (if any), description, LOC, autonomic signs (incontinence), postictal state (drowsiness, disorientation, headache, muscle fatigue), any injuries.
        2. Remain with client during seizure.

3. Alter environment to promote safety—move objects away from client to avoid injury.
4. Loosen tight clothing—maintain patent airway but do not insert any object into mouth; turn head to side.
5. Call for assistance if respiratory distress noted or if another seizure occurs before complete recovery—may indicate status epilepticus, which is a medical emergency.
6. Administer anticonvulsants on regular schedule to maintain therapeutic blood levels (see Table 36-5).

B. Assess mental status frequently.
1. Reorientate frequently, provide calendar and clock.
2. Restrain only if necessary to protect from injury.
3. Provide quiet environment—limit visitors, reduce extraneous noise and lighting, and limit approaches to client.

C. Assess neurological status—take appropriate nursing action related to deficit.
1. Hemiplegia.
    a. Consult rehabilitation service for physical therapy and occupational therapy.
    b. Obtain appropriate assistive devices (e.g., overhead trapeze, walker, cane).
    c. Teach client and family transfer techniques.
    d. Assist client with ambulation and transfers from affected side.
2. Visual deficit.
    a. Diplopia—recommend patch for one eye.
    b. Visual field defect.
        (1) Place objects on unaffected side.
        (2) Teach scanning technique.
        (3) Approach client from unaffected side.
3. Sensory deficits.
    a. Teach to test for potential environmental dangers (e.g., water temperature) with unaffected side.
    b. Teach to inspect skin in area of decreased sensation.
    c. Teach importance of frequent position changes to avoid skin breakdown.
4. Speech or language dysfunction.
    a. Listen patiently for client to express self.
    b. Consult speech therapist and include family in session.
5. Cognitive dysfunction.
    a. Discuss cognitive problem with client and family.
    b. Consult neuropsychologist for formal testing to determine deficits more specifically.
    c. Suggest vocational alternatives—consult social worker for assistance.
    d. Repeat information to client as needed.

II. Interventions to decrease incidence and severity of symptoms unique to brain tumors.
A. Administer steroids as ordered for cerebral edema.
1. Taper dosage when no longer needed.
2. Administer additional medication (famotidine [Pepcid], ranitidine [Zantac], cimetidine [Tagamet]) to prevent gastic irritation.
3. Teach side effects—increased appetite, fluid retention, irritability, and increased potential for infection.

B. Administer analgesics as needed for headache (usually extra-strength acetaminophen is sufficient).
C. Teach anticonvulsant medication schedule for maximum effectiveness with min-

imal side effects. (Take all of phenytoin dose at bedtime and follow seizure precautions [Table 9-9]).

    D. Instruct about use of diary for memory-impaired client.

III. Interventions to monitor for unique side effects of treatment for brain tumors.

    A. Assess neurological status and vital signs frequently after craniotomy; report any changes to physician immediately.

    B. Position client with supratentorial craniotomy with head of bed elevated 20 to 30 degrees.

    C. Position client with infratentorial craniotomy with bed flat; avoid pressure on operative site.

    D. Maintain neck in alignment to maintain adequate blood flow through carotid arteries.

    E. Monitor ICP via pressure monitor.

        1. Maintain ICP less than 20 mm Hg with mannitol, dexamethasone (Decadron), and hyperventilation.

        2. Measure and record output from Jackson-Pratt drainage tube and ventriculostomy.

    F. Monitor fluid balance and record.

        1. Monitor electrolyte values, especially sodium (client is prone to dehydration, especially when osmotherapy is used).

        2. Colloids rather than crystalloids are used for clients with hypovolemia to reduce risk of cerebral edema from intravascular shift to tissues.

    G. Assess client for thrombophlebitis—calf redness and tenderness and/or increased calf size.

        1. Encourage client to wear antiembolic stockings throughout hospital stay.

        2. Encourage postoperative ambulation as soon as possible.

    H. Assess incisional area for drainage, redness, tenderness, or edema; instruct client to keep area clean and dry and to clean with half-strength hydrogen peroxide daily after discharged until staples or sutures removed.

    I. Monitor bowel elimination; administer stool softeners on regular schedule and suppositories and laxatives as needed to avoid constipation and straining at stool (straining increases ICP).

IV. Interventions to enhance adaptation and rehabilitation.

    A. Provide information and resources to client and family about brain tumors and treatment.

    B. Initiate referral of client and family to individual psychologist or group therapy for counseling as indicated.

    C. Consult rehabilitation services for outpatient care for individual's specific neurological deficit.

    D. Consult social service department about financial counseling and home health services if needed; assist in completing Social Security Administration Disability Insurance forms if appropriate.

    E. Provide information about subsequent treatment (radiation therapy, chemotherapy).

V. Interventions to incorporate client and family in care.

    A. Assess client and family knowledge about disease, diagnostic tests, treatment, and expected outcome; discuss with family potential care problems in future and ability to meet care demands.

    B. Teach family about specific focal deficit and interventions to assist individual to work toward self-care.

C. Provide preoperative information, including information about hair shaving, head dressing, tubes, antiembolic stockings, and intensive care routines.

D. Provide resource (name of nurse and work phone number) for information and assistance after discharge and as disease progresses.

E. Provide information about client's particular behavioral, cognitive, and memory problems.

F. Teach client and family about discharge medications.

EVALUATION OF CLIENT AND FAMILY OUTCOMES

I. Identify type of cancer and rationale for treatment.
   A. Discuss verbal and written information about brain tumors and ask appropriate questions about the disease and treatment.
   B. Explain principle of increasing growth of tumor plus edema in a closed space and resultant pressure affecting brain function.
   C. Verbalize understanding of role of surgery followed by radiation therapy and chemotherapy in the treatment of brain tumors.

II. List signs and symptoms of immediate and long-term side effects of disease and treatment.
   A. Headache.
   B. Seizures.
   C. Hydrocephalus.
   D. Increasing ICP.
   E. Focal neurological deficits.
      1. Motor deficits.
      2. Sensory deficits.
      3. Speech and language problems.
      4. Visual deficits.
      5. Cognitive deficits.

III. List self-care measures to decrease incidence and severity of symptoms associated with disease and treatment.
   A. Discuss role of steroids and analgesics, including dosing schedule for relief of headache.
   B. List possible alterations in life-style (e.g., limit alcohol intake, reduce stress, get adequate rest) that may reduce risk of seizures and subsequent injury; verbalize understanding of route and schedule of anticonvulsants.
   C. List symptoms (excessive sleepiness, nausea and vomiting, or increase in frequency and severity of headache) to report promptly to physician.
   D. Demonstrate use of prescribed assistive devices for mobility problems.
   E. Verbalize understanding of importance of speech therapy for rehabilitation.
   F. Demonstrate scanning technique to compensate for visual field defect.
   G. Verbalize purpose of wearing eye patch for diplopia.
   H. Discuss role of maintaining daily diary to assist with short-term memory deficit.
   I. Demonstrate method to inspect skin daily in areas of decreased sensation.

IV. Describe schedule and procedures for routine follow-up.
   A. Neurological examination 1 to 2 weeks after craniotomy.
   B. CT, MRI, and/or neurological examination after radiation therapy.
   C. CT, MRI, or neurological examination every 2 months.
   D. If chemotherapy given, blood work before treatment and as indicated by drugs given; MRI or CT before treatment and after two chemotherapy cycles and then based on response and neurological status.

V. List signs and symptoms of recurrent disease.
  A. Deteriorating neurological status (usually recurrence of original presenting symptoms).
  B. Increase in frequency and intensity of headaches.
  C. Increasing periods of confusion.
  D. Nausea and vomiting.
  E. Decreasing LOC.

VI. Identify community resources to meet unique demands of CNS disease, treatment, and survivorship.
  A. Local support groups.
  B. Local rehabilitation hospital groups for brain-injured clients.
  C. Self-help references:
    1. Mace, L. and Rabins, P. (1981). *Thirty-Six Hour Day*. Baltimore: Johns Hopkins University Press. A family guide to caring for persons with Alzheimer's disease, related dementing illnesses, and memory loss in later life.
    2. Lohmann, J. (1989). *Gathering a Life*. Santa Barbara, Calif.: John Daniel and Company. A journal written by wife of brain tumor client.
  D. National associations and registries:
    1. National Brain Tumor Foundation
       323 Geary Street, Suite 510
       San Francisco, CA 94102
       (415)296-0404.
       Informational booklets, support information, client phone Support Line, and conferences; booklet; *Support Groups for Brain Tumor Patients and Families in North America*.
    2. American Brain Tumor Association (Formerly the Association for Brain Tumor Research)
       3725 North Talman Avenue
       Chicago, IL 60618
       (312)286-5571.
       Booklets, information on treatment options, newsletter, support group listings.
    3. National Familial Brain Tumor Registry (NFBTR)
       The Johns Hopkins Oncology Center
       600 N. Wolfe Street, Room 132
       Baltimore, MD 21205
       (301)955-0227.
       A tumor registry for families with two or more first-degree relatives or husbands and wives who have a primary brain tumor.

Spinal Cord Tumors

THEORY

I. Physiology and pathophysiology associated with spinal cord tumors.
  A. Anatomy of the spinal cord.
    1. Description of spinal cord (Figures 36-7 and 36-8).
      a. Cord body.
        (1) Begins at brainstem.
        (2) Extends through spinal foramina of vertebrae.
        (3) Extends to L1-L2 vertebral level.

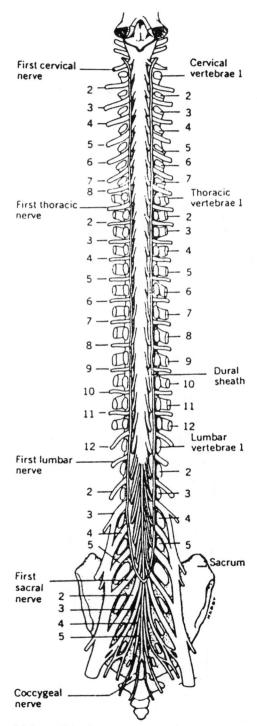

Figure 36-7 Spinal cord lying within the vertebral canal. Spinal nerves are numbered on the left side; vertebrae are numbered on the right side. *(From Chaffee, E.E. & Lytle, I.M. [1980].* Basic Physiology and Anatomy. *Philadelphia: J.B. Lippincott Co.)*

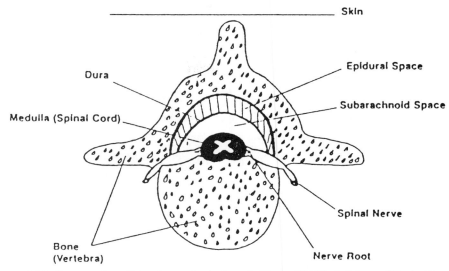

Figure 36-8 Cross section of vertebra and spinal cord. *(From [1991]. A Primer of Brain Tumors. Chicago: Association for Brain Tumor Research.)*

    b. Spinal nerves.
        (1) Thirty-one pairs, one pair for each segment of cord.
        (2) Exit from central cord at intervals.
        (3) Each nerve has a dorsal and ventral root:
            (a) Ventral-anterior—called *efferent* or *motor fibers.*
            (b) Dorsal-posterior—called *afferent* or *sensory fibers.*
  2. Identification of critical adjacent structures.
    a. Vertebral column.
        (1) Thirty-three vertebrae joined by ligaments.
        (2) Bony structure encasing and protecting cord.
        (3) Divisions—7 cervical, 12 thoracic, 5 lumbar, 5 sacral (fused), 4 coccygeal (fused).
    b. Intervertebral disks—cartilage pads separating vertebrae, allowing flexion of cord.
    c. Meninges—layers of tissue that surround cord and brain.
    d. Cerebral spinal fluid (CSF)—fluid that bathes and cushions the cord; all contained within the meninges.
    e. Vertebral blood vessels—supply from vertebral and spinal arteries.
B. Primary spinal cord functions.
  1. Cord body—carries fiber tracts to convey sensory, motor, and autonomic pulses between brain and body.
  2. Spinal nerves (Tables 36-8 and 36-9).
    a. Afferent fibers—carry sensory impulses from sensory receptors of the body to the cord.
    b. Efferent fibers—carry impulses from the cord to the muscles and glands of body.
C. Changes in function associated with spinal cord tumors.
  1. Cord compression.
    a. Minimal room for displacement.
    b. Mechanical pressure on neuronal elements.
  2. Damage to nerve roots and occlusion of spinal blood vessels.
  3. Progressive neurological deficits.

Table 36-8
SENSORY NERVE ROOTS AND AREA INNERVATED

Dorsal (Sensory) Spinal Root	Area of the Body Innervated
C-2	Back of the head
C-4	Around lower neck and upper thorax in the form of a collar
C-6	Radial aspect of lower arm and thumb
T-1	Upper chest and lower arm on side of small finger (includes small finger)
T-4	Nipple line
T-10	Umbilical region
L-1	Groin region
L-3	Kneecap
L-5	Anterior lower leg and anterior foot
S-3	Medial thigh
S-4, S-5	Perianal region

Modified from Hickey, J.V. (1986). *The Clinical Practice of Neurological and Neurosurgical Nursing* (2nd ed). Philadelphia: J.B. Lippincott Co., p. 41.

D. Metastatic patterns.
1. Some primary CNS tumors seed along the spinal cord.
2. Metastatic spinal cord tumors.
   a. Most commonly occur in thoracic area.
   b. Twenty-five percent of all spinal cord tumors are metastatic from cancers originating outside the CNS.
E. Trends in epidemiology.
1. No general statement can be made about spinal cord tumor changes in incidence over time.
2. Characteristics of tumors (Table 36-10).
   a. Location in relation to the dura:
      (1) Extradural—usually secondary or metastatic.

Table 36-9
MOTOR NERVE ROOTS AND MUSCLE ACTION

Ventral (Motor Nerve Roots)	Action of Muscles Innervated
C-5, C-6	Moves shoulders and flexes elbow
T1-7	Controls intercostal muscles
T6-12	Controls abdominal muscles
L1-3	Flexes hip
L-5, S-1	Everts foot
S-1, S-2	Plantar flexes foot
S3-5	Controls perianal muscles

Modified from Hickey, J.V. (1986). *The Clinical Practice of Neurological and Neurosurgical Nursing* (2nd ed). Philadelphia: J.B. Lippincott Co., p. 42.

Table 36-10
LOCATION AND ORIGIN OF SPINAL NEOPLASMS

Location and Origin	Percentage of All Cases
Extradural (45%)	
Metastatic (solid tumors)	25
Sarcoma	7
Lymphoma	4
Myeloma, chloroma	5
Other	4
Intradural (55%)	
Extramedullary (33%)	
Neurofibroma	12
Meningioma	15
Congenital tumors (epidermoid, 3.6%)	5
Other	1
Intramedullary (22%)	
Glioma (ependymoma, 5.3%; astrocytoma, 4.7%)	14
Vascular tumors	6
Other	2

Modified from Walker, M. (1982). Brain and peripheral nervous system tumors. In J.F. Holland & E. Frei, III (eds). *Cancer Medicine*. Philadelphia: Lea & Febiger, p. 1625.

    (2) Intradural—tumors of cord, nerve roots, or coverings of cord.
  b. Location in relation to vertebral and functional level.
  c. Classification by histology:
    (1) Neurofibroma.
      (a) Common primary cord tumor.
      (b) Benign by histology.
      (c) Unresponsive to radiation.
    (2) Meningioma.
      (a) Common primary cord tumor.
      (b) Benign.
      (c) Originates from dural coverings.
    (3) Ependymoma.
      (a) May occur in multiple locations along the cord.
      (b) Benign by histology.
    (4) Astrocytoma.
      (a) May be benign or malignant, depending on grade.
      (b) Most malignant by histology of all cord tumors.
    (5) Metastatic.
      (a) Most commonly originates in lung, breast, prostate, or kidney.
      (b) Invades bone and predisposes to pathological fractures.
      (c) Very painful.
II. Principles of medical management.
  A. Screening and diagnostic procedures.
    1. General procedures.
      a. Spine films.
      b. Computed tomography (CT).

       c. Lumbar puncture.

       d. Magnetic resonance imaging (MRI).

       e. Spinal angiography.

   2. Specific procedures unique to the spinal cord (see Tables 36-3 and 36-4).

       a. CT myelography.

       b. Electromyography (EMG).

B. Staging methods and procedures.

   1. Clinical neurological status (e.g., impairments).

   2. Invasion into adjacent structures.

C. Treatment strategies.

   1. Surgery.

       a. Surgical resection.

          (1) For biopsy only or partial or total tumor removal.

          (2) Indicated if resection will not cause further neurological deficits.

       b. Decompressive laminectomy.

          (1) Indicated when tumor compression is causing progressive neurological deficits.

          (2) Decompresses bony structures to provide more room for cord and nerve roots.

       c. Potential surgical complications.

          (1) CSF leak.

             (a) CSF seeps through small opening in dura.

             (b) Primary concern—increased risk of meningitis.

             (c) Treatment—lumbar drain inserted to relieve pressure.

             (d) Drain removed after few days when drainage decreased and dura has sealed.

          (2) Infection.

          (3) Hematoma.

          (4) Motor and/or sensory loss.

          (5) Disruption of graft or fusion.

   2. Radiation.

       a. Treatment of choice after surgery.

       b. Indicated for incompletely resected tumors and/or highly malignant tumors.

       c. Dose.

          (1) Entire cord—4000 rads in 5 weeks.

          (2) Cord segments—5000 rads in 5 weeks.

       d. Toxicities.

          (1) Delayed radiation myelopathy, producing neurological deficits that begin 6 to 12 months after radiation is completed.

          (2) Skin irritation.

       e. Quickly reduces tumor, providing pain relief.

   3. Chemotherapy.

       a. Intrathecal to treat some tumors.

       b. Systemic for metastatic disease.

   4. Overall treatment strategies.

       a. Local control of tumor.

       b. Preserved or improved neurological function.

D. Trends in survival.

   1. General survival for all cases by stage.

       a. Metastatic tumors—persons usually die from other systemic disease.

       b. Benign tumors—may recur or cause neurological deficits, but clients live for many years.

c. Malignant gliomas of the cord—death within 2 years even with surgery and radiation.
2. Determinants of survival.
   a. Histology—benign tumors rarely cause death, but malignant tumors do cause death.
   b. Location of tumor—high cervical cord tumors at or above C4 cause respiratory difficulties.

DATA COLLECTION

I. Pertinent personal and family history (risk factors).
   A. History of neurofibromatosis (Von Recklinghausen's disease).
      1. Neurofibromas—common.
      2. Higher risk of developing astrocytoma in brain or spinal cord.
   B. Report of neck or back pain.
   C. Report of sensory loss, especially for pain and temperature sensations.
   D. Report of motor weakness in an extremity.
   E. Report of bladder and/or bowel dysfunction.

II. Physical examination.
   A. Early signs and symptoms.
      1. Sensory impairment.
         a. Slow progression—begins unilaterally in an arm and leg and continues to spread upward to level of tumor.
         b. Sensory deficits—pain and temperature.
            (1) Coldness.
            (2) Numbness and tingling.
      2. Motor impairment.
         a. Develops in conjunction with sensory impairment.
         b. Paresis, clumsiness, spasticity, and hyperactive reflexes.
         c. Ataxia and hypotonia.
         d. Positive Babinski sign.
      3. Severe pain.
         a. Localized or diffuse.
         b. May be radicular.
            (1) Runs through the distribution of the sensory nerve root.
            (2) Caused by irritation or tension on the nerve.
            (3) Knifelike or dull ache, with episodes of sharp, piercing pain.
      4. Bowel and bladder dysfunction.
         a. Urinary retention.
         b. Constipation.
   B. Late signs and symptoms.
      1. Sensory deficits related to touch, vibration, and position sense.
      2. Motor impairment (spasticity, flaccid paralysis).
      3. Bowel and bladder incontinence (loss of sphincter control).
      4. Intractable pain.

III. Laboratory data unique to spinal cord tumors.
   A. CSF—for cytology.
   B. CSF—for elevated protein level.

ASSOCIATED NURSING DIAGNOSES

I. Impaired mobility related to hemiparesis, spasticity, ataxia, and/or paralysis.

II. Potential for injury related to sensory loss.

III. Alteration in comfort related to pain from nerve compression by tumor.

IV. Potential for infection related to bladder dysfunction or laminectomy.

V. Potential for impaired bowel elimination.

VI. Potential for sexual dysfunction related to neurological deficits.

NURSING PLANNING AND IMPLEMENTATION

I. Interventions to maximize safety for client and family.
   A. Assess baseline neurological status (motor, sensory, and bowel and bladder); report changes to physician.
   B. Provide appropriate devices to assist client with mobility (cane, walker, wheelchair); teach proper use.
   C. Assist client to decrease risk of injury from altered sensory input.
      1. Teach client to check position of affected limbs visually.
      2. Teach client to check skin integrity daily, especially in affected areas.
      3. Teach client to check temperature with unaffected extremity before applying heat or cold to affected area.
      4. Teach client to use heating or cooling devices with extreme caution.
   D. Assess urinary elimination pattern.
      1. Maintain intake and output record.
      2. Assess for bladder distention.
      3. Request order for intermittent catheterization if urinary retention becomes a problem.
   E. Assess for thrombophlebitis and take measures to prevent.
      1. Use antiembolic stockings preoperatively, intraoperatively, and postoperatively until ambulating often.
      2. Ambulate postoperatively as allowed.

II. Interventions to decrease incidence and severity of symptoms unique to spinal cord tumors.
   A. Assist client to maintain range of motion (ROM) and mobility.
      1. Consult physical therapist.
      2. Perform ROM exercises on all joints three or four times a day.
      3. Reposition every 2 hours with correct body alignment.
      4. Use support devices to maintain positioning.
   B. Assess bowel elimination pattern and institute bowel program.
      1. Auscultate for bowel sounds.
      2. Increase fiber in diet.
      3. Institute bowel program specific to client.
         a. Daily stool softener.
         b. Bisacodyl (Dulcolax) suppository every 2 to 3 days if no bowel movement.
         c. Mild laxative if suppository is not effective.
   C. Administer analgesics on regular schedule for pain control.

III. Interventions to monitor for unique side effects of treatment for spinal cord tumors.
   A. Reposition client every 2 hours after laminectomy.
      1. Thoracic or lumbar—bed flat; log roll.
      2. Cervical:
         a. Head of bed elevated, with small folded towel under head to maintain alignment; no flexion.

b. Collar or supportive device (Halo) on at all times.
B. Observe incision and dressing for bloody or serous drainage and/or for edema in incisional area; report to physician.
C. Maintain aseptic care of lumbar drain.
  1. Monitor temperature every 4 hours.
  2. Assess for neck stiffness.
  3. Note and record amount, color, and clarity of CSF from lumbar drain.
D. Medicate with muscle relaxants for postoperative muscle spasms.
E. Assess skin integrity in area of radiation.

IV. Interventions to enhance adaptation and rehabilitation.
A. Consult rehabilitation service (physical therapy, occupational therapy, and support services).
B. Discuss potential sexual dysfunction with client and significant other; offer information to assist with problems (see Chapter 7).
C. Teach self-catheterization.

V. Interventions to incorporate client and family in care.
A. Teach transfer techniques with assistive devices.
B. Teach principles of maintaining ROM; teach ROM exercises to continue at home.
C. Teach about possible injuries caused by limitation of mobility and/or decreased sensation and methods to prevent injury.
D. Provide information about counseling or support groups at rehabilitative facilities.

EVALUATION OF CLIENT AND FAMILY OUTCOMES

I. Identify type of cancer and rationale for treatment.
A. Verbalize understanding of histology and location of tumor and the resulting impact on function.
B. Verbalize understanding of role of surgery to remove tumor bulk to reduce pressure on cord.
C. Verbalize understanding of the purpose of radiation therapy—to reduce tumor size to remove pressure from cord, reduce risk of recurrence, and control pain.

II. List signs and symptoms of immediate and long-term side effects of spinal cord tumor and treatment.
A. Sensory impairment.
  1. Pain.
  2. Temperature.
  3. Touch.
  4. Vibration.
  5. Position sense.
B. Motor impairment.
  1. Hemiparesis.
  2. Hyperactive reflexes.
  3. Spasticity.
  4. Ataxia.
  5. Flaccid paralysis.
C. Pain.
  1. Diffuse or localized.
  2. May be radicular.
D. Bowel and bladder dysfunction.
  1. Urinary retention.
  2. Constipation.
  3. Incontinence.

E. Sexual dysfunction.
  1. Specific dysfunction related to cord level of tumor.
  2. Male—inability to attain erection.
  3. Female—inability to experience orgasm.

III. List self-care measures to decrease incidence and severity of symptoms associated with spinal cord tumors and treatment.
  A. Verbalize understanding of measures to prevent injury caused by motor and/or sensory loss.
  B. List measures to maintain ROM and maximize mobility.
  C. Verbalize understanding of analgesic medications—how and when to use; list possible toxicities.
  D. List steps of individualized bowel regimen.
  E. Identify resources to assist with problems related to sexual dysfunction.

IV. Demonstrate skill in self-care demanded by structural or functional effects of spinal cord tumor and treatment.
  A. Demonstrate self-catheterization technique and describe catheterization schedule after discharge.
  B. Demonstrate ability to use mobility-assistive devices.
  C. Demonstrate skin assessment with mirror in difficult-to-see areas of decreased sensation.

V. Describe schedule and procedure for routine follow-up.
  A. After laminectomy—1 to 2 weeks for suture removal and neurological assessment; then neurological examination in 1 month.
  B. Followup—weekly during radiation therapy and immediately after completion of therapy.
  C. MRI, CT, CT myelography—as indicated by clinical status and histology of tumor.

VI. List signs and symptoms of recurrent disease.
  A. Worsening neurological status.
  B. Increasing pain.
  C. New neurological deficits originating at a different level of the cord.

VII. Identify potential community resources to meet unique demands of spinal cord tumor, treatment, and survivorship.
  A. Local rehabilitation facilities—continued therapy and support services.
  B. State vocational rehabilitation office.

BIBLIOGRAPHY

Apuzzo, M.J. (ed) (1990). *Malignant Cerebral Glioma*. Park Ridge, Ill.: American Association of Neurological Surgeons.

Cammermeyer, M. & Appledorn, C. (eds) (1990). *Core Curriculum for Neuroscience Nursing* (3rd ed). Park Ridge, Ill.: American Association of Neuroscience Nurses.

(1987). *Coping With a Brain Tumor*. Chicago: Association for Brain Tumor Research.

Gilman, S., Bloedel, J., & Lechtenberg, R. (1981). *Disorders of the Cerebellum*. Philadelphia: F.A. Davis Co., pp. 333-372.

Hickey, J.V. (1986). *The Clinical Practice of Neurological and Neurosurgical Nursing* (2nd ed). Philadelphia: J.B. Lippincott Co.

Hochberg, F., Toniolo, P., & Cole, P. (1990). Nonoccupational risk indicators of glioblastoma in adults. *J Neuro-oncol 8*(1), 55-60.

Kornblith, P., Walker, M., & Cassady, J.R. (1987). *Neurologic Oncology*. Philadelphia: J.B. Lippincott Co.

Mahaley N.S, Jr., Mettlin, C., Natarajan, N., Laws, E.R., Jr., & Peace, B.B. (1989). National survey of patterns of care for brain-tumor patients. *J Neurosurg 71*(6), 826-836.

Menkes, J. (1985). *Textbook of Child Neurology*. Philadelphia: Lea & Febiger, pp. 531-589.

Mitchell, M.S. (1989). *Neuroscience Nursing: a Nursing Diagnosis Approach*. Baltimore: Williams & Wilkins.

Patchell, R.A., Tibbs, P.A., Walsh, J.W., Dempsey, R.J., Marayama, Y., Kryscio, R.J., Markesberry, W.R., MacDonald, J.S., & Young, B. (1990). A randomized trial of surgery in the treatment of single metastases to the brain. *N Engl J Med 322*(8), 494-500.

Robinson, C., Roy, C., Sr., & Seager, M. (1991). Central nervous system tumors. In S. Baird, R. McCorkle, & M. Grant (eds). *Cancer Nursing: A Comprehensive Textbook*. Philadelphia: W.B. Saunders Co., pp. 608-636.

Rowland, L.P. (ed) (1989). *Merritt's Textbook of Neurology* (8th ed). Philadelphia: Lea & Febiger.

Rudy, E.B. (1984). *Advanced Neurological and Neurosurgical Nursing*. St. Louis: C.V. Mosby Co.

Segal, F. (1988). *A Primer of Brain Tumors* (4th ed). Chicago: Association For Brain Tumor Research.

Shiminski-Maher, T. (1990). Brain tumors in childhood: implications for nursing practice. *J Pediatr Health Care 4*(3), 122-130.

Wegmann, J.A. & Hakius, P. (1990). Central nervous system cancers. In S.L. Groenwald, M.H. Frogge, M. Goodman, & C.H. Yarbro (eds). *Cancer Nursing: Principles and Practice* (2nd ed). Boston: Jones & Bartlett Publishers, pp. 751-773.

Woods, N. (1988). Alterations in human sexuality. In P. Mitchell, L. Hodges, M. Muwaswes, & C. Walleck (eds). *AANN's Neuroscience Nursing*. Norwalk, Conn.: Appleton & Lange, pp. 471-482.

37

HIV-Related Cancers

James Halloran, MSN, RN, OCN, ANP

THEORY

I. Human immunodeficiency virus (HIV) as a predisposing factor to cancer.
   A. Definition of HIV.
      1. Cytopathic retrovirus of lentivirus family.
         a. Causes chronic disease in host.
         b. Long incubation and gradual progression are typical.
      2. Structure.
         a. Core protein ribonucleic acid (RNA) genome—p24.
         b. Bilayered lipid envelope.
         c. Surface antigens—gp120, gp41.
            (1) gp120—attracted to CD4 surface marker on host cells.
            (2) Human cell with most abundant CD4—T lymphocyte; CD4 also prominent on macrophages and monocytes, microglial cells, Langerhans' cells, dendritic cells.
         d. Reverse transcriptase enzyme mediates transcription of viral ribonucleic acid (RNA) to deoxyribonucleic acid (DNA) in infected cell.
   B. Immunological structures.
      1. T lymphocyte.
         a. Stem cells from bone marrow mature in thymus, acquire surface markers, seed peripheral lymphoid tissue and circulation; approximately 80% of circulating lymphocytes are T cells.
         b. Pivotal agent in cell-mediated immunity; produces lymphokines, which regulate overall immune response, both promoting and inhibiting proliferation and differentiation of immunoactive cells and molecules.
         c. Protects against intracellular parasites and tumors; provides immunosurveillance; responsible for graft rejection; displays memory effect.
      2. B lymphocyte.
         a. Believed to mature in bone marrow; circulates to and seeds peripheral lymphoid germinal centers; 12% to 15% of circulating lymphocytes are B cells.
         b. Stimulated B cell produces plasma cells, which produce antigen-specific antibody.

    c. Protects against bacterial and viral infections.

    d. B memory cells provide anamnestic effect (stores template of specific antibodies).

  3. Lymphoid organs and circulation.

    a. Primary organs—bone marrow and thymus.

    b. Also included—lymphatic vessels, lymph nodes, spleen, and liver.

    c. Nonencapsulated clusters of lymphoid tissue are found around lining of aerodigestive tract.

    d. Lymph nodes are located at junction of lymphatic channels.

      (1) Small and bean shaped; store T and B cells and macrophages.

      (2) Lymphadenopathy (increase in size of lymph nodes) occurs when immune response is invoked by presence of antigen.

  4. Natural killer (NK) cells.

    a. Large granular lymphocytes without surface markers of T or B cells.

    b. Primary function is cytotoxicity; target tumor and virally infected cells.

    c. Nonspecific action; no memory function.

C. Physiological basis of HIV infection and HIV-related cancers.

  1. HIV effect on T4 lymphocytes.

    a. HIV binds to CD4 surface marker on T4 cells.

    b. Fusion and release of viral RNA into host cells.

    c. Viral RNA is transcribed to DNA through action of reverse transcriptase and is integrated into host nuclear DNA; viral particles also are found in host cell cytoplasm.

    d. May remain dormant for variable period, or immediate viral production by infected cell may occur.

    e. Newly produced virion buds from surface of infected cell and infects other cells.

    f. Host cells eventually are depleted.

  2. HIV effect on immune system.

    a. Progressive infection leads to qualitative and quantitative T4 lymphocyte dysfunction, with resultant defect in both cellular and humoral immunity as immunoregulatory function of T4 cells is gradually impaired.

      (1) Progressive destruction of T cells results from viral replication in host.

      (2) HIV may cause polyclonal B-cell activity (also may be due to coinfection with Epstein-Barr virus [EBV]).

      (3) Impaired immune function allows proliferation of malignantly transformed cells.

      (4) No conclusive data exist about quantitative changes in the T4 cell count and stage of disease.

    b. Cofactors in disease progression.

      (1) Definitive role of specific cofactors in disease progression is controversial; may be difficult to distinguish between comorbid infection and true causal relationship.

      (2) Infectious cofactors may include presence of cytomegalovirus (CMV), EBV, and other viruses.

      (3) Life-style factors may also influence course of infection; risk for disease progression increases in presence of inadequate nutrition, general poor health, smoking, activities that may result in infection with other strains of HIV.

  3. Clinical staging and classification of HIV infection.

    a. Infection with HIV produces a continuum of changes in health status.

    b. Clinical status may change rapidly in either direction.

Table 37-1
CENTERS FOR DISEASE CONTROL (CDC) CLASSIFICATION SYSTEM FOR HIV INFECTION

Group	Classification
I	Acute infection with HIV
II	Asymptomatic infection
III	Persistent generalized lymphadenopathy
IV (subgroups)	Other disease
A	Constitutional disease
B	Neurological disease
C-1	Specified secondary infectious diseases in CDC surveillance definition for AIDS (1987)
C-2	Other specified secondary infectious diseases
D	Secondary cancers
E	Other conditions

    c. Knowledge of disease stage guides selection of therapeutic intervention and psychosocial support.

    d. Two major systems for classifying HIV disease—Centers for Disease Control (CDC) system and Walter Reed System.

      (1) Purposes of CDC classification system:

        (a) Provides surveillance definitions to guide epidemiological data collection.

        (b) Serves as vehicle for reporting clinical experience rather than as method to monitor individual status (Table 37-1).

      (2) Walter Reed Staging System.

        (a) Based on clinical presentation of individual client.

        (b) Designed to correlate with progressive immune dysfunction.

        (c) Six criteria:

          (1) HIV antibody positivity.

          (2) Chronic lymphadenopathy.

          (3) Absolute T4 helper cell count.

          (4) Delayed hypersensitivity (skin anergy).

          (5) Oral thrush.

          (6) Opportunistic infection(s) and/or malignancy.

        (d) Excludes neurological symptoms (Table 37-2).

    4. Malignant disease as a result of HIV infection.

      a. Impaired immune surveillance function and polyclonal B-cell activity lead to growth of malignantly transformed cells.

      b. Kaposi's sarcoma and B-cell lymphomas—most frequent malignant disease in HIV-infected clients.

      c. Distinguished by abnormal sites of presentation, poor duration of response to therapy, presence of comorbid opportunistic infection.

II. HIV-related Kaposi's sarcoma (KS).

  A. Definition/pathogenesis: soft-tissue malignancy characterized by malignant growth of reticuloendothelial cell origin in HIV-infected persons.

Table 37-2
WALTER REED STAGING SYSTEM FOR HIV INFECTION

Stage	HIV Antibody Status	Chronic Lymphadenopathy	CD4 Count	Skin Test	Oral Thrush	Opportunistic Infection
0	Negative	—	>400	WNL	—	—
1	Positive	—	>400	WNL	—	—
2	Positive	Present	>400	WNL	—	—
3	Positive	+ / −	<400	WNL	—	—
4	Positive	+ / −	<400	Partial anergy	—	—
5	Positive	+ / −	<400	Complete anergy	Yes	—
6	Positive	+ / −	<400	Partial/complete anergy	+ / −	Yes

WNL, *within normal limits*; + / −, may or may not be present.

B. Cause.
  1. Before HIV, pandemic KS occurred primarily in elderly males of Mediterranean origin (classic or non-African KS) and in persons receiving post–organ transplant immunosuppressive agents (transplant-associated KS).
  2. In clients with HIV-related KS (epidemic KS) malignantly transformed cells reproduce unchecked as a result of underlying immune defect.
    a. HIV-associated *tat* gene is thought to promote growth of KS lesions.
    b. Use of nitrite inhalants ("poppers") may be related to development of KS in HIV-infected people.
C. Appearance and metastasis of HIV-related KS.
  1. Classic presentation includes skin lesions, ranging from pink to purple to brownish, flat or raised, which are painless and do not blanch with pressure.
  2. HIV-related KS may present as skin lesions or may appear first in any other organ system.
  3. Classic KS is typically indolent, whereas HIV-related KS may be very aggressive and progress rapidly.

III. HIV-related lymphoma.
  A. Definition/pathogenesis: majority of clients present with B-cell tumors of high-grade histological type.
    1. Extranodal involvement is common; primary gastrointestinal (GI) or central nervous system (CNS) lymphoma and bone marrow involvement are common.
    2. Lymphoproliferative conditions seen less frequently in HIV-infected persons include Hodgkin's disease, multiple myeloma, and B-cell acute lymphocytic leukemia.
  B. Cause.
    1. EBV, direct effect of HIV, or activation of c-*myc* oncogene may play causative role.
    2. Lack of effective T-cell mediated imunoregulation allows polyclonal B-cell activity.
  C. Appearance and metastasis—CNS, GI tract, and bone marrow involvement are more frequent in HIV-infected persons; virtually every organ system may be involved.

1. CNS lesions may cause changes in cognitive function, memory loss, decreased attention span, headaches, personality change, focal neurological deficits, or generalized seizure activity.
2. GI tract lesions may cause malabsorption, diarrhea, constipation, or focal or diffuse abdominal discomfort or may present as asymptomatic abdominal mass.
3. Blood counts are usually normal despite bone marrow involvement.

IV. Principles of medical management.
   A. Diagnostic tests.
     1. Diagnosis of HIV infection is usually made on basis of positive antibody test.
       a. Enzyme-linked immunosorbent assay (ELISA) test for antibody to HIV is used for screening—high sensitivity and specificity in populations at risk.
       b. If ELISA test is positive, test is repeated; if second test is positive, confirmatory Western blot is conducted on same specimen.
       c. Other tests to demonstrate infection with HIV—polymerase chain reaction (PCR; a gene amplification technique) or viral culture.
     2. Diagnosis of HIV-related KS or lymphoma—similar to testing done for same conditions when not related to HIV infection; because of the wide variance in presenting symptoms, the workup in the HIV-infected person may be more aggressive or comprehensive than in the uninfected person.
       a. Once tissue diagnosis of KS lesions has been confirmed, the physician may elect not to biopsy new skin lesions; visceral lesions may be biopsied if the risk-to-benefit ratio permits.
       b. Brain biopsy may be performed to establish differential diagnosis between CNS lymphoma and other opportunistic infections; constitutional symptoms such as night sweats may relate to infection with *Mycobacterium avium-intracellulare,* and CNS symptoms may relate to cerebral toxoplasmosis.
       c. Because of the risk associated with brain biopsy, a trial of radiotherapy may be undertaken without tissue biopsy.
         (1) Response is seen with lymphoma, whereas toxoplasmosis will not respond to radiotherapy.
         (2) Alternatively, some physicians may choose to treat for toxoplasmosis (especially if the client has a previous history) and observe for response. sponse.

   B. Staging methods and procedures.
     1. Staging for HIV-related lymphoma typically follows the same schema for non–HIV-related lymphoma (e.g., the Ann Arbor Staging System) (see Chapter 38).
     2. No universally accepted staging system for HIV-related KS has been identified; schema used include parameters of cutaneous, lymph node, and visceral involvement and the occurrence of "B symptoms" (fever, chills, night sweats, diarrhea, unintentional weight loss).
     3. Because HIV-related malignancies may present at abnormal sites, diagnostic imaging and/or endoscopic examinations may be more extensive than in HIV-negative persons.

   C. Standard therapies.
     1. Treatment of HIV-related cancers is based on approaches used for uninfected persons, but the underlying immune deficiency, presence of other opportunistic infections, administration of other medications, and generalized poor health status may require dose reduction, scheduling modifications, and/or selection of alternative approaches.

2. Surgery.
    a. May be used to remove KS lesions that interfere with function or appearance such as gingival or upper aerodigestive tract lesions, those obstructing lymphatic flow on the gingiva, or those in cosmetically sensitive areas such as the head and neck; surgical approaches may be limited by the anatomical location of the lesion or client's poor overall health that precludes use of general anesthesia.
    b. Generally not used in clients with HIV-related lymphoma.
3. Chemotherapy.
    a. May be necessary to adjust dosage based on response, tolerance, co-morbidity, contraindication to agents being used to treat other conditions.
    b. HIV-related KS may be treated with single or multiple agents.
        (1) Etoposide may be used as either first-line or salvage therapy.
        (2) Combination approaches include use of vinca alkaloids (especially vinblastine) and bleomycin, vinblastine and methotrexate, vinblastine and doxorubicin, or bleomycin with or without dacarbazine.
    c. HIV-related lymphoma is treated with combination chemotherapy, using cyclophosphamide, vincristine, methotrexate, etoposide, cytosine arabinoside, bleomycin, and steroids; use of methotrexate, bleomycin, and doxorubicin, cyclophosphamide, vincristine, and dexamethasone (M-BACOD) is common.
        (1) Primary CNS lymphoma is usually resistant to systemic chemotherapy.
        (2) Intrathecal administration of chemotherapy may be considered.
4. Radiotherapy.
    a. KS lesions are typically radiosensitive.
        (1) Effective short- to moderate-term local control may be achieved, especially for cosmetic effects or relief of lymphedema caused by lymphatic lesions.
        (2) The aggressive nature of epidemic KS precludes radiotherapy with curative intent.
    b. HIV-related lymphoma may respond to radiotherapy, but control of high-grade tumors is poor; low-grade tumors may be controlled for several months to years.
5. Biological response modifiers.
    a. α-Interferon, with or without concomitant zidovudine (AZT), has been approved as treatment for HIV-related KS; the efficacy of other biological response modifiers is being evaluated.
    b. Other biological response modifiers are being evaluated as treatment for the underlying HIV infection, but they generally are not used to treat HIV-related lymphomas.
6. Combined-modality treatment is not well documented as therapy for HIV-related malignancies; synergistic therapeutic and side effects must be weighed carefully.

D. Prognosis.
1. Survival in persons with HIV-related malignancies depends on multiple factors, including degree of immunosuppression, presence of opportunistic infection(s), nutritional status, location of presenting lesion, life-style, and availability and accessibility of adequate care.
2. HIV-related KS.
    a. In the absence of other major opportunistic infections, clients with HIV-related KS have survived for several years.
    b. In clients with GI tract lesions or B symptoms, survival time is shorter.

       c. Clients with prior or comorbid major opportunistic infection have the worst prognosis, with median survival time of less than 1 year.
    3. HIV-related lymphoma.
       a. Most clients present with high-grade, advanced-stage disease, with resultant poor prognosis; high histological grade, CNS primary tumor, prior persistent generalized lymphadenopathy, and incomplete response to chemotherapy are indicators of poor prognosis.
       b. Median survival time ranges from 4 to 10½ months; shortest survival time is with CNS primary tumor (median, 1 to 2 months); longest survival time is with low-grade lymphomas (12 months to 4 years).

DATA COLLECTION

  I. Clients at risk for HIV-related cancers.
    A. Individuals identified as HIV-positive.
    B. Risks for infection with HIV are highest among people who have:
      1. Been sexually active with more than one partner since 1978.
      2. Used needles to inject illicit drugs or had sex with someone who does.
      3. Received blood or blood products or organ transplant between 1978 and 1985.
      4. Been born to HIV-infected mothers.
      5. Been exposed to HIV in other ways such as through accidental needle stick.

  II. Pertinent history—requires tact and sensitivity on the part of the nurse when inquiring about sensitive topics such as sexuality and illicit drug use.
    A. Inquire about sexual and drug use history.
      1. Unprotected (i.e., without a condom) vaginal or rectal intercourse (highest risk).
      2. Sharing of needles for drug injection, especially in areas of high incidence of HIV infection (major risk); persons with substance abuse disorders may also be at high risk for sexual transmission from engaging in high-risk sex while intoxicated or in "survival sex" (engaging in sex to obtain money, drugs, food, or other needs).
      3. Homosexual or bisexual males may be reluctant to acknowledge sexual activity with other males; use tact and a nonjudgmental approach.
      4. Women may be unaware of bisexual behavior of partner or deny such behavior.
      5. History of one or more sexually transmitted diseases (syphilis, gonorrhea, herpes, chlamydia, hepatitis, genital warts) indicates higher risk.
    B. Inquire about history of blood, blood product, or organ transplantation.
      1. Since 1985 all blood and blood products in the United States have been tested for the presence of HIV antibodies; transfusions received in other countries may not have been tested.
      2. Since the early 1980s clotting factors used by hemophiliacs have been treated to kill HIV.
    C. Among children, determine HIV status of mother; children born to mothers infected with HIV have a 30% to 50% chance of being infected.
    D. Inquire about changes in mental status, memory, attention span, or personality; family members or significant others may recognize these changes before the client does; include these findings in data collection.
    E. Ask if the person has been tested for the presence of HIV antibody and what the result was.
      1. Because of social stigma attached to HIV infection and discrimination against HIV-infected people, the person may be reluctant to acknowledge having been tested or the result.
      2. Explain that information about HIV status may be important in determining a diagnosis and treatment plan.

3. Legal restrictions and requirements relative to HIV infection vary among states; the ethical obligation of the nurse to maintain client confidentiality is universal.

III. Physical examination.
  A. Signs and symptoms may vary in intensity, may wax and wane over time, but are usually progressive.
  B. Inspect the skin.
    1. Include gingiva and oral cavity, skin folds, plantar surfaces, scalp, and nares; KS lesions can appear anywhere on the body.
    2. Integumentary changes in a client known as infected with HIV may indicate opportunistic infection and should be reported to the attending physician, and/or the client should be referred for further workup.
    3. KS lesions may be purple to pink to brown, flat or raised, do not blanch with pressure, and are usually painless unless in a sensitive anatomical area.
    4. Despite appearance, KS lesions do not bleed easily.
    5. Lymphedema may result from obstruction of lymph flow by neoplastic growth.
  C. Assess the thorax and abdomen.
    1. Lesions in the lungs can cause rales, wheezes, or cacophonous breath sounds.
    2. Cardiac involvement occurs and can cause muffled heart tones or other abnormal heart sounds, palpitations, or chest pain.
    3. Evaluate abdomen for tenderness, masses, hyperactive bowel sounds, hepatic or splenic enlargement.
  D. Neurological and mental status examination can reveal changes caused by CNS lesions, opportunistic infections, or HIV-related dementia.
    1. Obtain baseline examination for comparison.
    2. Assess memory, gait, pupillary response, appearance, behavior, speech, affect, sensorimotor activity, presence of chronic headache, lightheadedness, dizziness, photophobia, syncope, paresthesias.
    3. Findings may vary day to day.
    4. Include findings obtained from family, caregiver, and significant other(s).
  E. Other signs and symptoms to assess—unintentional weight loss, diarrhea or constipation, fever, chills, night sweats, lymphadenopathy.

IV. Evaluation of laboratory data.
  A. Laboratory studies related to neoplastic processes are the same as those for clients with same pathology who are not infected with HIV.
    1. Hematological values may be skewed in presence of HIV bone marrow invasion; white cell count or platelet count may be elevated or reduced.
    2. Schedule of routine testing may differ from that used among non–HIV-infected individuals.
  B. Studies to monitor HIV infection.
    1. CD4/T4 lymphocyte count decreases over time at a median rate of 10 cells per month as a result of the progressive destruction of T4 cells by HIV; may be used to quantify the relative immunocompetence of the host, with lower values reflecting decreased immune response.
    2. Virally infected cells produce β_2-microglobulin; increasing serum levels indicate progressive infection.
    3. HIV core antigen p24 serum levels increase with progressive infection.
      a. Levels of β_2-microglobulin and p24 may decrease in end-stage disease.
      b. Decreases may be due to depletion of target cell population rather than to improvement of immune function.

ASSOCIATED NURSING DIAGNOSES

I. Potential for infection.

II. Body image disturbance.

III. Decisional conflict.

IV. Fatigue.

V. Altered nutrition: less than body requirements.

VI. Altered thought processes.

NURSING PLANNING AND IMPLEMENTATION

I. Interventions to maximize safety for client/significant other.
   A. Ensure environmental safety for clients experiencing sensorimotor changes (e.g., provide adequate lighting, especially at night).
   B. Instruct client about avoidance of potential environmental sources of opportunistic infection such as animal waste from pets or uncooked, undercooked, or improperly stored food.
   C. Teach techniques to reduce possibility of HIV transmission.
      1. HIV is transmitted through blood and semen; use a latex condom during every episode of vaginal, rectal, or oral intercourse, with a condom-compatible, water-based lubricant to reduce risk (petroleum-based lubricants or cosmetic creams weaken the condom, increasing the chance of breakage during use).
      2. Do not share toothbrushes, razors, other personal care items.
      3. For cleanup of emesis or other body fluid spills, wear gloves and use a solution of one part household bleach to 10 parts water.
      4. Insist that healthcare workers and volunteer caregivers follow universal precautions as recommended by CDC to reduce the risk of occupational exposure to HIV (Table 37-3).

II. Interventions to decrease incidence and severity of symptoms associated with disease or treatment.

Table 37-3
BODY FLUIDS IN UNIVERSAL PRECAUTIONS (CDC)

Body Fluids to Which Universal Precautions Apply	Body Fluids to Which Universal Precautions DO NOT Apply (unless contaminated by blood)
Blood; any secretion or excretion contaminated with blood	Urine
Cerebrospinal fluid	Feces
Semen; vaginal secretions	Vomitus
Synovial fluid	Perspiration
Amniotic fluid	Nasal secretions
Pericardial fluid	Tears
Pleural fluid	Sputum or saliva (except in dental practice)
Peritoneal fluid	

A. Teach (or refer for teaching) ways to enhance appearance such as use of covering cosmetics to hide KS lesions in cosmetically sensitive areas; use of scarves or other clothing to cover swollen lymph nodes; use of clothing appropriate to changing body mass with weight loss.

B. Instruct to use nonsteroidal anti-inflammatory agents rather than aspirin or acetaminophen, which may interfere with platelet function, to control fevers, minor aches, and pains (unless otherwise instructed by physician).

C. Encourage to establish routine of regular rest periods and to schedule activities in accordance with energy level.

D. Monitor nutritional status.
   1. Teach techniques to increase nutritional intake (e.g., use of supplements, keeping ready-to-eat foods available, eating smaller and more frequent meals).
   2. Provide or encourage frequent oral hygiene.

E. Teach appropriate techniques for care of skin in areas being treated with radiotherapy (see Chapter 20).

F. Assess knowledge or use of experimental and/or alternative treatment regimens.
   1. Determine and assess client knowledge of any contraindications that may exist between prescribed therapies and those obtained outside usual healthcare channels.
   2. Some experimental agents become available before receiving full Food and Drug Administration approval through "parallel track" programs, which allow use of drugs outside the clinical trial setting.
   3. Alternative therapies available through various sources (such as "buyers' clubs") may be used by clients.
      a. Ascertain all treatment regimens client is using, regardless of the source.
      b. Monitor interactions between multiple forms of therapy.
      c. Assist client with the process of evaluating alternative therapies in terms of effectiveness, side effects, costs, and safety.

III. Interventions to monitor for sequelae of disease and treatment.
   A. Provide teaching about myelotoxic side effects of chemotherapy and signs and symptoms of infection such as acute temperature elevation, appearance of suppurative lesions, bleeding.
   B. Assess anorectal skin integrity in clients with diarrhea; teach appropriate skin care.
   C. Instruct client to report changes in sense of touch, peripheral tingling, or numbness (may be side effect of vinca alkaloid chemotherapy or due to HIV infection).

IV. Interventions to monitor response to medical management.
   A. Assess and document location, appearance, size of KS lesions and/or lymphadenopathy or other tumor effects (abdominal masses, oral lesions).
   B. Monitor for changes in size or appearance of lymphomatous lesions.
   C. Obtain baseline and ongoing evaluation of mental status, performance status, and self-care ability.
   D. Assess nutritional status and document changes.
      1. Maintain serial record of body weight, with client wearing approximately same clothing with each recording.
      2. Document presence of dysphagia and changes in appetite or taste, which may result from oral lesions or as a side effect of treatment.

V. Interventions to enhance adaptation and rehabilitation.
   A. Use notes, phone calls, or other reminders for appointments and medication administration times (may also use a pillbox with built-in alarm).

1. Provide written instructions with frequent repetition and reinforcement included.
2. Provide instruction to caregivers and significant others if client experiences mental status changes.
   B. Refer client and significant other(s) to community agencies, civic organizations, or churches for assistance with social entitlement programs, peer support, and other available services such as home meal delivery.
   C. Refer for physical and/or occupational therapy to assist to learn adaptive techniques to cope with sensorimotor deficits.
   D. Encourage discussion about client's wishes for use of resuscitative measures.
      1. Facilitate decision-making process by establishing atmosphere of trust and acceptance, providing accurate information, respecting client choices.
      2. Ensure that client's wishes are properly documented and communicated to health care providers.

VI. Interventions to incorporate client and significant other in care.
   A. Recognize that client's family of choice may differ from biological family of origin.
      1. Determine and follow client's expressed wishes regarding who is to receive what kind of information, who will be allowed visitation in hospital, and which terms to use to describe relationship (e.g., lover, partner, friend).
      2. Assist or refer for assistance with execution of durable power of attorney, will, and other necessary legal documentation.
   B. Assess resources and coping strategies of client and significant other.
      1. Determine past experience with HIV disease; in areas of high-incidence, multiple losses may occur without adequate time for effective grieving.
      2. Consider that significant other with HIV disease may experience symptoms that limit ability to provide care.
      3. Recognize that a significant other who is not infected with HIV may experience feelings of guilt, uncertainty about own health, concern for the future.
      4. Monitor for indications of maladaptive coping strategies, especially if a history of substance use disorder is present; assist with learning alternative behaviors to manage stress and cope.
      5. Assess knowledge and/or use of alternative therapies.
   C. Include persons identified by client as significant others in teaching and care decisions when appropriate.

EVALUATION OF CLIENT AND SIGNIFICANT OTHER OUTCOMES

I. Identify the presence of HIV infection, specific malignancy, and rationale for treatment.

II. Identify immediate and long-term side effects of disease and treatment—exacerbation of immune suppression by myelotoxic therapies, side effects specific to agents used, skin changes caused by radiotherapy.

III. Identify self-care measures to decrease incidence and severity of symptoms associated with disease and treatment—maintenance of adequate rest and nutrition, monitoring body temperature, scheduling of activities to minimize fatigue, use of appropriate skin care techniques, use of prescribed antiemetic agents, or other techniques for symptom management.

IV. Demonstrate skills in self-care demanded by structural or functional effects of disease—use of written reminders for routine activities and appointments, use of pillbox with alarm or other means to manage multiple drug administration, use of cosmetic or other means to disguise lesions.

V. Describe schedule and procedures for follow-up care, which will vary according to condition.

VI. List signs and symptoms of recurrent disease—growth of old or appearance of new KS lesions, increasing lymphadenopathy or lymphedema, return or exacerbation of sensorimotor changes, increase in rate of weight loss, change in elimination pattern, exacerbation of prior symptoms.

VII. Identify community resources to meet demands of disease, treatment, and survivorship—local acquired immunodeficiency syndrome (AIDS) service organizations, church or civic organizations, American Cancer Society, hospice organizations, self-help groups such as Alcoholics Anonymous or Narcotics Anonymous when appropriate, local credit bureau or other financial services or planning agency, social service program offices such as Social Security.

BIBLIOGRAPHY

Cohn, J.A. (1989). Virology, immunology, and natural history of HIV infection. *J Nurse Midwife 34*(5), 242-252.

Cremer, K.J., Spring, S.B., & Gruber, J. (1990). Role of human immunodeficiency virus type 1 and other viruses in malignancies associated with acquired immunodeficiency disease syndrome. *J Natl Cancer Inst 82*(12), 1016-1024.

DeVita, V.T., Hellman, S., & Rosenberg, S.A. (eds) (1988). *AIDS: Etiology, Diagnosis, Treatment and Prevention* (2nd ed). Philadelphia: J.B. Lippincott Co.

Doll, D.C. & Ringenberg, Q.S. (1989). Lymphomas associated with HIV infection. *Semin Oncol Nurs 5*(4), 255-262.

Ensoli, B., Barillari, G., Salahuddin, S.Z., Gallo, R.C., & Wong-Staal, F. (1990). *Tat* protein of HIV-1 stimulates growth of cells derived from Kaposi's sarcoma lesions of AIDS patients. *Nature 345*(6270), 84-86.

Flaskerud, J.H. (1987). AIDS: neuropsychiatric complications. *J Psychosoc Nurs Ment Health Serv 25*(12), 17-20.

Gallo, R.C. & Nerurkar, L.S. (1989). Human retroviruses: their role in neoplasia and immunodeficiency. *Ann NY Acad Sci 567,* 82-94.

Gallucci, B. (1987). The immune system and cancer. *Oncol Nurs Forum 14*(6, suppl), 3-12.

Glasner, P.D. & Kaslow, R.A. (1990). The epidemiology of human immunodeficiency virus infection. *J Consult Clin Psychol 58*(1), 13-21.

Grady, C. (1988). HIV: epidemiology, immunopathogenesis, and clinical consequences. *Nurs Clin North Am 23*(4), 683-696.

Grady, C. (1988). Host defense mechanisms: an overview. *Semin Oncol Nurs 4*(2), 86-94.

Hall, J.M., Koehler, S.L., & Lewis, A. (1989). HIV-related mental health nursing issues. *Semin Oncol Nurs 5*(4), 276-283.

Halloran, J.P. Jr., & Hughes, A.M. (1991). Knowledge deficit related to prevention and early detection of HIV disease. In J.C. McNally, E.T. Somerville, C. Miaskowski, & M. Rostad (eds). *Guidelines for Oncology Nursing Practice* (2nd ed). Philadelphia: W.B. Saunders Co., pp. 47-54.

Halloran, J., Hughes, A., & Mayer, D.K. (1988). Oncology Nursing Society position paper on HIV-related issues. *Oncol Nurs Forum 15*(2), 206-217.

Horowitz, M.E. & Pizzo, P.A. (1990). Cancer in the child infected with human immunodeficiency virus. *J Pediatr 116*(5), 730-731.

Jacob, J.L., Baird, B.F., Haller, S., & Ostchega, Y. (1989). AIDS-related Kaposi's sarcoma: concepts of care. *Semin Oncol Nurs 5*(4), 263-275.

Krigel, R.L. & Friedman-Kien, A.E. (1990). Epidemic Kaposi's sarcoma. *Semin Oncol 17*(3), 350-360.

Krigel, R.L., Laubenstein, L.J., & Muggia, F.M. (1983). Kaposi's sarcoma: a new staging classification. *Cancer Treat Rep 67*(6), 531-534.

Krown, S.E., Gold, J.W., Niedzwiecki, D., Bundow, D., Flomenberg, N., Gansbacher, B., & Brew, B.J. (1990). Interferon-alpha with zidovudine: safety, tolerance, and clinical and virologic effects in patients with Kaposi sarcoma associated with the acquired immunodeficiency syndrome (AIDS). *Ann Intern Med 112*(1), 812-821.

Lange, J.M.A., de Wolf, F., & Goudsmit, J. (1989). Markers for progression in HIV infection. *AIDS 3*(suppl 1), S153-160.

Lovejoy, N.C. (1988). The pathophysiology of AIDS. *Oncol Nurs Forum 15*(5), 563-571.

McArthur, J.H., Palenicek, J.G., & Bowersox, L.L. (1988). Human immunodeficiency virus and the nervous system. *Nurs Clin North Am 23*(4), 823-841.

McMahon, K.M. & Coyne, N. (1989). Symptom management in patients with AIDS. *Semin Oncol Nurs 5*(4), 289-301.

Moran, T.A. (1988). Cancers in HIV infection. In G. Gee & T.A. Moran (eds). *AIDS: Concepts in Nursing Practice*. Baltimore: Williams & Wilkins, pp. 123-140.

Redfield, R.R., Wright, D.C., Tramont, E.C. (1986). The Walter Reed staging classification for HTLV-III/ LAV infection. *N Engl J Med 314*(2), 131-132.

Scherer, P. (1990). How HIV attacks the peripheral nervous system. *Am J Nurs 90*(5), 66-70.

Siegal, B., Levinton-Kriss, S., Schiffer, A., Sayar, J., Engelberg, I., Vonsover, A., Ramon, Y., & Rubinstein, E. (1990). Kaposi's sarcoma in immunosuppression. Possibly the result of a dual viral infection. *Cancer 65*(3), 492-498.

Tirelli, U., Vaccher, E., Rezza, G., et al. (1989). Hodgkin's disease in association with acquired immuno-deficiency syndrome (AIDS). A report on 36 patients. *Acta Oncol 28*(5), 637-639.

Ungvarski, P. (1988). Assessment: the key to nursing an AIDS patient. *RN 51*(9), 28-34.

Vlahov, D. (1989). AIDS: overview, immunology, virology, and informational needs. *Semin Oncol Nurs 5*(4), 227-235.

38

Lymphomas

Joyce Alexander, MN, RN, OCN

THEORY

I. Physiology and pathophysiology of the lymphatic system.
  A. Components of the lymphatic system—lymphocytes; epithelial and stromal cells.
    1. Primary lymphoid tissues—thymus and bone marrow.
    2. Secondary lymphoid tissues—lymph nodes, tonsils, adenoids, spleen, and Peyer's patches of gut.
      a. Lymphatic precursors arise from pluripotent stem cells in marrow.
      b. Carried through the blood to the lymph nodes and spleen.
      c. Proliferate and differentiate on contact with antigens.
  B. Functions of the lymphatic system.
    1. Recognition of self- and non–self-antigens.
    2. Development of antigen receptors to respond to antigen challenges.
    3. Destruction of non–self-antigens.
    4. Development and proliferation of memory cells.
  C. Pathological changes associated with cancer.
    1. Increased number of immature lymphoid cells infiltrate lymphoid tissues.
    2. Decreased number of functional immunocompetent cells.
    3. Decreased ability of the body to recognize and destroy foreign substances.
  D. Types of lymphoma (Table 38-1).
    1. Hodgkin's disease.
    2. Non-Hodgkin's lymphoma.

II. Principles of medical management.
  A. Diagnosis—biopsy of enlarged lymph node.
  B. Staging methods and procedures:
    1. Ann Arbor staging system (see Appendix).
    2. Staging procedures:
      a. History and physical examination.
      b. Radiographic examinations—chest x-ray, intravenous pyelogram, lymphangiogram, computed tomographic (CT) scan.
      c. Pathological examinations—bone marrow biopsy, biopsy of enlarged lymph nodes, surgical specimens from exploratory laparotomy.

Table 38-1
CLINICAL FEATURES OF THE LYMPHOMAS

Hodgkin's Disease	Non-Hodgkin's Lymphoma
Lymph node disease "centripetal"; tends to be in axial lymph nodes	Lymph node disease "centrifugal"; noncontiguous
Epitrochlear nodes, Waldeyer's ring; testicular and gastrointestinal sites uncommon	More common involvement of epitrochlear nodes, Waldeyer's ring, testes, and gastrointestinal tract
Mediastinal presentation in 50% of clients	Mediastinal presentation less common (~20%) Distinct syndrome of T-cell lymphoblastic lymphoma with mediastinal presentation, most commonly in second and third decades
Abdominal nodal involvement uncommon in asymptomatic clients but common in older clients or when fever or night sweats present	Abdominal lymph node involvement common
Commonly localized; contiguous nodal disease	Rarely localized nodal disease (<10%)
Bone marrow involvement uncommon	Bone marrow involvement common
Liver involvement uncommon; when present, spleen usually involved; is rare without fever or night sweats	Liver commonly involved in follicular lymphoma; rare in diffuse lymphoma

Modified from DeVita, V.T., Jr., Jaffe, E.S. and Hellman, S. (1989). Hodgkin's disease and the non-Hodgkin's lymphoma. In V.T. DeVita, Jr., S. Hellman, & S.A. Rosenberg (eds). *Cancer Principles & Practice of Oncology* (3rd ed). Philadelphia: J.B. Lippincott Co., p. 1702.

C. Treatment strategies.
  1. Hodgkin's disease—determined by the stage of disease and physiological status of the client.
    a. Localized disease—radiation therapy.
    b. Disseminated disease—combination chemotherapy alone or combination radiation therapy and chemotherapy.
      (1) Nitrogen mustard, vincristine, procarbazine, and prednisone (MOPP).
      (2) BCNU (bischloroethylnitrosourea [carmustine]), cyclophosphamide, vinblastine, procarbazine, and prednisone (BCVPP).
      (3) Doxorubicin, bleomycin, vinblastine, and DTIC (dacarbazine) (ABVD).
    c. Salvage treatment.
      (1) Relapse after radiation therapy alone—combination chemotherapy.
      (2) Relapse after chemotherapy—different chemotherapy regimen and/or bone marrow transplant.
  2. Non-Hodgkin's lymphoma—treatment determined by histology, stage, and physiological status of client.
    a. Localized disease:
      (1) Favorable histology (nodular)—radiation therapy.
      (2) Less favorable histology—radiation therapy and adjuvant chemotherapy.
    b. Disseminated disease (stages III and IV).
      (1) Indolent, asymptomatic disease or client in poor physiological condition—single-agent treatment, with or without prednisone.

(2) Aggressive histology:
- (a) Doxorubicin, cyclophosphamide, vincristine, and prednisone (CHOP).
- (b) Cyclophosphamide, nitrogen mustard, vincristine, procarbazine, and prednisone (C-MOPP).
- (c) Bleomycin, doxorubicin, cyclophosphamide, vincristine, and prednisone (BACOP).
- (d) Methotrexate, doxorubicin, cyclophosphamide, vincristine, prednisone, and bleomycin (MACOP-B).

D. Trends in survival.
1. Dramatic improvement in survival rate in the past 20 years among clients with Hodgkin's disease, with 70% to 90% of clients with early stage (I or II) disease surviving 5 years.
2. Complete remission achieved in 80% of clients receiving combination chemotherapy.
3. Of those clients achieving complete remission, 75% are cured of disease.
4. Clients with non-Hodgkin's lymphoma have a worse prognosis in general.

DATA COLLECTION

I. Pertinent personal and family history.
   A. Age.
      1. Peak incidence of Hodgkin's lymphoma—20 to 40 years of age.
      2. Peak incidence for non-Hodgkin's lymphoma—60 to 69 years of age.
   B. Family history of Hodgkin's disease in sibling—relative risk, 7.1 times greater than usual.
   C. Chronic immunosuppression.
   D. Epstein-Barr virus associated with Burkitt's lymphoma in Africa.
   E. History of lymph node enlargement that does not resolve over 4 to 6 weeks.
   F. Presence of B symptoms:
      1. Fever.
      2. Anorexia with weight loss.
      3. Night sweats.
      4. Itching.

II. Physical examination
   A. Palpation of enlarged lymph nodes—discrete, hard, fixed, matted, or spherical node(s) greater than 1 cm in diameter.
   B. Palpation of liver and spleen.

III. Evaluation of laboratory data.
   A. Abnormal peripheral hematological values—complete blood count, white blood cell count, and platelet count.
   B. Elevated liver and kidney function studies—blood urea nitrogen, creatinine, alkaline phosphatase, protein electrophoresis, and uric acid levels.
   C. Sedimentation rate.

IV. Radiographic data.
   A. Chest x-ray examination.
   B. Intravenous pyelogram.
   C. Lymphangiogram.
   D. Abdominal CT scan.

ASSOCIATED NURSING DIAGNOSES

I. Anxiety.

II. Knowledge deficit.

III. Alteration in protective mechanisms.

IV. Body image disturbance.

V. Sexual dysfunction.

VI. Alteration in comfort.

NURSING PLANNING AND IMPLEMENTATION

I. Interventions to maximize safety for the client (see Chapter 7—thrombocytopenia, leukopenia, and anemia).

II. Interventions to decrease the incidence, severity, or complications associated with disease and treatment.
   A. See Chapter 7—itching and fever.
   B. See Chapters 19, 20, 21, and 24.
   C. See Chapter 8—spinal cord compression and superior vena cava syndrome.
   D. See Chapter 9—tumor lysis syndrome and hypercalcemia.

III. Interventions to enhance adaptation and rehabilitation.
   A. Monitor hormone levels (thyroid-stimulating hormone, follicle-stimulating hormone, luteinizing hormone, testosterone) and suggest hormone replacement as needed.
      1. Evaluate signs and symptoms related to estrogen deficit in women—hot flashes, irritability, vaginal dryness, or discomfort with vaginal intercourse.
      2. Evaluate signs and symptoms related to testosterone deficit in men—decreased libido.
      3. Evaluate signs and symptoms related to hypothyroidism in client receiving mantle radiation—lethargy, constipation, cold intolerance, menorrhagia, slowing of intellectual and motor activity, weight gain, dry skin, and deepening of voice.
   B. Provide information about support groups in local community.
   C. Provide counseling about childbearing after treatment.
      1. Childbearing can occur after treatment for lymphomas.
      2. Long-term data on Hodgkin's disease survivors indicate:
         a. Pregnancy is less likely to occur than before treatment.
         b. Increased abortion rates and fetal abnormalities occur in clients receiving combination radiation therapy and chemotherapy.

EVALUATION OF CLIENT AND FAMILY OUTCOMES

I. Describe personal risk factors for lymphoma.

II. Discuss rationale, schedule, and personal demands of treatment and follow-up plans.

III. List potential side effects of disease and treatment.

IV. Describe self-care measures to decrease the incidence, severity, and complications of treatment.

V. Demonstrate competence in self-care measures demanded by structural or functional effects of treatment.

VI. Specify symptoms to report immediately to the health care team:
   A. Fever of 101° F or greater.
   B. Recurrence of night sweats.
   C. Weight loss of 5 pounds in 1 week.
   D. Marked decrease in urinary output.
   E. Recurrence of itching.

BIBLIOGRAPHY

Averette, H.E., Baike, G.M., & Jerrell, M.A. (1990). Effects of cancer chemotherapy on gonadal function and reproductive capacity. *CA* 40(4), 199-209.

Bakemeier, R.F., Zagars, G., Cooper, R.A., Jr., & Rubin, P. (1983). The malignant lymphomas. In P. Rubin (ed). *Clinical Oncology: a Multidisciplinary Approach* (6th ed). New York: American Cancer Society, pp. 346-369.

DeVita, V.T., Jr., Jaffe, E.S., Mauch, P., & Longo, D.L. (1989). Lymphocytic lymphomas. In V.T. DeVita, Jr., S. Hellman, & S.A. Rosenberg (eds). *Cancer: Principles & Practice of Oncology* (3rd ed). Philadelphia: J.B. Lippincott Co., pp. 1741-1798.

Hellman, S., Jaffe, E.S., & DeVita, V.T., Jr. (1989). Hodgkin's disease. In V.T. DeVita, Jr., S. Hellman, & S.A. Rosenberg (eds). *Cancer: Principles & Practice of Oncology* (3rd ed). Philadelphia: J.B. Lippincott Co., pp. 1696-1740.

Roush, G.C., Holford, T.R., Schymura, M.J., & White, C. (1987). *Cancer Risk and Incidence Trends: the Connecticut Perspective*. Washington, D.C.: Hemisphere Publishing Corp.

Site-Specific and TMN Staging

STAGE-GROUPING IN CARCINOMA OF THE LUNG

Stage	Description
I	
Tis, N0, M0	Carcinoma in situ
T1, N0, M0	A tumor that can be classified T1 without any metastasis or with metastasis to the
T1, N1, M0	lymph nodes in the ipsilateral hilar region only; or a tumor that can be classified
T2, N0, M0	T2 without any metastasis to nodes or distant metastasis.
	NOTE: TX, N1, M0 and T0, N1, M0 are also theoretically possible, but such a clinical diagnosis would be difficult if not impossible to make. If such a diagnosis is made, it should be included in Stage I.
II	
T2, N1, M0	A tumor classified as T2 with metastasis to the lymph nodes in the ipsilateral hilar region only.
III	
T3 with any N or M	Any tumor more extensive than T2; or any tumor with metastasis to the lymph
N2 with T or M	nodes in the mediastinum or with distant metastasis.
M1 with any T or N	

From American Joint Committee for Cancer Staging & End Results Reporting (1983). *Manual for Staging of Cancer*. Chicago: The Committee.

TNM DEFINITIONS

T—Primary Tumors

T0   No evidence of primary tumor

TX   Tumor proven by cytology but not visualized

Tis   Carcinoma in situ

T1   Tumor that is 3.0 cm or less without evidence of invasion of a lobar bronchus

T2   Tumor more than 3.0 cm in greatest diameter or tumor of any size that invades the visceral pleura or, with its associated atelectasis or obstructive pneumonitis, extends to the hilar region; no pleural effusion

T3   Tumor of any size with direct extension into an adjacent structure or demonstrable bronchographically to involve a main bronchus less than 2.0 cm distal to the carina; any tumor associated with atelectasis or obstructive pneumonitis of an entire lung or pleural effusion

N—Regional Lymph Nodes

N0   No demonstrable metastasis to regional lymph nodes

N1   Metastasis to lymph nodes in the peribronchial and/or the ipsilateral hilar region (including direct extension)

N2   Metastasis to lymph nodes in the mediastinum

M—Distant Metastasis

M0   No distant metastasis

M1   Distant metastasis such as in scalene, cervical, or contralateral hilar lymph nodes, brain, bones, lung, liver

From American Joint Committee for Cancer Staging & End Results Reporting (1983). *Manual for Staging of Cancer*. Chicago: The Committee.

STAGING OF BREAST CANCER

Stage	Description
0 Tis, N0, M0	Carcinoma in situ
I T1, N0, M0	Tumor 2 cm or less in greatest dimension; axillary nodes negative; no evidence of distant metastasis
II T1, N1, M0 T2, N0, M0 T2, N1, M0	Tumor 5 cm or less in greatest dimension; axillary nodes may be positive but are not fixed to one another; no evidence of distant metastasis
III T1, N2, M0 T2, N2, M0 T3, N0, M0 T3, N1 or N2, M0 Any T, N3, M0 Any T4, any N, M0	Tumor may be greater than 5 cm and may be fixated to underlying pectoral fascia or chest wall; axillary nodes may be positive and fixed to one another; internal mammary nodes may be positive; no evidence of distant metastasis
IV Any T, any N, M1	Any combination of tumors and node involvement with evidence of distant metastasis; includes metastasis to supravicular lymph node(s)

From American Joint Committee for Cancer Staging & End Results Reporting (1983). *Manual for Staging of Cancer*. Chicago: The Committee.

STAGING OF RENAL CELL CANCER

Stage	Description
I	Tumor is confined to the kidney; perinephric fat, renal vein, and regional nodes show no evidence of malignancy
II	Tumor involves the perinephric fat but is confined within Gerota's fascia; renal vein and regional nodes show no evidence of malignancy
III	Tumor involves the renal vein or regional nodes, with or without involvement of the vena cava or perinephric fat
IV	Distant metastases secondary to renal cell carcinoma present on admission or histological involvement by tumor of contiguous visceral structures

From American Joint Committee for Cancer Staging & End Results Reporting (1983). *Manual for Staging of Cancer*. Chicago: The Committee.

TNM CLASSIFICATION SYSTEM FOR RENAL CELL CARCINOMA

Primary Tumor (T)

TX	Minimum requirements cannot be met
T0	No evidence of primary tumor
T1	Small tumor, minimal renal and caliceal distortion or deformity; circumscribed neo-vasculature surrounded by normal parenchyma
T2	Large tumor with deformity and/or enlargement of the kidney and/or collecting system
T3a	Tumor involving perinephric tissues
T3b	Tumor involving renal vein
T3c	Tumor involving renal vein and infradiaphragmatic vena cava

NOTE: Under T3, tumor may extend into perinephric tissues, into renal vein, and into vena cava as shown on cavography; in these instances, the T classification may be shown as T3a, b, and c or some appropriate combination, depending on extension—for example, T3a,b is tumor in perinephric fat and extending into the renal vein.

T4a	Tumor invasion of neighboring structures (e.g., muscle, bowel)
T4b	Tumor involving supradiaphragmatic vena cava

Nodal Involvement (N)

The regional lymph nodes are the para-aortic and paracaval nodes; the juxtaregional lymph nodes are the pelvic nodes and the mediastinal nodes

NX	Minimum requirements cannot be met
N0	No evidence of involvement of regional nodes
N1	Single, homolateral regional nodal involvement
N2	Involvement of multiple regional or contralateral or bilateral nodes
N3	Fixed regional nodes (assessable only at surgical exploration)
N4	Involvement of juxtaregional nodes

NOTE: If lymphography is source of staging, add "l" between "N" and designator number; if histological proof is provided, "+" if positive, and "−" if negative. Thus Nl2 indicates multiple positive nodes seen on lymphography and proved at operation by biopsy.

Distant Metastasis (M)

MX	Not assessed
M0	No (known) distant metastasis
M1	Distant metastasis present; specify sites according to the following notations:

PUL—Pulmonary	MAR—Bone marrow
OSS—Osseous	PLE—Pleura
HEP—Hepatic	SKI—Skin
BRA—Brain	EYE—Eye
LYM—Lymph nodes	OTH—Other

NOTE: Add + to the abbreviated notation to indicate that the pathology (p) is proven

From American Joint Committee for Cancer Staging and End Results Reporting (1983). *Manual for Staging of Cancer.* Chicago: The Committee.

BLADDER CANCER STAGING SYSTEMS

1946 Jewett-Strong	1952 Jewett	1952 Marshall		1974, TNM Clinical	Pathologic
		0	No tumor definitive specimen	T0	P0
			Carcinoma in situ	TIS	PIS
			Papillary tumor and invasion		
A	A	A		T1	P1
			Invasion of the lamina propria		
B	B1	B1	Superficial	T2	P2
	B2	B2	Deep — Muscle Invasion	T3A	P3
C	C	C	Invasion of perivesical fat	T3B	
		D1	Invasion contiguous viscera	T4A-B	P4
			Pelvic nodes		N1-3
		D2	Distant metastases		M1
			Nodes above the aortic bifurcation		N4

From deKernion, J. (1980). Bladder cancer. In C. Haskell (ed). *Cancer Treatment*. Philadelphia: W.B. Saunders.

STAGING OF PROSTATE CANCER

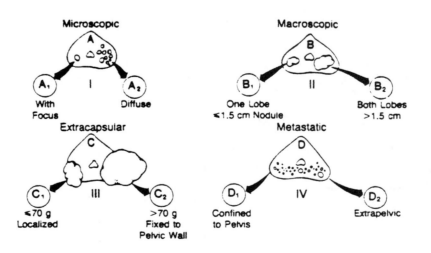

From Gittes, R.F. (1991). Carcinoma of the prostate. *NEJM* 324:236-245.

CLINICAL STAGING FOR CERVICAL CANCER (FIGO*)

Stage	Description
0	Carcinoma in situ, intraepithelial carcinoma
I	Carcinoma confined to the cervix (extension to the corpus should be avoided)
IA	Preclinical carcinomas of the cervix (diagnosed only by microscopy)
IA1	Minimal microscopically evident stromal invasion
IA2	Lesions detected microscopically that can be measured, showing no more than a 5-mm depth of invasion when taken from the base of the epithelium and no more than 7 mm of horizontal spread
IB	Lesions of greater dimensions than stage IA2, whether seen clinically or not
II	Involvement of the vagina but not of the lower third or infiltration of the parametria but not out to the side wall
IIA	Involvement of the vagina but no evidence of parametrial involvement
IIB	Infiltration of the parametria but not out to the side wall
III	Involvement of the lower third of the vagina or extension to the pelvic side wall; all cases with hydronephrosis or nonfunctioning kidney unless known to be from another cause
IIIA	Involvement of the lower third of the vagina but not out to the pelvic side wall
IIIB	Involvement of one or both parametria out to the side wall or hydronephrosis or nonfunctioning kidney
IV	Extension beyond the true pelvis
IVA	Involvement of the mucosa of the bladder or rectum
IVB	Distant metastasis

*FIGO: International Federation of Gynecology and Obstetrics.

STAGING FOR ENDOMETRIAL CARCINOMA (FIGO*)

Stage	Description
0	Atypical hyperplasia or carcinoma in situ
IA	Tumor limited to the endometrium
IB	Invasion to less than one half of myometrium
IC	Invasion to more than one half of myometrium
IIA	Endocervical glandular involvement only
IIB	Cervical stromal invasion
IIIA	Invasion of serosa and adnexa and/or positive peritoneal cytology
IIIB	Vaginal metastases
IIIC	Metastases to pelvic and/or para-aortic lymph nodes
IVA	Invasion of bladder and/or bowel mucosa
IVB	Distant metastases, including intra-abdominal and/or inguinal lymph nodes

*FIGO: International Federation of Gynecology and Obstetrics.

STAGING FOR OVARIAN CANCER (FIGO*)

Stage	Description
I	Growth limited to the ovaries
IA	Growth limited to one ovary; no ascites; no tumor on the external surface; capsule intact
IB	Growth limited to both ovaries; no ascites; no tumor on the external surfaces; capsules intact
IC	Either stage IA or IB tumor but with tumor on surface of one or both ovaries, with capsule ruptured, with ascites present containing malignant cells, or with positive peritoneal washings
II	Growth involving one or both ovaries with pelvic extension
IIA	Extension and/or metastases to the uterus and/or tubes
IIB	Extension to other pelvic tissues
IIC	Either stage IIA or IIB tumor but with tumor on the surface of one or both ovaries, with capsule(s) ruptured, with ascites present and containing malignant cells, or with positive peritoneal washings
III	Tumor involving one or both ovaries, with peritoneal implants outside the pelvis and/or positive retroperitoneal or inguinal nodes; superficial liver metastasis equals stage III
IIIA	Tumor grossly limited to the true pelvis, with negative nodes but histologically confirmed microscopic seeding of abdominal peritoneal surfaces
IIIB	Tumor of one or both ovaries, with histologically confirmed implants of abdominal peritoneal surfaces, with none exceeding 2 cm in diameter; nodes are negative
IIIC	Abdominal implants greater than 2 cm in diameter and/or positive retroperitoneal or inguinal nodes
IV	Growth involving one or both ovaries with distant metastases; if pleural effusion is present, cytology must be positive to allot a case to stage IV; parenchymal liver metastasis equals stage IV

*International Federation of Gynecology and Obstetrics.

STAGING SYSTEM FOR TESTICULAR CARCINOMA

Stage	Description
A	Tumor is confined to the testicle; no evidence of spread beyond the confines of the scrotum
B1	Evidence of *minimal* retroperitoneal lymph node metastases, determined either by retroperitoneal lymph node dissection or lymphangiography (less than six positive nodes, well encapsulated)
B2	Evidence of moderate retroperitoneal lymph node spread (more than six nodes)
B3	Massive retroperitoneal lymph node involvement, usually a palpable mass on physical examination but without evidence of spread above the diaphragm (may invade contiguous structures directly)
C	Metastatic tumor noted above the diaphragm or to solid visceral organs (liver, brain, or bone)

From Smith, R.B. (1985). Testicular cancer. In Haskell, C. (ed). *Cancer Treatment* (2nd ed). Philadelphia: W.B. Saunders Co.

STAGING OF COLORECTAL CANCER

Definitions

Primary tumor (T)

TX	Primary tumor cannot be assessed
T0	No evidence of primary tumor
Tis	Carcinoma in situ
T1	Tumor invades submucosa
T2	Tumor invades muscularis propria
T3	Tumor invades through muscularis propria into subserosa or into nonperitonealized pericolic or perirectal tissues
T4	Tumor perforates visceral peritoneum, or directly invades other organs or structures

Lymph node (N)

NX	Regional lymph nodes cannot be assessed
N0	No regional lymph node metastasis
N1	Metastasis in one to three pericolic or perirectal lymph nodes
N2	Metastasis in four or more pericolic or perirectal lymph nodes
N3	Metastasis in any lymph node along course of a major named vascular trunk

Distant metastasis (M)

MX	Presence of distant metastasis cannot be assessed
M0	No distant metastasis
M1	Distant metastasis

Stage Grouping

0	Tis	N0	M0
I	T1	N0	M0
	T2	N0	M0
II	T3	N0	M0
	T4	N0	M0
III	Any T	N1	M0
	Any T	N2	M0
	Any T	N3	M0
IV	Any T	Any N	M1

Histopathological Grade (G)

GX	Grade cannot be assessed
G1	Well differentiated
G2	Moderately well differentiated
G3	Poorly differentiated
G4	Undifferentiated

From American Joint Committee on Cancer (1988). *Manual for Staging of Cancer* (3rd ed). Philadelphia: J.B. Lippincott Co.

STAGING SYSTEM FOR PENILE CANCER

Stage	Extent of Disease
I	Tumor limited to the glands or prepuce
II	Tumor extending onto shaft of penis
III	Tumors with regional lymph node metastases that are operable
IV	Tumors involving adjacent structures or with inoperable lymph node metastasis or distant metastases

From Paulson, D.F., Perez, C.A., & Anderson, T. (1985). Cancer of the urethra and penis. In V.T. DeVita, Jr., S. Hellman, & S.A. Rosenberg (eds). *Cancer Principles & Practice of Oncology*. Philadelphia: J.B. Lippincott Co., p. 967.

STAGING OF ANAL CANCER

Definitions

The following is the TNM classification for the staging of cancers that arise in the anal canal only. Cancers that arise at the anal margin are staged according to cancers of the skin.

Primary tumor (T)

TX	Primary tumor cannot be assessed
T0	No evidence of primary tumor
Tis	Carcinoma in situ
T1	Tumor 2 cm or less in greatest dimension
T2	Tumor more than 2 cm but not more than 5 cm in greatest dimension
T3	Tumor more than 5 cm in greatest dimension
T4	Tumor of any size invades adjacent organ(s) (e.g., vagina, urethra, bladder; involvement of the sphincter muscle(s) *alone* is not classified as T4)

NOTE: The adjacent organs involved with tumor should be specified.

Regional lymph nodes (N)

NX	Regional lymph nodes cannot be assessed
N0	No regional lymph node metastasis
N1	Metastasis in perirectal lymph nodes(s)
N2	Metastasis in unilateral internal iliac and/or inguinal lymph node(s)
N3	Metastasis in perirectal and inguinal lymph nodes and/or bilateral internal iliac and/or inguinal lymph nodes

From American Joint Committee on Cancer. (1988). *Manual for Staging of Cancer* (3rd ed). Philadelphia: J.B. Lippincott Co.

STAGING OF ANAL CANCER *Continued*

Distant metastases (M)

MX   Presence of distant metastasis cannot be assessed

M0   No distant metastasis

M1   Distant metastasis

Stage Grouping

Stage 0	Tis	N0	M0
Stage I	T1	N0	M0
Stage II	T2	N0	M0
	T3	N0	M0
Stage IIIA	T4	N0	M0
	T1	N1	M0
	T2	N1	M0
	T3	N1	M0
Stage IIIB	T4	N1	M0
	Any T	N2, N3	M0
Stage IV	Any T	Any N	M1

Histopathological type

This staging classification applies to all carcinomas that arise in the colon and rectum.

Sites of distant metastasis

Pulmonary	PUL
Osseous	OSS
Hepatic	HEP
Brain	BRA
Lymph nodes	LYM
Bone marrow	MAR
Pleura	PLE
Peritoneum	PER
Skin	SKI
Other	OTH

STAGING OF HEAD AND NECK CANCER

Primary Tumor (T)

TX   Primary tumor cannot be assessed

T0   No evidence of primary tumor

Tis   Carcinoma in situ

T1   Tumor 2 cm or less in greatest dimension

T2   Tumor more than 2 cm but less than 4 cm in greatest dimension

T3   Tumor more than 4 cm in greatest dimension

NOTE: The larynx and maxillary sinus have a T designation that is at considerable variance to this one, but most of the sites use this system as a general guide; all N classifications are the same.

Regional Lymph Nodes (N)

NX   Regional lymph nodes cannot be assessed

N0   No regional lymph node metastasis

N1   Metastasis in a single ipsilateral lymph node; 3 cm or less in greatest dimension

N2   Metastasis in a single ipsilateral lymph node; more than 3 cm but not more than 6 cm in greatest dimension; in multiple ipsilateral lymph nodes, none more than 6 cm in greatest dimension; in bilateral or contralateral lymph nodes, none more than 6 cm in greatest dimension

N2a   Metastasis in a single ipsilateral lymph node between 3 and 6 cm in greatest dimension

N2b   Metastasis in multiple ipsilateral lymph nodes; none more than 6 cm in greatest dimension

N2c   Metastasis in bilateral or contralateral lymph nodes; none more than 6 cm in greatest dimension

N3   Metastasis in a lymph node more than 6 cm in greatest dimension

Distant Metastasis (M)

MX   Presence of distant metastasis cannot be assessed

M0   No distant metastasis

M1   Distant metastasis

Stage Grouping

Stage	T	N	M
Stage 0	Tis	N0	M0
Stage I	T1	N0	M0
Stage II	T2	N0	M0
Stage III	T3	N0	M0
	T1, T2, or T3	N1	M0
Stage IV	T4	N0, N1	M0
	Any T	N2, N3	M0
	Any T	Any N	M1

From Sievers, A.E.F. & Donald, P.J. (1989). Staging system for head and neck cancer. *J Soc of Otorhinolaryngol Head-Neck Nurses.*

TNM CLASSIFICATION OF BRAIN TUMORS

Primary Tumor (T)

TX   Primary tumor cannot be assessed

T0   No evidence of primary tumor

Supratentorial Tumor

T1   Tumor 5 cm or less in greatest dimension; limited to one side

T2   Tumor more than 5 cm in greatest dimension; limited to one side

T3   Tumor invades or encroaches on the ventricular system

T4   Tumor crosses the midline, invades the opposite hemisphere, or invades infratentorially

Infratentorial Tumor

T1   Tumor 3 cm or less in greatest dimension; limited to one side

T2   Tumor more than 3 cm in greatest dimension; limited to one side

T3   Tumor invades or encroaches on the ventricular system

T4   Tumor crosses the midline, invades the opposite hemisphere, or invades supratentorially

Regional Lymph Nodes (N)

This category does not apply to this site.

Distant Metastasis (M)

MX   Presence of distant metastasis cannot be assessed

M0   No distant metastasis

M1   Distant metastasis

Histopathological Grade (G)

GX   Grade cannot be assessed

G1   Well differentiated

G2   Moderately well differentiated

G3   Poorly differentiated

G4   Undifferentiated

Stage Grouping

Stage IA	G1	T1	M0
Stage IB	G1	T2	M0
	G1	T3	M0
Stage IIA	G2	T1	M0
Stage IIB	G2	T2	M0
	G2	T3	M0
Stage IIIA	G3	T1	M0
Stage IIIB	G3	T2	M0
	G3	T3	M0
Stage IV	G1, G2, G3	T4	M0
	G4	Any T	M0
	Any G	Any T	M1

From Beahrs, O.H., Henson, D.E., Hutter, R., et al. (1988). *Manual for Staging of Cancer* (ed 3). Philadelphia: JB Lippincott Co., pp. 249-254.

ANN ARBOR STAGING SYSTEM FOR LYMPHOMAS

Involvement	Systemic Symptoms	Stage
Single lymph node region	No	IA
	Yes	IB
Two or more lymph node regions: same side of diaphragm	No	IIA
	Yes	IIB
Lymph node regions both sides of the diaphragm	No	IIIA
	Yes	IIIB
Disseminated—organs outside lymphatic system; may include lymph nodes	No	IVA
	Yes	IVB

From Bakemeier, R.F., Zagars, G., Cooper, R.A., Jr., & Rubin, P. (1983). The malignant lymphomas. In P. Rubin (ed). *Clinical Oncology: A Multidisciplinary Approach* (6th ed). New York: American Cancer Society.

Index

Note: Numbers in *italics* refer to illustrations; numbers followed by t refer to tables.

Beta radiation, 321, *325*
Beta-hCG (chorionic gonadotropin [beta subunit]), 48t
Biochemical studies, in cancer diagnosis, 273-274, 291
Biological markers, 46, 47t–53t
Biological response modifier therapy, definition of, 346
    for breast cancer, 420
    for HIV-related Kaposi's sarcoma, 559
    for ovarian cancer, 461
    implications of, 346-357, 348t–355t
    nursing planning and implementation of, 355-357
Biological risk factors, 36-37
Biomedical effects, of cancer survivorship, 258-259
Biopsy, 303-304
    cervical, 452, *453*
    excisional, 303, 309, 310t, 503
    fine needle, 303
    in breast cancer, 417
    incisional, 303, 309, 310t, 503
    needle, 309, 310t
    needle core, 416t
    open, 416t
    punch, 303
    stereotactic, brain tumors and, 528, *529*, 530t–531t, 532t
Biotherapy, 346-357
Bisacodyl (Dulcolax), 550
Bis(chloromethyl)ether (BCME), 34t
Black Americans, access to health care and, 200
    cancer incidence and, 198, 296
    perception of cancer among, 202
Bladder, 45
Bladder cancer, 435-442
    medical management of, 436-438
    nursing planning and implementation for, 439-442
    physiology and pathophysiology of, 435-436
    rehabilitation issues in, 216t
    staging of, 576t
    survival rates for, 438, 438t
Bladder incontinence, 126
Bleomycin (Blenoxane), 338t
Blood, autologous, 374
    whole, 375t
Blood capillaries, metastasis via, 266-267
Blood chemistry, 50t–51t
Blood component therapy, 374-377, 375t
Blood pressure, activity and, 119t
Blood transfusion, reactions to, 376
Blood-brain barrier, 522
Blurred vision, 72, 75
Body image, 130-132
    head and neck cancer and, 514
Bone malignancies, 216t
Bone marrow donor, 359
Bone marrow transplant, 359-369
    allogeneic, 359, 363
    autologous, *361*, 363, 420
    complications associated with, 364t–365t
    leukemia and, 482, 483t
    nursing planning and implementation for, 366-369
    stages of, *360*
    syngeneic, 363
Bone scans, 503
Bowel and bladder program, 161, 162t
Bowel incontinence, 127
Brachytherapy, 322, 506
Brain, 522-526, *526*
Brain tumors, 522-543, 528
    epidemiology of, 527-528
    functional changes associated with, 526-527

Brain tumors *(Continued)*
    medical management of, 528-537
    metastatic patterns of, 527
    pediatric, 528
    physiology and pathophysiology of, 522-528
    risk factors for, 537-538
    staging methods of, 528
    surgery for, 528-534
    survival rates for, 535-537, 537t
    TNM classification of, 583t
Brainstem, 522, 526
Brainstem tumors, 537
Breach of duty, liability and, 253
Breast, anatomy of, 413, *414*
    clinical examination of, 44t, 46, 55, *56*
    fibrocystic changes in, 421
    lymphatic drainage from, *414*
    mammography of, 55, 199-200, 201, 416
Breast biopsy, 416t
Breast cancer, 197, 413-427
    adjuvant chemotherapy and endocrine therapy for, 417t, 419
    early detection of, 199, 201
    epidemiology of, 415
    histological types of, 415t
    history of, 421
    hormonal therapy for, 419-420
    incidence of, 195, *295*, 296
    medical management of, 416-420
    metastasis and, 413-415, 422
    nursing planning and implementation for, 422-425, *423*
    physiology and pathophysiology of, 413-415
    publications about, 426
    radiation therapy for, 419
    rehabilitation issues in, 216t
    risk factors for, 420-421
    signs and symptoms of, 421-422
    staging of, 417, 574t
    surgery for, 418t
    survival rate for, 297
    treatment strategies for, 417-420
Breast reconstruction, 418-419
Breast self-examination (BSE), 55, *56*, 416
    after mastectomy, 424
Breslow's measurement, 491
Bronchoscopy, 406t
Bruce Medical Supply, 520
BSE (breast self-examination), 55, *56*, 416
    after mastectomy, 424
Burnout, 230-231
    definition of, 231
    home care provider and, 212
    professional, 231
        in oncology unit, 209
Busulfan, 37

Cadmium, 34t, 446
Calcitonin, 49t, 185t
Calcium, 50t
    levels of, regulation of, 183-187, *184*
Cancer, 279, 401-571. See also specific anatomic site, e.g., *Breast cancer.*
    current statistics for, 295-298
    definition of, 265-268
    diagnosis of, 272-282
        factors affecting, 25-30, 29t
    early detection of, 199-202
    education of persons at-risk for, 62
    epidemiology of, 287-299

Carcinogens *(Continued)*
    carcinogenesis and, 268-272
  linked to kidney cancer, 432
  synergistic effects of, 37
Carcinoid syndrome, 274t
Carcinoma. See also *Cancer* entries.
  basal cell, 488, 489, 493-494, 495-496
  classification of, 279
  squamous cell, 279, 489, 490, 493, 495-496
Carcinoma in situ (CIS), 266, 451
Cardiac system, 45
Cardiac tamponade, 165-168
Cardiovascular system, 258
Carotid artery, rupture of, 514-516
Case manager, in oncology health care setting, 205
Catalogue of Federal Domestic Assistance (CFDA), 228t
Catheter(s), arterial, 394, 395t
  venous, 394, 395t
CAUTION (Cancer's Seven Warning Signals), 44
CD4 lymphocyte, HIV infection and, 240, 241
CDC. See *Centers for Disease Control (CDC)*.
CEA (carcinoembryonic antigen), 48t, 273
Cefazolin sodium, 378t-379t
Cefotaxime sodium, 378t-379t
Cefoxitin sodium, 378t-379t
Cell(s), abnormal differentiation of, 275-276
  division of, 329-330
  kinetic studies in, 274-277
  proliferation of, radiation exposure and, 269
Cell cycle, 330
  antineoplastic therapy and, 329, *330*, 331-332
  radiation exposure and, 269
Cell cycle-nonspecific chemotherapy agents, 332
Cell cycle-specific chemotherapy agents, 331
Cell membrane, changes in, 273-274
Cell-mediated immunity, 346
Cell-to-cell recognition and adhesion, defect in, 274
Centers for Disease Control (CDC), classification system of, for HIV infection, 241, 556, 556t
  guidelines of, for HIV-positive health care workers, 240
  occupational health hazards and. See *Occupational health hazards*.
  recommendations of, for handwashing, 367t
Central nervous system, 216t
Central venous access devices (CVAD), 14t
Cephalosporins, 378t-379t
Cephalothin sodium, 378t-379t
Cephamandole, 378t-379t
Cerebellum, 522, 526
Cerebral angiography, brain tumors and, 528, 530t-531t, 532t
Cerebral blood vessels, 522
Cerebral dominance, 525
Cerebral hemispheres, lobes of, *523*
Cerebrospinal fluid (CSF), 522, *523*, 545
  brain tumors and, 539
  leak of, surgery for spinal cord tumors and, 548
Cerebrum, 522, 525-526
Certification, 222, 237
Cerubidine (daunorubicin), 339t
Cervical biopsy, 452
Cervical cancer, 451-457
  chemotherapy for, 454
  early detection of, 199, 201
  medical management of, 452-454
  metastatic patterns of, 451
  nursing planning and implementation for, 455-456
  physiology and pathophysiology of, 451-452

Cervical cancer *(Continued)*
  radiation therapy for, 454, 456
  recurrent, 454
  staging of, 452-453, 577t
  survival rates for, 454, 454t
  treatment strategies of, 453-454
  trends in epidemiology for, 451-452
Cervical intraepithelial neoplasia (CIN), 451, *453*
Cervicography, 44t, 57, 452
Cervix, anatomy of, 451
  cervicography of, 44t, 57, 452
Cesium-137, half-life of, 326t
CFDA (*Catalogue of Federal Domestic Assistance*), 228t
Chaplain, in oncology health care setting, 205
Chemical dependency, in health care workers, 255-256
Chemicals. See also specific agent.
  carcinogenic, 270t, 271
  unproven, in cancer care, 372
Chemoprevention, breast cancer and, 420
Chemotherapy, 329-340. See also *Antineoplastic therapy*.
  adjuvant, 305, 309-310
    for breast cancer, 417t, 419
    for ovarian cancer, 461
  atypical toxicities of, 338t-339t
  combined with surgery, 313
  constipation and, 120
  effect of, on wound healing, 312
  for brain tumors, 534-535
  for cervical cancer, 454
  for colorectal cancer, 473-474, 478
  for HIV-related Kaposi's sarcoma, 559
  for lung cancer, 407-408
  for malignant melanoma, 492
  for nonmelanoma skin cancer, 492
  for penile cancer, 467
  for renal cell cancer, 432
  for spinal cord tumors, 548
  for testicular cancer, 464
  leukopenia and, 106
  nursing planning and implementation for, 336-339
  role of, in cancer care, 331
  side effects of, 283
    potential, 333t
  stomatitis, esophagitis, and mucositis and, 111
  thrombocytopenia and, 109
  types of, 331-335
Chest x-ray, of head and neck cancer, 502
  of lung, 57
Chewing tobacco, 36
Children, cancer in, 296, 480, 528, 533, 537, 538, 539t
  survival rate for, 297-298
Children in Hospitals Inc., 252t
Chloromethyl methyl ether (CMME), 34t
Cholesterol, 50t
Chondrosarcoma, 280
Chorionic gonadotropin (beta subunit) (beta-hCG), 48t
Chromium, 34t
Chromosome(s), abnormal arrangements of, 272-273
  deletion of, 273
Cigarette smoking. See *Smoking*.
CIN (cervical intraepithelial neoplasia), 451, *453*
Cine-esophagography/barium swallow, 503, 505t
Circulation, of blood, 146-154
  anemia and, 146-148
  edema and, 148-151
  effusion and, 151-154
  fluid imbalance and, 148-154
CIS (carcinoma in situ), 266, 451
Cisplatin, 338t